Pulse Diagnosis in Early Chinese Medicine

This is a study of the earliest extensive account of Chinese pulse diagnosis, or more accurately, the examination of *mai*. Dr Hsu focuses on Chunyu Yi, a doctor of the early Han, and presents the first complete translation into English of his Memoir which appears in *The Records of the Historian* by Sima Qian (d. ca 86 BCE). This Memoir contains twenty-five medical case histories, and constitutes a document of enormous importance to the history of medicine in China.

The analysis covers the first ten medical cases and their rich vocabulary on touch, as used in Chinese pulse diagnosis. The patients treated were mostly nobility of the kingdom of Qi in eastern China, who suffered from the indulgences of court life and were treated with early forms of decoction, fomentation, fumigation, acupuncture and moxibustion. To date there is no book on early China of its kind.

ELISABETH HSU is Reader in Social Anthropology at the University of Oxford. Previous publications include *The Transmission of Chinese Medicine* (Cambridge, 1999) and *Innovation in Chinese Medicine* (Cambridge, 2001).

University of Cambridge Oriental Publications   68

Pulse Diagnosis in Early Chinese Medicine

A series list is shown at the back of the book

Pulse Diagnosis in Early Chinese Medicine:

The Telling Touch

With an annotated translation of the Memoir of Chunyu Yi (*Canggong zhuan*) in the 105th chapter of *The Records of the Historian* (*Shi ji*, ca 86 BCE) by Sima Qian, and an anthropological analysis of the first ten medical case histories

ELISABETH HSU

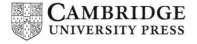
CAMBRIDGE
UNIVERSITY PRESS

CAMBRIDGE
UNIVERSITY PRESS

University Printing House, Cambridge CB2 8BS, United Kingdom

One Liberty Plaza, 20th Floor, New York, NY 10006, USA

477 Williamstown Road, Port Melbourne, VIC 3207, Australia

314-321, 3rd Floor, Plot 3, Splendor Forum, Jasola District Centre, New Delhi - 110025, India

79 Anson Road, #06-04/06, Singapore 079906

Cambridge University Press is part of the University of Cambridge.

It furthers the University's mission by disseminating knowledge in the pursuit of education, learning and research at the highest international levels of excellence.

www.cambridge.org
Information on this title: www.cambridge.org/9781108468633

© Faculty of Oriental Studies, University of Cambridge 2010

First published 2010
First paperback edition 2018

A catalogue record for this publication is available from the British Library

ISBN 978-0-521-51662-4 Hardback
ISBN 978-1-108-46863-3 Paperback

For my mother Ruth (1929–64)

CONTENTS

LIST OF TABLES, BOXES AND MAPS

PREFACE

When, in October 1986, on my first day at Cambridge, I was asked during the welcome party: 'And what will the theme of your thesis be?', I was embarrassed not to know. I had graduated from Biology, disillusioned; turned away from Development Studies, dismayed; and after a year of travelling and searching, decided to enrol in Social Anthropology, General Linguistics and Chinese Studies, which I did for a year before attending the postgraduate course on General Linguistics that began with said welcome. Through reading Joseph Needham's works, I thereupon found Chunyu Yi's Memoir in the 105th chapter of Sima Qian's *Shi ji* (*The Records of the Historian*), which is the first dynastic history of the unified Chinese empire, dating to ca 86 BCE. It contained twenty-five medical case histories. This, I thought, was 'doable' in a Master's thesis.

However, twenty years later I find myself still puzzling over the same text. The time has come to admit that with the material at hand it cannot be conclusively decoded. What then is the contribution of this book to scholarship? First, an attempt has been made to contribute to Chinese medical history with a solid piece of research that attends to questions of methodology and language. Although Yi's Memoir cannot be classified as a medical treatise and although it is part of a dynastic history, it remains an immensely important text for understanding early Chinese medicine. It is in fact the earliest extant text, which contains a reasonably extensive account of Chinese pulse diagnosis, and also reports fairly frequently on, depending on their definition, 'acupuncture and moxibustion' and treatment with 'decoctions'. As Yamada Keiji points out, pulse diagnosis and decoctions have ever since been intrinsic to Chinese medical practice.

Second, a text critical method, 'text structure semantics', was developed for decoding the medical case histories recorded in this text, which, as will be demonstrated in this study, are formulaic. The future will show whether this method can be used for decoding other formulaic premodern scientific texts written in a highly elaborate if not technical vocabulary. The aim was to understand Yi's rationale in a way that tries to avoid anachronism and ethnocentricity. The detailed word-for-word analysis is meant to make transparent why certain decisions of translation were made, and also to highlight the range of ambiguities intrinsic to any interpretation of the text.

Third, this study addresses theoretical concerns in medical anthropology by questioning widely held assumptions about illness causation and by highlighting new avenues for thinking about diagnostic procedures. With its focus on tactility during the diagnostic process, the study aims to contribute to the anthropology of sensory experience. The more than forty verbs of touch investigated relate tactile qualities to body internal processes, often in iconic and indexical ways, to use C. S. Peirce's terminology.

Needless to say, this book has seen many reincarnations. The MPhil thesis in General Linguistics 'Lexical Semantics and Chinese Medical Terms' of 1987, conducted under the supervision of Stephen Levinson, was getting dusty when Sir Geoffrey Lloyd read it in 1991 and enthusiastically encouraged me to do an annotated translation of Yi's Memoir. I was then in the final stages of my doctoral studies in Social Anthropology on Traditional Chinese Medicine in the People's Republic of China. I was fluent in modern Chinese, but felt I barely had any knowledge of literary Chinese. Nathan Sivin too emphasised my then limited linguistic fitness in both English and literary Chinese and, in recognition of the importance of this text, published a piece on it himself (Sivin 1995a). Sir Geoffrey nevertheless encouraged me with the motto 'learning by doing'. So, I applied for and received a one-year grant from the National Science Foundation of the United States at the Needham Research Institute in Cambridge, a Charitable Trust adjunct institution to the University, which Geoffrey Lloyd aimed to enliven with innovative scholarship. He probably had in mind an enlightened essay in the style of sophisticated English scholarship, yet was soon to realise that I was an obstinate Chinese and hopeless Swiss perfectionist, trained six and a half years in the humanistic tradition of German philology at high school. The study grew from an unpublished annotated 100-page translation of the 25 medical cases in 1995, to a 400-page Habilitationsschrift in Sinology at the University of Heidelberg in 2001, to this embarrassingly long tome of 200,000 words in 2007.

The translation could never have been done without the most generous help and basic training received from specialists in Chinese Studies, mostly at Cambridge. The very early days had seen the help of Ma Boying, who was a visiting scholar at the Needham Research Institute in the mid-1980s and of Ma Kanwen, who then still oscillated between German and Anglo-Saxon countries. It also benefited from weekly tutorials with Robert Neather on literary Chinese grammar and grammatical particles. Most important, however, was Mark Lewis' critical review of the entire first and second typed out draft translations of the twenty-five cases in 1995. He cracked so many nuts, it has been difficult to acknowledge each in the text. Eventually, however, Michael Loewe became the most constant support for over a decade and answered hundreds of questions on endless details. His bibliographic guide to early Chinese studies makes the entry into this field possible for latecomers, and the transcription of the names of the Japanese commentators in chapter 9 relies entirely on his expertise. Most memorable are our weekly sessions in his study at Granchester, in July 1995, where we scrutinised the names, titles and residence places of Yi's clientele, which inspired him to write his 1997 essay.

At the University of Zurich, where I was employed as Assistant Lecturer in Social Anthropology from 1992 to 1996, Robert Gassmann, as Sinologist mentor to the stipend from the Boral Stiftung, which gave me dispensation from my teaching for nine months, commented extensively on the final 1995 version. Catherine Despeux provided few but excellent comments, as did Donald Harper, who continued to provide occasional but decisive support. To my surprise Lisa Raphals, with whom I shared the office at the Needham Research Institute in summer 1995, as well as an enthusiasm for the text, published more or less verbatim an early draft of my three tables with the clientele's names and the names and causes of their disorders in 1998.

In the late 1990s, while I was Chiang Chingkuo Teaching and Research Fellow in the History of Chinese Science and Technology at the Faculty of Oriental Studies of the University of Cambridge, Charles Aylmer of the University Library's Aoi Pavilion provided most crucial support with bibliographical problems. John Moffett at the Needham Research Institute was also most helpful, particularly in recent years. The seminars I then organised for the Institute gave me an opportunity, when no other speaker could be found, to present select cases to a lively and critical audience. Christopher Cullen, Vivienne Lo, Kim Taylor and several temporary research and visiting fellows provided vital help and necessary challenges. Furthermore, the case histories were presented to clinicians: Dorin Ritzmann, Carsten Flohr and, later, Jeffery Aronson.

The 1995 translation formed the basis for securing further funding from the Swiss National Foundation in 1999–2001, for a Habilitationsschrift in Medical Anthropology, which was made possible with the support of Hans-Rudolf Wicker and Wolfgang Marschall, Professors in Social Anthropology at the University of Berne. When the situation in Berne changed, it was a stroke of luck that in 2001 Rudolph Wagner agreed to examine the study as a Habilitationsschrift in Sinology. My curriculum vitae and former publications were scrutinised, I was grilled for a whole day over the telephone during my stay at the Max Planck Institute for Social Anthropology in Halle, and had to travel to Heidelberg to give a seminar, which resulted in a heated three-hour debate from 7 to 10 pm at night. Sinologists at their best! The examination procedure took over a year, during which regulations changed, requiring me to teach the equivalent of a one-semester-long course on literary Chinese, in addition to the usual oral examination, in my case, on modern Chinese Studies. The former was one of the most memorable teaching experiences I have ever had, reading Wang Chong's 'Empty Talk about Dragons' and the 'Uselessness of Ritual' with brilliant students; the latter was one of the worst examinations I ever passed. Finally, in December 2002, the process came to a dignified end with my 'Antrittsvorlesung in der alten Aula' on 'Der Ertastete Koerper' (published as 'Tactility and the Body in Early Chinese Medicine' in 2005).

The saga continued after I had become Lecturer in Medical Anthropology at the University of Oxford when, in 2003, William Nienhauser searched for someone to do the translation of the entire *Shi ji* 105. Coincidently I found myself again generously funded by the Chiang Chingkuo Foundation, having been invited as international expert into a group of Taiwanese anthropologists working on the senses in medicine. It allowed me to attend a conference at the University of Wisconsin on the translation of the *Shi ji* in September 2004, during which I received detailed feedback, in particular from Hans van Ess and Tsai-Fa Cheng. Most importantly it permitted me to employ a research assistant, Yanxia Zhang. Old files were retrieved, Chinese characters retyped, new bibliographical references added, comments incorporated from Rudolf Pfister, Paolo Santangelo, Roel Sterckx, Leslie de Vries, Yili Wu and many others, among them Hermann Tessenow and Wang Zilan, who helped with computer searches. In 2005 the penultimate version of the translation of Yi's Memoir was presented in Robert Chard's reading seminars at the Institute of Chinese Studies of the University of Oxford, where several important issues were clarified and some later followed up by Brandon Miller and Ka Tam. As the end was in sight, Sir Geoffrey, who had initiated the project, kindly provided pertinent critique on the versions of summer 2005 and 2006.

Finally, thanks go to my lifelong friends and loved ones, to Benjamin, who appreciated the case histories as short stories and poetry, to Robert, who checked the entire Habilitationsschrift for its clarity in English but missed so many typos, and also to those who found it hard to see me spending long hours with this text instead of them; to my parents and to my three brothers, Martin, Andrew and Peter, who saw me through some of the most difficult episodes of my life. While I could never have completed this study without the assistance and support of the above colleagues, friends and family, and many more whom I have not mentioned by name, I take full responsibility for this text and translation.

NOTE ON TRANSCRIPTIONS IN *PINYIN*

Pre-modern Chinese is transcribed, character by character, in single syllables; standard modern Chinese is given, as usual, in multisyllabic words.

ABBREVIATIONS

CSJC	*Cong shu ji cheng* 叢書集成
CY	*Ciyuan* 詞源
HDNJSW	*Huangdi nei jing Su wen* 黃帝內經素問
HYDCD	*Hanyu dacidian* 漢語大詞典
HYDZD	*Hanyu dazidian* 漢語大字典
MWD	Mawangdui manuscripts 馬王堆
MWD YY	Mawangdui 'Yinyang shiyimai jiujing' 陰陽十一脈灸經
MWD ZB	Mawangdui 'Zubi shiyimai jiujing' 足臂十一脈灸經
OED	Oxford English Dictionary
SBBY	*Si bu bei yao* 四部備要
SBCK	*Si bu cong kan* 四部叢刊
SKQS	*Si ku quan shu* 四庫全書
ZJS	Zhangjiashan manuscripts 張家山
ZJS MSSW	Zhangjiashan 'Maishu 脈書 shiwen'
ZJS YSSW	Zhangjiashan 'Yinshu 引書 shiwen'
ZHYH	*Zhonghua yaohai* 中華藥海
ZYDCD	*Zhongyao dacidian* 中藥大詞典

I
Framing the field

1

Introduction

Pulse diagnosis was the aspect of Chinese medicine most admired in Europe as selected extracts of medical treatises became available in translation from the late 17th century onwards. Du Halde said with admiration: 'In effect, their able physicians predict pretty exactly all the Symptoms of a disease; and it is chiefly this that has rendered Chinese Physicians so famous in the World.'[1] To the present day, pulse diagnosis is met with fascination and disbelief.[2] This book concerns the earliest account of medical practices that pertain to Chinese pulse diagnosis.

The earliest extensive account of Chinese pulse diagnosis, or more accurately, the examination of *mai* 脈 (vessels, pulses, channels) is contained in a biography of a doctor of the Han dynasty (206 BCE – 220 CE), who lived in the period immediately following the first unification of the Chinese empire. He was called Chunyu Yi 淳于意. Since he was an official in the kingdom of Qi 齊 before devoting himself entirely to the study of medicine in 180 BCE, he was also known by his title of office 'Master of the Granary' (Canggong 倉公). His biography comprises two introductory sections about his life, twenty-five medical case histories and eight questions and answers on his medical rationale and its transmission. The biography or, rather, the 'Memoir' (*liezhuan* 列傳), constitutes the second part of the 105th chapter in the *Records of the Historian* (*Shi ji* 史記, ca 86 BCE) by Sima Qian 司馬遷 (?145–ca 86 BCE) and complements that of the legendary physician Bian Que 扁鵲, his three medical case histories and six principles of medical ethics.[3] Throughout Chinese medical history, Bian Que was venerated for his knowledge of *mai*, but, as this study will show, Chunyu Yi's Memoir provides more detail on the innovative method of examining *mai*.

---

[1] Du Halde (1735:184). On the reception of Chinese pulse diagnosis in Europe, see Grmek (1962).

[2] On pulse diagnosis in the Greek and East Asian imagination, see Kuriyama (1986, 1987, 1995b, 1999).

[3] *Shi ji* 105 is called 'Memoir of Bian Que and the Master of the Granary' (Bian Que Canggong zhuan 扁鵲倉公傳); translated into English by Hsu and Nienhauser (in press).

3

The concept of *qi* 氣, which related to airs, vapours and breaths as well as impulsions, irritations and resonances, was central to Chunyu Yi's diagnostic practice and therapy, as was the concept of the 'viscera' (*zang* 藏). The form of pulse diagnosis that Yi practised relied on examining the *mai* on the body surface to identify qualities of *qi* coming from internal viscera. His method of 'examining *mai*' (*zhen mai* 診脈) is often paraphrased as consisting of *qie mai* 切脈 (also called *qiemo*), which probably means 'to palpate' *mai*, or, perhaps, more specifically, to 'press' onto them (as if cutting through them). This study will treat *qie mai* as a pulse diagnostic method that relies on touch. It will investigate how the heightened sense of tactility that it entailed was intricately related to the specific conceptions of body and personhood intrinsic to Yi's medical practice, which, in turn, was based on a subtle understanding of the complexities of illness events and on a unique mode of tackling the question of illness causation. In particular, it will highlight that *qi* gained centrality in medical reasoning as physicians became interested in the management of psychological aspects of personhood, and as emotions became medicalised.

As Yi's Memoir represents a document of similar importance to the history of medicine in China as did the *Epidemics* in the Hippocratic corpus to Greek medicine or the Ebers papyrus to Egyptian medicine, this book also contains the first complete translation into English of the Memoir of Chunyu Yi (*Canggong zhuan* 倉公傳; see chapters 7, 8 and 9).[4] Contemporary scholarship generally considers its composition to have been completed by ca 86 BCE. Accordingly, it can be viewed as a document that pre-dates the final compilation of the *Yellow Emperor's Inner Canon* (short: *Inner Canon*; *Huangdi nei jing* 黃帝內經).[5] Even though this study demonstrates that its textual history is far more complicated, Yi's Memoir remains of primary importance to the study of early developments leading to the foundations of the medical rationale today called 'Chinese medicine'. The Memoir furthermore tells us about the transmission of medical knowledge and practice, names a variety of 'medical' treatises[6] and throws light on early developments in the history of Chinese therapeutics, in particular, of

---

[4] On its textual history, see Hulsewé (1993).

[5] The *Huangdi nei jing* is generally considered the earliest and most important canonical work of Chinese elite medical knowledge. More than half its material dates from between the third century BCE and before 260 CE (Keegan 1988:17). It is to be assumed that several books by this title were in circulation in antiquity and that the earliest version of the extant compilation probably dates from the first century CE (Unschuld 2003:5), which in its extant form is the heavily revised edition from the Song dynasty (960–1279 CE) (Sivin 1993). In its extant form it consists of two books, the *Su wen* (Basic Questions) and *Ling shu* (Divine Pivot), but the same materials are organised differently in the *Huangdi nei jing Tai su* (Grand Basis). On 'canonical' medicine, see ch. 1, n. 9.

[6] Keegan (1988), Sivin (1995a). 'Medicine' is used in a wide sense here and elsewhere in this study, designating practices thought to enhance a person's aliveness. In the early Han, they ranged from the calisthenic, dietetic and sexual arts to prognosticatory and mantic techniques for determining a person's constitution, afflictions and life span.

decoctions, acupuncture and moxibustion.[7] Diagnosis based on *mai* and *se* 色 (colour/complexion) and therapeutics through administration of decoctions, acupuncture and moxibustion have remained the distinctive features of elite medical practices in China for two millennia. While Yi's body conceptions and therapeutic interventions show continuities with those recorded in the early medical manuscript literature,[8] they are framed in a more elaborate medical rationale, which in general, however, pre-dates that of the canonical 'medicine of systematic correspondences'.[9]

The Memoir is of interest to the anthropologist, social and medical historian not least because of the genre in which it records medical knowledge: in twenty-five medical case histories or, in Yi's own terms, 'examination records' (*zhen ji* 診籍). These records provide unparalleled detail on medical practice in antiquity, from diagnostic procedure to therapeutic intervention. The doctor meticulously records the name of the disorder, its concomitant signs and symptoms, explains how the disorder was contracted, and gives reasons why he came to this diagnosis. Most importantly, he prognosticates whether or not the disorder will lead to death. His predictions are always correct; ten cases end in death, the other fifteen involve therapeutic interventions which are always successful, such as the ingestion of broths, the application of poultices, fumigation, needling and cauterisation. The doctor often details stages in the course of the illness or, if he applies treatment, of betterment. His terminology is technical, and he clearly has a complex understanding of medical disorders. He also reports on medical disputes, which throw light on forms of argumentation and scientific debate in antiquity.[10] Since medical knowledge is presented in narrative form, the Memoir also has a literary value that is as yet insufficiently explored.

One crucial finding of this study is that the case histories are formulaic. This applies in particular to cases 1–10. The formulaic features are found in recurrent phrases, which can be interpreted to concern different aspects of a patient's disorder (*bing* 病), namely (1) the name of the disorder, (2) the cause of the disorder and (3) the diagnostic quality indicative of the disorder.[11] The other fifteen cases exhibit more variation but nevertheless can be shown to have the same formulaic features. By contrast, Bian Que's three medical cases and the case on the premature death of a certain

---

[7] Yamada (1998). 'Decoctions' are remedies made by simmering herbal, animal or mineral ingredients in water, decanting the liquid and ingesting it (see case 5, line 7); 'acupuncture' is needle therapy applied within a cosmological schema, e.g. *yin yang*; moxibustion is cauterisation with crushed *Artemisia vulgaris* leaves. See ch. 7, sections 4.2, 4.4 and 4.7.

[8] Discussed in detail in chapters 3 and 4.

[9] The term was coined by Unschuld ([1980]1985), on the basis of Porkert (1974), in light of the pervasive reasoning in terms of so-called 'five phases' or 'five agents' (*wu xing* 五行) that is particularly prominent in the *Su wen*. See p. 23. 'Canonical' refers to all those medical works, which in Imperial times were called 'canons' (*jing* 經), like the *Huangdi nei jing, Zhen jiu jia yi jing, Mai jing, Nan jing*; it is not accorded the meaning it has in Christian doctrine. On 'canons', see Chan (1998:304–5).

[10] Lloyd (1996).   [11] See p. 112 and tables 2–4.

King Wen 文, recorded in the last section of Yi's Memoir, do not fit this formula.

The finding that the case histories are formulaic is central to their interpretation in this study. As the text reports in a learned vocabulary on many bodily processes and medical interventions with which a contemporary reader is not familiar, its terminology can easily be misinterpreted if one unguardedly imputes to it ideas of medical reasoning known from the *Inner Canon* and other texts of the received medical literature. This study takes advantage of the text's formulaic structure and focuses in each case history on those clauses that are linguistically marked and hence considered rhetorically relevant. By ordering these clauses into three long paradigmatic lists of (1) the compound words designating the names of the disorder, (2) the phrases outlining the causes given for each illness occurrence and (3) the rather lengthy explications on mostly tactile qualities of *mai*, it became possible to systematically compare and contrast them with each other. The aim of using this text structural method was to counter the problem of every historian and ethnographer, which is to be anachronistic and ethnocentric. The study thus represents a sustained effort to account for the conceptions of body and personhood, illness and illness causation in accordance with the weighting of the premodern Chinese narrator(s).

The text also mentions signs and symptoms of illness events, sometimes even as constituents of the compound words that formed the names of the disorders. However, generally these signs and symptoms were not part of the rhetorically marked formulae. Rather, they were mentioned here and there in passing. In other words, they were considered concomitant aspects of the illness but in the narrator's view not features of primary importance for the assessment of the illness event, as they are in contemporary 'differential diagnosis'. Previous studies of the Memoir have focused mostly on these concomitantly mentioned signs and symptoms in their assessment of the disorders described. This reflects the anachronistic concerns of contemporary biomedical doctors but does not do justice to the multilayered meanings of a learned ancient terminology. Thus, the two previous translators of this Memoir into German and French, respectively, F. Hübotter and R. Bridgman, who were physicians by training, identified the disorders in terms of biomedicine.[12] In a similar vein, Joseph Needham and Lu Gweidjen focused mostly on signs and symptoms, giving retrospective biomedical diagnoses.[13] Their guesses were sophisticated but highly speculative, and they revealed little about the early Chinese medical rationale underlying the case histories.

This study is anthropologically framed in that it seeks to explore conceptions of body and illness, diagnosis and treatment implicit to the culture

---

[12] Hübotter (1927), Bridgman (1955).
[13] Lu and Needham (1967 and 1980:106–13). See also Needham *et al.* (1970) and Needham and Lu (1999).

and society so vividly depicted in this Memoir. Inspired by recent studies on the anthropology of the body,[14] interpretive/critical medical anthropology,[15] and their application to Chinese cultures,[16] this study explores meanings in relation to other aspects of the practices described and refrains from equating specific bodily processes with their supposed contemporary correlates. For instance, *dong mai* 動脈 is not, in a decontextualised way, translated as 'beating vessel/pulse' and interpreted as 'pulsating artery'.

From an anthropological viewpoint, the diagnostic practices are informed by sophisticated theorising that has to be understood in its own terms and which is misrepresented by such labels as 'primitive magic', 'occult thought' and 'natural philosophy', notions that implicitly claim superiority of occidental rationality and reason. From the perspective of the social historian, the field of medical diagnosis grew out of the prognosticatory sciences, which were practised by retainers that local nobility entertained in the Warring States (475–221 BCE) and early Han.[17] In Yi's Memoir, pulse diagnosis clearly is a form of pulse prognosis.

Ultimately, this study also contributes to the anthropology of sensory experience by viewing the body techniques of physicians and their medical rationale as a cultural elaboration of a specific mode of perception.[18] It concerns science in the widest sense, where science is understood as a field of enquiry that takes seriously the perception of the external world and explores it in a systematic fashion as any formulaically structured enquiry does.[19] Furthermore, it concerns science in that it deals with the practice of learned knowledge with layers of meaning that in antiquity as well were intelligible only to those initiated into the social group that cultivated it.[20]

The terminology on which this study focuses concerns verbs of touch,[21] which interpret tactile experience within a culture-specific frame of learned knowledge.[22] These terms are often common words in literary Chinese, but in this text are used in a technical sense. The vocabulary is technical, but not in the sense that is typical of the modern sciences (with narrow definitions of word meaning that should prevent ambiguity). Rather, the physicians used common words in a special sense, and the special sense in which they used these terms in medicine often showed continuities with other

---

[14] e.g. Scheper-Hughes and Lock (1987), Duden ([1987]1991), Leslie and Young (1992), Shilling (1993), Csordas (2002), Lock and Farquhar (2007).

[15] e.g. Lindenbaum and Lock (1993), Good (1994), Nichter and Lock (2002), Lambek and Antze (2003).

[16] e.g. Kleinman (1980), Ots (1990a), Farquhar (1994, 2002), Hsu (1999), Scheid (2002); Bray (1997), Kuriyama (1999), Furth (1999).

[17] e.g. Sivin (1995b and 1995d), Major (1993), Li Jianmin (2000).

[18] e.g. Howes (1991, 2004), Ingold (2000), Geurts (2003), Bendix and Brenneis (2005).

[19] e.g. Granet (1934), Needham (1956), Lloyd ([1966]1992).

[20] e.g. Woolgar (1988), Latour ([1993]2006), Mol (2003).

[21] Literary Chinese grammar classifies them as 'static verbs' rather than 'adjectives', e.g. *jian* 堅 'to be firm' rather than 'firm'.

[22] On tactility, see e.g. Boyle (1998), Harvey (2003), Classen (2005); after Montagu (1971).

fields of specialised knowledge among court retainers. Nevertheless, they also created new terms and neologisms and sometimes made attempts to give definitions, for instance, of *qi*, or of the tactile perception of a particular pulse quality.

The qualities of touch encountered in the context of pulse diagnosis were elicited through specific bodily techniques that are, however, barely described in the text studied, and must be inferred or accepted as an unknown given. Tactile perception is notoriously difficult to put into words, and in Chinese pulse diagnosis has been conveyed in metaphors and similes, compound words and single-syllabic static verbs. This tactile terminology is enormously rich and fertile: in it we find implicitly contained conceptions of body and universe, causation of and recovery from illness.

This study is based primarily on an investigation of what linguists and semanticists call 'sense relations', a linguistic method for deriving word meaning from the systematic comparison of the contexts in which a term is mentioned.[23] It does not provide the reader with much evidence of the referential meaning of the terms in their specialised usage, simply because one cannot know it on the basis of the textual information at hand.[24] Well aware of the limitations of semantics, this textual study has also taken account of speech act theory and pragmatics,[25] not least because the terms studied occur in utterances that are recorded in case histories where people are in social interaction with each other.

The study certainly builds on the philological method but goes beyond it by taking a more general text critical approach to the exploration of word meaning. This is achieved by taking account of the overall structure of the text when researching the meaning of one particular term, by paying attention to the multiple layers of meaning contained in texts of compilations, and by noting instances of humour and irony.[26] Critical textual studies have opened up new horizons on how to read ancient esoteric texts, and one of the key findings is that these texts are generally compilations of short primary texts. Word meaning can critically change when one puts aside the idea that long texts were composed by one single author and instead reads a long text as a compilation of short texts.[27]

The method of 'text structure semantics' developed in the course of this study is a tool, it is hoped, which may prove useful for future meaning-oriented explorations of formulaic texts. The method was applied to the exploration of the meaning of terms that are polysemous or multivocalic

---

[23] e.g. the rough pulse is the 'opposite' of the slippery pulse.
[24] e.g. what does a 'rough' pulse feel like?
[25] Sense and reference highlight different aspects of word meaning but are not entirely independent of each other (Kempson 1977, Lyons 1977, Cruse 1986). On pragmatics, see Levinson (1983). On registers of speech, see Boyer (1990).
[26] On humour, see, e.g., Harbsmeier (1989), Pfister (2002).
[27] e.g. Keegan (1988), Kern (2002).

(which can be read with specific but distinctively different meanings in different contexts), and vague or general (which regardless of context always have a wide range of meanings). The formulaic structure of the text thus was crucial for identifying which terms designated a name of a disorder and which verbs described a tactile quality during the diagnostic procedure. However, given the complexities of the terms studied, with their many ambiguities and implicit connotations, the meanings identified must be understood to relate just to this particular text.

The study could have examined the literary style of early medical case records with a focus on narrative theory. It could have discussed the epistemological question relevant to the philosophy of science of 'Thinking in cases'[28] or 'Thinking with cases',[29] which explores the quality and validity of knowledge that is generated through individual case studies. It could have scrutinised pressing questions of Chinese historiography that concern the significance of these medical cases in Sima Qian's monumental history of the Han empire. Or, it could have centred on the innovative therapeutic methods mentioned in this Memoir.[30] These, and further questions,[31] will be addressed tangentially. The study's focus is on diagnosis as encompassed by a complex medical rationale and by body techniques involving touch.

---

[28] Forrester (1996).   [29] Furth *et al.* (2007).   [30] Yamada (1998).
[31] e.g. Lloyd (unpubl.) 'Why Case Histories?' 32 p.

2
The questions

Chunyu Yi relies on the two pillars of so-called 'Chinese medicine': pulse diagnosis and decoctions (or 'proto-decoctions'; *tang* 湯).[1] He also makes therapeutic use of 'needling' (*ci* 刺) and 'cauterising' (*jiu* 炙). Since he applies these methods within an elaborate framework of medical reasoning, one can regard needling and cauterising as early forms of acupuncture and moxibustion.[2] Although Yi is the one who meticulously reports on the examination of *mai*, Bian Que was celebrated as the founder of their study.[3] *Shi ji* 105 was known if not memorised by scholar-physicians for centuries to come; and although perhaps hardly understood in its original sense, it lived on in their minds.

Due to the technicality of the vocabulary and considerable medical speculation, the text is extremely difficult to understand. As already mentioned, two physicians have translated the Memoir into a Western language: F. Hübotter into German and R. Bridgman into French.[4] Both translations represent a remarkable achievement for their times, but recent research in anthropology and history brings questions of a different sort into play.

These questions concern, first, the notions of *mai* (vessels/pulses) and the terminology used for expressing the qualities of tactile perception after examining *mai*; second, conceptions of *qi* and the body in the late Warring States and Han; and, third, illness causation, and whether diagnosis must always be directed at identifying the cause of a medical disorder.

Tactility in diagnosis

A new reading of the early manuscript literature reveals that the term *mai* has a remarkable history in the Warring States and early Western Han (206

---

[1] Yamada (1998).

[2] Hsu (2007a). The term *zhen jiu* 'acupuncture and moxibustion' occurs in the Memoir's section 4.2, see ch. 7, n. 66.

[3] Li Bozong (1990).

[4] Hübotter (1927), Bridgman (1955), the latter with an apparatus on medical contents. More recently, Sivin (1995a) translated extracts from the Memoir's introductory parts and the interrogation sections 4.5–4.7 into English.

BCE–9 CE) before it starts to be explored tactually (see pp. 26–8). In fact, the word 'pulse' as an approximate translation for the tactually explored *mai* evokes the wrong connotations, because it makes us think of pulsations and the heartbeat. Accordingly, Du Halde said that the Chinese were able 'By the Beating of the Pulse only to discover the Cause of Disease, and in what Part of the Body it resides'.[5] However, a more careful reading of their medical texts reveals that Chinese physicians were not merely interested in 'Beatings of the Pulse', nor were they searching for the 'Cause of the Disease' in past events. Rather, as will be argued here, their pulse diagnosis attended to the present.

The tactile experiences for distinguishing different *mai* are very subtle. Ethnographic fieldwork revealed that the procedure of examining *mai* puts the doctor into a position of great uncertainty.[6] From the standpoint of pragmatics, the generating of uncertainty between the healer and his clientele is one of the main achievements of divinatory practices.[7] Why generate uncertainty, one may ask, during a process in which an illness is to be named and labelled, i.e. in a diagnostic process that aims at establishing certainty? As medical anthropology emphasises, diagnosis is a complex process, which involves the negotiation of social relations,[8] takes account of economic constraints,[9] local histories and politics,[10] and searches for culturally acceptable forms of expression and interaction.[11] In biomedicine, diagnosis requires investigation into the past and identification of the cause of the patient's condition. However, as medical anthropologists point out, diagnosis also critically accounts for the present and for situational circumstance, and it names the condition examined often strategically in light of the treatment available. This is so in biomedicine as well as among so-called 'folk healers', even if the respective medical ideologies may disclaim it.[12]

A diagnostic procedure that generates uncertainty brings into play the present. Furthermore, it opens up a space for thinking about the future and the choices of treatment available. The creation of uncertainty thus enhances the practitioner's and patient's attentiveness to situational circumstance. Anthropologists have emphasised how social, cultural, economic, as well as historical and political, processes shape such situations. There has been a tendency, however, to underplay the bodily processes of the patients and

---

[5] Du Halde (1735:184).

[6] The fieldwork was undertaken in Kunming city, Yunnan province, People's Republic of China, 1988–9. See Hsu (1999).

[7] Whyte (1997).   [8] e.g. Lock (1993), Samuelsen and Steffen (2004).

[9] e.g. Scheper-Hughes (1992), Farmer (1999).   [10] e.g. Young (1995), Davis (2000).

[11] e.g. Laderman and Roseman (1996), Lewis (1999).

[12] Nichter (1996:120–3) highlighted the strategic aspects of illness labelling and, in contradistinction to 'disease taxonomies', spoke of 'illness task-onomies'. Kleinman (1988:16) highlighted that strategic thinking applies also to biomedical diagnoses, e.g. health insurance reimbursements. Also, the availability of lithium multiplied diagnoses of the bipolar disorder.

practitioners in such circumstances due to the dichotomy intrinsic to Western scholarship, which takes biomedicine as authority on bodily processes and the social sciences as authority on those that are not bodily. Inroads towards overcoming this dichotomy have been made within the fields of the anthropology of the body and also the anthropology of the senses and emotions.[13]

Foucauldian approaches to the anthropology of the body emphasise how the social is inscribed in the body, how institutional objectives are internalised by the subject and how power is everywhere, above and below, precisely because individuals have internalised the dominant discourse in a given society.[14] Phenomenological approaches, by contrast, foreground that the body is a generative principle. It is the starting point of any form of human experience, and cross-cultural variation arises from culture-specific elaboration of these bodily experiences common to humankind. Human existence is experienced primarily in and through the body.[15] The tension between these two theoretical approaches is partly resolved by practice theory, which reminds us that these processes happen in dynamic social fields, and involve actors – with specific tastes and dispositions – in negotiation with each other.[16] This provides the basis for the exploration of sensory experience pursued in this study.

Sensory perception and emotion, as experienced by individuals through their bodies, is culturally mediated and socially learnt. Case histories record subjective experiences that are instantiated in particular moments. Each is unique, and yet, seen together, they shape and are shaped by social and cultural processes among a certain group of people. These experiences are simultaneously social and bodily. The anthropology of sensory experience emphasises that the sensorial medium through which the external world is experienced shapes the way in which the person relates to it. Touch might be key to sensing feelings.

Pulse diagnosis generates in the medical practitioner an uncertainty that differs from the technique of a diviner who throws beads or lays out cards, in that this uncertainty is mediated through a sophisticated body technique that involves touch. Touch causes presence; a tap on one's arm catches one's attentiveness. Touch makes real; talk may be flattery, visual cues an optical illusion, odours are notoriously ephemeral and taste notoriously subjective (even if it is a socially learnt and sociologically distinct subjectivity), yet touch imbues events and things with veracity. Touch causes closeness, even intimacy; a physician feels the pulse and the patient feels closeness, opens

[13] This point was already argued in early works on the anthropology of emotions, e.g. Heelas and Lock (1981), Rosaldo (1980), Myers (1979).
[14] e.g. Foucault ([1963]1989, [1975]1979, [1976]1990), Lock and Kaufert (1998).
[15] e.g. Merleau-Ponty ([1945]1962), Csordas (1994), Lambek and Strathern (1998).
[16] e.g. Bourdieu ([1979]1984, 1991). See also Harker *et al.* (1990), Jenkins ([1992]2002) and Reckwitz (2002).

up, unravels personal stories. A physician's touch may calm a patient, transmit tranquility and increase confidence. The physician's active touch of intruding with his hand into the patient's intimate sphere furthermore asserts authority, even if it is at the most distant part of one's extremities, the wrist that can be stretched out far.[17] The presence that touch evokes, the sense of veracity, the combination of simultaneous intimacy and authority by the physician who takes the pulse must have marked the process of tactually exploring *mai*, also in antiquity.

The question arises as to whether this understanding of touch was shared by Chinese physicians in antiquity whose diagnostic procedure involved tactility. Why would physicians start to engage in a tactile exploration of *mai*, rather than in a visual, auditory or olfactory one? Why did they develop body techniques that could elicit different tactile qualities, which provided guidance in naming disease? Considering that Yi palpated *mai* in the context of deciding whether or not he should deliver treatment to a patient or whether the patient would die anyway, one wonders which tactile qualities of *mai* would interest him.

For making prognostications of death, one could say from an empiricist viewpoint that heart arrhythmias, which can be felt in the pulse, sometimes indicate imminent death. Without denying the pragmatically appealing aspect of this biomedical explanation, it does not explain how the Chinese physicians themselves thought about tactility and what the advantages were that they saw in tactually exploring *mai*. In this context, we are reminded of an important source of medical knowledge for Yi. As we will see when we come to Yi's prime medical authority 'Qi ke' (on p. 67), physicians had become interested in the visceral states of their patients by the early Han. As this study will show, their body technique of tactually exploring *mai* informed them on qualities of *qi*; *qi* that came from the viscera.

In cross-cultural perspective, the viscera are often viewed as the seat of emotion. Indeed, in ancient China the heart was the one viscus that was seat of emotion, cognition and moral sensitivities. The pre-dynastic and Han literature amply attests to this.[18] However, in Yi's Memoir two viscera are affected in those case histories that mention strong emotions and feelings: the heart (case 2) and the liver (case 6). These two viscera, as will be shown in more detail particularly with regard to case 2, may well attest to a conception of a bipartite body, with the heart above and the liver below the diaphragm (*ge*). Perhaps a body inhabited by two viscera pre-dated the body with the five viscera known to us from canonical doctrine?

Cross-culturally, feelings are often framed in terms of tactually felt warmth and coldness. In pre-dynastic China, they were primarily associated

---

[17] See references in ch. 1, n. 18, and Immerwahr (1978) and Mazis (1979).
[18] e.g. Graham (1989:25) emphasises the heart as seat of cognition, but it was also of morality and all emotion.

with the dynamics of *qi*,[19] and expressed in the language of *qi* and *yin yang*. Interestingly, Yi was able to perceive *qi* tactually through the innovative method of palpating *mai*. In Europe, tactility directs one's attention to the emotional dimension of human existence,[20] to which, it appears, members of the middle and upper classes pay particular attention, often in a verbose vocabulary.[21] Perhaps this applies to Eastern as to Western sensibilities, to ancient as to modern times. Perhaps Chinese physicians of the nobility, who started to attend to the psychology of their clientele, for this reason developed tactile techniques of diagnosis. Perhaps their idea that visceral distress can generate illness arose from their conception of the viscera as, primarily, the seat of emotion.[22]

Conceptions of the body: architectural body, sentimental body and body ecologic

This brings us to the second major theme of this book, namely *qi* and the 'viscera' (*zang*) in Yi's medical rationale and how they are related to his conceptions of the body. In this context, it is important to signal that the idea that the viscera gained prominence in medical language because they were conceived as the seat of emotion and, presumably, as storage places of *qi* (dynamics of which related to emotional processes) points to an entirely new way of thinking about *qi* and the viscera.

Historians of the Chinese sciences have it that in Han Chinese medicine *qi* is the transformative stuff that permeates the universe and that the notion of the 'five viscera' (*wu zang* 五藏) is derived from observations of proto-chemistry and empirical physiological observation.[23] Yet this study argues that in the late Warring States and early Han the notion of *qi* primarily related to body internal processes of breathing and feeling, and that the viscera – first, solely the heart,[24] then the heart and liver – gained centrality in medicine as physicians attended to the psychological aspects of personhood expressed in the language of *qi*, and medicalised emotion.

This argument results from extended research on Yi's Memoir, as in the course of this study it became apparent that a certain word was used in

---

[19] See Csikszentmihalyi (2004:101–60; 102, 147, 152, 156) on *Mengzi*'s 'systematic psychology', movements of *qi* affecting the heart, filial piety and righteousness.

[20] Mazis (1979).

[21] In the USA, as Kleinman (1980:172) puts it, 'middle-class Caucasians' 'psychologise' distress, while 'lower class' 'blue-collar workers' 'somatise' psychological problems.

[22] This critiques research that conceives of them primarily as 'proto-anatomical entities' or 'somatic' entities.

[23] On this understanding of *qi*, see Sivin (1987:46–53); on proto-chemistry, see Needham (1956:244); on an example of an empirical observation that links the stomach to digestion, see Unschuld (2003:130).

[24] In early manuscript texts, *qi*, or rather, various graphs interpreted as loanwords for *qi*, are mentioned in the context of the emotions (Puett 2004:45) and the 'heart' (Harper 2001:104/5).

different senses, sometimes within the same case history. It was thus necessary to differentiate whether the word (or phrase) in question alluded to a framework that conceptualises the body with reference to a rather static 'bodily architecture', as known through a rich vocabulary of bodily structures, or in regard to one that stresses seasonal change and humoral transformation. The latter body conception, elsewhere referred to as the 'body ecologic', prevailed in Chinese medical history for two thousand years, and often mentioned *qi* in its account of the seasonality of illness.[25]

Based on recent text critical studies which emphasise the composite character of learned texts, it was possible to identify text passages, buried among others in canonical texts and in Yi's Memoir, that referred to yet another body conception, namely the 'sentimental body'. These passages, which mentioned as two main sentiments grief/joy and anger in heart and liver, accounted for feelings in a visceral language and stressed psychological aspects of personhood (see also pp. 34–40). On reflection, it may not be surprising that a study on tactility should find in the 'sentimental body' a generally overlooked body conception of early Chinese medical history. This 'sentimental body', which is crucial for understanding Yi's medical rationale, throws new light on the history of the concepts *qi* and *zang* (viscera).

To be sure, the 'architectural body', the 'sentimental body' and the 'body ecologic' are not concepts that the ancient physicians themselves embraced. Rather, they provide a heuristic conceptual framework for the interpretation of word meaning in Yi's Memoir. They arose in the course of a close reading of his case histories, which revealed that recurrently encountered terms for body parts had different shades of meaning and were sometimes used in a slightly different sense. For instance, the term *xin* 心 meaning 'the heart' may be used in a body architectural way to refer to the internal cavity inside the chest; if it is used in the context of speaking of strong emotions and alludes to the 'sentimental body', however, it may connote grief or delight (or any other emotion); and in many canonical texts that mention the 'five viscera' (*wu zang* 五藏) and allude to the 'body ecologic', it connotes the season summer, the cardinal direction of the south, the colour red, heat and fire. Context may bring into play a different connotation of the very same term. Having said this, the term *xin* 心 usually has all these connotations, even in contemporary contexts. With this in mind, it should be clear that this study makes no attempt to argue that the 'architectural body', the 'sentimental body' and the 'body ecologic' outline different stages in the history of the Chinese medical body.

---

[25] On the 'body ecologic', see Hsu (1999:78–83, 2003, 2007b). In Hsu (2007b), I outlined the 'body ecologic' as a methodology, namely the genealogical approach, for investigating body concepts that reflect a concern with ecological change (e.g. the hot and cold). But in this study, the 'body ecologic' refers to body conceptions concerned with ecological change.

The question of illness causation

The third major topic of this study concerns the question of illness causation. In Du Halde's above quote (on p. 3), it is said that pulse diagnosis disclosed 'the Cause of Disease, and in what Part of the Body it resides'. In his view pulse diagnosis provided information on the cause of an illness and the body part in which it resided. His comment implies that diagnosis requires knowing the illness cause. However, as this study will show for Yi's cases 1–10, it is not the cause that is relevant for naming the disorder, but rather the tactile qualities felt by the doctor at the time of making a diagnosis.

The idea that illnesses have causes has a long history in European thought. In Du Halde's time, Aristotle's four causes were central to causal explanation, also in medicine. They were the material, formal, final, and efficient cause, whereby 'the matter corresponds to what a thing is made of, the form to the characteristic features that make it the thing it is, the final cause is its function or the good it serves, and the efficient selects what brings it about'.[26] This shows that European physicians of scholarly medicines had elaborate ideas about causation, but as Geoffrey Lloyd thereupon comments: 'Of these four, only the efficient cause looks like a cause in any ordinary English sense.' In other words, reasoning that alluded to Aristotle's four causes was heavily loaded with culture-specific meanings. No attempt is made to elucidate those here, but the above gives a hint of how fraught the notion of 'cause' is in occidental traditions of thinking.

The biomedical sciences grew out of Galenic and scholastic medical learning, even if their ideologies today emphasise the contrary by underlining the contrast between the 'traditional' and 'modern'. From the historian's viewpoint, it is not surprising to find that the biomedical sciences too consider the cause important for identifying disease. There is continuity in Europe between the 'modern' forms of medicine and the 'traditional' ones, and there are differences. David Hume (1711–76) is generally hailed as the philosopher who narrowed down the notion of cause by stressing that causes have effects and that causes must temporally precede effects. He used the mechanical metaphor of one billiard ball hitting another, thereby bringing it into motion at the speed and angle effected by the speed and angle with which it was hit.[27] That a cause precedes its effect seems a platitude today. However, if one takes account of the Aristotelean causes mentioned above, which were still in circulation in the eighteenth century, one understands that Hume's description of causes as having effects relates to what Lloyd calls the 'ordinary English sense of cause'.

The above should highlight how culture-specific the preoccupation with causation is to European medicines, modern and traditional. As Emiko

---

[26] Lloyd (1995:538).   [27] Hume ([1748]1999).

Ohnuki-Tierney has long pointed out in her ethnography on medical plural-ism in Japan, this need not be so in every cultural setting: 'We cannot assume *a priori* the presence of causal notions in every medical system, just because it is the central issue in biomedicine.'[28] In a similar vein, Robert Pool pro-vides an ethnographic vignette on how mystified the Cameroonian respon-dent is by the ethnographer's interest in illness causation.[29]

It is just possible that Du Halde's sentence quoted above, as a product of cultural translation, implicitly equates the European preoccupation of finding the 'cause of disease' with the Chinese one of identifying 'the part of the body' in which the disorder resides. In other words, Chinese physi-cians, rather than seeking the cause of an illness, which is found in the past history of the patient's life, made it their diagnostic task to locate the dis-order somewhere inside the body and determine within which of the dif-ferent potentially affected body parts it might reside. In other words, observed manifestations of the illness were not explained through the patient's past history, i.e. by causes that precede effects, but through the interpretation of synchronously given signs, i.e. signs elicited from investi-gating the body surface which were thought to indicate pathological pro-cesses inside the body. Based on such an investigation that in a synchronous way linked the outwardly perceived processes to postulated internal ones, the physician would name the patient's condition.

The emphasis on investigating synchronous signs for identifying the name of the disorder has a long history in China. Porkert contrasted the causal-analytic thinking in biomedicine with the inductive-synthetic thinking in Chinese medicine.[30] His analysis built on Western scholarship that contrasts reasoning in terms of correlative cosmologies with causal reasoning. Porkert emphasised difference, and did not make any suggestion that the inductive-synthetic reasoning represented an early stage in the history of civilisation nor that causal-analytic reasoning was its apex. And yet it is a widespread view that establishing analogies between macrocosmic and microcosmic processes, as done within the framework of correlative cosmologies, is an early form of causal reasoning.[31] Put crudely, the view is that the ancients, like bad statisticians, believed that all correlations were manifestations of causal relations.

The idea that correlative cosmologies represent an early stage of human thought typically found in literate ancient civilisations builds on empiricist and rationalist debates in Western scholarship. Causal reasoning is consid-ered superior to correlative thinking. It is the prerequisite for rational thought, generally considered the mode of thinking that has led to great progress in science and technology, which, in turn, has led to, and legitimises, the current world order.

---

[28] Ohnuki-Tierney (1984:85).   [29] Pool (1994).   [30] Porkert (1974).
[31] Farmer, Henderson and Witzel (2000).

Since the notions of causality and rationality are inextricably linked to the legitimation of medical intervention, any discussion pertaining to ideas of illness causation in contemporary medicine is fraught with problems affecting its legitimacy. Physicians of the Western and Eastern traditions, both eager to legitimise their own learning, have mutually accused each other of not accounting for illness causation. Thus, Western physicians in the early twentieth century claimed that Western medicine alone investigated causation, and they accused Chinese physicians of attending to synchronous signs and symptoms only, as one does in the framework of correlative cosmologies. Chinese physicians, by contrast, accused Western physicians of being body- and symptom-oriented in an unacceptably narrow and materialistic way, while they themselves, due to the subtle connections that correlative cosmologies highlight, had the intellectual framework to find those causes of the illness that really mattered.[32]

Anthropologists took the opposite stance to the above physicians. In a well-meaning attempt to credit other peoples with legitimate ways of thinking and the faculty of causal reasoning, they widened the notion of cause to frame non-Western practices and ideas in logical and rationally intelligible ways. However, they discussed under the rubric 'illness causation' rather different questions. Thus, W. H. R. Rivers was interested in the question of why a certain treatment is delivered and not another, and found that treatment choices were informed 'by definite ideas concerning the causation of disease'.[33] His point was that the peoples in question were perfectly rational, they could think logically and were capable of causal reasoning, they just built on the wrong assumptions. E. E. Evans-Pritchard, by contrast, addressed the question 'Why me? Why now?' and focused on indigenous attributions of causation that modern science can only explain in terms of 'coincidence'.[34] Both wrote on 'illness causation', but they set out to explain rather different aspects of other peoples' medicines.

Gilbert Lewis notes that causal reasoning in medicine is closely related to the question: what counts as evidence in diagnosis?[35] Practitioners are confronted with daily life problems, yet in their explanations often allude to variables outside everyday life experience and perception. What goes beyond immediate perception is considered a 'causal explanation'. To a certain extent, one might say, anthropologists have been quick to link evidence in diagnosis given in a register of speech that goes beyond that used in daily life to 'causal explanation'.

However, evidence in diagnosis need not, by definition, be linked to a Humean cause–effect relation of the condition presented, where the cause temporally precedes the effect. This is what emerges with great clarity from Yi's case histories. Yi found diagnostic evidence in signs that are synchro-

---

[32] Unschuld (1992).   [33] Rivers (1924:28).
[34] Evans-Pritchard (1937:63–83).   [35] Lewis (1975:223).

nous to the complaint. Naturally, one may object to this on the grounds that these signs are, in fact, indicative of causes. However, this objection is problematic insofar as the rephrasing of synchronous signs as indicative of causes may be nothing more than a well-meant ethnocentric legitimation for a medical rationale that, if one looks carefully, is not actually concerned with causes preceding effects.

One may point out that Yi wrote medical case histories, and that therefore he was undeniably interested in the patient's past history. If the cause of the illness is essential to the identification of illness, which is an age-old assumption in European thinking, and if causes precede effects, which is not the Aristotelean but the Humean understanding of cause, it follows logically that a physician interested in making a diagnosis should investigate the past to find the cause and hence focus on the history of the illness. A biomedical anamnesis is indubitably set up with the intention to find the cause of the illness, which should provide the key for naming the illness. However, it would be wrong to deduce from biomedical conventions that the writing of medical case histories by definition indicates that any physician who writes case histories searches for the cause of the illness. Medical case histories, as recorded in the *Epidemics* in Greek antiquity, were not written with the intention to find the cause of the illness in the patient's past history, quite simply, because the Greeks did not have a Humean concept of cause. More importantly, as Lloyd points out, the thrust of the authors of the *Epidemics* was to identify individual misfortune in account of 'constitutions' in the atmosphere at large.[36] From this follows that if a physician writes case histories, this is not evidence enough for being preoccupied with finding causes that precede effects in the Humean sense.

In all twenty-five case histories Yi rhetorically marks aspects of the patient's disorder that can be interpreted to refer to the 'cause' of the disorder. However, in many cases it was impossible to correlate the cause with the name of the disorder. Rather, as Yi himself indicates in a phrase he recurrently uses, he has other means of recognising and naming the disorder. The means whereby he recognised it consisted of examining *mai*. His pulse diagnostic techniques allowed him to elicit different tactile qualities. To be sure, when I began this study it was not clear whether the verbs of touch with which he assessed these qualities were relevant to his diagnosis. It was through the method of so-called 'text structure semantics' (see part III) that it became evident that they were crucial for naming the disorder.

What is important here is that the tactile qualities elicited through examining *mai* are synchronous signs and that these were relevant for naming a disorder. Yi reports on the causes of the illness, which no doubt are an important feature of his narrative but, as the method of 'text structure

[36] Lloyd (1983:32).

semantics' shows, his diagnostic method does not accord them much relevance within his medical rationale. Rather than turning to the past and searching for causes in history, Yi is preoccupied with investigating the present. One could object that Yi draws out a medical ideology, i.e. that what he says he does is not what he actually does. For instance, in the process of taking the pulse his patients may have confided past experience in him of equal importance for reaching the results that his ideology ascribes to pulse diagnosis. The point I make here is that Yi's medical ideology is that the means whereby he recognises an illness consists in investigating synchronous events, and not in interpreting the past events that brought on the illness (like Humean causes bring on effects).

The idea that illnesses are considered to reside in certain body parts recasts the question of illness causation as an enterprise that makes spatial entities, rather than past events, responsible for the condition of the patient. The question that then arises is how space is related to time. There may be a connection between past events and currently affected body parts. Yi does not refer to demons and ghosts as causes of the illness, although he makes use of demonological terms; he speaks of illnesses 'visiting' (*ke*) body parts and body parts acting as 'hosts' (*zhu*) of the illness.[37] Possibly, at some stage in China's medical history, the cause of the illness was attributed to demons who were understood to visit body parts that acted as hosts to them and were thereby harmed by them. Regardless of such hypothetical medical history implicit in Yi's terminology, let us reiterate that the medical ideology he adheres to gives priority to synchronicity: outwardly perceptible signs indicate which body parts are internally affected.

Correlative thinking emphasises synchronicity: Ågren, for instance, points out that the *Inner Canon* focuses on synchronic correlations, while the *Treatise on Cold Damage Disorders* (*Shang han lun*) of 196 CE stresses that illnesses go through stages.[38] The former was held in high esteem in China, the latter in Japan; and Japan much more readily embraced Western medicine and Western notions of causality, which locate causes of illnesses in the past. One therefore wonders why doctors like Yi and the authors of the *Inner Canon* insisted on a medical ideology of investigating synchronous signs. The rationalist viewpoint that correlative thought is typical of an earlier stage in the evolution of humanity, which in the post-Enlightenment period culminates in the triumph of rationality, clearly is unappealing in this context. A more interesting question is what does correlative thought do which causal reasoning cannot achieve? Above we noted that touch was a sense *par excellence* for causing presence, and here we note that diagnostic ideology emphasises attentiveness to synchronous qualities. Evidently,

[37] e.g. case 1 (line 19) and case 5 (line 3). Please note that references of this kind often imply extended discussion of the terms mentioned. Page references are given in the summary of cases 1–10 on pp. 103–8. For instance, the term 'host' in case 1 (line 19) is discussed on p. 132.

[38] Ågren (1986).

both Yi's bodily techniques for eliciting diagnostic signs and his medical ideology stressed synchronicity. Why?

The generation of synchronicity between different aspects of the universe is closely related to a specific concept of personhood and self. We are reminded that the self is not an unproblematic given. De Martino, who wrote on what he called 'primitive magic', suggested that for patients treated by primitive magic, it is the 'reality of presence' that is a problem, presence being 'something to be aimed for, a task, a drama, a problem'. Illness and its treatment become an issue of the existential drama concerned with the mastery and consolidation of 'the elementary being-in-the-world or presence of the individual'. Treatments that focus on synchronicity are concerned with the 'risk and redemption of presence'.[39]

De Martino wrote in the early twentieth century and, in the *Zeitgeist* of his time, contrasted primitive magic that consolidates the individual's presence in therapy with modern medicine which foregrounds knowing and knowledge. Needless to say such an opposition between magical treatment and scientific medicine is uninteresting because it distorts reality, i.e. the 'consolidation of presence' may be as indispensable an aspect of successful treatment in modern medicine, particularly in so-called 'difficult cases', as may be 'knowledge' in magic.[40] Albeit in some respects dated, De Martino's study is relevant here as it points to the dimension of the self and its being-in-the-world. It highlights that therapy can be designed so as to manipulate the self and its presence in the world.

Yi makes connections between affected body parts of the patient and qualities he perceives on the body surface. He reports on a world of movements and transformations. Illnesses are not entities that can be expelled like demons in exorcistic practices. Rather, aspects of the body that are affected by illness are transformed into other things or forces, often fluids that are subsequently exuded, vomited or excreted. The drama of the self and its being-in-the-world is phrased as one of movements and transformations within and outside the body. The notion central to these processes is *qi*.

---

[39] De Martino ([1948]1988:92, 147).   [40] Hsu (2005b).

3

Diagnosis and medicine in the Warring States and the early Han

Chunyu Yi's method of examining *mai* built on medical knowledge of the Warring States and early Han known to us primarily from manuscript texts unearthed in the 1970s and 1980s. After presenting a synopsis of the literature and an overview of the medical landscape, three early manuscript texts that contain passages on the diagnostic investigation of *mai* are briefly mentioned. They highlight that diagnosis in the late Warring States and early Han involved a variety of sensory modes, while Yi relied particularly in cases 1–10 on a tactile method remarkable for its explicit identification of the qualities of *qi* as an aspect of the *mai*.

Literature review

This study elucidates the medical rationale in *Shi ji* 105 by comparing it to the manuscript literature that in recent decades has been unearthed from tombs closed in the Warring States (475–221 BCE), Western Han (206 BCE–9 CE) and Eastern Han (25–220 CE). Among these tombs are most notably those dating to the Western Han in Mawangdui, tomb 3 (168 BCE), near Changsha, in Hunan province, and in Zhangjiashan, tomb 247 (mid-second century BCE), at Jiangling, in Hubei province.[1] Studies on these manuscripts concern so-called 'magical therapies' and drug-based recipes,[2] nurturing life practices and the gymnastics of 'guiding and pulling',[3] the sexual arts,[4] and the study of *mai* (vessels, pulses).[5] The texts devoted to the study of *mai* are

---

[1] For transcription of the Mawangdui (MWD) manuscripts on themes classified as medical, see Mawangdui Hanmu boshu zhengli xiaozu (1985). For translation of all those, see Harper (1998, 1982). For a concordance with variant graphs, see Emura (1987). For comparison of the Mawangdui vessel texts with *Ling shu* 10, and translation of these three texts, see Keegan (1988: chapter 3, 114–66, and appendix 2, 265–344) and Han Jianping (1999). For a freely edited and richly annotated version, see Ma Jixing (1992). For the Zhangjiashan 'Maishu' and Zhangjiashan 'Yinshu', see Jiangling Zhangjiashan Hanjian zhengli xiaozu (short: ZJS MSSW 1989), Zhangjiashan Hanjian zhenglizu (ZJS YSSW 1990), Gao Dalun (1992) and Zhangjiashan 247 hao Hanmu zhujian zhengli xiaozu (ZJS 2001); see also Ma Jixing (1992:58–172).
[2] Harper (1982, 1998), Yamada (1998).   [3] Lo (2001).
[4] Harper (1998), Pfister (in press).
[5] Keegan (1988), Harper (1998), Han (1999), Li Jianmin (2000).

the so-called Mawangdui 'Model for the Study of Mai' (Maifa 脈法) and the Zhangjiashan 'Document on the Study of Mai' (Maishu 脈書), part 3, as well as the 'Cauterisation Canon of the Eleven Mai of Foot and Forearm' (Zubi shiyimai jiujing 足臂十一脈灸經) and the 'Cauterisation Canon of the Eleven Yin and Yang Mai' (Yinyang shiyimai jiujing 陰陽十一脈灸經),[6] of which the latter parallels the Zhangjiashan 'Maishu', part 2. To those texts may be added the lacquer figurine from Yongxing, tomb 2 (before 118 BCE), in the Mianyang district of Sichuan province, which shows red lines on black ground, presumably *mai*.[7]

It is the case that correlative cosmology in terms of the 'five agents' (*wu xing* 五行) is mentioned in Western Han manuscripts as it is in *Shi ji* 105, but it does not figure very prominently in these documents. This suggests that by the second century BCE medical reasoning in terms of the five agents was neither widely accepted nor very elaborate.[8] In Yi's Memoir, correlative cosmology in terms of the five agents is invoked particularly in the context of diagnosis by means of 'colour/complexion',[9] as in case 15, which mentions yellow as a colour that correlates with the stomach.[10] However, Yi's reasoning explicitly alludes to correlations of the five agents only in cases 15 and 21, and only once mentions the term 'five viscera', in case 3 (line 15).

Correlative cosmology was central to hemerological texts (which outline time periods of good and bad fortune), pre-dating the above Western Han manuscript finds. Thus, manuscripts on divinatory practices involving propitiation and exorcism have been unearthed from Baoshan, tomb 2 (ca 316 BCE), in Hubei, and manuscripts on correlative-cosmology iatromancy (the art of predicting medical events) from Jiudian, tomb 56 (late fourth century BCE), at Jiangling, and from Shuihudi, tomb 11 (ca 217 BCE), in Yunmeng,

---

[6] All titles of these texts are modern. The latter are given as Mawangdui 'vessel texts', i.e. MWD ZB and MWD YY (of the latter there are two versions in manuscript form; references are to no. 1, unless otherwise stated). Harper (1998:23) dates their script to 215 and 205–195 BCE. Han (1999:99–100) suggests the MWD 'Maifa' was written in the Qin dynasty (215–206 BCE) and the ZJS 'Maishu' in the early Han.

[7] He and Lo (1996).

[8] This is in line with recent research in Chinese Studies on five agents doctrine in political history (e.g. Loewe 2004:496–7). Queen (1996) has shown that the chapter in Dong Zhongshu's (?179–?104 BCE) *Chun qiu fan lu* 春秋繁露 (Luxuriant Dew of the Spring and Autumn Annals) on the five agents, which was thought to date to the second century BCE, in all likelihood was composed in the Eastern Han.

[9] In Yi's Memoir only cases 12, 15, 17 and 21 mention *se*: case 12 mentions *yan se* 顏色 'complexion', case 17 *tai yang se* 太陽色 'the colour of the major *yang*', case 21, which alludes to a correlation of the five grains and five viscera, has *gu se* 固色 'solid colour' (see pp. 30–3). On case 15, see main text.

[10] In canonical doctrine, yellow (*huang* 黃) correlates with the spleen (*pi* 脾), of which the stomach is the outer aspect. Blue-green (*qing* 青) with the liver (*gan* 肝), red (*chi* 赤) with the heart (*xin* 心), white (*bai* 白) with the lungs (*fei* 肺), and black (*hei* 黑) with the kidneys (*shen* 腎). See *Su wen* 5, pp. 20–21.

both also in Hubei province.[11] Furthermore, two hemerological manuscripts were found in Fangmatan, tomb 1 (230–220 BCE), in Tianshui, Gansu province, among which a text known for its 'Spell binding' (Jie 結) that exorcises illness-harbouring demons is particularly well known.[12]

Two further manuscript finds have been relevant for the interpretation and translation of *Shi ji* 105, primarily because of the drugs they list, which partially parallel the extant *materia medica* (*ben cao* 本草) of the Eastern Han. One was unearthed from Shangudui, tomb 1 (ca 165 BCE), in Fuyang, Anhui province, with a text on 'The Myriad Things' (Wanwu 万物) that, *inter alia*, lists drugs used for medical purposes.[13] The other, with extensive lists of drugs, was found in a tomb (first century CE) near Wuwei in Gansu province.[14]

The above manuscripts,[15] and a few others,[16] are relevant to the study of Warring States and Han medicine and related fields of learned knowledge. To this list should be added the Dunhuang medico-religious manuscripts of medieval times from the sixth to eleventh centuries CE,[17] and recent studies on them in Western languages.[18] Following David Keegan's study of esoteric texts and their structure, which he links to their particular mode of transmission,[19] these medieval manuscripts are best read as compilations that assembled primary texts of the Han period in a modular fashion.[20] Since this mode of transmission results in texts within which the smallest textual units are preserved fairly intact, it would appear justifiable to use medieval texts, judiciously read, for elucidating Han conceptions of the body. In spite of this, this study will take account of medieval medical manuscripts only in a few critical cases.

Scholarly tools for text critical analysis have been found in numerous dictionaries, including specialist medical dictionaries; in computerised versions of the standard dynastic histories, the medical canons and the early manuscript literature; in the concordances of pre- and Han dynastic works by D. C. Lau and of the *Inner Canon* by Ren Yingqiu 任應秋;[21] as well as in the bibliographical guide to early Chinese texts by Michael

---

[11] Harper (2001). For transcription of the Baoshan, Jiudian and Shuihudi manuscripts, see Hubeisheng Jingsha tielu kaogudui (1991), Hubeisheng wenwu kaogu yanjiusuo (1995), Shuihudi Qinmu zhujian zhengli xiaozu (1990).

[12] For transcription of 'Spell binding', see Gansusheng wenwu kaogu yanjiusuo, Qinjian zhengli xiaozu (1989). For translation, see Harper (1996).

[13] The manuscripts include also texts on hemerology, astrology, the physiognomy of dogs, and breath cultivation. For transcription, see Fuyang Hanjian zhenglizu (1983, 1988).

[14] For transcription, see Gansusheng bowuguan and Wuweixian wenhuaguan (1975).

[15] Given also in Unschuld and Zheng (2005).

[16] See Harper (1998:30–36).   [17] Ma Jixing *et al.* (1998), Cong Chunyu (1994).

[18] Kalinowski (2003), Lo and Cullen (2005), Despeux (in press).

[19] Keegan (1988) points to texts 1 compiled in texts 2.   [20] Hsu (in press c).

[21] See ch. 1, n. 5. Wang Bing (fl. 762) is considered to have interpolated chapters 66–71, 74; and in parts 5 and 9. See Porkert (1974), Ren (1982), Ma (1990), Despeux (2001), Unschuld, Zheng and Tessenow (2003), Feng (2003).

Loewe.[22] Translations of and extensive studies on early and medieval Chinese medical texts of the received tradition have increased in the last two decades.[23] Moreover, some recent studies, which discuss antiquity as part of a larger project within the history of Chinese medicine, are innovative for the ways in which they have addressed questions of social history and anthropology.[24]

A brief note on the medical landscape

The above manuscript finds highlight that in the late Warring States and Han, literate groups of medical practitioners could be found in many different places in China, ranging from Hunan province in the South to Gansu in the North, from Sichuan in the West to Anhui in the East. Despite the spatial distances between the archaeological sites and the temporal gaps, spanning a period of over five hundred years, and despite notable differences in vocabulary and script, the manuscripts suggest that there was a field of transregional exchange, also in medicine.

The medical landscape was populated by practitioners of different creeds, some of whom conversed with each other in a more sophisticated vocabulary than others. Some were literate, wrote and recited texts; others undoubtedly were not (although the latter is based on an assumption rather than unambiguous archaeological evidence). Yi's movements, even if the place names had been edited into the Memoir in the early first century BCE (see pp. 52–7 and ch. 9), would suggest that people displaced themselves frequently, sometimes over great distances. There were medicines for protection during travel.[25] Yi wandered among the feudal lords and treated their dependents but the norm seems to have been that physicians were kept at court, like other retainers. Although the arts they practised and proscribed have been called 'occult' or 'magical', one has to keep in mind that the techniques were those of the elite. Cross-culturally, they compare with the taste of the elite, its sense of rank and distinction and its embodied sensitivities.

Despite variation in medical texts and techniques, there are striking continuities. For instance, the same medical terms resurface in a variety of manuscript texts and, as we will see, also in Yi's Memoir and the received canonical medical literature. Most conspicuous in this respect is the concept of *mai*, which figures centrally in the Mawangdui vessel texts, the Zhangjiashan 'Maishu', the *Divine Pivot* (*Ling shu* 靈樞), chapter 10, and Yi's case

---

[22] Loewe (1993).
[23] Unschuld (1986a, b, 2003), Despeux (1985, 1987), Obringer (1997), Wilms (2002), Feng (2003).
[24] Ma Boying (1994), Sivin (1995c), Lloyd (1996), Kuriyama (1999), Otsuka *et al.* (1999), Hsu (2001c).
[25] MWD 'Yangsheng fang' (1985:116, S194ff.).

histories. Strictly speaking, there is no evidence to suggest that Yi conceived of the *mai* as routes on the body surface as they are described in the Mawangdui vessel texts and drawn out as red lines on the Mianyang figurine. However, considering the many textual parallels between these manuscript texts and *Ling shu* 10, and between Yi's Memoir and the *Inner Canon* in general, one is led to assume that Yi had a similar understanding of them. The innovative aspect of the *mai* in Yi's Memoir is that they connect with the viscera, as they do in *Ling shu* 10 but generally not in the early manuscript texts. Even if a closer look at the Mawangdui vessel texts reveals only a few connections (in one text one *mai* connects to the 'liver', in the other, one *mai* arguably to the 'kidneys' and two to the 'heart', see p. 42), no early medical manuscript text explicitly refers to *qi* flowing inside the *mai*.

The argument

It appears that Yi's Memoir is the earliest extant document in which the *mai* connect to the viscera and *qi* is recurrently encountered as an aspect of *mai*. This raises the question of why and how *qi* came to be perceived as flowing in the *mai*. Rather than viewing *qi* as an intrinsic aspect of *mai* since time immemorial, this study suggests that in the Warring States *qi* referred to an internal aspect of personhood, eventually thought to be stored in the viscera, and that it was only when the internal aspects of personhood were put in connection with *mai,* as in Yi's Memoir, that physicians started to conceive of *qi* as an aspect of the *mai*. The viscera, rather than gaining importance within medicine as proto-anatomical entities, may have become medically significant as storage places for feelings and *qi*. Introducing a visceral language into medicine is likely to have been attractive to physicians attending to an elite clientele who had become interested in the link between emotion and illness. This historical process can be paraphrased either as a 'psychologising of medicine' or a 'medicalisation of emotion'. Yi's Memoir gives us a glimpse into some of the changes that it entailed within medical rationale.

Three early manuscript texts on the diagnostic investigation of *mai*

There are three manuscript texts of the second century BCE that concern methods of investigating *mai* for diagnostic purposes. None of them contains conclusive evidence that *qi* was thought to circulate in the *mai*,[26] and therefore they cannot be used as counterevidence to the above argument. The longest manuscript text on *mai*, the Zhangjiashan 'Maishu', part 3, section 7, concerns the identification of disorders by means of 'inspecting /

---

[26] Harper (1998:81, in a comment on ZJS 'Maishu', says: 'To paraphrase, health depends on the condition of vapour [*qi*] in the vessels [*mai*].' However, this statement is not based on textual evidence; the ZJS 'Maishu' does not explicitly say that there is *qi* in the *mai*.

investigating / divining *mai*' (*xiang mai* 相脈) and 'looking at *mai*' (*shi mai* 視脈).[27] If one interprets the terms *xiang* 相 and *shi* 視 in a narrow sense, this method relied primarily on a visual inspection of *mai* but not exclusively, as it also mentions tactile explorations of *mai*. However, one can also read *xiang* and *shi* in a general sense, meaning 'to divine' and 'to investigate' regardless of any sensory mode.

Another manuscript text is the Mawangdui 'Maifa' and the corresponding Zhangjiashan 'Maishu', part 3, section 6.[28] A literal reading that is informed by the anthropology of the senses suggests that the opening lines in this text contain an implicit contrast between visual and aural modes of knowing. This is said in awareness that aural perception often implied perception per se and the term *ting* 聽 (lit. to hear, to listen) was often used in the sense of 'attentively perceiving'.[29] It was perhaps in this general sense that the graph *ting* 聽 conventionally was used as a substitute for *sheng* 聖, meaning 'sage' in early manuscript texts.

The above two manuscript texts have in common that they claim to be about the study of *mai*. They are not concerned with the prognostication of death but with the identification of 'disorders' (*bing* 病), states of 'being exuberant' (*you guo* 有過) and '*qi* that rises' (*qi shang* 氣上). Finally, the Mawangdui 'Zubi vessel text' contains a passage that concerns the prognostication of death by attending to signs of various kinds. Among those belong signs elicited through a tactile exploration of *mai*, namely 'stroking *mai*' (*xun mai* 循脈).[30]

A novel translation, motivated by sensory concerns, of these three passages in the early medical manuscripts is presented in a collection of essays on 'bodies in resonance' (*shentigan* 身體感) with other bodies, objects and things.[31] Important here is merely that the manuscript texts mention different sensory modes of investigating *mai*.[32] Yi's tactile method was an

---

[27] See ZJS MSSW (1989), ZJS 'Maishu' (2001:245), and Gao (1992:104), who divides part 3 into 7 sections. For conventional translations, see Harper (1998:213–18), Lo (2001), Pfister (in press: vol.1, chs. 2.3.4), Hsu (2001b, 2005a).

[28] MWD 'Maifa' (1985:17). ZJS MSSW (1989), ZJS 'Maishu' (2001:244), and Gao (1992:86), For conventional translations, see Ma (1994:276), Harper (1998:213).

[29] e.g. *Zhou li* (Rites of Zhou), *juan* 35, p. 873c, 'Qiu guan si kou' 秋官司寇, 'Xiao si kou' 小司寇.

[30] MWD ZB (1985:234). For translation, see Ma (1992:204) and Harper (1998:200).

[31] Hsu (2008b).

[32] Perception in diagnosis, as in daily life, rarely relies on one sense alone and the *Nei jing* also points to different sensory modes. Verbs that primarily related visual perception but sometimes were used in a more general sense were 'to inspect' (*xiang*), 'to look at' (*shi*), 'to observe' (*guan* 觀), 'to see signs' (*hou* 候), 'to be an eyewitness' (*du* 睹 or 覩) and 'to arbitrate over colour' (*bian se* 辯色). Others, which often have a notable semantic stretch, include to 'listen and hear' (*ting* 聽), 'to listen or smell' (*wen* 聞), 'to manifest / perceive / experience / feel' (*xian* 見), 'to get' (*de* 得). In the *Nei jing*, many verbs concerned primarily tactile qualities such as 'to tap' (*tan* 彈), 'to palpate' (*an* 按), 'to stroke [horizontally?]' (*xun* 循), 'to press [cutting vertically?]' (*qie* 切), 'to hold' (*ju* 舉), 'to touch' (*men* 捫) and 'to grasp' (*chi* 持). Verbs describing the cognitive processes of a diagnosis were 'to investigate' (*cha* 察), 'to scrutinise' (*shen* 審), 'to divine' (*zhan* 占) and 'to examine' (*zhen* 診). The list is not comprehensive.

innovation intricately related to body conceptions and medical practice that accounted in sophisticated ways for the complexities of illness and personhood.

In this context, it is worth noting that already in Han times different sensory modes were thought to relate to different aspects of the body. Thus, *Huainanzi* 1, which according to the interpretation offered here discusses visual, auditory and tactile perception in a sequence, states 'form' (*xing* 形) can be seen, 'sound' (*sheng* 聲) heard and the 'body' (*shen* 身) known by stroking it:

> Now, the Formless is the great forefather of creatures,
> the Soundless is the great ancestor of sounds ...
> Therefore, you look at it and cannot see its form,
> you listen to it and cannot hear its sound,
> you stroke it but cannot obtain its body.[33]

> *fu wu xing zhe, wu zhi da zu ye,* 夫無形者 物之大祖也
> *wu yin zhe, sheng zhi da zong ye.* 無音者 聲之大宗也 ...
> *shi gu shi zhi bu jian qi xing,* 是故視之不見其形
> *ting zhi bu wen qi sheng,* 聽之不聞其聲
> *xun zhi bu de qi shen.* 循之不得其身

Based on the *Huainanzi* that states that *xing*-form is known through vision, *sheng*-sound through auditory perception, and the *shen*-body through tactile exploration, one is inclined to infer that Yi was interested in the *shen*-body. However, Yi's Memoir provides no cues on this.

What stands out clearly in Yi's Memoir is that his method of 'examining *mai*' (*zhen mai* 診脈) involved an innovative form of active touch: *qie mai* or *qiemo* 切脈, 'palpating' or 'pressing onto the *mai*'. In case 1, Yi then remarks that he 'got' (*de* 得) a certain quality of *qi*. One surmises that he 'got to feel' this quality, although in most other cases he is not as explicit (see box 1 on p. 348). Yi generally identified *qi* as coming from one of the viscera, and other aspects of the body interior. This raises the question of the significance *qi* had for Yi, particularly in diagnosis, and why his tactile procedure led to the perception of *qi*.

---

[33] *Huainanzi* 1, p. 86. The commentary quotes *Shuo wen* 12A, p. 30a: 'To stroke means to rub' (*shun mo ye* 揗摩也). Translation based on Pregadio (2004:101), but, for his third phrase: 'You follow it and cannot get to its person', an entirely new reading is given.

4

Conceptions of the body in the Warring States and the early Han

Key to understanding *qi* in Yi's case histories is that in the nurturing life texts of the Warring States and early Han *qi* was conceived of as a body internal phenomenon, an experiential reality, an inner, invisible aspect of human existence. The bodily form, by contrast, which together with *qi* made up personhood, was outwardly visible. This understanding of *qi* in early nurturing life texts, early medical manuscripts and some passages of the canonical medical texts that may reflect these early medical ideas differs from that of the contemporary practitioner and the historian familiar with canonical Chinese medical texts.[1]

The firm, hard and solid were seen as positive attributes of the outward form, which, in turn, was likened to a fresh plant, with shiny, glossy leaves and stems full of water, hard from high turgor, or to a polished stone, luminescent like jade (the hardest stone). Such a firmed-up body form was thought to provide an abode for *qi*. The body internal *qi* and regular breathing contrasted with the capricious outdoor winds.

Outward form and inward *qi* (*xing zai wai, qi zai nei* 形在外 氣在內)

Nurturing life practices were thought to firm up the outward 'form' (*xing* 形). According to the Mawangdui 'Shiwen' 十問, they resulted in the form becoming hard (*xing nai gang* 刑[形]乃剛).[2] Such a firmed-up body form provided a shelter for *qi*, as outlined in the *Guanzi* 官子 (Master Guan), 'Nei ye' 內業 (Inner Life):[3]

---

[1] Lo (2001) also noted that *qi* plays a more central role in the nurturing life texts than in the Mawangdui vessel texts, where *qi* mostly refers to distinct processes, breathing, farting, coughing, etc.: 'When able to defecate and pass vapour [*qi*, i.e. intestinal gas] there is welcome relief' (*de hou yu qi ze die ran shuai* 得後與氣則怢然衰), 'ailing from hunger; [insufficiency of] vapour; a tendency to become angry' (*bing ji, qi [bu zu], shan nu* 病飢, 氣[不足], 善怒). See MWD YY (1985:11, 12), Harper (1998:208, 210). For 'heavenly *qi*' (*tian qi* 天氣) and 'earthly *qi*' (*di qi* 地氣), see MWD 'Yinyangmai sihou'(1985:21). On early conceptions of *qi*, see Hsu (2007c).

[2] MWD 'Shiwen' (1985:152, S99).

[3] *Guanzi* 5.49, 'Nei ye', p. 2b; translation by Rickett (1998:43), with minor modifications.

With the heart fixed within,	*ding xin zai zhong* 定心在中
sight is clear, hearing distinct,	*er mu cong ming* 耳目聰明
the four limbs are firm and solid, and	*si zhi jian gu* 四肢堅固
become the abode for the quintessential.	*ke yi wei jing she* 可以為精舍
The quintessential is	*jing ye zhe* 精也者
the quintessence of *qi*.	*qi zhi jing zhe ye* 氣之精者也

Form and *qi* were seen as mutually complementary. The Mawangdui 'Shiwen' states the *xing*-form should become 'hard' (*gang* 剛), and the *Guanzi* speaks positively of the state in which the four limbs are 'firm' (*jian* 堅) and 'solid' (*gu* 固). This affirmation for the firm, solid and hard in nurturing life texts may appear odd to someone familiar with the canonical Chinese medical literature, where being hard, firm and solid often has negative connotations.

However, it is also positively valued in a few select passages of the *Inner Canon*. Thus, *Su wen* 3 speaks positively of 'bone and marrow [that] are firm and solid' (*gu sui jian gu* 骨髓堅固).[4] Furthermore, solidity can be a quality of *mai*, as in *Su wen* 46, where in winter (when everything is frozen hard) the *mai*, if 'solid' (*gu*), are considered healthy, and in *Ling shu* 10, where the *mai* that are 'not firm' (*bu jian* 不堅) entail pathological conditions.[5] In a similar vein, I have suggested translating a phrase in the Zhangjiashan 'Maishu', part 3, section 7, as a '*mai* that in its healthy state is solid' (*mai gu* 脈固).[6] Likewise, it is possible that in case 21 Yi mentions as a sign of health the 'solid colour' (*gu se* 固色), an expression which may have referred to the intensity of colour, although, as will be emphasised throughout this study, it is impossible to be certain about the referential meaning of such terms.[7] The above phrases all point to a body conception that positively values the maintenance of one's body form as an outer shell that is hard, firm and solid.

The body as polished stone or fresh plant

The term 'being solid' (*gu* 固) seems to derive from a lithic metaphor.[8] Nurturing life practices were directed towards achieving a body like a stone

---

[4] *Su wen* 3, p. 14. See also *Su wen* 3, p. 12: 'If one follows it [heaven], one's *yang qi* is solid' (*shun zhi, ze yang qi gu* 順之則陽氣固), and p. 15, 'if *yang* is dense, then it is solid' (*yang mi, nai gu* 陽密乃固). In *Su wen* 5, p. 20, 'not being solid' (*bu gu* 不固) is unhealthy. For *jian* (firm), see case 5 (line 15) and case 6 (line 3). For *gang* (hard), see case 6 (lines 14, 36).
[5] *Su wen* 46, p. 129, and *Ling shu* 10, p. 306.   [6] ZJS 'Maishu' (2001:245), Hsu (2008b).
[7] See also *Su wen* 39, p. 113: 'The five viscera and six cavities: [for determining] as to whether they are solid or exhausted there are parts [on the face?], look at their five colours' (*wu zang liu fu, gu jin you bu, shi qi wu se* 五藏六府 固盡有部 視其五色).
[8] Many have noted – foremost Rawson (1995), also Lo (2002) – how deeply valued 'stone' (*shi* 石) is in Chinese cultures, but none seems to have drawn attention to *gu* 固 as a cherished lithic quality.

in luminescence and solidity. Thus, in the context of discussing ways of solidifying the body, the Mawangdui 'Shiwen' explicitly mentions the luminescence of jade: 'The five viscera become solid and white, their jade colour doubles its glow' (*wu zang gu bai yu se chong guang* 五臟[藏]𩑾白, 玉色重光).[9] Although in medical texts *gu* 'solid, hard' often has negative connotations, the Mawangdui 'Shiwen' advocates solidifying one's body.

The Zhangjiashan 'Maishu', part 3, section 7, invokes a similar body conception that celebrates the firm and solid when it opposes 'being full' (*ying* 盈) to 'empty' (*xu* 虛), and 'being glossy and slippery' (*hua* 滑) to 'rough' (*se* 澀).[10] These oppositions are preserved in later medical texts,[11] although the full and slippery, which in this early medical manuscript text are positively valued, sometimes take on negative meanings.[12] A human being, like a fresh plant or a polished stone, in its desirable state has a bodily form that is full of life, firm and solid, with a glossy and shiny skin that is smooth and slippery.

No doubt, the full and shiny/glossy/slippery invoke the botanical metaphor Shigehisa Kuriyama mentioned in his discussion of 'colour' and 'blossoming' (*hua* 花), which likens the human body to a plant.[13] To be shiny and glossy (*hua*) and brim-full (*ying*) are mentioned as positive attributes of a plant in various non-medical texts,[14] although the latter term is used mostly as an attribute of the 'ten thousand things' (*wan wu* 萬物).[15] In a canonical medical text both terms occur in a simile that invokes the botanical imagery of stroking a (bamboo) rod.[16]

---

[9] MWD 'Shiwen' (1985:152, S101). Translation based on Harper (1998:411), but modified.

[10] ZJS (2001:245). Gao (1992:105) reads the graph in question as a loanword for *se* 澀, Harper (1998:217) suggests *shuai* 率, Pfister (2004 p.c.) considers the reading uncertain. Cognate to *se* 濇澀 is *se* 泣 that hinders the flow of blood. See *Ling shu* 81, p. 480, quoted on p. 124.

[11] e.g. for positive connotations of *hua*, see *Su wen* 28, p. 86: 'Hence if the five viscera, the bones and flesh are slippery/shiny and agreeable, one is able to live long' (*gu wu zang gu rou hua li, ke yi chang jiu ye* 故五藏骨肉滑利, 可以長久也), *Ling shu* 18, p. 325: 'As for a person in his prime, if *qi* and blood are abundant, his muscle and flesh are slippery/shiny' (*zhuang zhe zhi qi xue sheng, qi ji rou hua* 壯者之氣血盛, 其肌肉滑); *ying* generally has negative connotations, e.g. *Su wen* 18 (quoted in ch. 4, n. 16).

[12] The slippery then becomes indicative of pathological conditions of 'wind' (*feng* 風), e.g. *Su wen* 18, p. 55: 'If the *mai* is abundant, slippery and firm, the disorder is on the outside' (*mai sheng hua jian zhe yue bing zai wai* 脈盛滑堅者 曰病在外), *Ling shu* 8, p. 292: 'Lung *qi* . . . if it is replete, one wheezes. The chest feels full and one breathes while lying on one's back, facing upward [gasping for air]' (*fei qi . . . shi ze chuan he xiong ying yang xi* 肺氣 . . . 實則喘喝胸盈仰息). See also case 8 (line 12) and *Ling shu* 74, p. 454. 'Wind' is sometimes opposed to 'obstructions' (*bi* 痹) or 'accumulations' (*ji* 積) indicated by a rough pulse, e.g. *Su wen* 8, p. 28; 48, p. 136; 64, p. 178.

[13] Kuriyama (1995a, 1999:187).

[14] e.g. *Shi jing* edition called *Mao shi* 毛詩, p. 363: 'The leaves are firm, yet shiny/slippery and lustrous' (*ye jian er hua ze* 葉堅而滑澤).

[15] e.g. *Zhou yi*, 'Qian' 乾, p. 13.

[16] *Su wen* 18, p. 57: 'If the coming of the *mai* of an ailing liver is full and replete, yet slippery, as if one were stroking a long rod, one calls it a liver disorder' (*bing gan mai lai, ying shi er hua, ru xun chang gan, yue gan bing* 病肝脈來, 盈實而滑, 如循長竿, 曰肝病).

Fresh plants with high turgor are firm, and their opposite, which is the soft and rotten, is mentioned as a sign of death in the Mawangdui 'Yinyang-mai sihou' 陰陽脈死候: 'The three *yin* [*mai*], by putrefying the viscera and rotting the intestines, govern death' (*san yin fu* [*fu*] *zang lian* [*lan*] *chang er zhu sha* 三陰窅 [腐]臧[臟]煉[爛]腸而主殺).[17] In a similar vein, Yi speaks of a pathological process when in case 1 (line 41) he mentions 'spoilage' (*lan* 爛) of the 'flowing links' (*liu luo* 流絡). Again, we note similarities between the early manuscript literature and Yi's case material, insofar as the nega-tive value attributed to the spoilt and soft implicitly points to a body con-ception that celebrates not only the shiny and full but also the firm as a sign of aliveness.[18]

Various medical texts indicate that being full was a visible quality. One could see 'abundance' (*sheng* 盛) or 'emptiness/depletion' (*xu* 虛), 'exuber-ance' (*you guo* 有過 or *tai guo* 太過) and 'insufficiency' (*bu ji* 不及), 'bounty' (*you yu* 有餘) and 'dearth' (*bu zu* 不足).[19] The 'form' (*xing* 形), the *mai* and the 'links' (*luo* 絡) could be abundant or empty, exuberant or insufficient. Although occasionally similar qualities were attributed to *qi* in the *Inner Canon*, and sometimes also to the viscera and channels inside the body,[20] these qualities were often explicitly said to be visible from the outside. One could look at them (*shi* 視) and observe them (*guan* 觀).[21]

Another visible quality was *se*, which in Yi's Memoir means 'colour', but in pre-dynastic times was often a meaningful outward expression of one's inward states, as is the 'hungry air' or 'woeful mien'.[22] In the Mawangdui manuscript texts, *se* is mentioned about ten times. It generally refers to the complexion,[23] which can be either 'freshly white' (*xian bai* 鮮白) or 'mouldy black' (*yan* 黯).[24] Apart from occurring in idioms like 'jade colour' (*yu se* 玉色) and 'five colours' (*wu se* 五色),[25] it is also used in a wide sense, meaning

---

[17] MWD 'Yinyangmai sihou' (1985:21, S86).
[18] Compare with modern English where infirmity is an opposite of the firm.
[19] e.g. 'see the abundance' (*shi qi sheng zhe* 視其盛者) in *Su wen* 41, p. 118; and 'see the abun-dance on the ankle' (*shi fu shang sheng zhe* 視跗上盛者) in *Ling shu* 23, p. 341; 'see the emptiness/depletion' (*shi qi xu* 視其虛) in *Su wen* 31, p. 93; and 'see the empty/depleted links' (*shi qi xu luo* 視其虛絡) in *Su wen* 62, p. 168; 'see the exuberance of his channels in the *yang* sphere' (*shi qi jing zhi guo yu yang zhe* 視其經之過於陽者) in *Su wen* 60, p. 163; 'use the outside to know the inside, use the principle of observing exuberance and insufficiency' (*yi biao zhi li, yi guan guo yu bu ji zhi li* 以表知裡, 以觀過與不及之理) in *Su wen* 5, p. 23; 'see bounty and dearth' (*shi you yu bu zu* 視有餘不足) in *Ling shu* 5, p. 280.
[20] *Su wen* 62, pp. 168–9, concerns bounty and dearth of 'spirit' (*shen* 神), *qi*, 'blood' (*xue* 血), 'form' (*xing* 形) and 'will' (*zhi* 志) that are not reported to be visually perceived.
[21] e.g. *Su wen* 80, p. 253: 'Hence while examining [a patient] some look at the breathing and look at the intention' (*gu zhen zhi huo shi xi shi yi* 故診之或視息視意) or *Ling shu* 72, p. 450: 'Look out for the noxious and normal' (*shi qi xie zheng* 視其邪正), or *Su wen* 26, p. 86, quoted on p. 36; *shi* is being used here either in its narrow or its wide sense, see ch. 3, n. 32.
[22] Kuriyama (1999:174).
[23] Harper (1998:333, 357–8) translates it as 'complexion' in the MWD 'Yangsheng fang' 養生方 (1985:106, S36; 117, S205; 117, S208). See also MWD 'Zaliao fang' 雜療方 and 'Shiwen' (1985:126, S42; 145, S8).
[24] MWD 'Shiwen' and YY (1985:12, S64 and 145, S9).
[25] MWD 'Shiwen' (1985:152, S101; 145, S10).

'lust'.[26] In the *Inner Canon*, *se* is 'lustrous' (*ze* 澤) and 'tender' (*yao* 夭),[27] 'bright and not coarse' (*se ming bu cu* 色明不麤),[28] apart from referring to the five hues that correlated with the five internal viscera.[29] In contemporary Chinese medicine, *se* refers to the complexion, and in case 15, where Yi says 'When I looked at him, it was mortally yellow. When I inspected him, it was the deathly green of a straw mat' (*wang zhi sha ran huang, cha zhi ru si qing zhi ci* 望之殺然黃察之如死青之茲), there is little doubt he speaks of the complexion. In the *Inner Canon*, however, the eyes, ears, abdomen, body and head hair all could have colour,[30] and also *mai*. It is therefore not entirely clear whether when Yi says in case 19, 'At the above, the skin was yellow and coarse' (*shang fu huang cu* 上膚黃麤), he uses *shang* 上 in the sense of the head or face, the upper bodily cavity, i.e. chest area, or the skin's superficial layers.

Ling shu 10 clearly comments on the colour of *mai*: 'Whenever one examines the linking *mai*, if the colour of the *mai* is blue-green, then there is coldness and pain, if it is red, then there is heat' (*fan zhen luo mai, mai se qing, ze han qie tong, chi ze you re* 凡診絡脈 脈色青 則寒且痛 赤則有熱).[31] Blue-green *mai* (*qing mai* 青脈) were observed in front of the ear or on the forearm,[32] red *mai* (*chi mai* 赤脈) typically in the eyes.[33] With this in mind, Yi may be speaking of the colour of the *mai* called 'major *yang*' in case 17 when he says 'the colour of the major *yang* is dry' (*tai yang se gan* 太陽色 乾), although it is also possible that he meant the colour of the area at the temples called *tai yang*.[34]

In summary, the body was likened to a polished stone or fresh plant that was firm from high turgor, and had visible qualities of being luminescent, glossy and full. Further visible aspects were its colour and *mai*. They were an aspect of the outward visible 'form' (*xing*).

---

[26] MWD 'Tianxia zhi dao tan' (1985:165, S40); see Harper (1998:432).

[27] e.g. *Su wen* 19, p. 63.

[28] *Ling shu* 49, p. 401, where it also takes on qualities typically attributed to *mai*, such as floating (*fu* 浮) and sunken (*chen* 沉), dispersed (*san* 散) and united (*tuan* 摶). Diagnosis of *mai* and *se* had much in common; often the same static verbs assessed their qualities. See case 5 (lines 14–17) and case 7 (lines 17–19). See also case 7, n. 106.

[29] See p. 23 and ch. 3, n. 10.

[30] e.g. 'the five colours of the eyes' (*mu zhi wu se* 目之五色) in *Ling shu* 71, p. 447; 'the colours of the ears' (*er se* 耳色) in *Ling shu* 64, p. 432; 'the colour of the abdomen' (*fu se* 腹色) in *Ling shu* 57, p. 414; 'the colour of the head and body hair is lustrous or: the body hair is head-hair-like [i.e. fine, long, sturdy] and the complexion/colour lustrous' (*mao fa er se ze* 毛髮而色澤) in case 12; and also 'the colour of the body hair is not lustrous' (*mao se bu ze* 髦色不澤) in *Ling shu* 10, p. 305.

[31] *Ling shu* 10, p. 306. Consider also *Ling shu* 74, p. 454: 'Blue-green blood vessels are indicative of coldness inside the stomach' (*you qing xue mai zhe, wei zhong you han* 有青血脈者 胃 中有寒).

[32] See, for instance, 'the blue-green *mai* between the ears' (*er jian qing mai* 耳間青脈) in *Ling shu* 20, p. 332, and 'when on the forearm there is an increase of blue-green *mai*, one calls it...' (*bi duo qing mai, yue...* 臂多青脈曰...) in *Su wen* 18, p. 56.

[33] e.g. *Ling shu* 70, p. 444; an exception is *Su wen* 10, p. 36.

[34] See chapter 7, n. 32.

Inward feelings expressed in the language of *qi*

The visually comprehended 'form' contrasted with internal aspects of the body that could not be apprehended through vision directly, such as feelings and emotions, one's will and spirit, and *qi*. This difference between the visible and invisible aspects of human existence is reminiscent of modern medical oppositions, and may to a certain extent be intrinsic to any primarily visual comprehension of human existence. There is more to a person than the visually perceived physical body; this certainly is a cross-culturally valid experience.

Some texts in the *Inner Canon* emphasise *qi* as the atmospheric in the universe, and 'form' as the earthly manifestation of the spiritual or numinous, as does *Su wen* 66:[35]

> The numinous ... in heaven it becomes *qi*, on earth it turns into form.
> *shen ... zai tian wei qi, zai di cheng xing*   神 ... 在天為氣 在地成形

However, *Su wen* 66 belongs among the chapters that probably became incorporated into the *Su wen* in the Tang dynasty (618–907 CE), or later. Therefore the opposition of *xing* and *qi* that it advocates is best regarded as a later understanding of these two concepts.[36] The distinction between *xing* and *qi* that pre-dynastic and early dynastic texts on nurturing life practices invoke is a different one. It is one that emphasises the opposition between an outwardly visible 'form' and inwardly experienced aspects of personhood: *qi*.

This opposition is clearly stated in the above *Guanzi* passage (see p. 30). It is also variously mentioned in medical texts. Thus, *Su wen* 6 states:[37]

> *Qi* inside and the form outside mutually constitute each other.
> *qi li xing biao er wei xiang cheng ye* 氣裡形表而為相成也

In this context, we are reminded that the *Inner Canon* is a compilation of texts that span many centuries, and that what elsewhere has been called a 'modular reading' of esoteric compilations allows one to unearth in medieval and later compilations phrases dating to the late Warring States and early Han.[38] Depending on the period and place whence a certain passage in the compilation dates, a term has different shades of meaning. It is, of course, difficult to date phrases in a compilation. Grammar, textual markers, semantics and, in some rare cases, the underlying body conception implied by a certain clause may provide a hint. For instance, a body ecological understanding usually hints at changes in medical practice that took place

---

[35] *Su wen* 66, p. 182; translated by Hsu (1999:166–8).   [36] On its dating, see ch. 3, n. 21.
[37] *Su wen* 6, p. 25.   [38] See ch. 3, nn. 19 and 20.

in late Han and medieval times. When investigating word meaning, it is therefore important to consider the body conception to which the word alludes.

One may wonder what the attributes of *qi* inside the body were. When comparing the ways of the ancients with those of the people of its own times, *Su wen* 13 says of the latter:[39]

> Suffering from grief affects their internal parts,
> exerting their bodily form harms their external parts.
>
> *you huan yuan qi nei* 憂患緣其內
> *ku xing shang qi wai* 苦形傷其外

Su wen 13 highlights a contrast between the outward 'form' that is harmed by overwork, and feelings that affect one's innermost. *Su wen* 1 invokes a similar opposition between outward 'form' and inward feelings of the sages:[40]

> Externally they do not overwork their bodily form in daily chores,
> internally they are without the troubles of worrying and thinking.
>
> *wai bu lao xing yu shi* 外不勞形於事
> *nei wu si xiang zhi huan* 內無思想之患

So, physical toil affected the 'form', while troubling feelings and thoughts harmed one inside. *Su wen* 1 continues by invoking a contrast between outward 'body form' (*xing ti* 形體) and 'essences and spirits' (*jing shen* 精神):

> If the bodily structure of the form does not collapse,
> the essences and spirits are not dispersed [i.e. remain inside].
>
> *xing ti bu bi* 形體不敝
> *jing shen bu san* 精神不散

The contrast between 'form' (*xing*) and 'spirit' (*shen*) is also given in *Su wen* 9, which speaks of nine viscera, four 'viscera on the body form' (*xing zang* 形藏) and five 'viscera of spirit-matter' (*shen zang* 神藏).[41] The former are the corner of the head, the ears and eyes, mouth and teeth, and the centre of the chest (or other body parts, depending on the text in which they are mentioned); the latter invariably are the heart, lungs, spleen, liver and kidneys. If cross-culturally the viscera are the seat of emotion and feelings, it may not be surprising that in Chinese medicine the five internal viscera were associated with thinking and feeling and spirit: *shen*.

---

[39] *Su wen* 13, p. 41.   [40] *Su wen* 1, p. 9.

[41] See *Su wen* 9, p. 31, and 20, p. 65; Dunhang P3287, text 1, col. 2 (Ma *et al.* 1994:9); and P3477, text 1, col. 6–13 (Ma *et al.* 1994:153). In Chinese, the four 'form viscera' are *tou jiao* 頭角, *er mu* 耳目, *kou chi* 口齒, *xiong zhong* 胸中.

Su wen 62 opposes the 'form' (*xing*) to the 'will/intent' (*zhi*), when it dis-cusses first the spirits, then blood and *qi* and, finally, form and will/intent.[42] The title of *Su wen* 24, 'Xue qi xing zhi' 血氣形志, juxtaposes not only blood and *qi*, but interestingly also form and intent.[43] *Su wen* 26 implies that without knowing the internal emotional disposition one cannot correctly diagnose symptoms manifesting on the outward 'form':[44]

> Hence one calls it keeping the doors closed within,
> if without recognising the [internal] feelings/situation,
>   one looks at the noxious on the form.
>
> *gu yue shou qi men hu yan* 故曰守其門戶焉
> *mo zhi qi qing er jian xie xing ye* 莫知其情而見邪形也

Because this translation frames the text from *Su wen* 26 in regard to the 'sentimental body', it can posit semantic continuity for the term *qing* 情 (feelings).[45]

The aspects of the form that were outwardly visible were thus *mai* and *se*, bounty and dearth, exuberance and insufficiency.[46] The inward aspects of personhood were one's feelings and emotions, one's intent/will, one's spirits and the five viscera, which were called spirit viscera in some contexts, and, in all likelihood, were each conceived of as a seat of thought and emotion. To be sure, these explicit oppositions between externally visible form and inward feelings, thought, spirit and will/intent are given in the *Inner Canon,* while in the third and second centuries BCE, the manuscript texts merely speak of *xing* and *qi*. It is due to the above passages in the *Inner Canon* that I realised that *qi* was a term with connotations relating to a person's internal feelings and emotions, and not merely to breath or vapour, in the above *Guanzi* quote (on p. 30) and other pre- and early dynastic texts that invoke the opposition of *xing* and *qi*.

The sentimental body, *yin qi* and *yang qi*

The discussion of 'form' as an opposite to *qi* also has implications for the meaning of *qi*. It needs to be borne in mind that the notion of *qi* in medical texts of early dynastic times did not necessarily always have connotations

---

[42] *Su wen* 62, p. 167.
[43] *Su wen* 24, pp. 77–8. This title presumably translates into 'blood and *qi*' and 'form and intent', and not into 'blood *qi*' and the 'form's intent', because the chapter later discusses four combinations of either form or intent 'rejoicing' (*le* 樂) or 'suffering' (*ku* 苦). See also *Ling shu* 78, p. 472, with slight variations.
[44] *Su wen* 26, p. 82.
[45] Compare and contrast with Harbsmeier's translation (2004:76).
[46] 'Flesh' (*rou* 肉) was primarily tactually known, but the 'flesh of the form' (*xing rou*) may have been visually perceived, e.g. *Ling shu* 4, p. 275, or 61, p. 422.

of the atmospheric notion of *qi* that permeates the universe.[47] Rather, *qi* was often mentioned in the context of speaking about the internal aspects of personhood.[48] If the viscera were perceived as seats of emotion and thinking, as the term 'spirit viscera' may imply, and if emotion and psychological issues were expressed in the language of *qi*, as certainly was the case in the *Mengzi*,[49] the viscera may eventually have come to be conceived of as storage places of *qi*.

A text in *Ling shu* 6 relates the emotions to *qi*, and *qi* to the internal viscera. This passage distinguishes between two different aetiologies of illness, namely an ecological and emotional one:[50]

> Wind and coldness harm the form,
> while grief, fear, rage and anger harm *qi*.

> *Qi* harms the viscera, and thereby causes disorder in the viscera.
> Coldness harms the form, and thereby causes resonance in the form.
> Wind harms the sinews and *mai*, the sinews and *mai* then resonate.

> This is the resonance of the outer and inner [aspects of the body],
> form and *qi*

> *feng han shang xing* 風寒傷形
> *you kong fen nu shang qi* 憂恐忿怒傷氣

> *qi shang zang, nai bing zang* 氣傷藏 乃病藏
> *han shang xing, nai ying xing* 寒傷形 乃應形
> *feng shang jin mai, jin mai nai ying* 風傷筋脈筋脈乃應

> *ci xing qi wai nei zhi xiang ying ye* 此形氣外內之相應也

The above passage is made up of a duplet, a triplet and a summarising statement. It first mentions, as ecological aetiologies, external wind and coldness, which affect the outward aspect of the body, namely the 'form' (*xing*). Thereafter, it discusses the emotional aetiologies that harm *qi*, which in turn adversely affects the internal aspects of the body, the 'viscera' (*zang*).

With regard to numerology we note that the outward 'form' in *Ling shu* 6 is affected by two ecological forces, namely 'wind and coldness' (*feng han* 風寒), rather than the canonically known five as in the *locus classicus* for ecological aetiologies, *Su wen* 4 and 5.[51] It is well known that *Su wen* 4

---

[47] Practitioners and historians of Chinese medicine are familiar with sayings like '*yang* transforms into *qi*, *yin* becomes form' (*yang hua qi, yin cheng xing* 陽化氣 陰成形). This sentence is recorded in *Su wen* 5, p. 18, which like *Su wen* 66, belongs to the *Su wen* chapters that were incorporated in the Tang dynasty or later. On its dating, see ch. 3, n. 21.

[48] Hsu (2007c, in press a).

[49] Csikszentmihalyi (2004). See ch. 2, n. 19.   [50] *Ling shu* 6, p. 284.

[51] *Su wen* 4, p. 17, and *Su wen* 5, pp. 20–21.

and 5 speak of resonances between the five seasons and five viscera – this in contrast to *Ling shu* 6. Evidently, *Su wen* 4 and 5 as well as *Ling shu* 6 all allude to the ecological aetiology of illness. In *Su wen* 4 and 5 the ecological aetiology is all-embracing, and the atmospheric *qi* resonates with *qi* in the five viscera. However, apart from the external ecological aetiologies *Ling shu* 6 also mentions emotional ones that affect *qi* inside the body, and so affect the viscera. *Ling shu* 6 evidently alludes to a different body conception from *Su wen* 4 and 5. Historians of Chinese medicine generally understand *qi* in terms of the meanings it adopts in the 'body ecologic', i.e. with regard to a body conception informed by predominantly ecological aetiologies, as known from *Su wen* 4 and 5. However, *Ling shu* 6 alludes to a body conception that differentiates between inner and outer aspects of the body, which are affected by either outward ecological or inward emotional aetiologies.

The question then arises as to how seasonal resonances on the outward form were perceived. There were four seasons and, as Han Jianping suggests, there were initially only two pairs of *yin* and *yang mai*, which resonated with the four seasons.[52] Han's idea is appealing but the evidence in support of it is, strictly speaking, insufficient. Nevertheless, it is in line with at least three *Su wen* passages on *mai* that resonate with the seasons (none is so specific, however, to state that there were only four *mai*).[53] Furthermore, a book title mentioned towards the end of Yi's Memoir, 'The Doubling of Yin and Yang due to Resonances with the Four Seasons', suggests there were seasonal pathological states that consisted of a doubling of the *yin* or *yang* quality (see p. 67). It appears that visible qualities on the body surface could be perceived to 'double', such as in the Mawangdui 'Shiwen' the 'doubling of the glow' (*chong guang* 重光) (see p. 31).

If changes in qualities of the outward form could be visually perceived, how were emotional aetiologies recognised? And how were they considered to emerge in the first place? Here the Zhangjiashan 'Yinshu' is explicit. It states that illness arises from emotional upheaval:[54]

> The nobility contracts illness from disharmony in joy and anger.
> If one is joyful, then the *yang qi* augments,
> if one is angry, then *yin qi* augments.

---

[52] Han (1999:31).
[53] See *Su wen* 13, p. 42: 'Colour resonates with the sun, the *mai* with the moon' (*se yi ying ri, mai yi ying yue* 色以應日 脈以應月) and immediately thereafter: 'The outward changes of colour, and the *mai* that resonate with the four seasons' (*fu se zhi bian hua, yi ying si shi zhi mai* 夫色之變化 以應四時之脈). See also *Su wen* 57, p. 153, which differentiates between passageways inside the body that have a 'constant colour' (*chang se* 常色) and *yin* links and *yang* links on the body surface; the *yang* links change their colour in accordance with the seasons if they are healthy: if it is cold, they get blue-green and black, if hot, they get yellow and red.
[54] ZJS YSSW (1990:86), ZJS 'Yinshu' (2001:299).

> *gui ren zhi suo yi de bing zhe* 貴人之所以得病者
> *yi qi xi nu zhi bu he ye* 以其喜怒之不和也
> *xi ze yang qi duo, nu ze yin qi duo* 喜則陽氣多, 怒則隂[陰]氣多

The 'Yinshu' speaks of nobility. Perhaps, regardless of place and time, physicians attending to clientele in upper social strata pay particular attention to psychological disposition (see pp. 13–14). The 'Yinshu' does not, however, mention viscera, but *Ling shu* 66 connects emotional distress to visceral states:[55]

> If joy and anger are not regulated, then they harm the viscera.
> *xi nu bu jie, ze shang zang* 喜怒不節 則傷藏

The Zhangjiashan 'Yinshu', *Ling shu* 66, and also other texts, such as Yi's Memoir, mention only two emotions. This suggests the 'sentimental body' comprised two emotions only: joy/love and anger. These emotions were evidently framed in *yin yang* complementarities, which seem to have provided the predominant schema for conceptualising bodily processes before five agents doctrine became favourable. Thus, a text buried among others in *Ling shu* 67 says of the 'double *yang* person' (*chong yang zhi ren* 重陽之人):

> The one who augments *yang*, is often joyful,
> the one who augments *yin*, is often angry.
>
> *duo yang zhe, duo xi* 多陽者 多喜
> *duo yin zhe, duo nu* 多陰者 多怒

And *Su wen* 77 remarks:[56]

> Sudden anger harms *yin*,
> sudden joy harms *yang*.
>
> *bao nu shang yin* 暴怒傷陰
> *bao xi shang yang* 暴喜傷陽

The above four passages from the Zhangjiashan 'Yinshu', *Ling shu* 66, *Ling shu* 67 and *Su wen* 77 suggest that the totality of emotional life was expressed in an idiom of two feelings only, either joy/love or anger, originating either in the upper *yang* or lower *yin* sphere of the body. The suggestion that the feelings were initially housed in a bipartite body is also given through another text, which is framed in a numerology of five, but mentions only two emotions. This text in *Ling shu* 66 enumerates among the disorders that arise in the *yin* sphere the following five:[57]

> Grief and worry harm the heart,
> a doubling of coldness harms the lungs,
> rage and anger harm the liver,

[55] *Ling shu* 66, p. 437. [56] *Ling shu* 67, p. 440; *Su wen* 77, p. 247.
[57] *Ling shu* 66, p. 439.

drunkenness and sexual indulgence, and while sweating encountering the
winds, harms the spleen,

if one uses force excessively, such as after sexual intercourse when sweat
is exuded, such that one can bathe in it, then one harms the kidneys.

These are the illnesses that are generated by the internal and external
[aetiologies] and the three parts.

you si shang xin 憂思傷心
chong han shang fei 重寒傷肺
fen nu shang gan 忿怒傷肝

zui yi ru fang, han chu dang feng shang pi 醉以入房 汗出當風 傷脾
yong li guo du, ruo ru fang han chu xi, ze shang shen
用力過度 若入房汗出浴 則傷腎
ci nei wai san bu zhi suo sheng bing ye 此內外三部之所生病者也

This text of *Ling shu* 66 is of particular interest because the five above
aetiologies correlate with Yi's cases 2, 4, 6, 15 and 17. Relevant to the discussion
here is that only two of the five aetiologies refer to strong emotions:
'grief and worry' harm the heart, 'rage and anger' the liver. It is as though
the *yin yang* conception of the 'sentimental body' had been retained, with
the heart in the upper sphere and the liver in the lower one, although the
entire passage is framed by the numerology of five.

All passages cited so far invoke a bipartite body in the context of discussing
emotional aetiologies. In the manuscript literature, this body was an
undifferentiated bipartite entity, within which *qi* took on either *yin*- or *yang*-
qualities depending on whether it arose in the upper or lower internal
bodily spheres respectively. It is only in the *Inner Canon* that viscera are
mentioned in the context of discussing emotions.

Qi shang 氣上: a trigger of emotional distress?

Excerpts from the medical canons suggest the emotions affected the flow
of *qi. Su wen* 39 states: 'In cases of anger, *qi* rises' (*nu ze qi shang* 怒則氣上)
and 'In cases of anger, *qi* is contravective' (*nu ze qi ni* 怒則氣逆).[58] It thereafter describes all kinds of different movements of *qi* brought into motion
through feelings. *Su wen* 47 notes: 'In the case of great fright, *qi* goes
upward and does not come down' (*da jing, qi shang er bu xia* 大驚 氣上而
不下).[59] *Ling shu* 66 maintains that regardless of the particular emotion
which sets it into motion, *qi* will always start to rise and become contravective: 'If internally one is harmed by grief and anger, then *qi* rises and
becomes contravective' (*ruo nei shang yu you nu, ze qi shang ni* 若內傷於憂

---

[58] *Su wen* 39, p. 113.   [59] *Su wen* 47, p. 133.

怒則氣上逆).[60] Evidently, upward movement of *qi* was considered pathological, as is also evident in the Zhangjiashan 'Maishu', part 3, section 6, strip 57:[61]

> Thus, when *qi* ascends and does not descend,
> then look at the *mai* that has exuberance and
> cauterise it at the 'ring' [i.e. the waist].
>
> *gu qi shang er bu xia* 故氣上而不下
> *ze shi you guo zhi mai* 則視有過之脈
> *dang huan er jiu zhi* 當環而久[灸]之

This manuscript text does not explicitly speak of emotional distress but of rising *qi* that cannot be brought down again.[62] The upward movement of *qi* that it describes is identical to that in the above quotes from the *Inner Canon*. The above canonical passages all explicitly say that strong emotions bring *qi* into motion, while the Zhangjiashan 'Maishu', part 3, section 5, strips 54–5, puts the interrelation between emotions and *qi* the other way round: 'If *qi* is agitated, then there is grief' (*qi dong, ze you* 氣動則憂). It is *qi* in agitation that brings about grief, whereby 'grief' in this context may well be a generic term for emotional distress of any kind. Since the Zhangjiashan text is explicit that an agitation of *qi* was considered to bring about emotional distress (rather than vice versa), it is possible that in early medical manuscripts '*qi* that rises' (*qi shang*) implied an emotional affection. Notably, the 'disorder of *qi* being separated' (*qi ge bing* 氣鬲病) in Yi's case 2, which is marked by a pathological upward movement of food, *qi* and blood, is attributed to an emotional indisposition. To be sure, it concerns *qi* that rises and is trapped in the chest, not in the *mai*.

To summarise, in early nurturing life and medical contexts the body was visually comprehended. Physicians differentiated between an externally visible 'form' and internally invisible *qi*. The outward form resonated with ecological forces, such as wind and coldness, and the visible *mai* on the body surface were an aspect of this outward form that resonated with the four seasons. By contrast, the inner aspect of the 'sentimental body' comprised only two feelings, joy/grief and anger, in the upper *yang* and lower *yin* sphere, i.e. the spheres of heart and liver.[63] The textual evidence assembled would suggest that '*qi* that rises' (*qi shang*) and '*qi* that is agitated' (*qi dong*) were closely associated with emotional eruptions and upheaval.

---

[60] *Ling shu* 66, p. 439.
[61] ZJS 'Maishu' (2001:244). For the range of translations given for this passage, see ch. 3, n. 27.
[62] Compare to the English notion of 'being upset' and not 'calming down'.
[63] Accordingly, the liver is an internal abdominal body part in a bipartite body. Compare and contrast with Harper (1998:197). See also ch. 4, n. 65, and case 6, nn. 100 and 101.

The bipartite architectural body

The Mawangdui and Zhangjiashan vessel texts also imply a bipartite body. They generally do not allude to the sentimental body but to a bipartite bodily architecture. They imply a clear distinction between the lower and upper extremities. Thus, the 'Zubi vessel text' mentions first the six *mai* originating in the lower extremities, and then the five *mai* originating in the upper extremities. Although the 'Yinyang vessel text' mentions all *yang mai* 陽脈 first and all *yin mai* 陰脈 thereafter, it then enumerates them in clusters of three that imply a differentiation into lower and upper extremities. Evidently, both vessel texts implicitly allude to a bipartite architectural body along a vertical axis.

The vessel texts report on three *yang mai* of foot and forearm, but in the case of the *yin mai*, they attribute three to the foot and only two to the forearm. This apparently accords with the numerology of *yin* and *yang* in the Warring States: six was the standard number for *yang*, five for *yin*.[64] The foot minor *yin mai* was the only foot *mai* that was connected to an internal body part; it was the liver (*gan* 肝), according to the Mawangdui 'Zubi vessel text', or, arguably, the kidneys (*shen* 腎), according to the Mawangdui 'Yinyang vessel text'.[65] The major and minor *yin* of the forearm were both connected to the heart (*xin* 心), according to the 'Yinyang vessel text'.[66] Where the 'Zubi vessel text' mentions only one viscus in the body interior, the 'liver', the 'Yinyang vessel text' implies bipartition with arguably the kidneys connecting to the minor *yin mai* of the lower extremities and with the body architectural heart connecting to the major and minor *yin mai* of the upper extremities.

Apparently, vertical bipartition into upper and lower body parts also applied to the architectural body and not merely the sentimental body. However, while *yin* and *yang* were associated with the emotions seated in the lower liver and upper heart regions respectively in the sentimental body, they have different implications for the *mai* in the architectural body.[67] Incidentally, Yi's cases 1 and 2, which are in textual structure very similar to each other (particularly in lines 1–15), will be shown to concern

[64] Han (1999:17) cites the *Zuo zhuan* 左傳 and the *Guo yu* 國語. Despeux and Obringer (1997:32–3) provide further evidence on the numerology of five *yin* and six *yang* in early medicine.

[65] MWD ZB (1985:4, S13) and MWD YY (1985:12, S26). Harper (1998:197) follows Yamada that *gan* (liver) in MWD ZB designates not an internal viscus, but a location on the body surface. This may apply to the graph identified as kidneys (see case 6, n. 100), but not to that of the liver (see ch. 4, n. 63).

[66] Harper (1998:212, fn 5) notes the connection of the forearm's *yin mai* to the heart but goes no further. It is given in MWD YY but not in MWD ZB. The ZJS 'Maishu' parallels the MWD YY.

[67] *Yin* and *yang* are today associated with the course of the *mai* on the inner and outer sides of the extremities respectively; they may or may not have had this referential meaning in antiquity.

a disorder of the *yin*-liver situated in the interior of the body, and a disorder situated in the body part above the diaphragm, the architectural region of the heart that is *yang*. Yi's cases 1 and 2 thus form a duplet which echoes the bipartite architectural and sentimental bodies described above.

Finally, a passage in the medieval Dunhuang manuscripts deserves to be mentioned as it describes pathological conditions which come very close to those of cases 1 and 2. This textual parallel is for several reasons worth noting. First, it highlights striking parallels between the manuscript literature (P3287) and the received literature (Yi's Memoir on the one hand, *Su wen* 20 on the other). Second, it highlights how terse Yi's medical notes may have been before they became integrated into Sima Qian's narrative history. Third, it gives us further insight into how the bodily bipartition of the architectural body differs from the body ecologic, and throws light on a difficult passage in case 1 (lines 21–5). The Dunhuang text reads:[68]

> If the *mai* of the middle (*zhong*) part are at once dispersed, at once frequent,
> the passageways are in disarray, and one dies.
> If the *mai* of the upper (*shang*) part come in an alternating way, and are hooked,
> the disorder resides in the linking vessels.

> *Qi zhong bu mai zha shu zha shuo zhe* 其中部脈乍疏乍數者
> *jing luan yi, yi si* 經亂矣 亦死
> *Qi shang bu mai lai dai er gou zhe* 其上部脈來代而鉤者
> *bing zai luo mai ye* 病在絡脈也

This Dunhuang text associates the 'passageways' (*jing*) with the 'middle part' (*zhong bu*), and the 'linking vessels' (*luo mai*) with the 'upper part' (*shang bu*), and thereby invokes a body partition into two parts. It alludes to a partition along a vertical axis, similar to that invoked by the Zhangjiashan 'Yinshu' authors within the sentimental body or by the Mawangdui vessel text authors within the architectural body. As will be demonstrated in detail (on p. 166), it describes pathological processes that translate easily into those of Yi's cases 1 and 2 (lines 1–15).

Interestingly, the Dunhuang text does not oppose the 'lower' and 'upper' parts but mentions first the 'middle' and then the 'upper' parts. It thus parallels case 1, where the liver is associated with *zhong* 中, the 'middle' (rather than with the 'lower' part), and case 2, which clearly concerns a disorder in the 'upper' bodily cavity. The Dunhuang authors may have added a *bu* 部 'part' to *zhong* 中, which can also designate the body's 'interior', and conceived of *zhong bu* 中部 as 'middle part'. Their tripartite body

---

[68] The excursus into P3287, text 1, col. 26 (Ma *et al.* 1994:11), is justified because it parallels *Su wen* 20, p. 65, a well-known Han source on pulse diagnosis (Kuriyama 1999:39). Text critical studies suggest that Han texts have survived fairly unaltered in medieval compilations (e.g. Keegan 1988); the modifications are telling.

conception, which divided the body into an upper, middle and lower part, was much like that of the early Han physicians' bipartite body, organised along a vertical axis. The parallel text in *Su wen* 20, however, alludes to a concentric body conception:[69]

> If the interior part (*zhong bu*) is at once dispersed, at once frequent, one dies.
> If its *mai* alternates, and is hooked,
> the disorder is in the linking vessels.
>
> *Zhong bu zha shu zha shuo zhe* 中部乍疏乍數者
> *si* 死
> *Qi mai dai er gou zhe* 其脈代而鈎者
> *bing zai luo mai* 病在絡脈

Su wen 20 evidently understands *zhong bu* 中部 as 'interior part' and opposes it to 'linking vessels' on the body surface. It makes no reference to the 'upper body' part, as does the Duanhuang text. However, since the 'hooked' pulse is characteristically that of the heart (and the season summer, see p. 170), it is likely that the ancient source for this canonical text used the graph *shang* 'above' for designating the body architectural heart, but the *Su wen* editors dropped it as they may not have understood that the deictic *shang* was a noun designating a body part.

In Yi's Memoir, a similarly concentric body conception is implied in the latter parts of case 1 (lines 21–5), which oppose 'disorders of the passageways' (*jing bing*) to 'disorders of the linking vessels' (*luo mai you bing*). Lines 21–5 differentiate between 'internally induced' disorders, which arise in bones and marrow and cause disorders in the passageways, and 'externally induced' ones, which arise due to an indulgent lifestyle and adversely affect the linking vessels. In this respect, lines 21–5 have more in common with the concentric body conception in *Su wen* 20 than with the bipartite architectural body implied by cases 1 and 2 in their lines 1–15. This concentric body conception implicitly alludes to the medical rationale of the 'body ecologic' that was framed in wind physiologies and pathologies, where protection of the 'interior' from environmental invasions became a trope, and the concentric view of the body became predominant.

In summary, the early Han medical manuscript texts not only refer to a bipartite sentimental body but also allude to a bipartite architectural body. Both were aligned along a vertical axis, while the canonical body ecologic concentrically aligned layers of bodily tissue.

---

[69] *Su wen* 20, p. 65, does not mention the phrase 'the passageways are in disarray' (*jing luan*) that is given in the medieval Dunhuang text. Perhaps, the copyists of the *Su wen* no longer understood it.

5

Discussion

The above showed that early nurturing life practices of the nobility differentiated between an externally visible *xing*-form and internal *qi*. The external form should be firm and solid, luminescent and lustrous, like a fresh plant or a polished stone. Colour (*se*) and *mai* were outwardly visible aspects of the form; they could be lustrous or dry, blue-green or red, full or empty, smooth or rough. *Qi*, by contrast, was an internal, invisible aspect of human existence, among which belonged feelings and emotions, thought and intent.

Qi inside the 'sentimental body' had either *yin* or *yang* characteristics, dependent on whether it arose in the upper or lower bodily sphere. If agitated, it led to strong emotions of grief (or joy/love) and anger. The presence of *qi* in the 'sentimental body' was thus experienced primarily when one became emotional. It is therefore likely that physicians heeding emotional distemper became interested in the diagnosis of *qi*. Considering that feelings are expressed in a tactile language, certainly in Europe (see p. 14) if not cross-culturally, and considering that they might be accessible primarily through the tactile mode, it may not be coincidence that Yi's diagnostic method that allowed him to identify different qualities of *qi* was a tactile one. It went hand in hand with a change in body conception, which made *qi* central to the language of medical rationale.

In the extant literature, there is no conclusive evidence that in the Warring States *qi* was thought to move through *mai*. In the Mawangdui vessel texts of the early Han, *qi* is not explicitly said to flow in *mai*. *Qi* becomes an aspect of *mai* for the first time in Yi's Memoir. In particular, the formula in his cases 1–10 provides explicit reference to *qi* as an aspect of *mai*. His method of 'examining *mai*' (*zhen mai*) consisted of 'palpating' or 'pressing onto *mai*' (*qie mai*), sometimes at an 'opening' 口 (*kou*).[1] He also once 'stroked' (*xun* 循) an area called *chi* 尺 (foot), in case 19.[2] He provided no

---

[1] See case 3 (lines 14, 16), n. 62. See also p. 68.
[2] *Su wen* 28, p. 86, has *mai kou* and *chi*. See case 3, n. 65. *Ling shu* 74, p. 454, quoted on p. 299, compares qualities of *mai* with those of the skin at the *chi* area.

hints on the location of either. In later medical texts, the 'opening' was located at the wrist and the 'foot' occupied, as the word would imply, an area as long as a foot on the forearm.[3]

---

[3] See references quoted in case 3, n. 64 and n. 66. Yi did not refer to a 'foot inch method' (*chi cun* 尺寸), but perhaps his diagnostic techniques were an early precursor. Pulse diagnosis on the wrist at three positions of equal size, *cun guan chi* 寸關尺, became prominent only in medieval times (Hsu 2008a and in press b).

II
The Memoir of Chunyu Yi in *Shi ji* 105

6

Outline of the Memoir (*Canggong zhuan*)

Part II outlines the structure and contents of Chunyu Yi's Memoir. It begins with discussing the Memoir's overall structure and socio-historical framing before delving into questions of who the medical authorities Yi refers to were, and what their genres of learning. This brings to the fore an unexpected multivocality of the text: when an attempt was made to derive from his patients' names the socio-historical cadre in which Yi lived, the question arose as to whether these personages actually were his clients. This led to questions pertaining to the Memoir's author- and editorship. Not only the names of his clientele but also details of medical knowledge hint at different primary sources. Medical authorities other than Yi are frequently quoted, and even the book titles he mentions may be of multiple provenance. Despite its compelling narrative, the Memoir stands out for its multivocality. Like many texts of antiquity, it is best read as a compilation.

The overall structure of the Memoir

Yi's Memoir can be divided into four sections, of which the first two are biographical. They both report that he started studying with a new master, a certain Yang Qing 陽慶, in the eighth year of Empress Gao 高 (180 BCE), in Linzi 臨菑, the capital of the kingdom of Qi 齊. The first section is in the third person singular, and may have been written by the astrologer-historian Sima Qian himself or a member of his team. It stands out for the story it tells, with folkloric elements, which made it known beyond medical circles. In the fourth year of Emperor Wen 文帝 (176 BCE) Yi was accused by a patient he refused to treat. He was brought to Chang'an 長安, the capital of the Western Han empire, where he was about to receive punishment by mutilation, when his fifth daughter,[1] Tiying 緹縈, presented a document to the Emperor,[2] who thereupon felt pity and in that year rescinded

---

[1] According to section one, Yi and Yang Qing both had no sons; Yi had five daughters.
[2] Tiying's memorial to the Emperor was much celebrated in antiquity, praising her skills of argumentation, but in the Song and Ming, she was remembered primarily for her filial piety (e.g. *Tai ping yu lan* 415, Raphals 1998a: 47–8, 136).

punishment.[3] The second introductory section, which is given in the first person singular, as are the third and fourth sections, details some of the information previously provided, for instance, the titles of the books Yi received. The third section is the longest and contains twenty-five medical case histories; the fourth consists of eight questions and answers.

Yi was a Han official of the kingdom of Qi who learnt medicine late in life. The end of the second section states he was thirty-nine *sui* 歲, i.e. thirty-eight years old, after serving his master for three years. Accordingly, he was born in 215 BCE.[4] More relevant for medical history is when he wrote the case histories.[5] The date of his accusation, 176, given in the first section, is at variance with other passages of the Han dynastic histories, which report he was amnestied in 167.[6] One would assume the accusation and amnesty happened in the same year, although it is not impossible that Yi spent nine years in Chang'an awaiting punishment.

The first introductory section ends with the following statement: 'An Imperial edict summoned him [Yi] and enquired about that which made him treat illnesses and [prognosticate] death and life. The cases proven true, how many were they? The main names among them were which ones?' The second, third and fourth sections are best read as a response to this edict, reporting on events that presumably happened before the Emperor's amnesty in either 176 or 167.

There is some controversy about whether the issuing of the edict was actually related to the amnesty. Some Chinese scholars and the previous translators of the Memoir have suggested that it was, but contemporary Sinological scholarship has contested this.[7] However, Fan Xingzhun, in

---

[3] Three cases were exempted from mutilation. Zhang Shoujie quotes *Han shu* 23, p. 1098. 'Tattooing the face and cutting off the nose makes two, [cutting off] the left and right foot combined are one, altogether this makes three' (*qing yi er [yue] zuo you zhi [he] yi, fan san ye* 黥 劓二 [刖]左右趾[合]一 凡三也).

[4] Much scholarly ink has been spilt over Yi's date of birth. Both introductory sections say he started serving Master Yang Qing in 180 BCE, which, in the light of the above, was at thirty-six *sui*. This means he was born in 216, according to the commentators Xu Guang and Zhang Wenhu, and Bridgman (1955:66, n. 73) and He (1984). But Loewe (1997:307–8), following Wilbur (1943:289), gives 206, which incidentally is the founding date of the Han dynasty. Fan Xingzhun (unpubl.) and Lin (1984) give 205. Sivin (1995a:179) points out that thirty-nine *sui* means he was thirty-eight years old and gives 214. Based on Xu, Zhang, He, Bridgman and Sivin, Yi's date of birth is 215 BCE.

[5] Loewe (1997:301), in recognition of textual parallels (see ch. 6, n. 6), considers the amnesty to have taken place in 167 BCE, i.e. the thirteenth year of Emperor Wen. Bridgman (1955:64, n. 63) provides a plausible explanation for a scribal error, four (176 BCE) being mistaken as thirteen (167 BCE). One could argue that 176 is ruled out by the sentence in the end of section two that Yang Qing had died ten years earlier. However, the sentence is odd as it is not thematically embedded in context. It reads like a late interjection into a passage concerned, first, with Yi's three years of apprenticeship and, then, his age after its completion.

[6] *Shi ji* 10, pp. 427–8; *Han shu* 23, pp. 1097–8; and *Shi ji* 22, p. 1127.

[7] Commentator Chen Zilong sees a causal connection between the Emperor's amnesty and the Imperial edict, as do Hübotter (1927:5) and Bridgman (1955:25), but not Sivin (1995a:178). Although Loewe (1997:307) did not find textual evidence of an Imperial edict being sent out to Qi, an event well worth recording, he too argues that Yi's statement is not a defence against the criminal charges, not least because some dealings with people Yi records, in his view, must have taken place at a later date than the amnesty.

particular, is emphatic that the case material was written and stored in Chang'an,[8] which in his view was essential for Sima Qian to access it. All contemporary researchers agree that the Memoir contains edited primary materials. The question is just how creative the editor was. Some consider Sima Qian and his team to have recorded the source material fairly unchanged; others consider him to have composed it in a free writing style, elaborating on materials cursorily consulted rather than faithfully quoted.[9] In this study I found that incongruencies in medical rationale and terminology could be explained by considering *Shi ji* 105 to be based on different primary sources, which were selectively if not heavily edited and richly embellished.

The third section of the Memoir is by far the longest, and for the medical historian it is a treasure on medical knowledge and practice in antiquity. The twenty-five medical case histories record the patient's name, title of office (or relationship to a noble or king), and place of residence, much in the manner of the twenty-five legal case records of 217 BCE called 'Models for Sealing and Investigating' (Fengzhenshi 封診式).[10] However, unlike the 'Models for Sealing and Investigating', which concerned personages identified as mister or misses XY from village YZ and which were presented as hypothetical cases, Yi's medical case histories report on past events and can be read as concerning historical individuals. Given that in all twenty-five cases, either Yi's prognostications of death were accurate or his treatments led to a cure, one can say that he followed the instructions of the Imperial edict closely (if the above translation from the first introductory section is correct). If the case histories he recounted were chosen from a larger pool, as stated in the Memoir's section 4.1, they are best read as justifications for his medical practice.

The fourth section, which consists of eight questions and answers, discusses Yi's medical rationale, his medical training and his teachings to his followers. In several respects, this section does not tally with the previous ones. There are differences in linguistic particles, in details of medical theory, and in names of book titles and personages. For instance, in the response to question six when Yi reports on his teachers, he names a certain Gongsun Guang 公孫光 from the ward Tang 唐 in Zichuan 菑川 and Yang Zhongqian 楊中倩 from Linzi, who had an adult son called Yin 殷. If one identifies Yang Qing from the ward Yuan 元 in Linzi with Yang Zhongqian, as do the commentators,[11] section one that claims he had no sons and section four flatly contradict each other.

---

[8] Fan (unpubl.).

[9] Nienhauser (2004, p.c.) inclines towards the former view, van Ess (2006, p.c.) towards the latter. Puett (2001:141–76) notes Sima Qian said of himself he *zuo* 作 created the text. In my reading of Yi's Memoir, Sima Qian emerges as an 'author-editor' of terse primary medical materials which he presents in a formulaic but eloquent freestyle prose.

[10] Translated by McLeod and Yates (1981), Bodde (1982), Hulsewé (1985).

[11] e.g. *Shiki kokujikai*, p. 75.

In summary, narrative analysis can structure the Memoir into four sections: three are written in the first person singular; the first in the third person singular. The first reports on the famous event of Chunyu Yi's fifth daughter Tiying and her skills in argumentation, recorded also in other Han literature. The following three sections, written in the first person singular, are presented as a response to an Imperial edict. Both introductory sections mention 180 BCE as the year in which Yi started learning with his teacher Yang Qing and devoted himself full-time to medicine. This seems to me the most relevant date for the purposes of interpreting the medical rationale in the core texts of the Memoir.

After extensive research, I am inclined to consider cases 1–10 as elaborating on a fairly coherent primary source, perhaps a medical document of 176 BCE kept in the archives of Chang'an and written by the historical figure Chunyu Yi (if he ever existed and by that name). In the early first century Sima Qian presumably edited this primary document. Perhaps he also assembled around it the following fifteen cases, and perhaps also parts of the fourth section. Or, since those clearly build on materials from different sources, they were added incrementally over time. Fan Xingzhun suggests Sima Qian composed the first section – he praises the prose; perhaps it dates to an earlier period than most of section four, perhaps to a later one.[12]

The socio-historical framework

Chunyu Yi lived in the difficult times of the political division of the great kingdom of Qi in the Eastern part of the Han empire. He relinquished his office and started studying medicine with Yang Qing in 180 BCE, which incidentally was the year when the then King of Qi, Liu Xiang 劉襄, made a bid for the Imperial throne after elimination of the Lü 呂 family. The kingdom of Qi had earlier lost parts of its territory in 193, 187, 181, when in 178, during the first year of Emperor Wen's reign (179–156), it was further diminished with the establishment of the kingdoms of Chengyang 成陽 (178 BCE–9 CE) and Jibei 濟北 (178–176 BCE).[13] The most important division of the kingdom of Qi happened in 164 BCE, when Liu Jianglü 劉將閭 (reign 164–153) became king of a drastically reduced Qi. In that year, the kingdom of Jibei (164–86) was reinstalled, and four new kingdoms were created, namely those of Jinan 濟南, Zichuan 菑川, Jiaoxi 膠西 and Jiaodong

---

[12] Fan (unpubl.), but consider case 2, n. 66.

[13] The first Han Emperor Liu Bang 劉邦 (Gaodi or Gaozu; reign 202–195 BCE) made his son Liu Fei 劉肥 (201–188) King of Qi. At his death, Liu Fei was succeeded by his son Liu Xiang 劉襄 (188–178), who at his death was succeeded by his son Liu Ze 劉則 (178–164). As Liu Ze died without successor, his uncle, Liu Jianglü 劉將閭 (164–153), became King of Qi. Commentators have it that Yi served Liu Jianglü, but if the primary materials were heterogeneous, this is not compelling.

膠東 (all reign 164–153). In all these six kingdoms a son of Liu Fei 劉肥, the first King of Qi (reign 201–188) or grandson of Emperor Gao 高帝 (reign 202–195, the first Han emperor) was made king, and they were all one generation junior to Emperor Wen. This significantly weakened the political clout of eastern China. The rulers of the four latter kingdoms took part in an unsuccessful revolt in 154, together with those of the well-established kingdoms of Zhao 趙 and Chu 楚, under the leadership of the King of Wu 吳. They were all executed, and from 153 their kingdoms became commanderies administered by the central government. Only the kingdom of Zichuan was restored again as a kingdom in that very year, as Liu Zhi 劉志, who had been King of Jibei from 164–153, transferred to Zichuan (reign 153–129). Since the kingdoms of Qi and Jibei were dissolved in 126 and 86 BCE respectively, the kingdom of Zichuan, together with that of Chengyang, was the only one to survive to the end of the Western Han.[14]

Chunyu Yi treated mainly members of the nobility, mostly of the kingdom of Qi. He also treated two slaves, three female 'attendants' or 'concubines', a child, a 'wet-nurse', a woman from his home town and two men, one of whom he treated, as he explains in section 4.3, en route between Qi and Chang'an. In case 8, Yi mentions the Noble of Yangxu 陽虛 and in case 23, he refers to the time when the King of Qi was the Noble of Yangxu, which identifies the person in case 23 as Liu Jianglü 劉將閭 (but if the primary material was heterogeneous, not necessarily the one mentioned in case 8). In case 11, Yi alludes to 'the former King of Jibei', in cases 9 and 12, to 'the King of Jibei', and in cases 14 and 16, to 'the King of Zichuan'. Strictly speaking, none of these kings can be identified with certainty, but Michael Loewe, who assumes that the Memoir consists of one coherent text, suggests the former King of Jibei was Liu Xingju 劉興居 (reign 178–176), the King of Jibei was Liu Zhi 劉志 (reign 164–153) and the King of Zichuan was Liu Xian 劉賢 (reign 164–153).[15] In section 4.3, a certain King Wen is mentioned, identified by Chinese commentators as King Wen of Qi, who apparently died as an adolescent in 164.[16] Furthermore, Yi mentions in section 4.3 the Kings of Zhao, Jiaoxi, Jinan and Wu, who all participated in the revolt of 154 and were killed in 153. As Loewe notes,[17] it may not have been coincidence that Yi refused to treat them.

Taking into account the above, case 23 would have happened before 164, when Liu Jianglü was Noble of Yangxu, but reported thereafter, when he was King of Qi; cases 14 and 16 would refer to times after Zichuan became a kingdom in 164; and section 4.3, which mentions King Wen of Qi and the Kings of Zhao, Jiaoxi, Jinan and Wu, would concern events after 164 and

---

[14] Based on Twitchett and Loewe (1986:128–52) and Loewe (1997), but Loewe (2000; 2004:363, 383–4) modifies data of his own earlier publications (e.g. dates). For place names, see ch. 9.
[15] Loewe (1997).   [16] *Han shu* 14, p. 398, but Xu Guang gives 165 BCE.
[17] Loewe (1997:309).

Table 1: Names and titles of Chunyu Yi's clientele

1. Cheng 成, an Attending Secretary of Qi 齊[a]
2. The youngest son of all the infants of the middle son[b] of the King of Qi
3. Xun 循, the Prefect of the Gentlemen of the Palace of Qi
4. Xin 信, the Chief of the Palace Wardrobe of Qi
5. The queen dowager of the King of Qi
6. Cao Shanfu 曹山跗 of the ward Zhangwu 章武 in Qi
7. Pan Manru 潘滿如, the Commandant of the Capital of Qi
8. Zhao Zhang 趙章, the Chancellor[c] of the Noble of Yangxu 陽虛
9. The King of Jibei 濟北
10. The accredited wife[d] Chuyu 出於 of Beigong[e] 北宮, the Officer of Works at Qi
11. The wet-nurse[f] of the former King of Jibei
12. The King of Jibei's woman Shu 豎
13. The Palace Grandee of Qi
14. A concubine[g] of the King of Zichuan 菑川
15. The slave of a Member of the Suite of the Chancellor of Qi
16. The King of Zichuan
17. The queen's younger brother Song Jian 宋建, at the home of the elder brother of the King of Qi's Lady Huang[h] called Huang Zhangqing 黃長卿
18. Dame Han 韓, an attendant of the King of Jibei
19. Bo Wu 薄吾, a woman of the ward Fan 氾 in Linzi 臨菑
20. The Major from Chunyu 淳于 in Qi
21. Po Shi 破石, a Gentleman of the Palace of Qi
22. Sui 遂, the Attending Physician of the King of Qi
23. The King of Qi, formerly Noble of Yangxu
24. Cheng Kaifang 成開方 from the ward Wudu 武都 in Anyang 安陽
25. Xiang Chu 項處, a *gong sheng* dignitary[i] of the ward Ban 阪 in Anling 安陵

[a]The translation of the titles is based on Bielenstein (1980). For case 1: *shi yu shi* 侍御史 (*ibid.*: 9–10, 90, 160, n. 26); 3: *lang zhong ling* 郎中令 (*ibid.*: 106); 4: *zhong yu fu zhang* 中御府長 (*ibid.*: 188, n. 126); 5: *tai hou* 太后, title borne by the queen-wife of a deceased monarch, not an official title (not in Bielenstein); 7: *Zhong wei* 中尉 'commandant of the capital' (*ibid.*: 106); 10: *si kong* 司空 (*ibid.*: 16), not recorded for the Western Han, probably refers to a low-ranking official; in the Eastern Han *si kong* is a degradation of the 'Grand Minister of Works' (*da si kong*); 13: *zhong da fu* 中大夫 (*ibid.*: 25); 15: *she ren* 舍人 (*ibid.*: 23, 164, n. 92), *cheng xiang* 丞相: 105, 106, 188, n. 125); 18: *shi zhe* 侍者 'messengers' (*ibid.*: 110, 190, n. 143), here given as 'attendant', descriptive term, not a title; 20: *sima* 司馬 (*ibid.*: 94, 115); 21: *zhong lang* 中郎; note inversion to *lang zhong ling* in case 3; 22: *shi yi* 侍醫, not in Bielenstein.
[b]Alternative translations: Zhu Ying *er xiao zi* 'the small prince Zhu Ying' (Hübotter 1927:9), which is unlikely because Yi usually repeats the name of the patient and here only *xiao zi*. Or: *Qi wang zhong er* Zhu Ying 'the middle son of the King of Qi, called Zhu Ying', which is grammatically possible but semantically, in the light of age-sensitive epidemiological aspects, the above is more likely.
[c]In the Han *xiang* 相 is the regular term for officials of various types and duties, including the one who was responsible for managing the estates of a noble. Originally termed *ling* 令, their title was changed to *xiang*. See *Han shu* 19A, p. 740. Before 145 BCE, *cheng xiang* 丞相, as given in case 15, rather than *xiang* is the word for Chancellor.
[d]*ming fu* 命婦 'accredited wife, titled wife'. See HYDCD 3.285, based on *Li ji* 24, p. 1441. Taki Motohiro extensively comments on the ranks of the husband of a *nei* or *wai ming fu*. The problem is that an 'officer of works' is too low a rank for an official to have a *ming fu*. According to Chavannes (1897:519, 523), quoted in Bridgman (1955:82, n. 142), a *si kong* would only have been allowed to have a slave. Xu Guang points to another edition with *fu* as *nu* 奴 'slave'. This would also solve problems of medical rationale in regard of gender (see p. 330). On the other hand, a low-ranking official with an accredited wife may also be an editorially intended hint at the debauchery at Qi.
[e]Beigong 北宮 is a surname, according to *Shiki kokujikai*, p. 46, and Yamada (1998:118). The alternative translation is 'northern palace' – but was there a northern (and by implication southern) palace at Qi? See p. 330 for context and further discussion.
[f]*a mu* 阿母 means *ru mu* 乳母 'wet-nurse' according to Sima Zhen. See also *Shi ji* 30A, p. 1049. She must have had a status of respect, as Yi 'formally announces' *gao* 告 the name of the disorder.
[g]*mei ren* 美人 'concubine', frequently mentioned in *Shi ji*. See e.g. *Shi ji* 118, p. 3075.
[h]*Huang yi* 黃姬: 'concubine Huang' (Hübotter 1927:18).
[i]*gongsheng* 公乘 is an order of honour (Loewe 1960:97–174).

prior to 153, but, since Yi says he refused to treat them, was probably recounted after 154. Considering that the first King of Jibei was killed in 176, and Yi treated his wet-nurse in case 11, she must have been very old, or Yi treated her very early in his career. Or, Yi composed the text after Liu Bo 劉勃 (reign 152–151) died in 151, and referred to Liu Zhi as 'former King of Jibei'.[18] In summary, if one decides to take the kings as indices for dating Yi's medical activities, one can be certain that two cases were written after 164, one was written after 164 on events before 164, and section 4.3 after 154 on events prior to 153.

In spite of detailed calculations of this kind, it is uncertain whether all the individuals mentioned in the Memoir were people with whom the historical person, Chunyu Yi, if he ever existed, had dealings. As already mentioned, the source material for this Memoir may have been rather heterogeneous. Thus, the biographical information in sections one and four is partly incongruous. Furthermore, the medical rationale in cases 1–10 forms a unity. While closely related to the following fifteen cases, it is distinctive, despite internal variation (particularly cases 4 and 10). Naturally, the case histories may reflect accumulated records over several decades, during which Yi changed his ideas. It is more likely, however, that a fairly coherent elite medical document was written after the events in Chang'an, as *Shi ji* 105 seems to imply, in 176 BCE, and that it was selectively edited, creatively restructured, and supplemented by later source materials.

This heterogeneous primary source material may or may not have been edited so as to refer to politically known personages. The surnames and given names of several patients are unusual; they sometimes rhyme (cases 1–9/10) or are nicknames (cases 10/11–25). Thus, when Cheng 成 (*Dieng) got ill, Chang 昌 (*T'iang) was told this in case 1, then Xin 信 (*Dziwen) and Xun 循 (*Sien) got ill in cases 3 and 4, and Yi spoke to the Grand Coachman Rao 饒 (*Niog)[19] and the Clerk of the Capital Yao 繇 (*Diog) in case 7.[20] The accredited wife Exit-At 出於 (Chu Yu) had an illness at the exit in case 10,[21] the Cold Dame 韓女 (Han nü) suffered from internal coldness in case 18,[22] and Mr Damaged-on-a-Rock 破石 (Po Shi) fell on to a

[18] Xu Guang notes another edition has the King of Qi in place of the King of Jibei.

[19] *tai pu* 太僕 and *nei shi* 內史 (Bielenstein 1980:106).

[20] Karlgren (1957:216, 818a; 191, 724a; 127, 465f; 110, 384a; 300, 1164o; 294, 1144n). The rhymes in cases 1, 3 and 4 are not as compelling as that in case 7 (Rudolf Pfister, 2005 p.c.).

[21] Chu Yu causes problems to Zhang Shoujie, who considers Chuyu a personal name. Cui Shi interprets *chu yu* as *bing yu chu* 病於出 'The illness is at the exit', which points, in his understanding, to this person's disorder in the bladder. This is a pun, rather than a rhyme.

[22] *Han* 韓 (g'an) and *han* 寒 (g'an) have the same pronunciation (Karlgren 1957:57, 140h, and 58, 143a). See also Wu Rulun's (1840–1903) comment on *han* 寒 and *han* 韓 in Wang (1983:2908). 韓女 can mean either Han nü 'dame Han' (Hübotter 1927:18; Bridgman 1955:39) or Han Ru. The former is grammatically unusual, if not incorrect (Loewe, 1995 p.c.), but Han as surname and Ru as personal name is odd because Ru generally is a surname (HYDCD 4.255). Yi tends to repeat the full name, not title and name (except in case 2 and arguably case 20), but then *nü* is not a title.

rock in case 21.[23] In addition, the talented person Shu 豎 in case 12 had as surname a word of abuse, which for reasons that become apparent only after the decoding of the case history, may reflect a moral judgement. In antiquity legal case records did not always mention names. Perhaps this also applied to medical case records. Perhaps the rhymed names represent an editorial addition to early medical records which contained titles but not names (cases 1–9/10), while the puns were an integral part of the stories that provided the primary materials for the later case histories (cases 10/11–25).

Rather than relying on names that sometimes rhyme or are puns for dating the Memoir, one may want to turn to taboo names of emperors. This, however, is also not always a reliable method. Nevertheless, if one assumes that the most frequently mentioned book title 'Qi ke' 奇咳 stands for that of 'Qi heng' 奇恆 in the *Inner Canon*, the primary texts in sections two, three and four, which all mention 'Qi ke' at least once, must have been written during Emperor Wen's reign (179–156).[24]

In this context, it is worth noting that Yi may have had misgivings about the King of Qi's bid for the throne in 180 BCE. He was an official of Qi and resigned in that very year. In cases 1–10, the clientele he mentions is mostly nobility of Qi (in cases 1–7 and 10); he furthermore mentions a Noble of Yangxu in case 8 and the King of Jibei in case 9. These titles existed already in 176 (or 167). It is only cases 11–25 that mention the 'King of Zichuan' (the first of whom existed after 164), a 'former King of Jibei' (the first of whom existed after 164) and 'the King of Qi, at the time when he was Noble of Yangxu' (unambiguously identified as Liu Jianglü, reign 164–153). Cases 1–10 have in common furthermore a fairly homogeneous medical rationale and terminology as well as a rigorously endorsed formulaic structure. They also have a strikingly similar message when it comes to non-medical contents. All this points to cases 1–10 as being derived from one primary source, and to a large extent edited by one hand.

The suggestion that the Memoir consists of heterogeneous primary materials, assembled around one substantive document, and that all were selectively edited, may also explain why in section 4.3 the kings mentioned can be interpreted to reflect on a politically astute editor. It mentions neither the King of Zichuan, whose successor was still reigning then, nor the King of Jiaodong, territory over which Liu Che 劉徹 had reigned for four years prior to becoming Emperor Wu 武帝 (reign 141–87 BCE),

---

[23] *po* 'to damage', *shi* 'stone'; Po Shi fell from a horse onto a rock, injured his lungs, and died.

[24] In MWD 'He yinyang' (1985:155, S103–4), *chang shan* 常山 is given in place of *heng shan* 恆山 in the view of scholars who argue that *heng* 恆 was a taboo character (*hui* 諱) during the reign of Liu Heng 劉恆, i.e. Emperor Wen 文帝 (Rudolf Pfister, 2005 p.c.). If 'Qi ke' in *Shi ji* 105 replaces 'Qi heng', the primary material of sections two, perhaps three, and arguably four, dates to 179–156 BCE. For a critique of taboo name-based dating, see Soymié (1990).

when Yi says he refused to see four of the seven kings who revolted in 154. Moreover, while the introductory two sections focus on Yi's teacher Yang Qing from Linzi, the capital of the mighty kingdom of Qi in the early Han, section 4.6 narrates at length on Yi's teacher Gongsun Guang from Zichuan. Zichuan was the capital of the kingdom of Zichuan, which in contrast to Qi, was still thriving in 86 BCE. This story may have arisen and become part of the *Shi ji* in the first century, perhaps even after Sima Qian's death.

Finally, we need to address the question of why medical histories were included in this monumental work on the political history of the first Chinese empire. The Grand Historian hints on how they should be read in his closing statement to the Memoir. He comments on Yi's fate of being a great medical doctor unfairly accused of a crime by (mis-)quoting *Laozi* 老子: 'Beauty and goodness are instruments for [attracting] calamities' (*fu mei hao zhe, bu xiang zhi qi* 夫美好者 不祥之器).[25] This quote also applies to the famous Bian Que, who was killed ruthlessly by a despot. Some suggest that Sima Qian himself identified with this quote,[26] since he had been castrated as a form of punishment after taking sides in a political controversy during the reign of Emperor Wu. It may be for other than purely medical reasons that in Yi's Memoir about half of the cases are attributed to indulgence in 'wine' (three cases), 'women' (five explicitly stated and three inferred cases) or 'wine and women' (two cases). Cases 1–10, in particular, blame wine and women (except cases 2 and 4), which hints at debauchery among the nobility of Qi. Perhaps the Memoir contains a coded critique by both the early second-century medical author and the early first-century editor. Both had reason for it.

The narrative of the Memoir: a multivocalic text

The above has made a case for considering Yi's Memoir a text with at least two layers of composition, based on primary materials of the early second century that were edited in the early first century BCE. This section goes one step further and highlights that Yi's Memoir is not a text with one authorial voice. It is possible, if not likely, that the case histories of section three and the stories surrounding the transmission of medical knowledge in section four testify to a variety of local medical traditions. Multivocality of authorship is furthermore signalled by the various book titles mentioned in sections two and four, the different 'Models' (Fa 法) referred to particularly

---

[25] *Laozi* 31, p. 191 reads: *fu bing zhe, bu xiang zhi qi* 夫兵者 不祥之器. The idiom *fu bing zhe* 'weapons', sometimes given as *jia bing zhe* 佳兵者 'excellent weapons', is given as *mei hao zhe* 美好者 'beauty and goodness' in the *Shi ji*. Was a different *Laozi* edition then in circulation? Is this a scribal error? Or did Sima Qian intentionally alter the wording of the *Laozi*?

[26] e.g. Durrant (1995:120). The statement recurs in *Shi ji* 49, p. 1984, and 83, p. 2473.

in section three, the named and unnamed other doctors, and the multivocalic medical rationale of Yi himself. Regardless of whether or not there was a historical figure called Chunyu Yi, in *Shi ji* 105 he has become a personage, in whose name various local narratives have been assembled into an overarching meta-narrative.

The reader of *Shi ji* 105 has to develop a sensitivity for the possible multiple provenance of the primary texts, possible editorial modifications and not infrequent commentatorial interjections. The major primary document which provided the basis for cases 1–10 may reflect medical knowledge learnt between 180 and 177 BCE, while cases 11–25 and the eight questions and answers in section four may be based on stories reflecting later but related medical understandings from a variety of localities and time periods. Sima Qian may have edited these texts in his own prose, which reflects early first-century currents of medical knowledge. His text may have been further amended in medieval times; it certainly was subject to a commentatorial history of two thousand years.

The case histories themselves contain many voices. Yi frequently refers to other medical authorities and physicians. The medical authorities, either written texts or memorised sets of sayings, include the 'Model of/for [the Study of] the Pulse' (Mai fa 脈法), the 'Model for the Examination of the Pulse' (Zhen mai fa 診脈法), or the 'Model of [Diagnostic] Examination' (Zhen fa 診法); and the 'Model of Disorders' (Bing fa 病法) (discussed in the next section). These 'Models' were sometimes concerned with the prognostication of death, but not with the time span until death would occur. Yi furthermore mentions the 'Fen jie fa' 分界法 ('Model of Allotments up to the Boundary [indicative of Death]' or 'Model for [Calculating] the Limits of one's Share') and the 'Si fa' 死法 ('Model of [Imminent] Death'), concerned with calculating the time span before death. The prediction of the time span before death was an essential aspect of iatromantic practices in the fourth and third centuries BCE, although in those manuscripts the prognostication was framed in terms of correlative cosmology. It was often pentic, as it is in Yi's case 21.[27] The repeatedly mentioned 'Fen jie fa' in cases 1–10 is also framed in a pentic numerology as it predicts death with reference to 'five allotments' (*wu fen* 五分). The 'Si fa', mentioned in cases 11–25, makes predictions with reference to 'seasons' (*shi* 時). Interestingly, the 'Fen jie fa' is considered a form of 'divination' (*zhan* 占) in the *Inner Canon*,[28] while the seasonality sensitive reasoning of the 'Si fa' had become an integral aspect of pulse diagnosis by medieval times, in the Dunhuang manuscripts.[29] Apart from the 'Mai fa', 'Zhen mai fa', 'Zhen fa', 'Bing fa', 'Fen jie fa' and 'Si fa', Yi occasionally mentions a 'word of the Master' (*shi yan* 師言) for explaining minor aberrations from the predictions he made.

---

[27] Harper (2001).   [28] *Su wen* 19, p. 60.   [29] Hsu (in press b).

There is also the voice of a group of doctors Yi refers to as 'all the many doctors' (*zong yi* 總醫), an expression that he uses in such a dismissive way that it appears to allude to a status difference, as though they were common doctors. Yi refers seven times to the misdiagnoses of these doctors; they are always mistaken and in his recounting did not have his sophisticated nosological vocabulary (except in case 10, lines 3–4). In Yi's account of their diagnoses, they had only one concept for his differentiated account of body-internal processes, namely *zhong* 中. This can either be a noun that refers to an undifferentiated body 'interior' or a verb meaning 'to strike the centre', much like the verb *ru* 入 'to enter' that expresses an assault by outside forces. These forces are 'wind' (*feng* 風) and 'coldness' (*han* 寒) in cases 1–10, and 'heat' (*re* 熱) in a later case. Furthermore, these doctors mention *jue* 蹶, which probably meant to them the 'dull', the 'numb' or 'the stone'.

Three other doctors, whom Yi named or referred to by their titles and who can be shown to have practised medicine within a similarly elaborate medical framework, also appear in the narrative because Yi is in disagreement with them. Thus, in case 6, he accuses the Prefect Grand Physician[30] of the kingdom of Qi of causing an iatrogenic disorder that ends in death. The Prefect Grand Physician does not speak for himself, but from Yi's report on his treatment, it is possible to show that the disagreement arose from differences in medical rationale parallel to those between the two Mawangdui vessel texts. In case 20, a doctor named Qin Xin[31] 秦信 comments on Yi's practice in direct speech and predicts that the patient will die, which turns out to be wrong. Case 22 concerns Yi's disputation with the Attending Physician of the King of Qi called Sui 遂. It is framed in *yin yang* rationale and recorded in dialogue form. To back their arguments, both quote a variety of medical authorities: Bian Que, a 'Discourse' (Lun 論) and the above 'Method of Examination'. Qin Xin, Sui and Yi used similar medical terminology and hence probably belonged to closely related currents of scholarly medical learning, which in all likelihood was text-based.

Yi himself is multivocalic in that he alludes to different frameworks of medical reasoning. In case 5, for instance, he mentions in the name of the disorder the *pao* 脬 bladder, a term which emphasises its *yin*-qualities, but later he speaks of the *pangguang* 膀胱 bladder, associated with *yang*-qualities. Or, he may use the same term-*dan* 癉 as a condition of over-exertion once associated with perspiration (case 5), once with heat (case 6). Yi appears to be an eclectic, who assembles knowledge from different medical currents. This is how I have presented him previously.[32]

---

[30] *Tai yi ling* 太醫令 (Bielenstein 1980:50–51).

[31] *yi Qin Xin* 醫秦信 means 'Doctor Qin Xin', see *Yi shuo* 1, p. 10a, and Hübotter (1927:20). Bridgman's (1955:40) 'doctor Xin from Qin' translates *Qin yi Xin*.

[32] Hsu (2001a).

In recent research, I found that the *Shi ji* personage Yi sometimes makes claims that for a reader trained in Chinese medicine appear downright erroneous or at least improbable. Was this the work of a humorous editor or of a later commentator who made interjections that were somewhat medically incongruous? It appears that Sima Qian may not merely have added or selectively altered some names of Yi's clientele, but also edited the medical contents of the text in creative ways. Sima Qian no doubt had basic knowledge of medicine, presumably of teachings dating to around 100 BCE, but perhaps some subtleties of elite medical learning were lost on him? Also, might he have drawn indiscriminately on both elite and popular medical knowledge, as anyone does who is not a medical specialist?

Furthermore, the *Shi ji* has a long history of reception, with a wealth of commentators, who not only commented on the primary text but also on each other. In this study, which builds on the most comprehensive *Shi ji* edition to date, the *Shiki kaichû kôshô* of 1934 by Kametarô Takigawa 瀧川龜太郎, the commentatorial apparatus adds further layers of meaning to the text. Some passages in the main text read as though they were originally editorial comments on or commentators' elucidations to the text, but it is difficult to demonstrate this, even when textual irregularities are evident. Others read like interjections of commentators who had no sense for Yi's line of argumentation.[33]

In summary, if there was a historical figure Chunyu Yi, he was in all likelihood born in 215 BCE. His loyalties were perhaps with Empress Lü in whose administration he worked as an official before devoting himself full-time to medicine in 180, the year in which the King of Qi made a bid for the throne. He probably wrote the document in 176, based on medical knowledge learnt in 180–177, that provided the source material for the *Shi ji* cases 1–10, which in their extant form contain in places indices of early scholarly medical knowledge. The *Shi ji* personage Chunyu Yi, by contrast, refers to clientele living through the politically traumatic events in eastern China from 164 to 154/153. He appears to have written one long document, namely sections two, three and four of the Memoir. This *Shi ji* personage emerges as a vivid narrator, who mostly adheres to scholarly medical knowledge, but sometimes combines it with popular medical and non-medical knowledge, due to editorial interpolations and commentatorial interjections.[34]

The medical contents hint at a compilation from multiple sources of related but distinct currents of medical knowledge. While the overall nar-

---

[33] All comments to cases 1–10 were read but not all translated; some were paraphrased, some omitted. Commentators were often anachronistic. The names of the commentators are given in chapter 8.

[34] Consider *bu gu* 不鼓 'not drumming' (case 6, line 18), perhaps used in a popular medical sense, or *feng* 風 'wind', used in the sense of a life-engendering principle (case 9, line 3), and *yi* 遺 'remanent' (case 10, line 8), used in a non-medical sense.

rative is strikingly structured and coherent, closer scrutiny suggests it derives from multiple authors and primary sources that were subject to an editor who had an agenda other than a purely medical one. Furthermore, many commentators left their traces in the text. The text gives several medical specialists a voice and invokes numerous written or memorised medical authorities. The *Shi ji* personage Yi himself appears as an eclectic, who combined knowledge from different strands.

Finally, not only Yi's Memoir but the entire chapter of *Shi ji* 105 also emerges as a collation, since the sequencing of the two Memoirs may not reveal much about the date of their composition/compilation. Bridgman suggests, irrespective of Bian Que's traditional Zhou life dates, that his Memoir was composed in 90 BCE, and was more recent than Yi's.[35] He points out medical terms that occur in Bian Que's Memoir, but not in Yi's, such as the triple burner (*san jiao* 三焦). Yamada, in his study of Bian Que, also dates his Memoir around 100, and reiterates this in his more recent study when he says of the two Memoirs that they contain 'materials of entirely different natures'.[36] In narrative style, Bian Que's Memoir celebrates the fabulous and miraculous, while Yi's is formulaic and meticulous. The medical rationale in Bian Que's three cases is much more accessible to someone familiar with canonical medical texts than Yi's cases 1–10. Both contain the technical terminology known from the medical canons, but Yi's Memoir requires the reader to search for passages, which are not as well known in contemporary Chinese medical scholarship and often show striking parallels with early medical manuscripts. In summary, due to the multivocalic fabric of the text, the dating of *Shi ji* 105 becomes truly complex; it presumably compiles texts dating from between 176 and 86 BCE, and perhaps even later (see pp. 116–17), apart from copious interjections by later commentators.

Medical knowledge contained in quotes from medical authorities

This section will detail aspects of the medical knowledge contained in the quotes of 'Models' (Fa) that Yi mentions in his case histories and furnish us with evidence on the relative consistency in medical rationale of cases 1–10, although there are also important differences among them. Yi most frequently cites as medical authority the so-called 'Mai fa' (Model of the Pulse), namely in cases 1, 2, 4, 5, 6, 15 and 23 or the 'Zhen mai fa' (Model for the Examination of the Pulse) in case 21. The 'Mai fa' may have been a written text, like those in the Mawangdui and Zhangjiashan medical manuscripts on silk, bamboo strips and wooden plates.

The 'Mai fa' quotes in cases 1–10 all concern qualities of *mai* which provide indices for identifying the disorder (except arguably in case 4).

---

[35] Bridgman (1955:14).   [36] Yamada (1988) and (1998:36).

Three out of five cases mention a so-called 'host of the disorder': 'In cases where the *mai*, while being elongated, are strung – if it is not [the *mai*] that alternates in accordance with the four seasons – the host of the disorder resides in the liver';[37] 'in cases where the *mai* come frequently and swiftly, and leave with difficulty, but are not one [in unison], the host of the disorder resides in the heart';[38] 'In cases when, as one sinks [into the *mai*], it is very firm, and when, as one floats [on the surface of the *mai*], it is very tight, the host of the disorder resides in the kidneys'.[39] The 'Mai fa' in case 4 is anomalous in that it concerns a prognostication of death: 'In the case of a heat disorder, those whose *yin* and *yang* intermingle, die';[40] and in case 6 in that it names the disorder: 'In cases of the uneven and not drumming, the body form is fading away'.

With one exception,[41] I found parallels for the 'Mai fa' quotes in the received literature. This finding was crucial, for it demonstrated that even though the *Shi ji* personage Yi might be a construct of an editor with a primarily non-medical agenda, his main medical authority, the 'Mai fa', attested to canonical medical knowledge. The 'Mai fa' quotes constitute a recurrent element in his pattern of argumentation. They appear intrinsic to the prose of the *Shi ji* personage Yi, although the possibility cannot be discarded entirely that they were interjected by a later commentator.

The 'Mai fa' is also quoted in case 15 and the 'Zhen mai fa' in case 21. However, in contrast to cases 1–10, these quotes concern the prognostication of death, not the diagnosis of disease. Thus, in case 15, the 'Mai fa' is quoted in the context of explaining why the doctor prognosticated the time span before death, and in case 21, the 'Zhen mai fa', which opposes 'being smooth' (*shun* 順) to 'contravective' (*ni* 逆), is cited to comment on good and bad death.

In this context, it is interesting to note that in case 8 Yi quotes the 'word of the Master': 'A word of the Master says: "Those who accommodate with ease to cereals will live beyond the appointed time. Those who reject cereals will not reach it."' This comment appears like an orally transmitted 'hot tip' that a master who has experience in making predictions with the 'Mai fa' gives to his disciple with the intention of explaining an irregularity observed in medical practice. Case 15 contains a comment of a similar kind, almost verbatim, repeated in case 21: 'If there is additionally an illness, one dies in mid-spring. If there is [additionally] a favourable and smooth [condi-

---

[37] Case 1, paralleling *Mai jing* 3.1, p. 68.
[38] Case 2, paralleling *Su wen* 19, p. 59, and *Mai jing* 3.2, p. 72.
[39] Case 5, paralleling *Mai jing* 1.13, p. 25, and 6.9, p. 209, with modifications.
[40] Case 4, paralleling, for instance, *Su wen* 33, p. 96.
[41] Case 6. However, the version Xu Guang noted with the pulse quality 'dispersed' parallels *Su wen* 1, p. 9, quoted on p. 35, in that a form that 'fades away' (*bi* 敝) causes 'dispersal' (*san* 散).

tion], one reaches one [more] season.' Yi indicates in cases 8 and 21, but not case 15, that the comment was orally transmitted.

The 'Mai fa' is also mentioned in section four of Yi's Memoir. In section 4.1, it outlines its function for medical practice, in section 4.4, age-appropriate conduct. In section 4.1, Yi furthermore explains he drew up a table for recording his Master's practice and compared his findings with maxims from the 'Mai fa'. Incidentally, this statement reconfirms a finding I arrived at independently through textual analysis. This is that after quoting the 'Mai fa' in cases 1–10, Yi comments on it in another vocabulary. He thus appears to compare two teachings of pulse diagnosis, each with their own vocabulary. As already stated, the case histories started making sense once I understood that Yi's own words reflected different strands of medical knowledge and practice. However, in recent research, I was rather disconcerted to find that within a single case these teachings are framed in terms of an incompatible medical rationale and I wondered whether they dated from different periods, e.g. the early second versus the early first century BCE, and possibly sometimes even later. Such reasoning cannot reflect that of a historical person, even if he were extremely eclectic. It reinforces the idea that the *Shi ji* personage Yi and his reasoning might be the construction of a skilful editor.

The 'Mai fa' is not the only authority Yi quotes. As already mentioned, he repeatedly takes recourse to what in case 8 is called the 'Fen jie fa' (Model of Allotments up to the Boundary), which is used for making predictions of how much time is allotted to a patient before death. In cases 1, 6 and 8, Yi prognosticates the time span before death on the grounds of its rationale. Once the boundary is reached, one dies; this happens when all five allotments along the *mai* are closed. Each allotment equals a day, thus as long as the *mai* is barely closed, one still has five days to live. In the material from cases 1–10, the 'Fen jie fa' is used in a consistent way, and links the study of *mai* to the prognostication of death. In case 17, by contrast, reasoning in terms of *fen* is used for diagnostic purposes by means of colour: Yi inspects degrees of the withering of colour, measured along a gradient of presumably five degrees, and deduces from this the length of the time the patient had been suffering. We note once again consistency of medical rationale in cases 1–10, which contrasts with that recorded in cases 11–25.

Yi also refers to the above-discussed 'Si fa' (Model of [Imminent] Death) in case 12 and to a not further specified 'Fa' (Model) in case 15 for predicting the time span a patient can still live before dying, which takes seasons as basic units for calculation. Yi furthermore quotes two unspecified 'Fa' which allude to a numerology of three for making predictions of death; in cases 7 and 23, they predict death in thirty days and three years respectively. Finally, the 'Model of Disorders' (Bing fa) in case 9 and the 'Model of

[Diagnostic] Examination' (Zhen fa) in case 22 have in common that they both allude to *yin yang* physiology, and are not concerned with the prognostication of death.[42]

In section four, the 'Mai fa' is mentioned in the answers to questions one and four. Three further 'Fa' occur in section 4.7, but in a slightly altered sense. While almost all 'Fa' in the medical case histories refer to maxims for prognosticating death, for making diagnoses and for deciding strategies of treatment, the 'Fa' here seem to be concerned with therapeutic techniques only.[43] Perhaps the graph 法 should be read as *fa* rather than 'Fa' and understood to refer to techniques, namely massage techniques (*an fa* 案法),[44] techniques for administering drugs (*yao fa* 藥法) and techniques for determining the five flavours and blending the regulatory broths (*ding wu wei ji he ji tang fa* 定五味及和齊湯法).[45] In contrast to the 'Fa' maxims in the twenty-five case histories of section three, the *fa* in section four probably designate therapeutic techniques.

In summary, Yi quotes a variety of 'Fa' in the case histories, which presumably contained written maxims for prognosis, diagnosis and treatment. In section three 'Fa' appear to be texts, but in section four they probably designate therapeutic techniques. In cases 1–10, the 'Mai fa' is generally concerned with locating the host of the disorder in a viscus, in case 4 and cases 11–25 with the prognosis of death, and in section four with the workings of the universe at large, inclusive of the universal process of ageing. The parallels in the received medical literature to Yi's 'Mai fa' quotes in cases 1–10 provided certainty that at least his main medical authority survived in elite medical writings. This finding was vital to this study that set out to make sense of Yi's medical rationale.

Book titles and the transmission of learned practice and knowledge

The 'Mai fa' and other 'Fa' occur in the twenty-five medical case histories, which form section three of Yi's Memoir, but not in sections one, two and four (except for the few above occurrences). Instead, Yi provides long lists of book titles.[46] A close re-examination of those reveals that the ones mentioned in section two refer to a conception of body that diverges from that

---

[42] 'Model for Treatment' (Zhi fa 治法) is possible in case 6 (lines 7–8), but unlikely. See case 6, n. 115.

[43] Case 12 is an exception, if *an fa* 案法 is there translated as 'massage techniques'.

[44] *an fa* 案法 is *an fa* 按法 in *Yi shuo* 1, p. 11a; it parallels *an fa* 案法 'massage techniques' in case 12. Compare and contrast with HYDCD 1.633 and Sivin (1995a:181). This renders Taki Mototane's comment obsolete that *an fa* means 'Cha fa' 察法 (Model for Diagnosis).

[45] *he ji tang* 和齊湯 is not attested elsewhere, perhaps meant to be *huo ji tang* 火齊湯. See case 5 (line 5).

[46] See also Keegan (1988: *passim*) and Sivin (1995a).

alluded to in the book titles of section four. One can put this down to *variatio*. However, if one takes seriously the possibility that section two elaborates on a document written at an earlier point in time than section four (or, at least, the answer to question seven in section four), one can see trends in how medical rationale changed in the time period that elapsed between the composition of the primary texts that formed the basis for sections two and four of Yi's Memoir.

Thus, Yi mentions the 'Pulse Book' attributed to Huangdi and Bian Que (Huangdi Bian Que Mai shu 黃帝扁鵲脈書),[47] and arguably 'The Discourse on Drugs' (Yao lun 藥論) in sections one and two. They probably were written texts, not least because section two describes an event when the disciple refuses the mat before formally receiving books from his master, although, on reflection, it is not impossible that this scene was interjected by a commentator of the Eastern Han or later, as it is the only sentence in the entire Memoir that mentions *fang shu* 方書 (documents of formulae, recipes, techniques) and 'secret books of formulae' (*jin fang shu* 禁方書). They are: 'The Pulse Book', 'The Upper and Lower Canon',[48] 'Diagnosis by means of the Five Colours',[49] 'The Art of the Irregular and Regular',[50] 'Gauging and Measuring the External Anomalies of Yin and Yang',[51] 'The

---

[47] *Han shu* 30, p. 1776, lists a 'Bian Que nei wai jing' 扁鵲內外經 (Bian Que's Inner and Outer Canon).

[48] 'Mai shu' 脈書 is not attested in the *Nei jing*, but the 'Shang xia jing' 上下經 is. The 'Shang jing' and 'Xia jing' occur in *Su wen* 34, 44 (3x), 46, 77 and 46, 77, 79 (3x), 80 (2x), 81, according to Ma (1990:63–4), and clearly refer to a text in *Su wen* 34, p. 100; 44, p. 124; 46, p. 130; 69, p. 196. On specific translation problems, see ch. 6, nn. 55 and 57. It is odd that a book, *shu*, is divided into two canons, *jing*. In the light of this, it is possible, if not likely, that a commentator who was familiar with the *Su wen* interjected 'Shang xia jing'.

[49] 'Wu se zhen' 五色診, not attested in the received literature. Wang Shumin (1983:2902–3) refers to a parallel between the 'Bing fa' 兵法 (Military Model), which has 'Wu yin qi kai' 五音奇侅 (Five Tones and the Irregular and Regular), and the 'Mai fa' 脈法 (Model of the Pulse) with its 'Wu se zhen' 五色診 and 'Qi ke shu' 奇咳術 (Examination based on the Five Colours and the Art of the Irregular and Regular).

[50] 'Qi ke shu' 奇咳術, parallels to the received literature are indirect. *Qi ke* literally means 'unusual coughs', but according to Wang Shumin (1983:2902–3), *ke* 咳 can be substituted by several other characters which all mean 'extraordinary, irregular'. Bridgman (1955:209) considers Yi's source book 'Qi ke shu' 奇咳術 to be the 'Da qi lun' 大奇論, i.e. *Su wen* 48. There are tenuous thematic affinities between *Su wen* 48 and, in particular, case 7. Ando Koretora considers 'Qi heng' 奇恆 (The Irregular and Regular) a title of a text in *Su wen* 46, p. 128 and p. 130. See ch. 6, nn. 62–5. On rendering the title of 'Qi heng' as 'Qi ke', see ch. 6, n. 24.

[51] 'Kui du yin yang wai bian' 揆度陰陽外變. Taki Motokata points to *Su wen* 15, p. 45; 46, p. 130; 77, p. 248, where there are pairs of *kui du* and *qi heng*. In *Su wen* 46, 'Kui du' seems to be a title of a text: 揆度者 切度之也 'As to "Gauging and Measuring", it is about palpating [vessels] and measuring them out'. The same applies to *Su wen* 15: 揆度者 度病之淺深也 奇恆者 言奇病也 'As to "Gauging and Measuring", it measures out the depth of the disorders. As to '"The Irregular and Regular", it is about the unusual illnesses'. For *Su wen* 77, see ch. 6, nn. 67–8. See also *Su wen* 19, p. 60.

Discourse on Drugs',[52] 'The Deities of the Stone',[53] and 'The Secret Book on Joining Yin and Yang'.[54]

In section four, interestingly, similar but not identical titles are given, such as 'The Irregular and Regular', 'The Five Examinations' and 'The Model of the Drugs'. No 'Pulse Book' is mentioned, and in place of *mai* the terms *jing mai* 經脈 (channels) and *luo jie* 絡結 (links and knots) appear as distinctive concepts in the following book titles:[55] 'Channels: Above and Below',[56] 'Upper and Lower Channels'[57] and 'Irregular Links and Knots'.[58] In addition, two titles appear, namely the 'Discourse on the Contravective and the Smooth', which alludes to a universe permeated by the flow of *qi*,[59] and 'The Doubling of Yin or Yang due to Resonances with the Four Seasons',[60] which implies a body subject to seasonal change.

These book titles hint at changes in the conception of the body. In section two the notion of *mai* (vessels/pulses) is prominent, in section four that of *jing mai* (channels). In section four, but not in section two, one title alludes to flows and counter-flows of *qi*, one to the seasonality of illness. The fact that these two titles in section four allude to the flow of *qi* and stress seasonality could be interpreted as an insignificant *variatio*, but incidentally it underlines recently noted developments within the conceptual history of Han medicine towards an understanding of the universe as being permeated by *qi* (which is not explicit in medical thinking of the Warring States). Therefore, it is possible that the book titles in section two date to an earlier primary document than those in section 4.7.

As repeatedly seen, the Warring States' 'sentimental body' consists of an outward *xing*-form that needs to be kept firm in order to house *qi* inside; the body of the early second century BCE in its description of the visually

---

[52] 'Yao lun' 藥論 and *yao lun shu*, but *yao lun* in other parts of sections one and two means probably 'a structured analysis of drugs'.

[53] 'Shi shen' 石神 is 'Bian shi zhi shen fa' 砭石之神法 (The Divine Model for Stone Needling), according to Taki Motokata.

[54] 'Jie yin yang jin shu' 接陰陽禁書 concerns the sexual arts, according to Ando Koretora and Ando Masamichi.

[55] The one-syllabic *mai* and *luo* occur in sections two and three of Yi's Memoir, while *jing mai* (tracts or channels) and *luo mai* (reticular tracts, Sivin 1987:249) are frequent in the *Nei jing*. One can consider this a matter of *variatio*, but the differences are consistent and systematic: the two-syllabic terms in Yi's section four may well date to a later time than those in section two. In Yi's Memoir, *jing* are translated as 'passageways' and *luo* as 'links' to signal my uncertainty as to whether their structure is the same as that implied by *Ling shu* 10. See case 1 (line 19), and case 6 (line 19). For *luo jie*, see *Ling shu* 38, p. 373.

[56] 'Jing mai gao xia' 經脈高下.

[57] 'Shang xia jing mai' 上下經脈. Compare with *Su wen* 16, p. 49: *qi shang xia jing sheng* 其上下 經盛 'his upper and lower channels are abundant'; *shang xia jing* must refer to the channels here, not to a canon. Contrast with: 'Mai shu' 'Shang xia jing' in section two, discussed in ch. 6, n. 48.

[58] 'Qi luo jie' 奇絡結.   [59] 'Ni shun lun' 逆順論.

[60] 'Si shi ying yin yang chong' 四時應陰陽重.

perceived course of *mai* focuses on a sophisticated, structurally defined 'body architecture'; while the canonical 'body ecologic' emphasises seasonality dependent processes. In the extant *Su wen*, derived from a compilation presumably of the Eastern Han, such body ecological reasoning is framed in terms of the five agents. Yi, by contrast, only rarely reasons in terms of the five agents (ostensibly only in cases 12, 15 and 21). Instead, seasonality dependent pathologies are expressed in terms of a doubling of *yin* or *yang*, as indicated by the book title 'The Doubling of Yin and Yang due to Resonances with the Four Seasons'. This book title, which expresses awareness of the seasonality of illness but alludes to a numerology of two rather than five, invokes a conception of illness as arising from a doubling of *yin* or *yang*, which is consistent with that given in cases 2, 4, 6 and 22. However, while Yi's case histories in section three provide ample evidence that disorders arose due to a 'doubling' (*chong* 重) of certain qualities, they nowhere allude to the doubling of seasonality dependent qualities as given in section four (except arguably in case 4).[61]

'The Regular and Irregular' is the book that is most frequently mentioned in Yi's Memoir, namely in sections two,[62] three[63] and four.[64] Interestingly, 'Qi heng' is also the most frequently mentioned book title in the *Su wen*.[65] If these two book titles refer to the same book, which is likely,[66] it helps explain the similarities in medical rationale between Yi's Memoir and the *Su wen* insofar as, in both, *qi* and the viscera are central concepts.

In section two, the book title 'Gauging and Measuring the External Anomalies of Yin and Yang' is juxtaposed to 'The Art of Assessing the Regular and Irregular'.[67] In *Su wen* 77 the latter is called 'Assessing the

---

[61] Note the 'double *yang*' (*chong yang* 重陽; case 2, line 20), 'paired *yin*' respectively 'double coldness' (*bing yin* 并陰 respectively *chong han* 重寒; case 4, line 29), 'double diminishment' (*chong sun* 重損; case 6, line 37), 'double encumbrance' (*chong kun* 重困; case 22). Sivin (1995a:182, n. 20) is mistaken to consider 'doubling' irrelevant to early Han medical rationale.

[62] 'Qi ke shu' 奇咳術.

[63] Yi mentions a 'word' from the 'Irregular and Regular' ('Qi ke' *yan* 奇咳言) in case 24, in a passage that reads like an interjection, quoted on p. 68.

[64] 'Qi ke' 奇咳.

[65] 'Qi heng' 奇恆 is mentioned in *Su wen* 15 (3x), 19 (1x), 46 (2x), 47 (1x), 77 (1x), according to Ma (1990:63). It is probably a book title also in *Su wen* 11, p. 37: 'Qi heng' *zhi fu*, elsewhere translated e.g. as 'paraorbs' (Porkert 1974), and means 'The cavities mentioned in the book "Qi heng"' (they are the brain, marrow, bones, *mai*, gall bladder and womb). This is said in awareness that *qi heng* can also be a verb or attribute, see *Su wen* 11, p. 37; 15, p. 46; 77, p. 247; 80, p. 253.

[66] See ch. 6, n. 24 and n. 65.

[67] In *Su wen* 77, p. 248, the 'Upper Canon' and 'Lower Canon', 'Gauging and Measuring *yin* and *yang*' and 'Assessing the Irregular and Regular of the Five Central Ones [i.e. the Five Viscera]' are mentioned in sequence (if my translation is correct, which differs from Unschuld 2003:81). Variants of these titles are mentioned in the same sequence in Yi's Memoir (see p. 65).

Irregular and Regular of the Five Interior Ones [i.e. the Five Viscera]' (*Qi heng wu zhong* 奇恆五中).[68] This suggests the former book concerns external anomalies on the body surface, while the latter stresses the need to investigate internal processes. Indeed, the word from the 'Qi ke' that Yi quotes in case 23 also refers to the internal viscera: 'When the *qi* [coming] from the [different] viscera turn against each other, one dies' (*zang qi xiang fan zhe, si* 藏氣相反者 死).

Su wen 15 underlines the idea that 'Qi ke' was a text that emphasised the importance of recognising body internal processes for diagnosis: 'In order to endorse the technique of "The Irregular and Regular", one takes the major *yin* at its beginning' (*xing qi heng zhi fa, yi tai yin shi* 行奇恆之法 以 太陰始).[69] In this quote neither the term 'major *yin*' nor the word 'beginning' can be unambiguously determined. As will be suggested in case 5, the major *yin* refers to the most hidden and central body part, the womb, which may well reflect an early second-century body conception. The major *yin* is an attribute of the centrally located stomach in the Mawangdui 'Yinyang vessel text', in the parallel Zhangjiashan 'Maishu', part 2, and in canonical texts on the '*mai* of the true viscera' (*zhen zang mai* 真藏脈).[70] In the corresponding *Ling shu* 10, however, it does not correlate with the stomach but with the *mai* of the lungs, which is considered the first in the cycle of the twelve *mai*.[71] This shows that the major *yin* consistently refers to the body's most inner part, which, depending on fashion in medical current or time period, was considered the womb, stomach/spleen or lungs. The term *shi* 始 may refer to a temporal or spatial 'beginning'. According to modern Chinese commentators who point out that in the Mawangdui vessel texts a *mai* usually begins at the extremities, it is spatially defined, as is the 'inch opening' (*cun kou* 寸口). When in case 1 (line 29), Yi speaks of pressing onto the minor *yang* at its 'beginning' (*chu* 初), he probably also had this understanding of *mai* and their routing. Likewise, in cases 4 (line 33) and 5 (line 12), when Yi examines the 'opening' (*kou* 口) of the 'major *yin*', he probably follows the same rationale. He evidently endorses the teachings of 'Qi ke'! In summary, regardless of how one interprets 'major *yin*' and 'beginning', all interpretations suggest that 'Qi ke' stressed the importance of examining the state of the internal viscera.

The above would suggest that the books 'Qi ke' and 'Qi heng' attributed great importance to the investigation of the regularities and irregularities of visceral processes for diagnostic purposes. In line with 'Qi ke', Yi assesses the state of the viscera by investigating qualities of *qi* in cases 1–10. Yi's

---

[68] See *Su wen* 77 in ch. 6, n. 67. Contrast with *Su wen* 46, pp. 128, 130. In *Su wen* 77, there is a 'Qi heng wu zhong', in *Su wen* 46 a 'Qi heng yin yang', the former probably relates manifestations of illness to the body interior, the latter to the external regularity of seasonal change.

[69] *Su wen* 15, p. 46.   [70] MWD YY (1985:11), and also *Su wen* 11, p. 37; 19, p. 62.

[71] *Ling shu* 10, p. 299.

Memoir is the first extant document to give *qi* and the viscera a central position in medical reasoning. Without denying that the notion of *qi* was occasionally mentioned in pre-dynastic texts, it would appear that the prominence of *qi* in medicine arose as doctors became interested in examining the visceral states of their patients.

Genres of learned knowledge and practice

Yi's medical knowledge and practice derives from many different genres. 'Qi ke' is given as an 'art' (*shu* 術) in section two and a 'word' (*yan* 言) is quoted from it in case 23, but in *Su wen* 15, 'Qi heng' is a 'Model' (Fa) or technique (*fa*). 'Drugs' (*yao* 藥) are analysed in 'structured discourse' (*lun*) in sections one and two, but applied in 'techniques' (*fa*) in section four. The genre 'canon' (*jing*) is mentioned only once, in section two.[72] Depending on translation, the 'Mai shu' is a canon in two volumes. Or 'The Upper and Lower Canon' are separate books. Or, regardless of translation, 'Shang xia jing' may be a late commentatorial interjection.[73] 'Documents of formulae' (*fang shu*) are mentioned once, in section two, possibly also in an interjected sentence. Sections one and two mention a 'Mai shu', but the medical case histories in section three quote a 'Mai fa'. In fact, apart from the 'Mai fa', which is also mentioned twice in section four, none of the 'Fa' in the case histories is mentioned in the other sections. The sheer variety of medical genres suggests medical physicians like Yi were exposed to many masters and typically were eclectics. The slight variations in genre specific to sections hint again at the Memoir's composite character.

Of the different genres, only *lun* can be further elucidated. It generally refers to an 'ordered discourse, which sorts things into their grades or categories'.[74] The Mohist Canon advocated as first discipline such 'sorting out' (i.e. knowledge of how to connect names and objects); as second, ethics (i.e. knowledge of how to act); as third, the sciences (i.e. the knowledge of objects); and as fourth, 'argumentation' (*bian* 辯) (i.e. the knowledge of names). The *Zhuangzi* rejected disputation of posed alternatives, *bian*, and was in favour of *lun*.[75]

Yi's drug therapy may have been Daoist in orientation, as in sections one and two he speaks of structured arguments on drugs (*yao lun*), without detailing, however, whether those were framed in *yin yang*. In section three, structured analytical arguments on drugs typically involve reasoning in

[72] This is if one translates *jing* as 'passageway' in case 23, see table 4, n.f. On *jing* as 'canons', see ch. 1, n. 9.
[73] The first view is held by Takigawa in *Shiki kaichû kôshô* 105, p. 22, and Li (2003:19), the second by Sivin (1995a:179), for the third, see ch. 6, n. 48.
[74] Graham (1989:167).
[75] The *Zhuangzi* said *lun* involved a particular mindset (Graham 1989:192); *lun* typically consisted of structured analytical arguments (Robert Chard, 2005 p.c.).

terms of *yin yang*.[76] In case 22, Yi quotes from a 'Lun' and refers to *yin yang* reasoning in a dispute over the appropriate application of drugs. In cases 4 and 9, he administers drugs in a context where the condition of the patient is assessed in terms of *yin yang* (but not in cases 14, 18 and 23).[77]

The above suggests that in the context of drug therapy Yi engaged in structured analytical discourses in terms of *yin yang*. However, the concepts *qi* and *zang* (viscera), and *zhong* (interior), which are central to Yi's diagnostic methods, came from another textual source, in all likelihood the 'Art of Qi ke'. Yi assessed visceral states inside the body by identifying qualities of *mai* on the body surface. As he detailed in his own vocabulary, when he tactually explored *mai,* he felt *qi, qi* coming from the viscera (and other bodily aspects; see table 5). This was a highly innovative diagnostic practice, which drew on a novel understanding of body and illness. It was framed in the language of *qi* and *zang* (viscera), and laid the foundations of Chinese medicine for generations to come.

---

[76] Note parallel to the *Shang han lun* 傷寒論 of ca 196 CE: a *lun* on pharmacotherapy, framed in *yin yang* reasoning.

[77] As repeatedly seen, the medical rationale in cases 1–10 differs from that in cases 11–25.

7

Translation of the Memoir of Chunyu Yi

[Section 1; *Shiki kaichû kôshô* 105, pp. 19–22; *Shi ji* 105, pp. 2794–6]

Tai Canggong 太倉公 (The Great Granarian) was the Chief of the Great Granary of Qi 齊.[1] He was from Linzi 臨菑.[2] His family name was Chunyu 淳于, his personal name Yi 意. When he was young, he was fond of medical formulae and techniques. In the eighth year of Empress Gao 高后 [180 BCE], he took to yet another master, the *gong sheng* dignitary[3] Yang Qing 陽慶 of the ward Yuan from the same commandery. Qing was over seventy years old, and had no sons. He had Yi discard all his previous formulae. Instead, he took all his [own] secret formulae and handed them over to him [Yi]. He transmitted books on *mai* attributed to the Yellow Emperor and Bian Que. He examined illness by means of the five colours, recognised whether a person would die or live, judged over the doubtful and determined the curable. When it came to structured analytical discussions on drugs, he was highly refined. After receiving these teachings for three years, he [Yi] on behalf of other people treated illness and made decisions about death and life, which largely were proven true. In spite of this, he wandered around among the feudal lords, and did not treat his home as a home. Sometimes, he did not treat illness on behalf of other people, and among the families of the ill many bore a grudge against him.

In the midst of the fourth year of Emperor Wen 文帝 [176 BCE],[4] a person submitted a memorial to the Emperor that denounced Yi with the charge of a crime deserving punishment by mutilation, and Yi had to be transferred to the West and go to Chang'an. Yi had five daughters. As they followed

---

[1] *Tai cang zhang* 太倉長. He figures in *Shi ji* 10, pp. 427–8, as *tai cangling* 太倉令 'Prefect of the Great Granary' (Bielenstein 1980:43), as *Chunyugong* 淳于公 'Chief Chunyu' and as *tai canggong* 太倉公 'Chief of the Great Granary'. No personal name Yi 意 is given. Chunyu is a family name here, as in *Han shu* 93, p. 3730. In *Lun heng* 12, 'Xie duan', p. 567 (translation by Forke 1962:81), there is mention of a Chunyu De 淳于德, also rendered as 淳于意, whom Wang Shumin (1983:2901) identifies as the same person as Chunyu Yi 淳于意. In section 4.3, Yi says he changed his personal name; according to Loewe (1997:31), from Yi 意 to De 惪.
[2] For place names, see chapter 9.
[3] See table 1, n. i; compare and contrast with Sivin (1995a:179).
[4] For reasons to contest this date, see ch. 6, nn. 5–6, for reasons to adhere to it, see pp. 52 and 60.

71

him, they wept. Yi got angry and scolded them: 'I have fathered children, but have not fathered any sons. In times of crisis, no one can be made to serve me.' At this his youngest daughter Tiying 緹縈 felt distressed by her father's words. She thereupon followed her father to the West and submitted a document to the Emperor saying: 'As to your maid's father as an official, everyone in Qi praises him for being honest and fair. Now, he is tried by law and faces punishment by mutilation. Your maid feels palpable pain. Just as the dead cannot return to life, those who have received punishment by mutilation cannot re-attach [a lost member] again. Even if they wish to mend their conduct and renew themselves, it is entirely impossible to achieve it. Your maid wishes to offer herself by becoming a female slave in order to remit her father's crime deserving punishment by mutilation, and effect that he can change his conduct and renew himself.' When the document was given a hearing, the Emperor was saddened by its meaning. Indeed, the law of punishment by mutilation was rescinded in that year. Yi [thereupon] lived at home.[5] An Imperial edict summoned him and enquired about that which made him treat illnesses and [prognosticate] death and life. The cases proven true, how many were they? The main names among them were which ones?

[Section 2; *Shiki kaichû kôshô* 105, pp. 22–4, *Shi ji* 105, pp. 2796–7]

The Imperial edict enquired of the former Chief of the Granary, your servant, Yi: 'Among the formulae and skills you are good at and the kinds of illnesses you can treat, are there any books about them, do you have them or not? In each case, where did you receive instruction [on them]? You received instruction for how many years? When you tried them, were there any that were verified? From which prefecture and which ward were the persons [that you treated]? What were the disorders? When the medical treatment and drugs were finished, the appearance of those disorders, what was it like, in all cases? Be comprehensive and detailed in your answers.'

Your servant, Yi, replied saying: 'From the time when I, Yi, was young, I was fond of medicine and drugs. The formulae of medicine and drugs, when I tried them out, mostly were not verified [i.e. they were ineffective]. When the eighth year of Empress Gao [180 BCE] was reached, I succeeded in meeting as master, the *gong sheng* dignitary Yang Qing from the ward Yuan in Linzi. Qing was over seventy years old, but I, Yi, had the privilege to meet and serve him. He spoke to me, Yi, saying: 'Discard all your formula books. They are wrong. I, Qing, have inherited and been transmitted from the ancient predecessors the books on *mai* that are attributed to the Yellow Emperor 黃帝 and Bian Que 扁鵲, and how to examine illness by means of the five colours, how to recognise whether a person will die or live, how to

---

[5] House arrest is a form of punishment (Fan unpubl.), all the more since Yi previously wandered about.

judge over the doubtful, and how to determine the curable. When it comes
to the books on structured analytical arguments on drugs, they are highly
refined. My family is wealthy. I dearly love you. I wish to take my books of
secret formulae in their entirety and teach them all to you.' Your servant,
Yi, thereupon said: 'I am very fortunate. This is more than what I, Yi, had
dared to hope for.' Your servant, Yi, then refused the mat and venerated
him repeatedly. I formally received his "Pulse Book", "The Upper and
Lower Canon", "Diagnosis by means of the Five Colours", "The Art of the
Irregular and Regular", "Gauging and Measuring the External Anomalies
of Yin and Yang", "The Discourse on Drugs", "The Deities of the Stone"
and "The Secret Book on Joining *yin* and *yang*".[6] I received, read, understood and checked them, for about a year. In the following year, when I
tested them, there were effective ones. However, I still had not yet reached
expertise. Essentially, I served him [Qing] for about three years, then,
probing [the formulae I had received], I, on behalf of other people, delivered
treatment, examined illnesses and assessed whether they would live or die.
There were successfully experienced [i.e. effective], refined and excellent
ones. Now, Qing has already been dead for about ten years. In the year of
completing the three years [of study with him], your servant, Yi, was thirty-
nine years old.'

[Section 3; *Shiki kaichû kôshô* 105, pp. 24–52, *Shi ji* 105, pp. 2797–813]

[Case 1]

Cheng, an Attending Secretary[7] of Qi, himself said that he was ill; the head
hurt. Your servant, Yi, examined his *mai* and formally announced saying:
'The illness of your Excellency is bad, I cannot speak about it.' Then I went
outside and solely informed Cheng's younger brother Chang saying: 'This
one is ailing from a *ju*-abscess. It will erupt internally in the region of the
intestines and stomach. After five days, it will become a *yong*-clog swelling.
After eight days, he will vomit pus and die.' Cheng's illness was contracted
from wine and women. Cheng then died at the predicted time.

The means whereby I recognised Cheng's illness were that when your
servant, Yi, pressed onto his *mai*, I got *qi* [coming] from the liver. The *qi*
[coming] from the liver, despite being murky, was still. This is a disorder of
the interior being closed off. The 'Model for the Study of Mai' ('Mai fa')
says: 'In cases where the *mai* are elongated, yet strung, – if it is not [the
mai] that alternates in accordance with the four seasons –, the host of the
disorder resides in the liver.' When they [the *mai*] blend, then the passage-
ways/channels govern the disorder. If they alternate, then the linking vessels
are exuberant. In cases where, [while] the channels govern the disorder,

---

[6] For detailed discussion of each book title in sections two and four, see pp. 64–9.
[7] For the identification of Yi's clientele, see pp. 52–7 and table 1 on p. 54.

they [the *mai*] blend, one's disorder is contracted in the sinews and the marrow. In cases where, while alternating and being severed, the *mai* spout, one's disorder is contracted from wine and women.

The means whereby I recognised that after five days he would have a *yong*-clog swelling, and that after eight days he would vomit pus and die, were that at the time when I pressed onto his *mai*, the minor *yang*, [at the place] where it begins, was alternating. In cases of the alternating, the passageways are in disorder. If the disorder leaves, it overcomes the person, the person then leaves [i.e. dies].

When the linking vessels govern the disorder – at the time in question, the minor *yang*, [at the place] where it begins, was closed by one *fen* [degree]. Hence the interior was hot, but pus had not yet been emitted – if it [the closure] reaches five *fen*, then it gets to the boundary of the minor *yang*. If it [the predicted time] reaches the eighth day, then one spits pus and dies. Hence when it [the closure] was above two *fen*, pus was emitted, when it reached the boundary, there was a *yong*-clog swelling, when there was complete discharge, he died. If heat rises, then it heats up the *yang* brightness and spoils the flowing links. If the flowing links are agitated, then the nodes of the *mai* burst open. If the nodes of the *mai* burst open, then the spoilage disperses. Hence the links intermingled. The hot *qi* had already wandered upward and upon reaching the head, agitated [it]. Hence the head hurt.

[*Case 2*]

The youngest son of all the infants of the middle son of the King of Qi fell ill. They summoned your servant, Yi. I examined him and pressed onto his *mai*. I formally announced saying: 'It is a disorder of *qi* that is blocked. The illness makes a person feel upset and oppressed. Food does not go down. At times, one vomits froth.' The illness is contracted from infantile irritability and [involves] frequently rejecting food and drink. Your servant, Yi, immediately made for him a broth that causes *qi* to go downward and got him to drink it. On the first day, the *qi* went downward. On the second day, he was able to eat. On the third day, the illness was cured.

The means whereby I recognised the youngest son's illness were that when I examined his *mai*, it was *qi* [coming] from the heart. They were [or: it was] murky and hurried, yet [the condition was] transient. This is a disorder of the links becoming *yang*. The 'Maifa' says: 'In cases where the *mai* come frequently and swiftly, and leave with difficulty, but are not one [in unison], the host of the disorder resides in the heart.' In cases where the entire body is hot and the *mai* are abundant, it is a double *yang*. As for the double *yang*, it overturns [the governor of] the heart. Hence he was upset and oppressed. If the food had not gone down, then the linking vessels would have had excess. If the linking vessels had had excess, then the blood would have risen to get out. If the blood had risen to get out, he would have died. This is what a sad heart generates. The illness is contracted from being irritable.

[*Case 3*]

Xun, the Prefect of the Gentlemen of the Palace of Qi, fell ill. All the many doctors considered it a numbness that had entered and struck the interior, and needled him. Your servant, Yi, examined him and said: 'It is a welling amassment. It makes that the person is unable to urinate and defecate.' Xun said: 'I have not been able to urinate and defecate for three days!' Your servant, Yi, had him drink a broth [prepared by careful] regulation of fire. After drinking the first [dose], he was able to urinate. After drinking the second, he thoroughly relieved himself. After drinking the third, the illness was cured. The illness was contracted from women.

The means whereby I recognised Xun's illness were that at the time when I pressed onto his *mai*, at the right opening, *qi* was intense. The *mai* did not have *qi* [coming] from the five viscera. At the right opening, the *mai* were large, yet frequent. In cases of the frequent, the interior/central and lower parts are hot, yet welling. The left is for [diagnosing] the lower parts, the right for the upper parts. There was in all cases no response from the five viscera. Hence I said a welling amassment. The interior was hot. Hence the urine was dark.

[*Case 4*]

Xin, the Chief of the Palace Wardrobe of Qi, fell ill. I entered [the palace] to examine his *mai* and formally announced saying: 'It is the *qi* of a heat disorder. So, you sweat [as one does] from summer heat. The *mai* are barely weakened. You will not die.' I said: 'This illness is contracted when one formerly bathed in running water, while it was very cold, and once it was over, got hot.' Xin said: 'Yes, so it is. Last winter season, I was sent as an envoy to the King of Chu. When I got to the Yangzhou river in Ju county, the planks of the bridge were partly damaged. I then seized the shaft of the carriage. I did not yet intend to cross. The horses became frightened and [I] promptly fell. I was immersed in water, and almost died. Some officers then came to save me and pulled me out of the water. My clothes were completely soaked. For a short time my body was cold. and once it was over, it got hot like a fire. Up to today, I cannot be exposed to the cold.' Your servant, Yi, thereupon made for him a decoction [prepared by careful] regulation of fire, to drive away the heat. After drinking the first dose, the sweating came to an end. After drinking the second, the heat left. After drinking the third, the illness ceased. I then made him apply medicines. After about twenty days, his body was without illness.

The means whereby I recognised Xin's illness were that at the time when I pressed onto his *mai*, there was a paired *yin*. The 'Mai fa' says: 'In the case of a heat disorder, those whose *yin* and *yang* intermingle, die.' When I pressed on them [the *mai*], there was no intermingling, but a paired *yin*. In cases of the paired *yin*, the *mai* are smooth and clear, and [the patient] recovers. Although his heat had not yet gone completely, he was still going to live. *Qi* [coming] from the kidneys was sometimes for a moment murky, at the opening of the major *yin mai*, however, it was thin. This is a case of water *qi*. The kidneys certainly govern water. Hence by means of this I recognised it [the disorder]. If one neglects treating [such disorders] instantly, then they turn into chills and hot flushes.

[*Case 5*]

The queen dowager of the King of Qi fell ill. They summoned your servant, Yi. I entered [the palace] to examine the *mai*. I said: 'A wind-induced condition caused by overexertion is visiting the bladder. One has difficulties with defecating and urinating, and the urine is dark.' Your servant, Yi, had her drink a broth [prepared by careful] regulation of fire. After drinking the first dose, she immediately could urinate and defecate. After drinking the second, the illness ceased. She urinated as before. The illness was contracted because, while dripping with sweat, she went outside to dry up. In cases of drying up, after having removed one's clothes, the sweat dries in the sunlight.

The means whereby I recognised the illness of the queen dowager of the King of Qi were that when your servant, Yi, examined her *mai*, and when I pressed onto the opening of the major *yin*, it was damp. In spite of this there was wind *qi*. The 'Mai fa' says: 'In cases when as one sinks [into the *mai* or the flesh of the buttocks?], it is very firm, and when as one floats [on the surface of the *mai* or the buttocks?], it is very tight, the host of the disorder resides in the kidneys.' When I pressed onto the kidneys, it was the other way round. The *mai* was large, yet hurried. In cases when it is large, it is *qi* [coming] from the bladder. In cases when it is hurried, the interior has heat and the urine is dark.

[*Case 6*]

Cao Shanfu of the ward Zhangwu in Qi fell ill. Your servant, Yi, examined his *mai* and said: 'It is a lung consumption. In addition there are chills and hot flushes.' Forthwith, I informed the members of the household saying: 'He will die. Incurable. In accordance with what he needs, provide maintenance. A doctor should not treat this one.' The 'Model' says: 'After three days, he will be in a state that matches madness. In a frenzy, he will rise to walk about, desiring to run. After five days, he will die.' He then died at the end of the predicted time period. Shanfu's illness was contracted from being in great anger, and in this condition indulging in women.

The means whereby I recognised Shanfu's illness were that when your servant, Yi, pressed onto his *mai*, the *qi* [coming] from the lungs was hot. The 'Mai fa' says: 'In cases of the uneven and not drumming, the body form is fading away.' This one's [disorder in] the high one [among the five viscera] went the distant number. And the passageways were in disorder. Hence at the time when I pressed onto them [the *mai*], they were not only uneven, but also alternating. In cases when they are uneven, the blood does not reside in its proper place. In cases when they alternate, from time to time three strokes arrive together, at once hurried, at once large. This one's two linking vessels were severed. Hence he died, and was incurable.

As for the reason why there were in addition chills and hot flushes, it was said that this person had fainted. In cases of fainting, the body form has been fading away. In cases where the body form has been fading away, it is not fitting to apply cauterisation and needle therapy, and to make [the patient] drink potent drugs. At the time when your servant, Yi, had not yet come to make an examination, the Grand Physician of Qi had already examined Shanfu's illness. He cauterised his foot's minor *yang* vessel, and orally, he made him drink a bolus of *Pinellia*. The patient immediately discharged and got drained. The abdominal part of the interior was depleted. Moreover, he [the Grand Physician] cauterised the minor *yin* vessel. This harmed the hardness of the liver, causing a rupture deep inside. In this way, he [the Grand Physician] doubly diminished the *qi* of the patient. Hence there were additionally chills and hot flushes.

As for the reason why, after three days, he [Shanfu] was in a state that matches madness, a link of the liver – the connecting and binding knot – was severed off from the *yang* brightness beneath the nipples. Hence, when the link was severed, it opened up the *yang* brightness *mai*. When the *yang* brightness *mai* was damaged, then in a state that matches madness he [Shanfu] ran about. As for dying after five days, liver and heart are distant from each other by five degrees [*fen*]. Hence I said: 'After five days, it [the distance] is exhausted. Being exhausted, he will thereupon die.'

[*Case 7*]

Pan Manru, the Commandant of the Capital of Qi, fell ill with pain in the minor abdomen. Your servant, Yi, examined his *mai* and said: 'It is a conglomeration disorder of remanent accumulations.' Your servant, Yi, then said to the Grand Coachman Rao and to the Clerk of the Capital Yao: 'If the Commandant does not any further restrain himself from an indulgence in women, then he will die in thirty days.' After twenty-odd days, he passed blood and died. The illness was contracted from wine and women.

The means whereby I recognised Pan Manru's illness were that when I, your servant, Yi, pressed onto his *mai*, they were deep, small and soft, abruptly they were confused, this is *qi* [coming] from the spleen. At the right *mai*'s opening, *qi* arrived tight and small, it manifested as *qi* [coming] from conglomerations. They [the *mai*] took turns in mutually riding on each other. Hence [I said] he would die after thirty days.

In cases where the three *yin* are entirely united, it is according to the 'Model'. In cases where they are not entirely united, the decision resides within the 'intensive time span'. In cases where they once are united and once are alternating, [death] is near. Hence when the three *yin* struck, he passed blood and died as [said] above.

[*Case 8*]

Zhao Zhang, the Chancellor of the Noble of Yangxu, got ill. They summoned me, Yi. All the many doctors took it for a coldness in the interior. Your servant, Yi, examined his *mai* and said: 'It is the wind of the void.' In cases of the wind of the void, drink and food go down the throat, are immediately evacuated and not retained. The 'Model' says: 'Death occurs after five days.' However, it was after ten days that he eventually died. The illness was contracted from an indulgence in wine.

The means whereby I recognised Zhao Zhang's illness were that when your servant, Yi, pressed onto his *mai*, the *mai* came slippery. This is *qi* [coming] from the wind of the within. In cases where drink and food go down the throat, are immediately evacuated and not retained, according to the 'Model', death occurs after five days. All this concerns the above-mentioned 'Model for [Calculating] the Limits of one's Share'. [Zhao Zhang] eventually died after ten days. As for the reason whereby he exceeded the predicted time: this person liked to eat gruel, hence the viscera in the interior were replete. The viscera in the interior were replete, hence he exceeded the predicted time. A word of the Master says: 'Those who accommodate with ease to cereals will live beyond the appointed time. Those who reject cereals will not reach it.'

[*Case 9*]

The King of Jibei fell ill. They summoned your servant, Yi. I examined his *mai*. I said: 'A wind-induced numbness/inversion. The chest feels full.' Forthwith, I prepared a drugged wine. After drinking three times twenty litres, the illness ceased. He contracted it [the illness] from sweating and lying prostrate on the ground.

The means whereby I recognised the illness of the King of Jibei were that at the time when your servant, Yi, pressed onto his *mai*, it was wind *qi*. The *mai* [coming] from the heart was murky. According to the 'Model of Disorders', if one excessively makes one's *yang* enter, then, while the *yang qi* is exhausted, the *yin qi* enters. If the *yin qi* enters and expands, then, while the cold *qi* ascends, the hot *qi* descends. Hence the chest feels full. As for the sweating and lying prostrate on the ground, when I pressed onto his *mai*, the *qi* was *yin*. In cases of *yin qi*, the illness [must have] entered and struck the interior. In order to expel it, it [must] reach a degree of swishing water.

[*Case 10*]

The accredited wife Chu Yu of Beigong, the Officer of Works at Qi, fell ill. All the many doctors took it for a wind that had entered and struck the interior. The host of the disorder resided in the lungs [liver]. They needled her foot's minor *yang mai*. Your servant, Yi, examined her *mai* and said: 'She is troubled by *qi* – an amassment is visiting the bladder – and she has difficulties with urinating and defecating, and the urine is dark. When the disorder is exposed to cold *qi*, then there is remanent urine. It makes the person's abdomen swollen.' Chu Yu's illness was contracted from intending to urinate, but without having the chance to do so, indulging in sexual intercourse.

The means whereby I recognised Chu Yu's illness were that when I pressed onto her *mai*, they were large, yet replete. They came with difficulty. This is an agitation of the dull *yin*. In cases where *mai* come with difficulty, the *qi* of an amassment is visiting the bladder [or: went into the abdomen]. As to the abdomen, the reason why it became swollen: it is said that a link of the dull *yin* is knotted to the small abdomen. When the dull *yin* had excess, then the node of the *mai* got agitated. When it got agitated, then the abdomen became swollen. Your servant, Yi, then cauterised her foot's dull *yin mai*. The left and the right one, each at one place. Then, as there was no remanent urine anymore, her urine was clear. The pain in the small abdomen stopped. Forthwith, I additionally prepared the broth [prepared by careful] regulation of fire and had her drink it. After three days, the *qi* of the amassment dissipated. She instantly recovered.

[*Case 11*]

The wet-nurse of the former King of Jibei herself reported that her feet felt hot and full. Your servant, Yi, formally announced: 'It is a heat inversion.' Then I needled the heart of her feet, each at three places.[8] I pressed onto them [until] no blood came out. The illness immediately ceased. The illness was contracted from drinking wine and getting badly drunk.

[*Case 12*]

The King of Jibei summoned your servant, Yi. I examined the *mai*.[9] Among all the women and servants, I got to the woman Shu. Shu did not have an

---

[8] *zu xin* 足心 is an acupuncture *locus*, but can also refer to the central region of the foot sole.
[9] This seems to have been a measure of preventive health care (Bridgman 1955:84 n. 152).

[apparent] illness. Your servant, Yi, formally announced to the Chief of the Rear Palace:[10] 'Shu has a damaged spleen. She is not allowed to exert herself. According to the "Model", in spring she will vomit blood and die.' Your servant, Yi, spoke to the king: 'The concubine[11] Shu, what kind of skills has she got?' The king said: 'This one is fond of formulae, she has many performative skills and does what [I] approve of. The massage techniques are new.[12] Last year, I purchased her on the town market of the common people. She was 470 *wan*, an equivalent of four persons.'[13] The king said: 'Is it possible that she does not have an illness?' Your servant, Yi, replied: 'Shu's illness is grave, she is [in a state recorded] in the "Model of [Imminent] Death".' The king summoned [her] to inspect her. Her complexion had not changed. He believed that it was not so, and did not sell her to any noble's household. When spring came, she held the sword and accompanied the king when he went to the toilet. The king left. Shu remained behind. The king ordered someone to summon her. Just then, she fell flat by the toilet, vomited blood and died. The illness was contracted from dripping with sweat. In cases of dripping with sweat, according to the 'Model', one ails gravely within. The colour of body hair and head hair is lustrous.[14] The pulse is not weakened. This is indeed a disorder of closing off the interior.

[*Case 13*]

The Palace Grandee of Qi fell ill with a decaying tooth. Your servant, Yi, cauterised his left [hand's] *yang* brightness vessel.[15] Forthwith, I made a broth of *ku shen*.[16] Daily he rinsed his mouth with three *sheng*.[17] After about five to six days, the illness ceased. The illness was contracted from wind and sleeping with an open mouth, from eating and not rinsing the mouth.

[*Case 14*]

A concubine of the King of Zichuan was with child, but did not give birth. They came to summon your servant, Yi. Your servant, Yi, went [there]. I

---

[10] *yong xiang* 永巷, lit, 'long alley in the palace'. See *Shi ji* 79, p. 1406.

[11] *cai ren* 才人 title of a high-graded court woman, often a concubine. See *Shi ji* 118, p. 3079.

[12] *wei suo shi an fa xin* 為所是案法新. The slave was skilled in sexual techniques (Mark Lewis, 1995 p.c.).

[13] *cao ou* 曹偶 means *tong lei* 同類 'of the same kind' or, according to Sima Zhen, *deng bei* 等輩 'the same kind'. Therefore, *cao ou* is rendered here as 'an equivalent of'. This interpretation diverges from Bridgman (1955:35) and Wilbur (1943:288).

[14] Compare with *Ling shu* 10, p. 305, quoted in ch. 4, n. 30.

[15] *da* [rather: *shou*] *yang ming mai* 大[手]陽明脈 'the large [rather: hand's] *yang* brightness vessel' is in MWD YY (1985:11) called *chi mai* 齒脈 'vessel for [treating] the teeth'.

[16] *ku shen* 苦參 *Sophora flavescens* Ait. (ZYDCD: entry 2624).

[17] One *sheng* 升 in Han times was 199 cubic centimetres (Twitchett & Loewe 1986:xxxvii).

made a drink with a pinch of *lang dang*[18] medicine; with wine I made her drink it. Immediately she gave birth. When your servant, Yi, examined her *mai* again, they were hurried. In cases when they are hurried, there is a lingering illness. Thereupon, I made a drink with a dose of nitre.[19] I made blood come out.[20] The blood [drops] were like beans, in succession, five to six.

[*Case 15*]

The slave of a Member of the Suite of the Chancellor of Qi accompanied [his master who went] to court and entered the palace. Your servant, Yi, saw him eating outside the gate of the inner quarters.[21] When I looked at his complexion, I saw that he had the *qi* of an illness. Your servant, Yi, thereupon formally announced [this] to Eunuch Ping 平. Ping was fond of [the study of] *mai*. He had studied at the place of your servant, Yi. Your servant, Yi, thereupon showed him the illness of the slave of the Member of the Suite, and formally announced saying: 'This one has the *qi* of having damaged the spleen. When spring will arrive, the diaphragm will be blocked, and not connect. He will not be able to eat and drink. According to the 'Model', when summer arrives, he will discharge blood and die.' The Eunuch Ping thereupon went to formally announce to the Chancellor: 'The slave of your Excellency's Member of the Suite has an illness. The illness is grave. The period before he dies is counted in days.' His Excellency, the Chancellor, said: 'Sir, how do you know that?' [Ping] said: 'At the time when your Excellency had the court session and had entered the palace, the slave of your Excellency's Member of the Suite finished off a meal outside the gate of the inner quarters. I, Ping, and the Master of the Granary were standing [there]. Thereupon, he [the Master] showed [it] to me, Ping, and said: "If you are ill like this one, you will die."' The Chancellor, thereupon, after summoning the Member of the Suite and the slave, spoke to them saying: 'Master, does the slave have an illness or not?' The Member of the Suite said: 'The slave does not have an illness. His body is without pain.' As spring arrived, [the slave] indeed fell ill. As the fourth month arrived, he discharged blood and died.

The means whereby I recognised the slave's illness were that *qi* [coming] from the spleen completely overrode the five viscera. After damaging the

---

[18] *lang dang* 莨礴 is not mentioned in the standard dictionaries on Chinese drugs. *Ben cao gang mu* 17, pp. 1140–4, mentions *lang dang zi* 莨菪子 (seeds), ZYDCD (entry 0649) mentions as a synonym *tian xian zi* 天仙子 (seeds), ZYDCD (entries 3717 and 3718) and ZHYH (1993:1.1429) mention *lang dang ye* 莨菪葉 (leaves) and *lang dang gen* 莨菪根 (roots), all taken from *Hyoscyamus niger* L.

[19] *xiao shi* 消石 'nitre'. Its main chemical compound is KNO_3. According to ZYDCD (entry 3959), it is produced from *Caryopteris nepetaefolia* (Benth.) Maxim. See also *Ben cao gang mu* 11, pp. 649–55, and *Tai ping yu lan* 988.

[20] On bloodletting in early China, see case 1, n. 104.

[21] *gui men* 闺門 'the gate of the inner quarters' where the women lived.

parts,[22] it intermingled [with them]. Hence there was the colour of a damaged spleen. When I looked at him, [his complexion] was mortally yellow. When I inspected him, [it] was the deathly green of a straw mat. The many doctors did not recognise [this illness]. They took it for large worms. They do not recognise [i.e. have a concept of] a damaged spleen.

As for the means whereby [one recognises that], as spring arrives, there is death [and illness],[23] *qi* [coming] from the stomach was yellow.[24] In cases of a yellow [complexion], it is *qi* [coming] from the earth. Earth does not overcome wood.[25] Hence as spring arrives, death occurs.

As for the means whereby [one recognises that], as summer arrives, there is death, the 'Mai fa' says: 'If an illness is grave, but the pulses are smooth and clear, one says "the interior is closed off".' [In the case of] a disorder of the interior being closed off, the person does not recognise that which is painful. The heart is [serene][26] while there is no suffering. If there is additionally an illness, one dies in mid-spring. If there is a favourable and smooth [quality], one reaches one [more] season.

The means whereby [I recognised] that he [the slave] would die in the fourth month were that when I examined this person, the [*mai*] were favourable and smooth. If they are favourable and smooth, the person is still fat.[27]

The illness of the slave was contracted because, dripping with sweat, he frequently went outside. After roasting by the fire, he, in this condition, went outside and exposed himself to big winds.

[*Case 16*]

The King of Zichuan fell ill. He summoned your servant, Yi. I examined *mai* and said: 'An inversion above.[28] It makes one feel heavy. The head aches and the body is hot and makes the person feel upset and oppressed.' Your servant, Yi, forthwith took cold water and clasped it onto his head. I needled

[22] *bu* 部 refers to *se bu* 色部, parts on the face for colour diagnosis. See also case 17. For parallels, see e.g. *Ling shu* 49, p. 399.

[23] *si bing* 死病 'death and illness'. Taki Motokata considers *si* mistaken as the slave did not die in spring, but Yi is here concerned with prognosticating death and therefore *bing* must be mistaken.

[24] Note that the colour of the stomach is inspected; in canonical doctrine the spleen correlates with yellow (e.g. *Su wen* 5, p. 21), and the stomach is an outer aspect of the spleen (e.g. *Ling shu* 10, p. 301).

[25] Yi reasons in terms of the five agents but his reasoning is odd. Five agents doctrine discusses the cycle of overcoming in the affirmative: e.g. earth overcomes water. In that case, death/ illness would occur in late summer, not in spring. Possibly, Yi's rationale is that earth overcomes water, and that therefore the death/illness does not break out in winter, but since earth does not overcome wood, it will occur in spring.

[26] *ji* 急 is *hui* 慧 'to be bright, serene', says Ando Koretora.

[27] This and the previous paragraph contain the same terms as case 4 (line 30); the next paragraph has the same terms as case 4 (line 19).

[28] *shang* 上 is to be read in the third tone, says Zhang Shoujie; it is a noun rather than a verb (Catherine Despeux, 1995 p.c.).

his foot's *yang* brightness *mai*, the left and the right one, each at three [different] places. The illness instantly ceased. The illness was contracted by washing one's hair and, while it was not yet dry, going to sleep. I examined him as [said] above.

The means whereby [I recognised] that it was an inversion in the head was that the heat reached [downward] to the shoulders.

[*Case 17*]

At the home of Huang Zhangqing, the elder brother of the King of Qi's Lady Huang, there was wine and they invited guests. They invited your servant, Yi. All guests were seated, and one had not yet served the meal, when your servant, Yi, having looked at and perceived the queen's younger brother Song Jian, formally announced saying: 'Your Excellency has an illness. For four to five days, your Excellency has had pain in the lower back and in the sides. You are not able to bend forward and backward. Moreover, you cannot urinate. If you do not treat it immediately, the disorder will forthwith enter the urinary kidneys.[29] As long as it has not yet settled in the five viscera, treat it urgently. The disorder is now visiting the urine of the kidneys.[30] This is a so-called "obstruction of the kidneys".'[31] Song Jian said: 'So it is. I certainly have pain in the lower back and the spine. Four to five days ago, it was raining. All the servants of the Huang family saw at my, Jian's, home a square stone beneath the storehouse. They then played with it. I, Jian, indeed wished to imitate them. I imitated them, but was not able to lift it. Instantly, I put it back down. In the evening, the lower back and spine hurt. I could not urinate. Until now I have not recovered.' Jian's illness was contracted from being fond of lifting heavy [things].

The means whereby I recognised Jian's illness were that when your servant, Yi, saw his complexion/colour, the colour of the major *yang* was dry.[32] Above the part of the kidneys up to the boundary and [in the part] below the lower back, it was withered to [the degree of] about four *fen*.

---

[29] *ru shen* 溽腎 'urinary kidneys', which parallels *niao pao* 尿脬 'urinary bladder' in Yang Shangshan's comment to *Huangdi nei jing Tai su* 3, p. 143: *pang guang cheng niao, gu wei zhi pao, ji niao pao* 膀胱成尿 故謂之胞 既尿脬 'the bladder composes the urine, hence it is called *pao* bladder, then urinary *pao* bladder'. See also HDNJSW 70, p. 150: *shen . . . qi shi ru* 腎 其實溽 'the kidneys . . . when replete, are soaked'. [*Wang Bing zhu:*] *zhong you jin ye ye* 中有津液也 [Wang Bing comments:] 'In the interior there are fluids.' Alternative translation: *ru ru* 入溽 'to enter and soak', according to Wang Shaozeng (1994:97).

[30] *ru* 溽 should read *shu* 輸, according to Zhang Wenhu. Case 22 also mentions *shu*-loci.

[31] On *shen bi* 腎痹, see *Shuo wen* 7B, p. 31: '*bi* is a disorder of dampness' (*bi shi bing ye* 痹 濕 病 也) and *Su wen* 10, p. 36. See also *shi bi* 濕痹 'obstruction due to dampness' as a disorder of the major *yang* warp in *Jin gui yao lüe* 2, p. 61. It also concerns dysuria but with different symptoms.

[32] *tai yang* 太陽 'major *yang* area at the temples', if Yi talks about 'parts' (*bu* 部) of the face relevant for a diagnosis based on the inspection of colour. Alternative translation: 'the colour of the major *yang mai*', which correlates with the canonical bladder (Bridgman 1955:90 n195). See also p. 33.

Hence I recognised that his [illness] had started four to five days ago. Your servant, Yi, immediately prepared a softening broth,[33] and made him apply it. After about eighteen days, he recovered from the illness.

[*Case 18*]

Dame Han, an attendant of the King of Jibei, fell ill. The lower back and the back hurt, and intermittently felt hot and cold. All the many doctors took it for chills and hot flushes. Your servant, Yi, examined her *mai* and said: 'The private within is cold, the menses do not descend.' Forthwith, I fumigated [her] with medicines. Instantly, the menses descended. The illness ceased. The illness was contracted because she desired a man but could not get one.

The means whereby I recognised Dame Han's illness were that at the time when I examined her *mai*, when I pressed onto them, it was the *mai* [coming] from the kidneys. It was rough and discontinuous. As to the rough and discontinuous, its coming is difficult and hard. Hence I said: 'The menses do not descend.'

The *mai* [coming] from the liver was strung, it came out at the left opening, hence I said: 'She desires a man, but cannot get one.'

[*Case 19*]

Bo Wu, a woman of the ward Fan in Linzi, fell very ill. All the many doctors took it for an aggravated state of chills and hot flushes. [They thought] she was about to die, and did not treat her. Your servant, Yi, examined her *mai* and said: 'A conglomeration of *rao*-worms.'[34] When a conglomeration of *rao*-worms becomes an illness, the abdomen is large, above the skin is yellow and coarse,[35] and stroking it is tender to touch [lit. it feels like 'cucu'].[36] Your servant, Yi, made a drink with a pinch of daphne.[37] Instantly,

---

[33] *rou tang* 柔湯 'softening broth', a 'supplementing medicine' (*bu yao* 補藥), according to Ando Koretora. Not attested in canonical texts, but in case 22 the 'softening recipe' (*rou ji* 柔齊) has *yin*-qualities.

[34] *rao* 蟯 '*rao*-worms'. See commentary to *Shuo wen* 13A, p. 42b. MWD 'Recipes' (1985:55), Ma (1992:516–18). Not in *Nei jing*. On *rao jia* 蟯瘕 'conglomeration of *rao*-worms', see Fan (1989:339).

[35] *fu* 膚 'skin'. For the diagnostic practice of investigating the skin quality, see MWD 'Yinyang simaihou' (1985:21): *lie fu* 裂膚 'a splitted skin' indicates death. See also *Su wen* 18, p. 56. Note continuities in medical terminology and medical rationale: *shang* 上 may refer to the head, as in case 16; the yellow complexion may have prompted the many doctors to diagnose 'large worms' in case 15.

[36] *qi qi* or *cu cu* 戚戚 is onomatopoetic, like *qia qia* 合合 in case 7 (line 11). Wang Shumin (1983:2908) cites *Mengzi zhu shu* 1B.2670: *fu zi yan zhi, yu wo xin you cu cu yan* 夫子言之於我心有戚戚焉 'you described it for me and your words struck a chord in me' (Lau 1970:55–6) and Zhao Qi 趙岐 comments: *cu cu ran, xin you dong ye* 戚戚然 心有動也 '*cu cu*: in the heart there are movements', i.e. one feels tenderness.

[37] *yuan hua* 芫華 *Daphne genkwa* Sieb. et Zucc. (ZYDCD: entry 2135).

it expelled the worms that amounted to about a *sheng*.[38] The illness ceased. After thirty days, she was as before. The illness, i.e. the worms, was contracted from dwelling in the cold and damp. Cold and damp *qi* clusters, condenses, cannot escape and transforms into worms.

The means whereby your servant, Yi, recognised Bo Wu's illness were that when I pressed onto her *mai* and when I stroked over her *chi* area,[39] her *chi* was ropy, prickly and coarse,[40] while the body hair was beautiful, [like] cicada antennas.[41] This is [typical of] the *qi* of worms. Her colour [of the skin] was lustrous. The viscera in the interior did not have any noxious *qi* nor a grave illness.

[*Case 20*]

The Major from Chunyu in Qi fell ill. Your servant, Yi, pressed onto his *mai* and formally announced saying: 'If this will become an illness, it will be the wind of the void.[42] The appearance of the wind of the void is that food and drink go down the throat and are immediately evacuated through the behind. The illness was contracted, after stuffing oneself, by running swiftly.' The Major from Chunyu said: 'I went to the king's family to eat horse liver.[43] I really stuffed myself. When I saw the wine coming, I immediately ran away and dashed swiftly home. Instantly, I had ten attacks of discharging myself.' Your servant, Yi, formally announced: 'Prepare a rice porridge by careful regulation of fire [i.e. by simmering it over a small fire] and drink it. After seven to eight days, you will recover.' At the time, the physician Qin Xin was at the side. After your servant, Yi, had gone away, Xin spoke to the Chief Commandants of the Left and Right Pavilion saying: 'What does Yi consider the disorder of the Major from Chunyu to be?' They said: 'He considers it a wind of the void, [and believes that] it can be cured.' Xin then laughed and said: 'This is ignorance. The disorder of the Major from Chunyu [is such that], according to the "Model", he will die

---

[38] One *sheng* 升 in Han times was ca 0.2 litres (Twitchett & Loewe 1986: xxxvii).

[39] *chi* 尺 'foot' area, presumably the foot-long area on the forearm between elbow and wrist. See ch. 5, n. 3 and case 3, nn. 64 and 66.

[40] *suo* 索 'rough, ropy' can mean *jin* 盡 'exhausted' or *ku zao* 枯燥 'dried out', according to Fan (1989:344). Alternative translation: *chi suo* 尺索 'rope of the *chi* area', according to Zhang Shoujie, but no textual parallels have been found for this.

[41] *feng* 奉 'to offer or receive respectfully with both hands, to esteem'. Xu Guang mentions *zou* 奏 and *qin* 秦 in other editions. Sima Zhen reads *qin* 秦 as *qin* 螓 'cicada'. Mark Lewis (1995 p.c.) notes cicada are *chong* 蟲 and an (iconic) diagnostic sign of the disorder, which is caused by '*rao*-worms'.

[42] Parallels to the 'wind of the void' in case 8 concern the name of the disorder, the signs and symptoms, and implicitly its cause, as the patient dashed away when he saw that wine was being served, although the explicitly given cause differs. Its outcome is favourable, because the disorder was not yet fully developed.

[43] On the adversarious effects of eating horse liver, see *Han shu* 88, p. 3612. For parallels, see *Shi ji* 28, p. 1390, *Lun heng* 66, p. 1500, and *Long yu he tu* as recorded in the *Gu wei shu* 34B, p. 640.

after nine days.' Even so, after nine days he did not die. His family summoned your servant, Yi, again. Your servant, Yi, went to ask him. It was entirely as I, Yi, had diagnosed it. Your servant instantly prepared one dose of the rice porridge [prepared by careful] regulation of fire and made him apply it. After seven to eight days, the illness ceased.

The means whereby I recognised it were that at the time when I examined his *mai*, when I pressed onto them, they were entirely according to the 'Model'. His illness was placid/smooth. Hence he did not die.

[Case 21]

Po Shi, a Gentleman of the Palace of Qi, was ill. Your servant, Yi, examined his *mai* and formally announced saying: 'The lungs are injured, incurable. In ten days on *dinghai*,[44] he will pass blood and die.' Thereupon, after eleven days, while passing blood, he died. Po Shi's illness was contracted from falling off a horse onto his back hitting a rock.

The means whereby I recognised Po Shi's illness were that, when I pressed onto his *mai*, I got *yin qi* [coming] from the lungs. They came dispersedly, arrived by several routes and were not one. Moreover, colour rode on them [i.e. multiplied their effects].

The means whereby I recognised that he fell from the horse were that when I pressed onto them [the *mai*], I got the reversed *yin mai*. If the reversed[45] *yin mai* enters the empty place,[46] it rides on the *mai* [coming] from the lungs. In cases when the *mai* coming from the lungs are dispersed, the solid complexion is altered,[47] and rides on it.

The reason why he did not die within the predicted time is that a word of the Master says: 'The patient, if at ease with grains, will surpass the predicted time. If he rejects grains, then he will not reach the predicted time.' This person relished millet. Millet governs the lungs.[48] Hence he surpassed the predicted time.

As to the reason why he passed blood, the 'Model for Examining *Mai*' says: 'If, when one is ill, while one is resting, one is at ease in *yin* places, one will have a smooth death. If, while one is resting, one is at ease in *yang* places, one will die adversely.' This person liked to be quiet on his own, he was not hurried. Moreover, he sat peacefully for long [periods of time]. By resting his head on his hands at a table, he slept. Hence the blood flowed out downward.

---

[44] *ding hai* 丁亥 *ding* is the fourth of the ten celestial stems and correlates with fire, *hai* is the twelfth of the twelve celestial branches. See Harper (2001), who translated case 21.

[45] *fan* 番 means *fan* 翻 'to turn over' means *fan* 反 'to reverse', according to Ando Koretora. Not attested in the medical manuscript and canonical literature, but note parallel to *fan yang mai* 番陽脈 in case 25.

[46] See case 6, n. 117.

[47] See ch. 4, n. 7; *gu* 固 'certainly' (Harper 2001:118) is grammatically odd (Robert Chard, 2005 p.c.).

[48] In *Ling shu* 56, p. 413, the lungs correlate with 'yellow millet' (*huang shu* 黃黍).

[*Case 22*]

Sui,[49] the Attending Physician of the King of Qi, fell ill. He refined for himself the five minerals[50] and applied them.[51] Your servant, Yi, went there to tell him he was wrong. Sui spoke to Yi saying: 'I unworthy one have an illness. I would be very fortunate if you examined me, Sui.' Your servant, Yi, then examined him and formally announced saying: 'Sir, you ail from heat in the interior. The "Discourse" says: "If in the case of the interior being hot, one cannot urinate frequently, one is not allowed to apply the five minerals." The basic character of minerals as drugs is that they are refined and violent. Since you, Sir, have applied them, you cannot urinate frequently. Instantly, you should cease to apply them. The colour is [indicating] that you will develop a *yong*-boil.' Sui said: 'Bian Que says: "*Yin* minerals are used for treating *yin* disorders, *yang* minerals are used for treating *yang* disorders." With regard to medical minerals, there is regularity in terms of *yin* and *yang*, water and fire. Hence if the interior is hot, then one prepares a softening recipe of *yin* minerals to treat it. If the interior is cold, then one prepares a hardening recipe of *yang* minerals to treat it.' Your servant, Yi, said: 'What you are discussing, Sir, is far off the mark. Although Bian Que's word is like this, you still have to examine it with care, establish the measures of length and weight, set up compass and square, calibrate weight and scale [of a balance], combine the models of colour and pulse, of the outer and inner, of having excess or being insufficient, and of the smooth and contravective. You [have to] consider whether a person in moments of movement and rest is in mutual resonance with his breathing [rhythm]. Then only can you provide a structured analytical discourse. The "Discourse" says: "When a *yang* affection resides inside and a *yin* form resonates on the outside, do not add violent drugs and stone needles." If violent drugs enter and strike the interior, then the noxious *qi* gathers. And the clustered *qi* goes deeper and deeper. The "Model of [Diagnostic] Examinations" says: "If the second *yin* resonates with the exterior and the first *yang* joins with the interior, you are not allowed to use a hardening drug."[52] If a hardening drug enters, then it agitates the *yang*. The *yin* disorder is increasingly weakened and the *yang* disorder becomes increasingly conspicuous. The noxious *qi* flows about and causes a doubled encumbrance[53] in the *shu*-areas.[54] Being

---

[49] For unknown reasons, Sui is identified as Wang Sui in *Yi shuo* 1, p. 10b.

[50] *wu shi* 五石 'five minerals'. The *Bao pu zi*, p. 69, translation by Ware (1966:82), details them as cinnabar, realgar, arsenolite, laminar malachite and magnetite, but here the term probably is used in a generic sense. Note parallel to *Su wen* 40, quoted on p. 256.

[51] *fu* 服 'to apply externally' (case 17), 'to drink' (case 20), here probably 'to eat'. See also case 4, n. 5.

[52] *gang yao* 剛藥 'hardening drug', probably has *yang*-qualities.

[53] On doubling as a pathological principle, see ch. 6, n. 61.

[54] *shu* 俞 *shu-loci*. In *Su wen* 4, p. 16; 38, p. 110; 43, p. 122, *shu* 俞 are closely connected to the viscera, which appears to be relevant here and in case 17. The *Ling shu* has no *shu* 俞, only *shu* 輸 and *shu* 腧. The Mawangdui vessel texts do not mention *shu* 俞輸腧.

enraged makes it burst and become a *ju*-abscess.' Yi formally announced to him that [this would happen] after one hundred and a few days. Indeed, it became a *ju*-abscess erupting above the nipples, invaded the collarbone and he died. This is the general outline of our discourse. You must have a pattern. If a clumsy craftsman has one [point] that he does not master, the *yin-* and *yang*-qualities of the patterning are lost.

[*Case 23*]

Formerly, at the time when he was Noble of Yangxu, the King of Qi seriously fell ill. All the many doctors considered it *jue*-numbness. Your servant, Yi, after examining *mai*, considered it an obstruction.[55] The root resided underneath the right side, bulging like a cup turned upside down.[56] It made the person pant, burp[57] and unable to eat. Your servant, Yi, thereupon took gruel [prepared by careful] regulation of fire and had him drink [it]. After six days, the *qi* descended. I then had him once again eat eggs as medicine.[58] After about six days, the illness ceased. The illness was contracted from indulging in women. At the time when I examined him, I was not able to know the explanation in terms of the passageways.[59] I vaguely knew the place where the disorder resided.

[*Case 24*]

Your servant, Yi, formerly examined Cheng Kaifang from the ward Wudu in Anyang. Kaifang said of himself that he thought he was not ill. Your servant, Yi, told him that he was ill, suffering from talkative winds.[60] In three years, he would not be able to use his four limbs himself. [The illness] made the person become mute.[61] Once mute, one thereupon dies. Now, I hear that his four limbs cannot be used. While he has lost his voice, he has not yet died. The illness was contracted by frequently drinking wine, and then by exposing himself to strong wind *qi*.

The means whereby I recognised Cheng Kaifang's illness were that, when I examined him, his *mai* were modelling [processes recorded in] the 'Qi ke'

---

[55] *bi* 庫 'obstruction', see also case 17 and ch. 7, n. 31. For parallels to case 23, see *Su wen* 19, p. 61. See also *Su wen* 43 called 'Bi lun' (Discourse on Obstructions).

[56] *fu bei* 覆杯. Common imagery in medical texts, e.g. *Ling shu* 4, p. 277; 71. p. 447.

[57] *ni qi* 逆氣 'burping' rather than 'contravective *qi*', as it is mentioned among a series of symptoms.

[58] *wan yao* 丸藥 'medicine in form of pellets'. 垸 in MWD 'Recipes' (1985:26, 27, 56) is 丸, according to Ma (1992:326). MWD 'Recipes' (1985:71) has 丸. It is mentioned once in *Su wen* 40, p. 114, as a therapeutic measure, meaning eggs of sparrows.

[59] *jing jie* 經解 'an explanation that identifies the disorder in respect of a passage way', the alternative reading 'an explanation in terms of canonical writings' is unlikely.

[60] *ku ta feng* 苦沓風 verb and bisyllabic noun. HYDCD 5.941 glosses *ta* as talkative, repetitive, intermingling, united, sluggish, boiling, etc. and has an entry on *ta feng*: a 'talkative wind', 'intermingling wind' or 'sluggish wind'? *Yi shuo* 3, p. 46a, by contrast, has *ku ta feng*.

[61] *yin* 瘖 'to be mute' (Yu 1953:211).

(The Regular and Irregular).[62] A word says: 'When visceral *qi* becomes mutually inverted, one dies.' When I pressed onto them [the *mai*], I got the kidneys inverted to the lungs. The 'Model' says: 'In three years one dies.'

[*Case 25*]

Xiang Chu, a *gong sheng* dignitary of the ward Ban in Anling, fell ill. Your servant, Yi, examined *mai* and said: 'A male amassment.'[63] Male amassments reside beneath the diaphragm, but above join with the lungs. The illness was contracted from an indulgence in women. Your servant, Yi, told him to beware of engaging in activities of physical exertion. If he would engage in activities of physical exertion, he necessarily would spit blood and die. Chu later played the ball game *cu ju* 蹴踘. The lower back got numb and cold, he sweated profusely and then spat blood. Your servant, Yi, examined him again and said: 'Tomorrow evening at dusk you will die.' Thereupon, he died. The illness was contracted from women.

The means whereby I recognised Xiang Chu's illness were that, when I pressed onto his *mai*, I got the reversed *yang*. When the reversed *yang* entered the empty place, Chu died on the following day. In cases when [the *mai*] are once reversed and once link up, it is a male amassment.

[Section 4: *Shiki kaichû kôshô* 105, pp. 52–62, *Shi ji* 105, pp. 2813–17]

Your servant, Yi, said: there were many other instances when I examined the time limits [before death], discerned whether someone would live or die, treated and cured disorders. As it was a long time ago, I have partially forgotten them. I cannot remember them in their entirety. I do not dare to use them for my response [to your queries].

[*Section 4.1*]

Your servant, Yi, has been asked: among the disorders that you examined and treated, the names of the disorders were often the same, yet after examining them, they differed; some [people] died, others not.[64] Why?

The answer is: the reason why the names of the disorders are often similar in kind, one cannot know. Hence the ancient sages invented for [recognising] them the 'Mai fa'. By establishing measures of length and weight, setting up compass and square, calibrating weight and scale, applying the

---

[62] *fa* 法 'to model'.

[63] *mu shan* 牡疝 'male amassment', i.e. an amassment in the heart since the heart is the male viscus (*xin wei mu zang* 心為牡藏), according to Horikawa Sai. See striking parallels to *Su wen* 17, p. 52.

[64] These two accusations appear unjustified: the 'wind of the void' resulted in case 8 in death and was cured because it was not yet fully developed in case 20. The *ju*-abscess, mentioned in cases 1 and 22, was lethal. *Nei guan zhi bing* (case 1, 15) and *guan nei zhi bing* (case 12) were lethal, and had similar manifestations in cases 12 and 15.

ink of the marking-cord, regulating *yin* and *yang*, they discerned *mai* in man, and named them each. They [the *mai*] mutually resonate with heaven and earth, and threefold unite in man. Hence one discerns the hundred illnesses by means of differentiating between them [the qualities of *mai*]. For those who master [the art of] number,[65] it is possible to differentiate between them [the *mai*, and accordingly the disorders]. Those who do not master [the art of] number, consider them the same. In spite of this, there is more to the 'Mai fa' than can be verified. If one examines a sick person and by the means of measures differentiates between them [the disorders], then one can distinguish between those with the same name and name the place where the host of the disorder resides. Now, those whom your servant, Yi, examined, all have recordings of their diagnostic examination. The means whereby I discerned them [the *mai*, and accordingly the disorders] were that the formulae that I had received from the Master were just about reaching completion, when the Master died. Hence I tabled what he had examined, [his] prognostications of the time period [before death] and assessments of whether [a patient] would live or die. I contemplated over those instances that were failures and those that were a success, and I combined [all this] with the 'Model of the Pulse'. Hence by now I can recognise them [the disorders].

[*Section 4.2*]

Your servant, Yi, has been asked: among those for whom you prognosticated the time period of the disorder, and decided whether [a patient] would live or die, some cases were not in accordance with the prognostication. For what reason?

The answer is: in each of these cases drink and food, joy and anger had not been regular, some should not have ingested drugs, some should not have applied needles and cauterisation.[66] Hence they did not die within the prognosticated time period.

[*Section 4.3*]

Your servant, Yi, has been asked: now that Yi is able to recognise disorders and whether [a patient] will live or die, and to provide a structured analytical discourse on [how] drugs are applied to that which is appropriate, among all the nobles, kings and great ministers is there anyone, or not, who has formerly asked for Yi? And, at the time when King Wen was ill, why has one not requested Yi to examine and treat him?

---

[65] *shu* 數 lit. 'number' involved mastery of regular patterns, including prognostication, within any discipline (Ho 1991).

[66] *zhen jiu* 針灸 alternative translation: 'acupuncture and moxibustion', as defined in ch. 1, n. 7. Yamada (1998) considers *Shi ji* 105 the earliest text to refer to it. See, in particular, ch. 7, case 13. See also sections 4.4, 4.7.

The answer is: the King of Zhao, the King of Jiaoxi, the King of Jinan and the King of Wu all sent messengers to come and summon your servant, Yi. Your servant, Yi, did not dare to go [to them]. At the time when King Wen was ill, your servant Yi's family was poor. On behalf of other people, I wished to treat illness. I honestly feared that an official would assign me a government post and detain me, your servant, Yi. Hence I shifted my name and number to the left and right, did not cultivate a home for my livelihood, and went out to wander among the kingdoms. I sought out those who were expert in formulae and number, and served them for a long time. I have seen and served numerous masters, I have received all their essential effects, I have exhaustively [studied] the meaning of their formula books, and I have interpreted and analysed them. I lived in the fiefdom of Yangxu, and therefore served the Noble. When the Noble entered the [Imperial] court, I, your servant, Yi, followed him to Chang'an. Hence I was able to examine the illness of Xiang Chu in Anling, and of others as well.

[*Section 4.4*]

Your servant, Yi, has been asked: does he know the means whereby King Wen contracted the illness that has the appearance [i.e. the syndrome] of not being able to get up?

Your servant, Yi, answered: I did not see King Wen when he was ill, but I heard that King Wen was ill with panting, headaches and a vision that was unclear. Your servant, Yi, analysed it in my heart-mind. I considered him not to be ill. My opinion is that due to being fat, he accumulated his essences. The person's entire body could not stand being moved, and the bones and flesh did not mutually support each other. Hence he panted. A doctor should not treat this. The 'Mai fa' says: 'At twenty years of age, the *qi* of the *mai* should be hasty. At thirty, one should have a swift pace. At forty, one should sit down quietly. At fifty, one should lie down quietly. When sixty years are accomplished and above, *qi* should be stored deeply.' King Wen had not yet reached twenty years. Just then *mai qi* is hasty. However, he walked slowly. He did not resonate with the way of heaven and the four seasons. Later, I heard that a doctor had cauterised him and thereby aggravated his condition. This is a mistake in the analysis of disorders [i.e. in diagnosis]. Your servant, Yi, analysed it. My opinion was that while the spirit *qi* was contending [with the consequences of cauterisation], the noxious *qi* entered. Not even his youth could retrieve it [the spirit *qi*]. Hence he died. As to so-called *qi*, one should harmonise drink and food, and choose clear days for coach rides and walks to broaden the mind in order to adjust the tendons, bones, flesh, blood and *mai* for bringing *qi* into flow. Hence the age of twenty is called 'the disposition for change'. According to the 'Model', one should not apply stone needles and cautery.[67] Stone needling and cauterisation can result in *qi* being expelled.

[*Section 4.5*]

Your servant, Yi, has been asked: whence has Master Qing received them [his teachings] and was he known among the feudal lords of Qi, or not?[68]

The answer is: I do not know the teacher whence he received [them]. Qing's family was wealthy. He was expert in medicine, but unwilling to treat illness on behalf of other people. It must be for this reason that he was not known among them. Qing, moreover, formally announced to your servant, Yi, saying: 'Beware not to let my sons and grandsons know that you have studied my formulae.'

[*Section 4.6*]

Your servant, Yi, has been asked: why did Master Qing, upon meeting me, Yi, come to favour me, Yi, and why did he wish to teach me, Yi, all his formulae?

The answer is: your servant, Yi, had not heard that Master Qing was expert at formulae. The means whereby I, Yi, got to know Qing – given that I, Yi, when I was young had been fond of all activities concerned with formulae – were that when your servant, Yi, tried out his formulae, all of them were very effective, refined and excellent.[69] Your servant, Yi, had heard that Gongsun Guang of the ward Tang in Zichuan was fond of formulae transmitted from the ancients. Your servant, Yi, thereupon went to pay respects to him. I had the opportunity to see and serve him. I received the formulae that transform *yin* and *yang* and was transmitted spoken 'Models'. Your servant, Yi, received them all and wrote them down.[70] Your servant, Yi, wished to receive in their entirety all of his other refined formulae. Gongsun Guang said: 'My [knowledge of] formulae has been exhausted; it is not that I begrudge you anything. My body is already weakened, there is nothing I could any longer devote my activities to. These are the wonderful formulae that I received when I was young. In their entirety, I have given them to you. Do not take them to teach to anyone else.' Your

---

[67] On *bian jiu* 砭灸 'stone needles and cauterisation', mentioned also in section 4.4, and *zhen shi* 針石 'stone needles', see Yamada (1998).

[68] Sections 4.5–4.7 are based on a draft translation of 1995, but have been modified in the account of Sivin (1995a).

[69] This translation follows Hübotter (1927:27) in order to avoid a contradiction with section 1.

[70] These two sentences concern oral and literate transmission of 'formulae' (*fang* 方) and/or 'models' (*fa* 法).

servant, Yi, said: 'I have had the privilege to meet and serve you in your presence and in their entirety I have obtained [your] secret formulae. I am very fortunate. I would rather die than dare transmit them to anyone inappropriately.' For some time Gongsun Guang lived at leisure. When your servant, Yi, analysed the formulae in depth, I encountered a word that was the most refined in one hundred generations. Master Guang was delighted and said: 'You are certain to become the most skilled in the land. I have that which I am good at, but it is few and far between. A fellow[71] lives in Linzi. He is fond of formulae, I cannot compare with him. His formulae are most exceptional. They are not what ordinary people have heard about. When I was in my prime, I formerly wanted to receive his formulae. Yang Zhongqian was unwilling and said: "You are not the right person." I must go with you to see him. He will recognise that you are fond of formulae. This person has also reached old age. His family is well supplied and wealthy.' At the time, as we had not yet gone [there], just then the son of [Yang] Qing, a young man [named] Yin,[72] came to present a horse. Since Master Guang offered the horse to the king's place [of residence],[73] I, Yi, therefore was able to become friendly with Yin. Guang moreover entrusted me, Yi, to Yin saying: 'Yi is devoted to [the art of] number. You must treat him with care. This person is a sage master of techniques.' Then, he wrote a letter in order to entrust me, Yi, to Yang Qing. Hence I got to know Qing. Your servant, Yi, served Qing diligently. Hence he favoured me, Yi.

[*Section 4.7*]

Your servant, Yi, has been asked: have there ever been officials or commoners who have served him and studied his, Yi's, formulae and have they all obtained his, Yi's, formulae in their entirety or not? Which prefecture and ward were the persons from?

The answer is: Song Yi 宋邑 of Linzi. Yi 邑 studied [with me]. Your servant, Yi, taught him 'The Five Examinations'. It took more than a year. The King of Jibei sent the Grand Physicians Gao Qi 高期 and Wang Yu 王禹 to study [with me]. Your servant, Yi, taught them 'Channels: Above and Below' and 'Irregular Links and Knots'. On a regular basis, we analysed the places the *shu* inhabited, and in accordance with whether the *qi* would rise or descend, exit or enter, be noxious, [flow] contravectively or smoothly, equipped with the appropriate stone needles, we determined the locations

---

[71] *tong chan* 同產 'half-brother who has the same mother as oneself'. Probably, here simply a 'fellow'.

[72] *nan* 男 is a term that defines a man's state for purposes of taxation. It designates males aged twenty-three to fifty-six (or sixty?) with neither appointment as an official nor conferment of aristocratic rank (Loewe 1967:2.74). His name 殷 is pronounced as Yin or Yang. Distinguish between *zi nan* 子男 here and *nan zi* 男子 in case 18.

[73] If the offering was made to the King of Zichuan, it is not possible that Yi started to study with Yang Qing in 180, as said in the introduction. See also Bridgman (1955:100, n. 261).

for stone needling and cautery. It took more than a year. The King of Zichuan, from time to time, sent the Chief of [the Stable and] the Great Granary,[74] Feng Xin 馮信, for rectifying the formulae. Your servant, Yi, taught him techniques for delivering massage, 'The Structured Analysis of the Contravective and Smooth', techniques of administering drugs, and techniques for determining the five flavours and blending the regulatory broths. Du Xin 杜信, deputy of the household of the Noble of Gaoyong 高永,[75] was fond of [the art of] *mai* and came to study. Your servant, Yi, taught him 'The Upper and Lower Channels' and 'The Five Examinations'. It took more than two years. Tang An 唐安 of the ward Zhao 召 in Linzi came to study. Your servant, Yi, taught him 'The Five Examinations', 'The Upper and Lower Channels and Vessels', 'The Regular and Irregular' and 'The Doubling of Yin and Yang due to Resonances with the Four Seasons'. He has not yet completed [his studies], but has been appointed the Attending Physician of the King of Qi.

[*Section 4.8*]

Your servant, Yi, has been asked: is he able to examine disorders and make decisions about death and life completely without mistakes?

Your servant, Yi's, answer is: if I, Yi, treat a patient, I must necessarily first press onto his *mai*, then [only] do I treat him. If they are bad and contravective, he [or she] is incurable. If they are smooth, then I treat him [or her]. When the heart-mind is not attentive to the *mai*, what I prognosticate of death and life and [what] I regard as curable, I time and again get wrong. Your servant, Yi, cannot be perfect.

The Grand Historian says:

A woman, regardless of whether she is beautiful or ugly, once she lives in the palace [harem], is envied. A man, regardless of whether he has sagacity or is unworthy, once he enters court, is met with suspicion. Hence Bian Que, due to his arts, experienced calamity. Canggong, by contrast, although he concealed his traces and himself went into hiding, was about to be punished by mutilation. Tiying forwarded a document [to the Emperor], and the father thereby obtained peace in later life. Hence Laozi says: 'Beauty and goodness are the instruments for [attracting] calamities.' Isn't he speaking about Bian Que's and others' calamity? As for Canggong, one can say he came close to it.

---

[74] *Tai cang ma zhang* 太倉馬長. According to Taki Motohiro, the character *ma* must be mistaken. Feng Xin was from Linzi and became Chief of the Great Granary of Qi.
[75] Gaoyong was no fiefdom, says Liang Yusheng; it is not mentioned in the slightly more elaborate account of Duxin in *Yi shuo* 1, pp. 11b–12a.

8

Commentators and commentaries to the Memoir

The commentators quoted in Takigawa Kametaro's 瀧川龜太郎 edition *Shiki kaichû kôshô* 史記會注考證 (Examination of the Collected Commentaries to the Records of the Historian), 1932–34. Toyo Bunka Gakuin, Tokyo, are:

The compilers of the commentaries:

a) *jijie* 集解 commentary: Pei Yin 裴駰 (5th century), who quotes Xu Guang 徐廣 (325–425)
b) *suoyin* 索隱 commentary: Sima Zhen 司馬貞 (early 8th century)
c) *zhengyi* 正義 commentary: Zhang Shoujie 張守節 (preface 737)
d) *kaozheng* 考證 commentary: Takigawa Kametaro, who quotes the following commentators:

Japanese commentators:

(An)do Koretora [安]藤維寅 or 滕惟寅	扁鵲倉公傳割解
(An)do Masamichi [安] 滕正路, his son	扁鵲倉公傳割解補考, afterword 1770
Horikawa Sai 堀川濟	扁鵲倉公傳考異並備參, ca 1850
Kaiho Gembi 海保元備	扁鵲倉公傳統考, undated
Oka Hakku 岡白駒	史記觿, 1756
Taki Motokata 多紀元堅	扁鵲倉公傳
Taki Motohiro 多紀元簡, his son	扁鵲倉公傳補注, completed in 1810
Taki Mototane 多紀元胤	難經疏証, preface 1819 no reference to him as a compiler of a *Shi ji* commentary

Chinese commentators:

Chen Zilong 陳子龍 (1608–47) (with Xu Fuyuan 徐孚遠)	史記測義

Cui Shi 崔適	史記探源, publ. 1910
Dong Fen 董份	泌園集, publ. 1541
Li Li 李笠	史記訂補, publ. 1924
Liang Yusheng 梁玉繩	史記志疑, publ. 1787
	瞥記
Ling Zhilong 凌稚隆 (late Ming period)	史記評林
Qian Daxin 錢大昕 (1728–1804)	二十二史記異
	三史拾遺
	駕齊瀁新錄
Wang Niansun 王念孫 (1744–1832)	讀書雜志
	commentary to 淮南子
Wang Yinzhi 王引之 (1766–1834), his son	讀書雜志
Zhang Wenhu 張文虎 (1808–85)	校史記札記
	舒藝室隨筆
Zhang Zhao 張照 (1671–1741)	館本史記考證

Commentators cited by the commentators:

Fu Qian 服虔 (ca 125–95)	通俗文
Guo Pu 郭璞 (276–324)	commentary to the 山海經
	commentary to the 方言
Gu Yewang 顧野王 (519–81)	compiler of 玉篇
Ru Chun 如淳 (fl. 198–265)	commentary to the 漢書
Tao Hongjing 陶弘景 (456–536)	innumerous works, most
(cited as Tao Yinju 陶隱居)	likely to be quoted
	from 本草經集注
Xu Guang 徐廣 (325–425)	commentary to the 漢書
Yan Shigu 顏師古 (581–645)	commentary to the 漢書
Yang Xuancao 楊玄操 (7th–8th century)	黄帝八十一難經注

Further Commentators:

Duan Yucai 段玉裁 (1735–1815)	commentary to 說文解字
Gao You 高誘 (ca 168–212)	commentary to 淮南子
Wang Xianqian 王先謙 (1842–1918)	漢書補注, publ. 1900
Zhao Qi 趙岐 (d. 201)	commentary to 孟子

9

Map of Chunyu Yi's itineraries

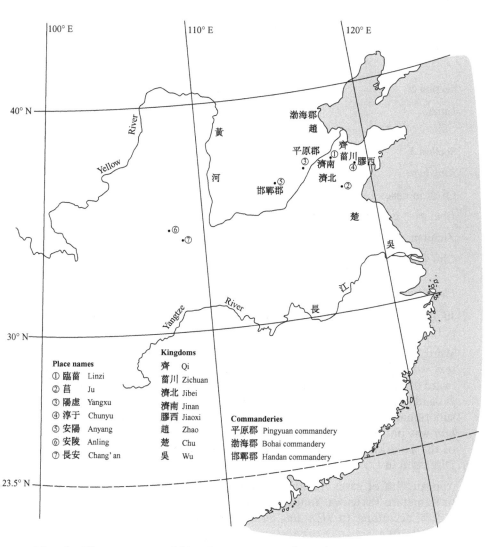

Map 1   Place names and kingdoms mentioned in Chunyu Yi's Memoir

Section 1:

Linzi 臨菑 was the capital of Qi 齊 at 36.9° N, 118.3° E (Tan 1991:19–20).

Qi 齊 was the most important kingdom in eastern China in the Warring States and early Han (roughly in the area of present-day province of Shandong 山東). In the mid-second century it was divided and much reduced (Twitchett and Loewe 1986: map 3 on p. 125 for 195 BCE and map 7 on pp. 146–7 for 143 BCE).

Chang'an 長安 was the capital of the Western Han (near present-day Xi'an 西安).

Section 2:

Linzi.

Section 3:

Kingdoms

Qi 齊 in cases 1–7 and 10, and in cases 13, 15, 17, 21, 22.

Jibei 濟北 is mentioned in cases 9, 11, 12, 18.

Zichuan 菑川 is mentioned in cases 14, 16.

Chu 楚 in case 4.

Place names

Ju 莒 of case 4 was in the kingdom of Chengyang 成陽 (*Han shu* 28B, p. 1635) at 35.3° N, 118.5° E (Tan 1991:19–20).

Ward Zhangwu 章武 of case 7. For *li* 里 as 'ward', see Bodde (1982:3). The text would appear defective since *li* requires a further specification, like 'ward of a prefecture'. Zhangwu 章武 is, in fact, the name of a 'county' (*xian* 縣) and a 'nobility' (*hou* 侯). It was a *hou* from 173–122 BCE; as a *xian* it was subordinated to Bohai 勃海 commandery. In pre-Imperial times, Zhangwu *hou* was part of Zhao 趙 kingdom, but it is uncertain whether it was part of the Han kingdom Zhao or Qi (*Han shu* 28A, p. 1579, 28B, p. 1655). Discussed in Loewe (1997).

Yangxu 陽虛 of cases 8 and 23 is Yangxu 楊虛 in *Han shu* 38, according to Kametaro Takigawa. Yangxu 楊虛 was part of the Pingyuan commandery 平原郡, according to *Han shu bu zhu*, 15.4b, at 36.6° N, 116.4° E (Tan 1991:19–20).

Linzi in case 19.

Chunyu 淳于 of case 20 is the name of a town east of Linzi at 36.5° N, 119.3° E (Tan 1991:19–20).

Anyang 安陽 of case 24 is difficult to locate since it is a popular place name. The Anyang most likely to be meant here is a few kilometres west of the modern Anyang in the province of Shanxi 山西, in what at the time was Handan 邯鄲 commandery, at 36.1° N, 114.3° E (Tan 1991:9–10). It is west of Yangxu, possibly on the route to Chang'an.

Anling 安陵 of case 25 was located in three possible places, according to Bridgman (1955:97, n. 238). Considering section 4.3, Anling situated in the north-west of Chang'an is the most probable; at 34.4° N, 108.8° E (Tan 1991: 15–16).

Section 4:

Kingdoms

Zhao 趙, Jiaoxi 膠西. Jiaonan 膠南, Wu 吳 (section 4.3) and Zichuan (sections 4.6 and 4.7), Jibei (section 4.7).

Place names

Linzi (sections 4.6 and 4.7).

III
Translation and interpretation of the medical case histories 1–10 in the Memoir of Chunyu Yi

Case 1: translation, p. 120

Critical evaluation of retrospective biomedical diagnoses, p. 122

The name of the disorder, p. 123
ju 疽 – *abscess (line 5) and yong* 癰 – *clog (lines 7, 26, and 39), p. 123*

The pulse qualities in the 'Mai fa' (lines 17–19), p. 126
chang 長 – *elongated (line 17), p. 126*
xian 弦 – *strung (line 17), p. 126*

Further pulse qualities (lines 20–5 and 30–2), p. 129
huo or he 和 – *blending* or *being harmonious (lines 20 and 22), p. 129*
dai 代 – *alternating (line 21), p. 130*
bing zhu 病主 – *the host of the disorder (line 19), p. 132*
jing zhu bing 經主病 *and jing bing* 經病 – *the channels govern the disorder*
and the passageways are in disorder (lines 20, 22, 30), p. 133

Text structure semantics, p. 135
zhuo 濁 – *murky (line 14), p. 135*
jing 靜 – *still (line 14), p. 138*
nei guan zhi bing 內關之病 – *'disorder of the interior being closed off' (line*
15), p. 139
Summary, p. 141

Prognosticating the day of death (lines 33–40), p. 142

Being exuberant (you guo 有過) *and heat that rises (re shang* 熱上) *in*
tubular structures (lines 20–1, 22–5, 33–5, 41–4, 45–6), p. 143

A note on the cause of the disorder (line 9), p. 146

Discussion, p. 147

Case 2: translation, p. 148

Critical evaluation of retrospective biomedical diagnoses, p. 149

Case 7: translation, p. 267

Critical evaluation of retrospective biomedical diagnoses, p. 268

The name of the disorder (line 4), p. 268
Introductory remarks, p. 268
jia 瘕 – *conglomerations in the Mawangdui and Zhangjiashan medical manuscripts, p. 269*
jia 瘕 – *conglomerations as chronic disorders, p. 274*
jia 瘕 – *a gender-specific disorder, p. 276*

Text structure semantics, p. 277
The pulse qualities given in Yi's own vocabulary (lines 9–14), p. 279
zhi 至 – *congested, to arrive or extremely (line 13), p. 281*
jin 緊 – *tight (line 13), p. 282*
xiao 小 – *small (line 13), p. 282*
shen 深 – *deep or very (line 10), p. 283*
xiao 小 – *small (line 10), p. 284*
ruo 弱 – *soft (line 10), p. 285*
Comparison of the pulse qualities (lines 10 and 13), p. 285
qia qia 合合 – *confused (line 11), p. 286*

The prognostication of death (lines 15–20), p. 288
yi ci xiang cheng 以次相乘 – *they took turns in riding on each other (line 15), p. 288*
san yin 三陰 – *the three yin? (line 17), p. 289*
bo 搏 *or tuan* 搏 – *to strike or to be united (lines 17, 18 and 19), p. 290*
Questions of timing (lines 17–20), p. 292

Discussion, p. 293

Case 8: translation, p. 294

Critical evaluation of retrospective biomedical diagnoses, p. 295

The name of the disorder, p. 295
dong feng 迥風 – *the wind of the void (line 4), p. 295*
han zhong 寒中 – *coldness in the interior (line 3), p. 298*

Text structure semantics, p. 298
hua 滑 – *slippery (line 12), p. 299*
nei qi 內氣 *or feng qi* 風氣 – *qi coming from within or from wind? (line 13), p. 299*

The prognostication of death (lines 7–8 and 14–16), p. 300

Discussion, p. 301

10

Text structure semantics

Shi ji 105 in Chunyu Yi's Memoir combines descriptive narrative, as is characteristic of the historiography in the *Zuo zhuan* (*Zuo* Tradition),[1] with elaborate medical speculation, as given in early medical manuscript texts, and thus provides us with the earliest extant medical case histories of individual patients. These also contain the earliest extant comprehensive account of Chinese pulse diagnosis. Perhaps this is not a coincidence.

Yi was interested in visceral states which, as argued above, may reflect the attention early Han physicians paid to the feelings and emotions of their elite clientele, i.e. they took individual psychology seriously, and in their view it affected visceral processes. In order to identify such body internal processes, they developed sophisticated tactile techniques, namely the examination of *mai* (*zhen mai*) and, in particular, *qie mai* (pressing onto *mai*). Their tactile exploration of the *mai* on the body surface, here interpreted as 'pulse diagnosis', resulted in the identification of different qualities of *qi* which they considered indicative of an individual's visceral states. Yi's rationale is grounded not only in the concepts *yin yang* and *mai*, as are the Mawangdui vessel texts, but also in 'viscera' (*zang*) and *qi,* as is the *Inner Canon*.

The key to making sense of Yi's case histories was the recognition that they are recorded in a formulaic fashion. This made it possible to develop the text critical method of 'text structure semantics', which is an interpretive method insofar as it assumes that linguistically marked clauses concern themes that the author(s)/editor(s) of a text consider important. Yi's case histories all concern *bing* (medical disorders). By attributing meaning to the repeated occurrence of certain rhetorical phrases, it was possible to identify three systematically discussed themes of *bing*: its 'name', 'cause' and 'quality'.

The overall theme of the case histories: *bing* 病 *(disorder)*

The opening statement in almost every case history is that a certain person is 'ill' (*bing*). Usually, Yi reports that so and so was ill and then adds that

---

[1] On the dating of *Zuo zhuan*, see Cheng (1993).

he was summoned to examine this person. Sometimes this opening statement is specified by the patient's subjective complaint: once the client
reports himself to be ill with a 'headache' (*tou tong* 頭痛) (case 1), once he
is ill with 'pain in the minor abdomen' (*shao fu tong* 少腹痛) (case 7), and
once he is reported to be 'ill' with a 'decaying tooth' (*zhu chi* 齲齒) (case
13).[2] Sometimes the condition of the 'illness' is modified and said to be
'serious' (*bing shen* 病甚), regardless of whether it is lethal (case 23) or can
be cured (case 19).[3]

In some cases, whether the condition described in the case history constitutes a *bing* or not appears controversial. In case 19, for instance, Yi
makes an extra note that worms can lead to an illness when he says 'A
conglomeration of *rao*-worms as a disorder ... [has the following specific
attributes]'.[4] One may wonder why Yi finds it necessary to make this statement. Since health workers encountered the belief that hookworms helped
the digestive process, even in twentieth-century China,[5] one may sympathise
with any doctor who stressed that worm infestations are pathological.

From the perspective of the anthropology of the body, the term *bing* is
generally understood to indicate disorder in the body politic. It implies that
illness arises from body parts in disarray and 'chaos' (*luan* 亂).[6] Historians
of Chinese medicine have consistently advocated as translation for *bing*
'disorder', but as seen above, *bing* also arises from infestations of parasites,
which are often linked to demonical attacks. Furthermore, as my research
into the more than sixty occurrences of *bing* in the *Zuo zhuan* has highlighted, *bing* can also mean disgrace or worry or refer to an individual's
utter state of distress, both physical and emotional. To date this connotation
of *bing*, which alludes to emotion and sentiment, has not been sufficiently
recognised. Yet systematic research into the *Zuo zhuan* has demonstrated
that while, indeed, in one third of its occurrences (ca twenty cases), *bing*
designates general disorder, impoverishment, famine or difficulty of a
kingdom or city, or of a people (sometimes as a causative), it refers to the
emotional state of a person who is aggrieved, often as a result of a previous

---

[2] Case 11 is an exception as the wet-nurse complains of heat in the feet, and not of an illness
(*bing*), but Yi says it is a disorder (*bing*) and names it. In case 20, the client considers himself
ill (*bing*), but Yi does not consider the condition to have yet developed into a full-fledged
disorder.

[3] Cases 11 and 14 do not mention *bing* in the opening sentence, but obviously conceived of
the complaint as *bing*. See ch. 10, n. 2 and n. 12.

[4] *rao jia wei bing* 蟯瘕為病. On *wei*, see Pulleyblank (1995:20, example 25). Yi later says 'ailing
from worms was contracted from ...' (*bing rao de zhi ...* 病蟯得之), although he usually does
not name the specific disorder in the formula 'the disorder is contracted from' (*bing de
zhi*) ... (see p. 112). Therefore, commentator Wang Niansun considers *rao* a scribal error,
but taking into account the above, it need not be.

[5] Lucas (1982:27). See also Geissler (1998a, b) and Ackerknecht (1947:143): 'Intestinal worms
among the African Thongas are not at all regarded as pathological. They are thought to be
necessary for digestion.'

[6] On *luan*, see Dunhuang text P3287 quoted on p. 43. On body political connotations of *bing*,
see Unschuld (1985) and Rosner (1991).

dispute, in one fourth of the cases (ca fifteen cases). Aggrievement was not taken lightly. In the *Zuo zhuan* the term *bing* designates a serious, sometimes even terminal condition, and *ji bing* 疾病 is always glossed as such.[7]

For the above reasons, translating *bing* as 'ailment' is inadequate for the *Zuo zhuan*, since the term 'ailment' generally conveys a sense of subjectively perceived, undefined conditions of unease or refers to superficial manifestations of a morbid condition. In the Mawangdui vessel texts and Yi's Memoir, even more so than in the *Zuo zhuan*, *bing* disorders are not unspecific 'ailments' but refer to nosological entities assessed in a learned language and framed in a sophisticated medical rationale.[8] Yi's rationale, as emerges from a careful analysis of his medical practice and his repeated reference to 'Qi ke' (see p. 68), ultimately was concerned with identifying visceral processes of the body's interior in terms of *qi*.

To be sure, no claim is made that the terms *ji* 疾 and *yi* 疫 referred to epidemics, seasonal and often infectious disease, and *bing* to emotional distress, but it is noteworthy that *bing* is consistently used in the elite medical manuscript texts on *mai* and in Yi's Memoir. The canonical medical literature uses *ji* and *bing* interchangeably, but early texts can make sharp distinctions between them: *ji* is 'point of origin of a morbid condition', *bing* its full-blown manifestation in an iatromantic Shuihudi manuscript from the early third century, a differentiation which applies also to Yi's case 22.[9] In Yi's case histories, *bing* predominantly belongs among Yi's vocabulary, but there are instances where a layperson uses it too. In case 15, the opposition between Yi's notion of *bing,* which accounts for the existence of latent conditions, and that of the layperson, who associates *bing* with consciously felt pain, becomes a matter of dispute. In case 20, the client reports he is 'ill' (*bing*) and another doctor also considers him 'ill' (*bing*), while Yi recognises that the condition is not yet so serious and that he merely 'is about to be ill' (*dang bing* 當病). In this context, Yi differentiates between the 'appearance' (*zhuang* 狀) of an illness, which in contemporary medical parlance translates into its 'signs and symptoms', and the disorder itself.

---

[7] *Bing* means 'disorder in a kingdom or city' in *Zuo zhuan*, pp. 1.282, 1.293, 1.306, 3.978, 3.1067, 4.1509, 4.1567, 4.1689, 4.1693, 'famine' in 2.761, and 'hardship among the people' in 3.957, 3.1089, 3.1157, 4.1417, 4.1726. It is a *causative* in 1.128, 1.247, 1.344, 1.387; and in 3.1095 for an individual. *Bing* refers to 'disgrace'; 'worry'; 'utter distress'; and 'aggrievement' of an individual in 1.315; 3.1137, 4.1288; 1.454, 2.630, 2.791–2.4.1294; and in 1.189, 2.707, 2.730, 3.926, 3.1095, 4.1239, 4.1291, 4.1486, 4.1694, 4.1733. Identified through the *Zuo zhuan* concordance by Lau and Chen (1992–). Thanks go to Bill Jenner, Robert Neather and John Moffett for the many hours spent with translating all passages. For more detail, see Hsu (2001a: ch.2); *ji* 疾 occurred too frequently in the *Zuo zhuan* to be studied in a systematic fashion.

[8] Harbsmeier's (2004:76) rendering of *qing* 情 in *de bing zhi qing* 得病之情 (*Su wen* 12, p. 40) as 'dynamic inner cause' recognises this but his claim that it is unrelated to feelings needs to be revised in light of the above finding that *bing* is a process/condition affecting the sentimental body.

[9] Harper (2001:112), Hsu (2001b:65).

To summarise, Yi as physician has a sophisticated concept of *bing*, but the term is also used by his clientele in a more general sense. It is the case that the manuscript texts on *mai*, which consistently refer to *bing*, go beyond investigating and treating only the visually perceived bodily 'form' (*xing*). Yet the *Zuo zhuan* and Yi's Memoir, perhaps not least due to their focus on human interaction and their narrative form, accord *bing* even more pronounced connotations of distress in account of inward aspects of personhood.

The marked aspects of *bing*: name, cause and quality

Which aspects of a pathological condition mattered to the *Shi ji* personage Yi, who identified *bing*?[10] In order to determine those aspects of *bing* that mattered to the narrator, aspects of the disorder that were introduced by recurrent phrases were investigated:

1.) a statement in the beginning of each case following the word:
   yue 曰 (I said), see table 1
2.) a statement following the phrase:
   bing de zhi 病得之 (the illness is contracted by), see table 2
3.) statements introduced by the phrase:
   suo yi zhi XY bing zhe 所以知 XY 病者 (the means whereby I recognised XY's illness were . . .), see table 3

Text structure semantics made possible the exploration of word meaning not only syntagmatically, as is usual when one reads a text, but also paradigmatically: each of the three above-mentioned aspects was put in a list and compared with twenty-four others. Aspect (1) concerns the 'name', (2) the 'cause' and (3) the 'quality' of the disorder (tables 2–4).[11] Based on text structure semantics it emerged that not the 'cause' of the disorder but the synchronous signs, i.e. the tactually felt 'qualities' of *mai*, each correlated with a constituent in the polysyllabic 'names' of the disorder. Synchronous signs, rather than past history, are pivotal to Yi's diagnosis.

The 'name' of the disorder

After stating in the opening sentence that the case history concerns the *bing* of an individual XY with title YZ from place Z, Yi states in the second sentence that he examined the patient. He then makes a diagnosis in that he 'says' the 'name' of the patient's condition. The only conditions that are

---

[10] The edited *Shi ji* cases are formulaic. Since cases 1–10 consistently report on the 'quality of the disorder' but not cases 11–25, the formulaic features are probably not merely the product of a creative editor. However, with the data at hand, it is impossible to know the structure of cases 1–10 in the presumed primary source of the early second century.

[11] 'Name', 'cause' and 'quality' are not the terms Yi uses, therefore they are in quotation marks.

Table 2: The 'name' of the disorder
Table 2 records the clauses introduced by the recurrent phrase *yue* 曰 (I said) . . .

1. this one is ailing from a *ju*-abscess (*ci bing ju ye* 此病疽也)
2. a disorder of *qi* that is blocked (*qi ge bing* 氣鬲病)
3. it is a welling amassment (*yong shan ye* 癰疝也)
   (the many doctors: numbness entered and struck the interior; *jue ru zhong* 厥入中)
4. it is *qi* of a heat disorder; so, you sweat [as] from summer heat
   (*re bing qi ye, ran shu han* 熱病氣也 然暑汗)
5. a wind-induced condition-of-overexertion is visiting the bladder
   (*feng dan ke pao* 風癉客胕)
6. it is wasting heat-due-to-overexertion in the lungs, i.e. a 'lung consumption'
   (*fei xiao dan ye* 肺消癉也)
7. it is a conglomeration of remanent accumulations (*yi ji jia ye* 遺積瘕也)
8. wind of the void (*dong feng* 迵風)
   (the many doctors: coldness in the interior, *han zhong* 寒中)
9. wind-induced numbness (*feng jue* 風蹶)
10. she is troubled by *qi* – an amassment is visiting the bladder – and has difficulties in
    urinating and defecating
    (*bing qi – shan ke yu pang guang – nan yu qian hou sou* 病氣 疝客於膀胱 難於前後溲)
    (the many doctors: wind entered and struck the interior, *feng ru zhong* 風入中)
11. it is a heat inversion (*re jue ye* 熱厥也)
12. Shu has a damaged spleen (*Shu shang pi* 豎傷脾)
13. —[a]
14. —
15. this one has the *qi* of having damaged the spleen (*ci shang pi qi ye* 此傷脾氣也)
    (the many doctors: large worms, *da chong* 大蟲)
16. an inversion above (*jue shang* 厥上)
17. . . . this is a so-called obstruction of the kidneys (. . . *ci suo wei shen bi ye* 此所謂腎痹也)
18. the private within is cold, the menses do not descend
    (*nei han, yue shi bu xia ye* 內寒月事不下也)
    (the many doctors: chills and hot flushes, *han re* 寒熱)
19. conglomeration of *rao*-worms (*rao jia* 蟯瘕)
    (the many doctors: aggravated state of chills and hot flushes, *han re du* 寒熱篤)
20. if it will become a disorder, it will be the wind of the void
    (*dang bing dong feng* 當病迵風)
21. the lungs are injured (*fei shang* 肺傷)
22. you ail from heat in the interior (*gong bing zhong re* 公病中熱)
23. [以為 replaces 曰] [I considered it] an obstruction (*bi* 痹)
    (the many doctors: numbness, *jue* 厥)
24. [謂之 replaces 曰] [I told him] he was ill, suffering from talkative winds
    (*wei zhi bing ku ta feng* 病 苦沓風)
25. male amassment (*mu shan* 牡疝)

[a]A dash means that the text provides no information in this slot for the name, cause or quality
of the disorder.

not named are those of a client who complains of being ill with tooth caries
(case 13) and a pregnant woman who cannot give birth (case 14).[12]

The 'names' of the disorders are mostly compound words. Since the text
structural features do not indicate when the theme introduced by the phrase

---

[12] Both are *bing*. In case 13, Yi says the 'illness ceased' (*bing yi* 病已), after five to six days of
treatment; in case 14, Yi mentions, after applying medicines which induce birth, a 'lingering
illness' (*yu bing* 餘病).

Table 3: The 'cause' of the disorder

Table 3 records the clauses introduced by the recurrent phrase *bing de zhi* 病得之 (the illness was contracted by/from) ...

1. wine and women
2. infantile irritability; it [involves] frequently rejecting food and drink
3. women
4. formerly bathing in running water while it was very cold, and once it was over, getting hot
5. while dripping with sweat, going outside to dry up. In cases of drying up, having removed one's clothes, the sweat dries in the sunlight
6. great anger, and in this condition indulging in women
7. wine and women
8. wine
9. sweating and lying prostrate on the ground
10. intending to urinate, but not having the chance to do so, and by indulging, in this condition, in sexual intercourse
11. drinking wine and getting badly drunk
12. dripping with sweat
13. wind, and sleeping with an open mouth; eating without rinsing the mouth
14. —
15. dripping with sweat and frequently going outside; having roasted by the fire, going outside and exposing oneself to big winds
16. washing one's hair and, while it is not yet dry, going to sleep
17. being fond of lifting heavy [things]
18. while desiring a man, not being able to get one
19. dwelling in the cold and damp
20. stuffing oneself and thereafter running swiftly
21. falling off a horse onto his back, hitting a rock
22. —
23. women
24. frequently drinking wine and exposing oneself to strong wind *qi*
25. women

'I said' ends, it is not always clear how long they are. They do not always have definite endings. Some 'names' can be interpreted to include a symptom-oriented description of the condition (e.g. cases 4, 10, 18), and, as in other scholarly cultures, are long and descriptive.[13] Others are not nouns but grammatically well-formed sentences, which do, however, mention a noun that can be interpreted as 'name of the disorder' (e.g. cases 1, 12, 15, 20, 22, 24).

The constituents[14] of the compound words comprise ecological variables such as wind (*feng* 風) and coldness (*han* 寒), heat (*re* 熱) and *qi*; cosmological notions like 'the void' (*dong* 迥) and 'the dull' (*jue* 蹷), which Yi also used in the sense of 'numbness' and 'inversion'. Some are verbs alluding to flows and fluxes in the body, such as 'welling' (*yong* 湧), 'being separated' (*ge* 鬲), 'remanent' (*yi* 遺) and what could be a verb but is here interpreted

---

[13] European botanical names were long and descriptive before Carolus Linnaeus invented the binomial system of naming (e.g. Atran 1990).

[14] Compound words are composed of 'constituents'. 'Any constituent part of a sentence that bears meaning ... will be termed a semantic constituent' (Cruse 1986:25ff.).

Table 4: The 'quality' of the disorder
Table 4 records the clauses introduced by the recurrent phrase *suo yi zhi XY bing zhe*
所以知 XY 病者 (the means whereby I recognised XY's illness were that)[a] ...

---

1. when I, your servant Yi, pressed onto his *mai*, I got the *qi* [coming] from the liver. The *qi* [coming] from the liver, despite being murky, was still. (Text continues in manner 1:[b] this is ...)
2. when I examined his *mai*, it was *qi* [coming] from the heart. Despite it being murky and hurried, [the condition was] transient. (Text continues in manner 1: this is ...)
3. at the time when I pressed onto his *mai*, at the right opening, *qi* was intense. The *mai* did not have *qi* [coming] from the five viscera. At the right opening, the *mai* were large, yet frequent. (Text continues in manner 2: in cases where they are frequent ...)
4. at the time when I pressed onto his *mai*, there was a paired *yin*. (Text continues in manner 3: the 'Mai fa' says ...)
5. when I, your servant Yi, examined her *mai*, and when I pressed onto the opening of the major *yin*, it was damp. In spite of this, there was wind *qi*. (Text continues in manner 3: the 'Mai fa' says ...)
6. when I, your servant Yi, pressed onto his *mai*, the *qi* [coming] from the lungs was hot. (Text continues in manner 3: the 'Mai fa' says ...)
7. when I, your servant Yi, pressed onto his *mai*, they were deep, small and soft, abruptly they were confused. (Text continues in manner 1: this is ...)
8. when I, your servant Yi, pressed onto his *mai*, the *mai* came slippery. (Text continues in manner 1: this is ...)
9. at the time when I, your servant Yi, pressed onto his *mai*, it was wind *qi*. The *mai* [coming] from the heart was murky. (Text continues in manner 3: the 'Bing fa' says ...)
10. when I pressed onto her *mai*, they were large, yet replete. They came with difficulty. (Text continues in manner 1: this is ...)[c]
11. —
12. —
13. —
14. —
15. sentence on colour.[d]
16. —
17. sentence on colour.
18. at the time when I examined her *mai*, when I pressed onto them, it was the *mai* [coming] from the kidneys. It was rough and discontinuous. (Text continues in manner 2: in cases where it is rough and discontinuous ...)
19. when I pressed onto her *mai* and stroked over her *chi* 尺 area, her *chi* was ropy, prickly and coarse, while the body hair was beautiful, [like] cicada antennas (Text continues in manner 1: this is ...)
20. at the time when I examined his *mai*, when I pressed onto them, they were entirely according to the 'Model'[e] His illness was smooth. (Text continues in manner 1: hence ...)
21. when I pressed onto his *mai*, I got lung *yin qi*. Their coming was dispersed; they arrived by several routes, and were not one. Moreover, colour rode on them. (Text continues in manner 4: the means whereby I knew ...)
22. —
23. at the time when I examined him, I was not able to know the explanation in terms of the passageways.
24. when I examined him, his *mai* were modelling [processes recorded in] the 'Qi ke'. (Text continues in manner 3: the word says ...) when I pressed onto them, I got the kidneys inverted to the lungs. (Text continues in manner 3: the 'Model' says ...)
25. when I pressed onto his *mai*, I got the reversed *yang*. (Text continues in manner 2: the reversed *yang* ...)

---

[a]Only sentences which mention *mai* are translated. Yi 'examines *mai*' (*zhen mai* 診脈), 'presses onto *mai*' (*qie mai* 切脈), twice 'presses onto the opening of the right [*mai*]' (*qie you* [*mai*] *kou* 切右[脈]口), once 'strokes the foot area' [perhaps, on the forearm] (*xun chi* 循尺).
[b]The text continues in the four following manners: (1) with a clause introduced by *ci* 此 'this is', or *shi* 是 'this is', or *gu* 故 'hence'; (2) with a clause introduced by the phrases like 'Mai fa' *yue* 脈法曰 'the "Model of the Pulse" says'; (3) with a clause introduced by the topic XY *zhe* 'in cases where XY', which reduplicates the last word of the previous sentence; (4) with a new theme.
[c]In cases 1–10 (except cases 2, 3, 4, 10), the self-reference is 'your servant, Yi'. This does not apply to any of the cases 11–25.
[d]See ch. 3, n. 9; ch. 4, n. 28; ch. 10, n. 24.
[e]Note textual irregularity: 'the means whereby I recognised it'.

as noun, 'accumulations' (*ji* 積). Other verbs include 'harming' or 'injuring' (*shang* 傷), which lead to death, as do 'wasting' (*xiao* 消) and 'being talkative' or 'sluggish' (*ta* 沓, both translations possible), while 'visiting' (*ke* 客) is temporary. Some refer to body parts, namely 'the private within' (*nei* 內), 'the interior/centre' (*zhong* 中), 'the above' (*shang* 上), the 'bladder' (*pao* 脬 or *pangguang* 膀胱), 'lungs' (*fei* 肺), 'spleen' (*pi* 脾) and 'kidneys' (*shen* 腎). Some are ideogrammatically marked by the illness radical no. 104, namely '*ju*-abscesses' (*ju* 疽), 'amassments' (*shan* 疝, also translated as 'tumours' or 'hernias'), 'conditions of overexertion' (*dan* 癉), 'conglomerations' (*jia* 瘕) and 'obstructions' (*bi* 痺). Only Yi, and no other doctor, mentions ideogrammatically marked names. Furthermore, only his names have as constituents specific viscera and *qi*.[15]

The disorder called *jue* 'numbness', 'inversion' and 'reversal' deserves particular attention because it is an important nosological term used in a slightly different sense by the many doctors, Yi and Bian Que. It is closely related to a form of needling and cauterisation that can be regarded a precursor to acupuncture and moxibustion. It involved 'needling' and 'cauterising' specific 'places' (*suo* 所). It has been suggested that in *Shi ji* 105 only *jue* conditions were treated by needling, but this is an unfounded overgeneralisation. Nor would it be correct to assume that *jue* conditions were by definition painful, and that needling was used primarily for treating pain, as it currently is in acupuncture.[16]

Yi's polysyllabic names are often unique to the *Shi ji*. Hence the idea arose as to whether they result from editorial and/or commentatorial emendations. If there was an early second-century medical document on which Yi's cases 1–10 elaborate, it may have recorded mostly monosyllabic names, as do the early medical manuscripts: *ju* 疽 (abscess); *qi ge* 氣鬲 (*qi* is blocked); *shan* 疝 (amassment); perhaps *shui re* 水熱 (water is hot); *dan* 癉 (condition of overexertion); *xiao* 消 (wasting); perhaps *jia* 瘕 (conglomerations); *dong* 迵 (the void); *jue* 厥 (numbness); *qi zhi fu* 氣之腹 (*qi* went to the abdomen). This hypothetical list of names was obtained by a very rigorous application of text structure semantics, which made minimal allowances for *variatio*, and imputed meaning into very slight differences in wording. The method produced reassuring findings insofar as the constituents subtracted out of the polysyllabic names showed recurrent features. They included body parts (such as the lungs, spleen and kidneys) that are non-deictic (as are e.g. 'the interior' or 'the above'); *qi* in the function of a semantic categoriser[17] (in cases 4 and 15); and for non-negligent reasons also 'wind' (in cases 8, 5 and 9).

---

[15] The named *bing* in the MWD and ZJS manuscripts are generally not written with the 104th radical. They mention neither viscera nor *qi*; seeming exceptions are debatable.

[16] See discussion of cases 3 (line 2) and 9 (line 3).

[17] 'Semantic categorisers' are 'elements [in a word] which indicate a general category' (Cruse 1986:33).

The 'cause' of the disorder

The phrase 'the illness is contracted by' introduces statements referring to what is here called 'cause of the disorder', although Yi himself does not use a term for 'cause'; *de* literally means 'to get, to attain'. In general, Yi mentions long-term circumstances that facilitated the emergence of a disorder, except in two cases which concern accidents (cases 4 and 21).[18] He points out, in particular, bad habits such as indulging in 'sexual intercourse' (*nei* 內), rendered here as 'women' in awareness that the term does not imply sexual orientation, and 'alcoholic beverages' (*jiu* 酒), rendered here as 'wine' because of their implications for rank and status, although Han fermentation technology probably produced a sort of millet beer.[19]

Yi's ideas of causation come close to other ancient nosologies and aetiologies as, for instance, to the ancient Greek *aitia*. Lloyd comments: 'Thus before *aitia* came to be used generally in the sense of "cause", it meant responsibility or blame, and the meaning of *to aition* is equivalent to "that which is responsible".' Physical causation is 'derived from the sphere of human responsibility'.[20] This understanding of 'cause' that comes close to 'blame' applies to all twenty-five case histories. The *Shi ji* personage Yi invariably makes his clients' conduct responsible for their medical disorders.

Considering that what here is called 'cause' comes close to 'blame', one cannot overlook that wine and/or women are blamed in eight out of the first ten cases, and that this points to debauchery. If cases 1–10 elaborate on an early medical document, it would be the historical figure Yi who bore a grudge against the nobility of Qi. If Sima Qian found this appealing for his own non-medical agenda, why would he have added the following fifteen cases, which blame wine and/or women in only five (see table 3) and barely concern Qi nobility (see table 1)? Was his, after all, not that keen a critique or were cases 11–25 added later, by one or several Han editors/commentators, well after his death?

The most frequently mentioned ecological cause is 'wind',[21] but it is mentioned in the text structural slot for 'causes' only in cases 11–25 and not as a 'cause' in cases 1–10. Interestingly, it is always given in combination with another 'cause' that blames the patient's conduct. Considering that wind is never mentioned on its own, the clauses on wind aetiologies which clearly allude to the body ecologic may have been later interjected. In this context, it is worth noting that cases 4 and 15 stand out for their body ecological illness aetiologies (perhaps due to later editorial or commentatorial

---

[18] The cause in case 17 is a habit, 'being fond of picking up heavy things' (*hao chi zhong* 好持重), not an accident of picking up too heavy a thing.

[19] e.g. Schafer (1977:119–22), Poo (1999).   [20] Lloyd (1983:29).

[21] On wind in ancient China, see case 5, n. 31. See also discussion of cases 5 (line 3), 8 (line 4), 9 (line 3).

additions?). In case 4, the patient had an accident of falling into cold water in winter, in case 15 the slave who got ill had roasted by the fire, until he was dripping with sweat, and then exposed himself to wind.

'Perspiration' (*han* 汗) is mentioned four times as 'cause' for the illness, in cases 5, 9, 12 and 15. This is surprising for perspiration is generally taken as a sign or symptom of an illness rather than its cause. Did Chunyu Yi confuse cause and symptom? In case 25, perspiration is mentioned as a symptom: as a consequence of physical exertion. However, even there it can be interpreted as a cause: it triggers vomiting blood, which leads to death. In case 15, as seen above, the sweating, no doubt, is related to body ecological considerations, but in the other three cases it points in the direction of physical toil, not from tilling fields or playing ball games, but from overexertion of another kind: in case 9, Yi explains that the King of Jibei who suffers from a 'wind-induced numbness' had 'excessively entered his *yang*'. Here, the 'cause' of the disorder, given as 'sweating and lying prostrate on the ground' quite unambiguously hints at sexual intercourse. In case 12, the 'talented person' Shu 豎, who as already mentioned has as a name a word of abuse, does what the King of Jibei approves of (*wei suo shi* 為所是). 'Profuse sweating' (*liu han* 流汗) causes her illness. Also in case 5, although it concerns a queen dowager, 'profuse sweating' points in the direction of sexual pleasures. In this context, it is noteworthy that Yi mentions perspiration as a 'cause' of the disorder in the case of a king, the slave of that king, and a queen dowager, i.e. individuals of high standing; he spoke in a coded way.[22]

To summarise, the 'cause of the disorder' sometimes correlates with the 'name', and sometimes with the 'quality' of the disorder. It also correlates with many concomitantly mentioned complaints and manifestations of the illness. The correlations are often tenuous, and sometimes can only be made indirectly by comparison with later medical writings. However, since in thirteen of the twenty-five cases the cause is wine and/or women (inclusive of those inferred from profuse sweating), and since the 'name' of the disorder in these thirteen cases differs in each, the 'cause' clearly cannot have determined the 'name' of the disorder.

The 'quality' of the disorder

Apart from the 'name' and 'cause', there is a third aspect of *bing*, particularly in cases 1–10, that is marked by a recurrent clause, above approximated as 'quality of the disorder'. This aspect of the disorder is introduced by the standard phrase 'the means whereby I recognised XY's illness were that …'. The phrase clearly indicates that the name-determining aspect of the disorder was to be found in the information that followed. In cases 1–10

---

[22] See discussion of cases 5 (lines 8–9) and 9 (lines 8, 22).

the statement that follows is: 'When I examined the vessels/pulses...' (*zhen qi mai* 診其脈), or a variant. The same applies to cases 18–21 and 24–25.[23] In cases 15 and 17, the phrase 'the means whereby I recognised...' introduces a statement about colour. Evidently, the *Shi ji* personage Yi considered the investigation of both *mai* and 'colour' relevant for naming the disorder. His case histories thus provide further evidence in support of arguing that the examination of *mai* and *se* (colour) arose in closely related circles of medical learning.[24]

The formula 'the means whereby I recognised the illness of XY were...' opens up the second part of the case history, which is often longer than the first. One would expect that after stating that he pressed onto *mai*, Yi describes the experiences he has. Since he generally 'pressed onto' (*qie* 切) the *mai* and once 'stroked' (*xun* 循) them, it is likely that he reported on a tactile perception. He sometimes gives qualifications of *mai* in terms of *qi*, sometimes with static verbs, but not with similes. It has been difficult to determine where Yi's discussion of the 'quality of the disorder' ended, but detailed comparison highlighted four recurrent patterns for opening the following paragraph (see table 4).

In cases 1 and 2, Yi states the interrelation between *mai* and *qi* most clearly: he palpates the *mai*, he senses the *qi* coming from one of the viscera and he characterises the qualities of this *qi* with different verbs. This seems to imply that Yi's pulse diagnosis is directed at identifying (a) whence *qi* comes and (b) what kind of (tactile) qualities it has. As will be shown in detail for each of the cases 1–10, the location whence *qi* comes as well as its qualities, determine Yi's naming of the disorder, i.e. his diagnosis.

In summary, the twenty-five case histories of the *Shi ji* personage Yi present the notion of *bing* (disorder) as one which comprises repeatedly recorded aspects, namely the 'name', 'cause' and 'quality' of the disorder. Since cases 1–10 consistently report on the 'quality of the disorder' but not the others, these systematically investigated aspects of *bing* are unlikely to be merely the product of a creative editor and may have been mentioned already in the presumed medical document of the early second century on which cases 1–10 may well elaborate. Based on text structure semantics, we note that for Yi it is not the 'cause' of the disorder but its 'quality' which is essential for determining the 'name' of the disorder. It is elicited in cases 1–10 through examining *mai*. Yi's medical ideology is that 'synchronous signs', i.e. tactually felt pulse qualities, are essential for diagnosis, not 'causes' in the patient's past history.

---

[23] Case 22 concerns a dispute between two doctors, not a diagnostic procedure. In case 23, Yi says he examined the client but does not specify how.

[24] Case 22 refers to *se mai* 'colour and pulse' as method of diagnosis. Note identical terms for assessing their qualities. See ch. 3, n. 9 and n. 10; ch. 4, n. 28; and case 7, n. 106.

11
Case 1

Translation (*Shiki kaichû kôshô* 105, pp. 24–7)

1. Cheng, an Attending Secretary of Qi, himself said that he was ill; the head hurt.
2. Your servant, Yi, examined his *mai* and formally announced saying:
3. 'The illness of your Excellency is bad, I cannot speak about it.'
4. Then I went outside and solely informed Cheng's younger brother Chang <u>saying</u>:

Name:
5. 'This one is ailing from a *ju*-abscess.
6. It will erupt internally in the region of the intestines and stomach.
7. After five days, it will become a *yong*-clog swelling.
8. After eight days, he will vomit pus and die.'

Cause:
9. <u>Cheng's illness was contracted from</u> wine and women.

10. Cheng then died at the predicted time.

Quality:
11. <u>The means whereby I recognised</u> Cheng's illness were that
12. when your servant, Yi, pressed onto his *mai*,
13. I got *qi* [coming] from the liver.
14. The *qi* [coming] from the liver, despite being murky, was still.
15. This is a disorder of the interior being closed off.
16. The 'Model for the Study of Mai' ('Mai fa') says:

1. 齋侍御史成自言病頭痛
2. 臣意診其脈告曰
3. 君之病惡不可言也
4. 即出獨告成弟昌曰
5. 此病疽也
6. 內發於腸胃之間
7. 後五日當臃腫
8. 後八日嘔膿死
9. 成之病得之飲酒且內
10. 成即如期死
11. 所以知成之病者
12. 臣意切其脈
13. 得肝氣
14. 肝氣濁而靜
15. 此內關之病也
16. 脈法曰

120

17. 'In cases where the *mai* are elongated, yet strung

17. 脈長而弦

18. – if it is not [the *mai*] that alternates in accordance with the four seasons –

18. 不得代四時者

19. the host of the disorder resides in the liver.'

19. 其病主在於肝

20. When they [the *mai*] blend, then the passageways/channels govern the disorder.

20. 和 即經主病也

21. If they alternate, then the linking vessels are exuberant.

21. 代 則絡脈有過

22. In cases where, [while] the channels govern the disorder, they [the *mai*] blend,

22. 經主病和者

23. one's disorder is contracted in the sinews and the marrow.

23. 其病得之筋髓裡

24. In cases where, while alternating and being severed, the *mai* spout,

24. 其代絕而脈賁者

25. one's disorder is contracted from wine and women.

25. 病得之酒且內

26. <u>The means whereby I recognised that</u> after five days he would have a *yong*-clog swelling, and

26. 所以知其後五日而臏腫

27. that after eight days he would vomit pus and die, were that

27. 八日嘔膿死者

28. at the time when I pressed onto his *mai*,

28. 切其脈時

29. the minor *yang*, [at the place] where it begins, was alternating.

29. 少陽初代

30. In cases of the alternating, the passageways are in disorder.

30. 代者經病

31. If the disorder leaves, it overcomes the person,

31. 病去過人

32. the person then leaves [i.e. dies].

32. 人則去

33. When linking vessels govern the disorder –

33. 絡脈主病

34. at the time in question, the minor *yang*, [at the place] where it begins, was closed by one *fen* [degree],

34. 當其時 少陽初關一分

35. <u>hence</u> the interior was hot, but pus had not yet been emitted –

35. 故中熱而膿未發也

36. if it [the closure] reaches five *fen*, then it gets to the boundary of the minor *yang*,

36. 及五分 則至少陽之界

37. if it [the predicted time] reaches the eighth day, then one vomits pus and dies.

37. 及八日 則嘔膿死

38. <u>Hence</u>, when it [the closure] was above two *fen*, pus was emitted,

38. 故上二分而膿發

39. when it reached the boundary, there was a *yong*-clog swelling,

39. 至界而臃腫

40. when there was complete discharge, he died.

40. 盡泄而死

41. If heat rises, then it heats up the *yang*
    brightness and spoils the flowing links.
42. If the flowing links are agitated, then the nodes
    of the *mai* burst open.
43. If the nodes of the *mai* burst open, then the
    spoilage disperses.
44. <u>Hence</u> the links intermingled.
45. The hot *qi* had already wandered upward and
    upon reaching the head, agitated [it].
46. <u>Hence</u> the head hurt.

41. 熱上 則熏陽明爛流絡

42. 流絡動 則脈結發

43. 脈結發 則爛解

44. 故絡交

45. 熱氣已上行
    至頭而動
46. 故頭痛

Interpretation

Case 1 begins with the patient Cheng declaring himself ill with a headache
(line 1). After examining *mai* (line 2), Yi refuses to speak to the patient
himself (line 3),[1] but tells his brother Chang the name of the disorder (lines
4–5) and outlines its future course, which, as he prognosticates, will end in
death (lines 6–8). He then announces the cause of the disorder (line 9), and
states that his prognostication was verified (line 10). The remainder is
medical speculation (lines 11–46).[2]

For explaining how he recognised the disorder, Yi first reports in his own
vocabulary on the qualities of *mai* he felt (lines 11–15). He then quotes the
'Mai fa' (lines 16–19), comments on it in yet another vocabulary (lines 20–
21), indicative of endogenous versus exogenous aetiologies (lines 22–5),
and explains how he recognised the disorder in its progressed stage by
reporting on a pulse quality (lines 26–9) indicative of death (lines 30–32).
After slightly modifying what he stated earlier (lines 33–5), he details how
he knew the time span before death (36–40) and outlines bodily processes
that end in death (lines 41–4). The last stanza provides a rationale for the
headache (lines 45–6).

Critical evaluation of retrospective biomedical diagnoses

This study, which searches for internal coherence even within a text as
multilayered as Yi's case histories, elucidates medical reasoning by

---

[1] Yi cannot speak about it; because the condition is 'unspeakably' bad, as e.g. in *Shi ji* 67,
p. 2218, or because, for reasons of medical ethics, it is 'inappropriate' to inform a patient
about his lethal condition?
[2] Takigawa differentiates between the 'statement' (*an* 案) (lines 1–10) and an ensuing 'discussion' (*lun* 論) (lines 11–46); the latter concerns the 'quality of the disorder'. For the full
names and dates of specific commentators to Yi's Memoir, see chapter 8.

investigating the semantics and pragmatics of Yi's terminology, with a focus on sense relations (rather than referential meaning) and connotations (rather than denotations).[3] The aim is to understand the medical rationale that framed these case histories. Previously, researchers have been interested primarily in the empirical reality of Yi's medical cases and provided retrospective biomedical diagnoses. However, retrospective diagnoses are notoriously speculative and add little to the ancient medical rationale contained in cases 1–10. Nevertheless, I will critically review these diagnoses at the beginning of each case for two reasons. First, they reflect the state of the art when I began my studies on Yi's Memoir in 1986. Second, they continue to be cited in the secondary literature without having been critiqued by recent scholarship.

Given the wealth of detail in Yi's case histories, one can understand why anyone would be tempted to make retrospective diagnoses. In addition to Yi's declaration of name, pulse qualities and cause of the disorder, which are central to his medical rationale,[4] the case histories often outline what appear to be different stages of the illness and sometimes mention signs and symptoms. The latter do not have much significance within Yi's intellectual project but, as became apparent in discussion with clinicians,[5] these signs and symptoms are crucial for differential diagnoses in biomedicine.

With regard to case 1, Bridgman suggests a peritoneal abscess of unknown origin which opens into the intestinal tract (perhaps appendicitis or a perforating ulcer?),[6] a well-known condition in medical history before laparotomies. Lu & Needham add that the perforation was perhaps 'due to heavy ascarid infestation',[7] and the clinicians I consulted confirm that amoebic and other parasitic infections cannot be ruled out entirely. One could object that a patient suffering from a peritoneal abscess would vomit blood rather than pus. Interestingly, the research on text structure semantics, presented in what follows, suggests vomiting blood is implied in case 1. However, differential diagnosis cannot explain the patient's headache.

The name of the disorder

ju 疽 – abscess (line 5) and yong 癰 – clog (lines 7, 26 and 39) *Ju*-'abscesses' and *yong*-'clogs' are often used in a similar sense but they are not synonyms. Although the phonographic part of both ideographs depicts much the same phenomenon, an obstruction,[8] each is distinctive: the *ju* ideograph is derived

---

[3] See ch. 1, n. 25.

[4] These aspects of the disorder are introduced by three recurrent phrases (see p. 112), underlined in translation (see e.g. p. 120).

[5] Personal communications with Dr med. Dorin Ritzmann in Zurich (1995–2001), Dr med. Carsten Flohr (2000) and Prof. Jeffery Aronson MD at the University of Oxford (2005).

[6] Bridgman (1955:69).   [7] Lu and Needham (1967:232).   [8] Karlgren (1957:32, 305).

from the depiction of a phallic-shaped ancestral tablet and the *yong* ideograph from that of a moat.[9] The Mawangdui 'Recipes' have separate entries on 'Ju-Abscess Disorders' (*ju bing* 疽[疽]病) and 'Yong-Clogs' (*yong* 癰).[10] Canonical medicine tends to classify them as either *yin* or *yang* disorders, and contemporary Chinese medicine generally considers *ju* deep-seated abscesses and *yong* superficial boils, although *yong* can also arise internally and *ju* present externally.[11] None of these distinctions applies to Yi's Memoir, however.

In case 1, Yi names the disorder a *ju*-abscess; after five days, i.e. in a progressed stage, it will manifest as a *yong*-clog swelling.[12] This is in line with *Ling shu* 81, entitled 'Clogs and Abscesses' (Yong ju 癰疽), where *yong*-clogs are given as manifestations of disorders called *ju*-abscesses: 'If a *yong*-clog erupts at A, its name is a B-*ju*-abscess' ([*yong*] *fa yu A, ming yue B ju* [癰] 發於 A 名曰 B 疽).[13] Elsewhere, *Ling shu* 81 explicitly says they arise from a coagulation of blood, in a long sentence on the origin of *yong*-clog swellings: 'If noxious coldness stays inside the links and channels, then blood coagulates; if blood coagulates, then there is no passage through; if there is no passage through, then the defensive *qi* returns home to it [the blood, which is constructive *qi*], and is not able to repetitively do its turns; hence there is a *yong*-clog swelling' (*han xie ke yu jing luo zhi zhong ze xue se, xue se ze bu tong, bu tong ze wei qi gui zhi, bu de fu fan, gu yong zhong* 寒邪客於經絡之中 則血泣 血泣則不通 不通則衛氣歸之 不得復反 故癰腫).[14] *Ling shu* 81 provides a hint that the *yong*-clog swelling in case 1 may have arisen from a coagulation of blood, although case 1 is framed neither in a complementarity of *yin yang*, constructive and defensive *qi*, nor the hot and cold.

Ju-abscesses were not always superordinate to *yong*-clogs, as they are in case 1 and in the above quote from *Ling shu* 81. Takigawa quotes the lexicographic work *Shuo wen jie zi* (Discussing Patterns and Explicating Characters, short: *Shuo wen*) of 121 CE, which defines a *ju*-abscess as an aggravated *yong*-clog condition: 'A *ju*-abscess is an old (chronic) *yong*-clog' (*ju jiu yong ye* 疽久癰也]).[15] However, this *Shuo wen* definition does not

---

[9] Harper (1998:290) on *yong*: 'Etymologically the word connotes a "walled-up" place where pus collects.'

[10] For *ju*-abscesses, see MWD 'Recipes' (1985:57–9), Harper (1998:276–9), Ma (1992:532–46). A *ju yong* is mentioned among these in strip 273. For *yong*-clogs, see MWD 'Recipes' (1985:67–8), Harper (1998:290–3), Ma (1992:591–600).

[11] e.g. *Zhongyi dacidian* (1995:1289). See also Yu (1953:126–7).

[12] *Yong* 癰 is *yong* 癰. Taki Mototane refers to variant characters in HDNJSW 40, p. 82, and *Zhen jiu jia yi jing* 11.9, pp. 1787–8. The characters he mentions differ slightly from those in the editions consulted.

[13] *Ling shu* 81, p. 480.

[14] *Ling shu* 81, p. 480. A variant is: 'When blood coagulates, it does not wander about' (*xue se er bu xing* 血泣而不行).

[15] *Shuo wen* 7B, p. 30.

apply to case 1, while it does to case 22: the patient in case 22 is a doctor called Sui, who suffers from heat in the interior. Yi first predicts that Sui will develop a *yong*-clog. The two doctors then get into a dispute, and thereafter Yi predicts that after a hundred plus days Sui will develop a *ju*-abscess, which will erupt in the region of the collarbone and precipitate his death. Clearly, the *Shuo wen* definition that chronic *yong*-clogs become *ju*-abscesses applies to case 22, but not to case 1.

Why is there a discrepancy between cases 1 and 22? It is of course possible that Yi used the terms *ju* and *yong* interchangeably. However, since the *Shuo wen* definition does not apply to *ju*-abscesses in the Mawangdui 'Recipes' either,[16] it is more likely that case 22 alludes to a medical understanding of *ju*-abscesses in line with the *Shuo wen*, and case 1 to one in line with the Mawangdui 'Recipes'. Cases 1 and 22 would then elaborate on primary texts from related but distinctive medical sources. Case 1 would allude to an understanding of *ju*-abscesses of the third and early second centuries BCE, similar to that in the Mawangdui manuscripts from before 168 BCE, and case 22 to a later one.

Interrelations between *yong*-clogs, 'pus' (*nong* 膿) and 'swellings' (*zhong* 腫), as given in lines 7–8, are also documented in other Han texts. Thus, the *Shuo wen* gives *yong*-clogs as swellings: 'A *yong*-clog is a swelling' (*yong zhong ye* 癰腫也).[17] The Mawangdui 'Maifa' associates them with pus: 'If a *yong*-clog swelling has pus, then . . .' (*yong zhong you nong* 壅腫有膿).[18] This is much elaborated in *Ling shu* 81, after the above quote (on p. 124). 'The cold *qi* transforms into heat, if the heat overcomes [it], the flesh rots, if the flesh rots, then it becomes pus' (*han qi hua wei re, re sheng ze fu rou, rou fu ze wei nong* 寒氣化為熱 熱勝則腐肉 肉腐則為膿).[19] Towards the end of case 1, Yi says heat causes pus (line 35) without, however, explicitly speaking of an initial coldness. Throughout the twenty-five cases, whenever Yi mentions heat, he generally does not explicitly allude to a hot–cold complementarity; this is in contrast to the *Ling shu*.

Vomiting pus is lethal, as Yi states in lines 8, 27, 37; commentator Ando Koretora confirms this by citing the [*Zhu*] *bing yuan hou lun* of 610 CE: 'If one vomits blood with pus, one cannot be cured' (*ruo tu nong xue zhe, bu ke zhi ye* 若吐膿血者 不可治也]).[20] This medieval text speaks explicitly of blood with pus, in contrast to case 1 and *Ling shu* 81, which have only 'vomiting pus' (*tu nong* 吐膿). Perhaps in Han times the idiom 'vomiting pus' meant 'vomiting blood with pus'.

In summary, *ju*-abscesses and *yong*-clogs both designate obstructions. In case 1, the *ju*-abscess figures as a superordinate term: after five days it manifests as a *yong*-clog swelling, whence three days later pus erupts, which

---

[16] Harper (1998:276). [17] *Shuo wen* 7B, p. 30.
[18] MWD 'Maifa' (1985:17); *yong zhong* is fairly frequent in the *Inner Canon*.
[19] *Ling shu* 81, p. 480. [20] *Zhu bing yuan hou lun* 33.42, p. 954.

in light of medieval texts may have been understood as pus mixed with blood. *Yong*-clog swellings develop pus, according to the Mawangdui 'Maifa', the *Inner Canon* and Yi's case 1. They arise from a coagulation of blood according to *Ling shu* 81. Heat produces pus, according to *Ling shu* 81, as it does in case 1 (line 35). However, where the *Ling shu* 81 conceives of heat as a response to an initial coldness, Yi does not speak of either heat or coldness in the opening lines 1–15 and later speaks only of heat, in lines 35, 41, 45.

The 'Mai fa' pulses

In cases 1–10, Yi reports on some qualities of *mai* in an unusual vocabulary (lines 11–15), while others, particularly those in the 'Mai fa' (lines 16–19), are familiar. Perhaps the 'Mai fa' terms are familiar to us because they were recorded in texts which later became canonised, and therefore handed down to us, while the qualities of *mai* in the unusual vocabulary relate to a rationale of pulse diagnosis that has since fallen into oblivion and therefore is difficult to understand? The text reads as though Yi was comparing knowledge of two different lineages of medical learning, which is confirmed in section 4.1 of *Shi ji* 105 by Yi saying: 'I tabled the recordings' (*biao ji* 表籍) and 'compared them to those given in the "Mai fa"' (*he 'Mai fa'* 合脈法). In case 1 Yi mentions six qualities of *mai*. Each is discussed separately in what follows. I begin with the two most familiar ones from the 'Mai fa': 'being elongated' and 'strung'.

***chang* 長 – elongated (line 17)**   'Being elongated' (*chang*) is not one of the twenty-four standard pulses in *Mai jing* 1.1 of the third century CE,[21] but one of the twenty-eight standard ones in contemporary Chinese medicine, paraphrased as 'harmonious and relaxed/slack' (*he huan* 和緩).[22] According to *Su wen* 17, 'if it is elongated, then *qi* is in control' (*chang ze qi zhi* 長則氣治);[23] if *qi* is regular, the person is healthy. This *Su wen* paragraph contrasts the long and short, high and low pulses, introduced by the opening statement that *mai* are a receptacle for blood (quoted on p. 249). Thus, although the above quote refers to *qi*, it does so in a paragraph on blood. 'Being elongated' may have been considered synonymous to *huo/he* (mixed/harmonious) on line 20, a term that often qualified blood.

***xian* 弦 – strung (line 17)**   'Being strung' (*xian*) belongs among the standard pulses both in *Mai jing* 1.1 and contemporary Chinese medicine. It is typically indicative of an impairment of the liver, apart from being the pulse

---

[21] *Mai jing* 1.1, pp. 1–3.   [22] *Zhongyi zhenduanxue* (Deng 1984:67–8).
[23] *Su wen* 17, p. 50.

which patients present in spring (the season that correlates with the liver), even if they have no liver condition. Commentator Taki Motohiro cites *Mai jing* 3.1: 'The spring-liver-wood-king, if his pulse is elongated, yet strung and thin, is called an "even pulse"' (*chun gan mu wang, qi mai xian xi er chang, ming yue ping mai ye* 春肝木王 其脈弦細而長 名曰平脈也]).[24] This sentence implies much the same as the 'Mai fa' in line 18, namely that an 'elongated yet strung' pulse indicates a healthy state in spring. *Su wen* 18 provides furthermore a parallel for the 'Mai fa' in lines 17 and 19: 'If in spring the stomach [pulse] is slightly strung, it indicates evenness [health]; if much of it is strung and little of it is stomach, it indicates a disorder of the liver; if it is strung without any stomach, it indicates death' (*chun wei wei xian yue ping, xian duo wei shao yue gan bing, dan xian wu wei yue si* 春胃微弦曰平 弦多胃少曰肝病 但弦無胃曰死).[25] The liver function is typically more pronounced in spring; a slightly strung pulse in spring is unproblematic, but a strung pulse on its own is indicative of death.[26]

Precisely speaking, the 'Mai fa' pulse is 'elongated, yet strung' (*mai chang er xian*). In contemporary Chinese medicine, this 'pulse image' (*mai xiang* 脈象) indicates that 'liver *yang* has bounty, *yang* is abundant, and the inside hot' (*gan yang you yu, yang sheng, nei re* 肝陽有餘 陽盛內熱).[27] Although the terms 'liver *yang*' and '*yang* abundance' are not part of Yi's vocabulary,[28] one is tempted to interpret the 'Mai fa' pulses accordingly as indicative of the heat in the interior (line 35) that rises and heats up the '*yang* brightness' (line 41), processes mentioned in the latter part of case 1.

For elucidating Yi's reasoning in the first part of case 1 (lines 1–15), let us further explore the pulse quality *xian*. It sometimes designates a 'string', sometimes the quality of a stretched out string, 'strung'. *Su wen* 19 describes it as 'straight and elongated', as one would expect the tactile qualities of a string to be. However, the same passage also paraphrases *xian* as 'slippery, while being tender and soft, light and empty', which appears to be the attribute of springtime when the ten thousand things come into being: 'The Yellow Emperor asked: "The *mai* of springtime is like a string, what is a string like?" Qibo responded: "The *mai* of springtime is the liver, the east is wood, it is the means by which the ten thousand things come into being, hence the coming of its *qi* is slippery, while being tender and soft, light and empty; it is straight and elongated, hence you call it strung; if [a *mai*] goes against this one, there is disorder' (*Huangdi wen yue: chun mai ru xian, he ru er xian? Qibo dui yue: chun mai zhe gan ye, dong fang mu ye, wan wu*

---

[24] *Mai jing* 3.1, p. 68. Zhang Shoujie cites another *Mai jing* quote (not located): 'If the pulse is elongated yet strung, the illness resides in the liver' (*mai chang er xian, bing yu gan ye* 脈長而弦 病於肝也).

[25] *Su wen* 18, p. 54. Zhang Shoujie cites excerpts from *Su wen* 22, pp. 70–71.

[26] *Su wen* 18, p. 54.

[27] *Zhongyi zhenduanxue* (Deng 1984:68).

[28] 'Liver *yang*' does not occur in the *Inner Canon*, and the few instances of '*yang* abundance' in the *Huangdi nei jing*, p. 1392, have barely any resemblance with case 1.

zhi suo yi shi sheng ye, gu qi qi lai, ruan ruo qing xu er hua, duan zhi er chang, gu yue xian, fan ci zhe bing 黃帝問曰 春脈如弦 何如而弦 岐伯對曰 春脈者 肝也 東方木也 萬物之所以始生也 故其氣來 耎弱輕虛而滑 端直以長 故曰弦 反此者病).[29] The 'straight and elongated' parallels pulse qualities given in tactile similes elsewhere in *Su wen* 19: 'When the *mai* of the true liver arrives, it feels taut in the interior and exterior, as if one were stroking the blade of a knife, or vigorously resistant, as if one were pressing onto the string of a lute ...' (*zhen gan mai zhi, zhong wai ji, ru xun dao ren, ze ze ran, ru an qin se xian* 真肝脈至 中外急 如循刀刃 責責然 如按琴瑟弦).[30] 'Stroking a blade', 'pressing onto the string of a lute', 'being straight and elongated' all allude to a distinctive tactile experience. They seem unrelated to the other pulse quality of the liver in the above *Su wen* 19 quote, which is 'slippery, while being tender and soft, light and empty'.

Perhaps the two different ways in which *xian* is paraphrased reflect different conceptions of the liver? Recent text critical research allows us to consider the possibility that these two qualities may testify to different currents of medicine, within which different attributes of the liver were emphasised, although they are mentioned in one and the same sentence.[31] The quality of being 'slippery, while being tender and soft, light and empty' may allude to the principle of unfolding life of a liver that correlates with the season spring in the body ecological reasoning of canonical doctrine. The tactile quality of stringiness, however, alludes to another body conception, scrutinised in what follows.

Su wen 48 alludes to stringiness by attributing the quality of a 'strung rope' to the womb: 'If the *mai* arrives like scattered leaves, this indicates that the liver *qi* is becoming depleted ... if the *mai* arrives like a strung rope, this indicates that the essences of the womb are insufficient' (*mai zhi ru san ye, shi gan qi yu xu ye ... mai zhi ru xian lü, shi bao jing yu bu zu ye* 脈至 如散葉 是肝氣予虛也 脈至如弦縷 是胞精予不足也).[32] In *Su wen* 48 the 'strung rope' is an attribute of the womb, although 'being strung' is generally an attribute of the liver.

What do womb and liver have in common? The answer may be that in an architecturally known body the liver/womb occupied a position in the interior/centre of the body.[33] The womb was known to generate life, as was the season spring. Perhaps the season spring, which is the period when life unfolds, was therefore put in correlation with the liver in later body ecological writings.

---

[29] *Su wen* 19, p. 58.   [30] *Su wen* 19, p. 62.

[31] Compilers considered it their task to juxtapose 'undecided controversies' (Kovacs and Unschuld 1998:19). See also Keegan (1988) and Hsu (in press b).

[32] *Su wen* 48, p. 136.

[33] On the womb, see discussion of case 5 (line 3). In *Su wen* 79, p. 250, 'strung' is a quality of the minor *yang* and also of the major *yang* and *yang* brightness.

In summary, in the *Nei jing* and *Mai jing* the 'strung' pulse generally is indicative of either a disorder in the liver or the normal pulse of spring, as it still is today. However, in *Su wen* 48, 'being strung' is a quality of the womb. Perhaps the 'string' invoked the umbilical cord as a metonym of the womb or, rather, as an indexical sign in terms of C.S. Peirce's theory of signs, whose theory will be applied to the discussion of all pulse qualities in this study.[34] The liver, much like the womb, had reproductive functions in canonical doctrine. Perhaps the 'strung', initially an indexical sign of the womb, therefore became a pulse of the liver.

Further pulse qualities (lines 20–25 and 30–32)

huo or he 和 – blending or being harmonious (lines 20 and 22)   There is some controversy over the length of the 'Mai fa' quote. Commentator Taki Motokata considers lines 17–21 to constitute the 'Mai fa' quote, but I suggest that the 'Mai fa' quote discusses the 'elongated yet strung' pulse only, on lines 17–19. Lines 20–25 thematically form a unity; they concern the qualities 'blending' (*huo/he*) and 'alternating' (*dai*) and allude to bodily processes that take place in tubular structures. They seem to postulate a hierarchical relation between *jing* (passageways, channels) located inside the body and *luo mai* (linking vessels) on the body surface. Moreover, lines 22–5 discuss pulse qualities in the light of the cause of the illness. This is unusual, as with the exception of case 9, lines 18–19, and case 18, Yi generally does not do so.

The graph 和, pronounced *he,* often means 'to harmonise' in canonical medical texts, but here it probably should read *huo,* meaning 'to blend' or 'mix', as it does in early medical manuscripts.[35] Case 1 appears to report on a tension expressed in the idiom 'murky yet still' in Yi's vocabulary (line 14), 'elongated yet strung' in the 'Mai fa' (line 17), and 'blending' as opposed to 'alternating' (lines 20–21) in yet another pulse diagnostic terminology. Perhaps *huo* refers to a smooth 'blending', which in other contexts means 'harmonising' (*he*), and *dai* to an abrupt 'alternation' of two qualities of *mai*. Perhaps *huo/he* indicates a mildly pathological condition, as it potentially does in *Su wen* 74: 'When it [*qi*] is mixed, even it out; when it is violent, weaken it' (*huo zhe ping zhi, bao zhe duo zhi* 和者平之 暴者奪之).[36] Here *huo* is indicative of a less acute condition than either *bao* (violent) in *Su wen* 74 or *dai* in case 1.

'Blending' indicates that passageways/channels govern the disorder. That these are thought to be linked to the liver in case 1, much like the 'sinews' (*jin* 筋) correlate with the canonical liver, can be deduced from the following

---

[34] Peirce (1932), see ch. 21, pp. 351–3.   [35] For *huo* 和, see Zhang (2000:203).
[36] *Su wen* 74, p. 237; translation is based on the gloss by Nanjing zhongyi xueyuan (1991:639). On *duo* 奪 'to faint', 'to collapse', see case 6 (line 26).

Su wen statement that 'blending' is indicative of liver impairments, which commentator Zhang Shoujie quotes: 'If one contracts the illness from the sinews, it is the blending of the liver' (*de bing yu jin, gan zhi huo ye* 得病於 筋 肝之和也). Commentator Kaiho Gembi rightly remarks that this quote cannot be found in extant *Su wen* editions. However, it provides a rationale for why 'blending' indicates a disorder governed by the 'passageways/ channels' (line 20), originating in 'marrow and sinews' (lines 22–3), as it suggests that at one stage in Chinese medical history both were considered aspects of the liver.[37] This is supported by the finding that in *Ling shu* 64 (quoted on pp. 145–6) *huo/he* qualifies blood, which according to canonical doctrine is stored in the liver.[38]

***dai* 代 – alternating (line 21)**   The pulse quality *dai* occurs in cases 1, 6 and 7, and in all three the patient dies. It is one of the standard pulses of *Mai jing* 1.1, of which Zhang Shoujie quotes a variant: 'If it comes frequently, but inmidst [of the movement] comes to a halt, and as it cannot turn round on its own, therefore is repeatedly agitated, it is called intermittent. In cases of the intermittent, death occurs' (*lai shuo er zhong zhi, bu neng zi huan, yin er fu dong, ming yue dai, dai zhe si* 來數而中止 不能自還 因而復動 名曰代 代者死).[39] It is usually translated as 'intermittent' or 'regularly interrupted' in medicine,[40] but in line with its literal meaning 'to substitute' or 'represent',[41] it is in this study rendered as 'alternating'. In case 6 (lines 22–3), Yi explicitly says that *dai* refers to 'alternating' tactile qualities of two (or three) *mai* out of sync, and in case 1 Taki Motokata quotes *Su wen* 79, where *dai* unmistakenly refers to an 'alternation': 'If one *yin* and one *yang* alternate and are severed, this is *yin qi* reaching the heart [centre] . . .' (*yi yin yi yang dai jue, ci yin qi zhi xin* 一陰一陽代絕 此陰氣至心).[42] *Su wen* 79 speaks of an alternation of *yin* and *yang*.

Having said this, the medieval Wang Bing (fl. 762 CE) glosses *dai* as 'intermittent' in his comment to the above *Su wen* 79: 'As to the intermittently interrupted, while being agitated, it inmidst [of the movement] comes to a halt' (*dai jue zhe, dong er zhong zhi ye* 代絕者 動而中

---

[37] *jing zhu bing* is here taken as a topic in the phrase *jing zhu bing [mai] he zhe*, which itself is a topic. Compare with case 2 (line 19): *zhou shen re* is a topic in the phrase *zhou shen re mai sheng zhe*, which is also a topic.

[38] *Su wen* 62, p. 167, states 'the liver stores blood' (*gan cang xue* 肝藏血).

[39] Compare and contrast with *Mai jing* 1.1, p. 3. Zhang Shoujie quotes it in an attempt to explain *dai* in line 18, erroneously, since *dai* in line 18 is used in a different sense.

[40] e.g. Wiseman (1990).

[41] Taki Motohiro notes that *dai* 'to represent', 'to alternate in accordance with' (line 18) is not to be confused with *dai* 'alternating' (line 21). This is further evidence for the 'Mai fa' ending with line 19.

[42] *Su wen* 79, p. 251, later states 'the disorder resides in the earth-spleen' (*bing zai tu pi* 病在 土脾). This suggests the body architectural *xin* was a space that later the canonical spleen and stomach inhabited. See also *Shuo wen* 10B, quoted on p. 162.

止也).[43] Wang Bing reads *dai jue* as a compound word. Given that Yi juxtaposes *dai* and *jue* 絕 (to be severed, to stop) in case 1 (line 24),[44] and says *dai* is indicative of a severance in case 6 (line 23), one wonders whether he may have used *dai* in the sense of 'intermittent' after all. An intermittent pulse is today indicative of 'depletion patterns' (*xu zheng* 虛證),[45] much in line with *Su wen* 17: 'If it [the pulse] is 'intermittent', then *qi* is weakened' (*dai ze qi shuai* 代則氣衰).[46]

Yi always mentions *dai* towards the end of a case history, as in case 7 or at the end of the first part of cases 1 (lines 1–32) and 6 (lines 1–24). In the second part of cases 1 and 6 the illness eventually ends in an affection of the *yang* brightness and death due to *yang* excess (rather than in a state of depletion). One could argue that the second parts of cases 1 and 6 were added by a creative commentator/editor who had little understanding for the conditions described in the first parts (which is not impossible). However it be, the *Shi ji* personage Yi considers *dai* indicative of death due to either weakness and wasting or excess and heat. Therefore, *dai* in canonical texts is here translated as 'intermittent' (and by implication weak), but not *dai* in Yi's narrative.

The above interpretation of *dai* as indicative of patterns of exuberance builds on Kaiho Gembi's remark that *mai* that 'alternate and are severed, yet nevertheless spout' (line 24) reflect that 'linking vessels are exuberant' (line 22).[47] To be sure, Kaiho Gembi may have made this remark to stress that *dai* is indicative of disordered 'linking vessels', rather than of exuberance. Ando Koretora certainly did so, when he quoted *Ling shu* 48: 'If it is intermittent, then take the blood-links' (*dai ze qu xue luo* 代則取血絡)[48] and *Su wen* 20 (quoted on p. 44). Evidently, the Japanese commentators considered *dai* indicative of disorders in the 'linking vessels on the body surface'.

However, in canonical texts, *dai* also indicates disorders in the bodily interior. For instance, in the above *Su wen* 20 quote the 'interior/central part' (*zhong bu*) is described in a wording similar to that for 'alternating' in case 6 (line 22), and as will be shown (on pp. 253–4), also elsewhere in the *Inner Canon*. In a similar vein, the pulse of the centrally positioned spleen is said to be intermittent in *Su wen* 23: 'The pulse of the spleen is intermittent' (*pi mai dai ye* 脾脈代也), and in *Ling shu* 4 the pulse of the yellow, which is the colour of spleen and stomach: 'As to the yellow, its

---

[43] HDNJSW 79, p. 199.

[44] The compound word *dai jue* hints at a possible medieval date of lines 22–5.

[45] *Zhongyi zhenduanxue* (Deng 1984:69–70).

[46] *Su wen* 17, p. 50.

[47] Kaiho Gembi considers this phrase synonymous with *dai* in case 6 (line 22). See also Osobe Yô (1994:66–7).

[48] *Ling shu* 48, p. 397. 'Links' evidently contained blood (see p. 144).

pulse is intermittent' (*huang zhe, qi mai dai* 黃者 其脈代).[49] Evidently, *dai* is also indicative of disorders in the interior.

In line with the above canonical medical texts, and contrary to the Japanese commentators' viewpoint, Yi reports that, at the time when he pressed onto *mai*, the minor *yang* was 'alternating' (lines 28–9), at the place where it begins (*chu*),[50] and since this is later interpreted as meaning that the minor *yang* was then closed by one *fen* (line 34), which is indicative of the interior being hot (*zhong re*; line 35), the minor *yang* must have connected to the body's interior (*zhong*).

This precipitates questions over the connotations of the 'interior/centre' (*zhong*). In discussion of the 'strung' pulse, liver and womb were suggested to be located centrally inside the architectural body (pp. 127–9), in discussion of the 'alternating' pulse in *Su wen* 79 in the body architectural heart (p. 130) and in *Su wen* 23 in the canonical spleen (p. 131), and now, in case 1 (lines 34–5), the minor *yang* appears to be connecting to the interior: is this not a contradiction? The answer to this must be that at an early stage in Chinese medical history the bodily interior was a fairly undefined body architectural space, in some contexts inhabited by the liver/womb, in others by the heart/lungs. It was only in canonical doctrine that five well-defined interdependent viscera occupied the interior. The spleen was probably the last of the five to be canonised (see p. 133) and, interestingly, took on the most central position.

In summary, the pulse quality *dai* consistently indicates death, in Yi's Memoir, and likewise in canonical and contemporary medicine. Its standard translation is 'regularly interrupted', which indicates depletion. However, in Yi's cases 1 and 6, *dai* is also mentioned in a context of death due to exuberance and heat, and therefore it is translated as 'alternating'. While Japanese commentators consider *dai* indicative of disorders in the linking vessels on the body surface, it is obvious from both Yi's cases and canonical texts that *dai* also indicates disorders in the body's interior.

Finally, a further problem needs to be highlighted. Yi once says *dai* indicates that 'linking vessels are exuberant' (*luo mai you guo*; line 21), once that 'passageways are in disorder' (*jing bing*; line 30). To solve this seeming contradiction, the notion of *jing* (passageways, channels) and related concepts need to be examined.

bing zhu 病主 – **the host of the disorder (line 19)**   The 'Mai fa' phrase *bing zhu zai gan* 病主在肝 (line 19) comes close to *gan zhu bing* 肝主病 in contemporary medicine, which generally is translated as: 'The liver governs the disorder'. However, *zhu* 主 need not necessarily be a verb and could be a

---

[49] *Su wen* 23, p. 76, and *Ling shu* 4, p. 276.
[50] *chu* 初 can be noun or verb 'to begin'. Kaiho Gembi takes it as a noun: 'the place where the *shao yang* vessel begins' (*shao yang chu wei* 少陽初位). See *tai yin shi* on pp. 68–9 and *kou* in case 3 (lines 14, 16) and case 3, n. 62.

noun: 'The governor of the disorder resides in the liver', 'the governor of the liver is ill'. The noun *zhu* meaning 'governor' would then refer to an administrative function within the body politic. Paul Unschuld, in particular, emphasises administrative metaphors of Han medicine.[51] Yet *zhu* also means 'host' and *bing zhu* may have had more religious connotations.[52] Just as ancestor tablets are hosts to ancestors, body parts may have been hosts to illnesses. This understanding of *zhu* as 'host' would emphasise continuities between sickness and ancestors, ghosts and demons, and their movements and erratic presence among humans.

In case 1, *bing zhu* (the host of the disorder) is said to reside in the liver, in case 2 in the heart, in case 5 in the kidneys, and in case 10 in the lungs. It may not be coincidence that Yi mentions the 'host of the disorder' with regard to four viscera only, and not with regard to the fifth, the spleen. The concept *bing zhu* may have been grounded in a demonological understanding of illness causation, prominent in pre-Imperial China, which lost in importance during the Han, at the time when the spleen became one of the five viscera.[53]

jing zhu bing 經主病 and *jing bing* 經病 – the channels govern the disorder and the passageways are in disorder (lines 20, 22, 30)

After speaking of *zhu* (host, governor) as a noun in the 'Mai fa' (line 19), Yi mentions it again in the following stanzas, as a verb or noun, probably rather a verb, in the idioms *jing zhu bing* (line 20) and *luo mai zhu bing* (line 33), meaning 'the channels govern the disorder' and 'the linking vessels govern the disorder'. The idea that *jing* and *luo* (channels and links) are bodily entities known primarily through their function of 'governing' (*zhu*) has striking parallels with *Ling shu* 3: 'Skin, flesh, sinews and *mai*, each has its place, but speaking of channels and links, each has that which it governs' (*pi rou jin mai, ge you suo chu zhe, yan jing luo, ge you suo zhu ye* 皮肉筋脈 各有所處者 言經絡 各有所主也]).[54] Skin and flesh, sinews and *mai* allude to an architectural body within which they occupy certain locations, while channels and links are known primarily through their function within the body politic.

Yi also speaks of *jing bing* (line 30). He thus mentions two idioms, *jing zhu bing* and *jing bing*. Unless one assumes that *jing zhu bing* and *jing bing* have different meanings, the text contains blatant contradictions.[55] One

---

[51] Unschuld (1985). See also Despeux and Obringer (1997:32–3).

[52] Machle (1992:377).

[53] For liver, heart and kidneys, see p. 62, for the lungs, see case 10 (line 3). For further evidence that the spleen was the fifth and last viscus to be added to the above four, see Hsu (2007b).

[54] *Ling shu* 3, p. 273.

[55] In lines 20–21, 'blending' indicates that *jing zhu bing* (and 'alternating' that the 'linking vessels are exuberant'), but in line 30 'alternating' indicates *jing bing*. This suggests *jing zhu bing* and *jing bing* have distinct if not opposite meanings. Note furthermore, *jing zhu bing* indicates that a, say, congenital illness has been contracted in the sinews and marrow which is not lethal (lines 22–3), but *jing bing* is a terminal disease (lines 30–2).

could of course say that *jing bing* is part of an interpolated phrase that makes no sense (lines 30–32), as does Kaiho Gembi.[56] He suggests the statement 'in cases of the alternating' (*dai zhe*; line 30) ends with 'the linking vessels govern the disorder' (*luo mai zhu bing*; line 33), a statement which would parallel line 21: 'If they alternate, then the linking vessels are exuberant'. However, *jing bing* is also mentioned in case 6 (line 19), in a comparable context of medical reasoning. Moreover, it parallels the idiom 'the passageways are in disarray' (*jing luan*) in the Dunhuang manuscript P3287 discussed on p. 43, which has striking parallels to case 1. It makes more sense to read line 30 as an intact text. Lines 31–2 may have been interjected by a commentator to elucidate line 30 such that, in the extant text, lines 30–32 form one stanza on one theme: death.

The above contradictions can be solved by suggesting that the notion *jing* was used in different senses in lines 20–25 and 30–32, say, in a narrow sense in line 22, and in a wide one in line 30. Perhaps it should be translated as 'channels' and 'passageways' respectively. Thus, *jing* on line 22 in the clause *jing zhu bing* (the channels govern the disorder) is an opposite of *luo mai* (linking vessels), as it is in canonical texts.[57] It is used in a narrower sense than *jing* on line 30 in the clause *jing bing* (the passageways are in disorder). When the passageways are in disorder, a disorder may (a) transition from one body part to another, perhaps in a passageway deep inside the body (case 6, line 19) and (b) affect the linking vessels on the body surface, which perhaps were conceived of as a subordinate aspect of the superordinate passageways (cases 1 and 6).[58] This interpretation, which postulates that *jing* was used once in the narrow sense of canonical 'channels' and once in the wide sense of pre-canonical 'passageways' in stanzas of presumably different textual provenance, if not time periods, dissolves the contradictions.

---

[56] Case 1, lines 30–2, *jing bing bing qu guo ren ren ze qu* 經病病去過人人則去, make no sense to Kaiho Gembi, but Osobe Yô (1994:78) points to *Su wen* 20, pp. 64–6, and to the *Cha bing zhi nan* 察病指南 (not located). He comments: 'If that which governs the disorders of the twelve channels has left the human realm and reached the heavenly realm, one calls it "man then left"' (*shi er jing suo zhu zhi bing qu guo ren bu zhi tian bu wei zhi ren ze qu* 十二經所主之病去過人部至天部謂之人則去). The heavenly realm is the heart; heart and liver are separated from each other by five *fen* (see case 6, line 44).

[57] In *Su wen* 62, p. 170, and *Ling shu* 81, p. 286, the 'tiny, second-generation vessels' (*sun mai* 孫脈), 'linking vessels' (*luo mai* 絡脈) and 'channels' (*jing mai* 經脈) stand in a hierarchical relation to each other; from small to large, from outside to inside.

[58] *jing* 經 can be understood either way in line 20. As the text reads now, lines 20 and 21 form a duplet, and *jing* 經 accordingly means 'channels' as opposed to 'linking vessels', but note irregularity in grammatical construction (the particles *ji* 即 and *ze* 則). Perhaps line 20 once stood on its own, reading *huo ji jing bing* 和即經病, where *jing* referred to 'passageways', which like 'sinews' were considered an aspect of the liver.

Text structure semantics

Applied to Yi's case histories, text structure semantics postulates that the pulse qualities given in his vocabulary, which are introduced by the phrase 'the means whereby I recognised the illness', each correlate with one of the constituents in the name of the disorder, which is mentioned after the phrase 'I said'. This means '*qi* [coming] from the liver' (line 13) should explain why Yi named the disorder a '*ju*-abscess' (line 5). In the first instance, such a correlation seems implausible, but as we will see, it starts making sense if one develops a body architectural understanding for the liver, which likens it to the centrally located womb with reproductive capacities.

zhuo 濁 – **murky (line 14)** 'Being murky' (*zhuo*) is often contrasted with 'being clear' (*qing* 清), and seems primarily to have referred to the quality of water, as for instance in the *Shi jing*: 'Look at that spring water, now it is clear, now it is muddied' (*xiang bi quan shui, zai qing zai zhuo* 相彼泉水載清載濁).[59] It is an opposite not only of 'being clear', but also of 'being cool'. *Ling shu* 40 states: 'The clear fills the *yin*, the murky fills the *yang*' (*qing zhe zhu yin, zhuo zhe zhu yang* 清者注陰 濁者注陽).[60] Probably, *qing* that fills *yin* means 'clear' as well as 'cool', as the term *yin* implies the cool and lowly. This is reinforced by *Ling shu* 34: 'Cool/clear *qi* resides in the *yin*, murky *qi* in the *yang*' (*qing qi zai yin, zhuo qi zai yang* 清氣在陰 濁氣在陽).[61] *Ling shu* 1 also underlines this: 'Now whenever *qi* resides in the *mai*, the noxious *qi* resides above, the murky *qi* resides in the middle, and the cool *qi* resides below' (*fu qi zhi zai mai ye, xie qi zai shang, zhuo qi zai zhong, qing qi zai xia* 夫氣之在脈也 邪氣在上 濁氣在中 清氣在下).[62] Cool/clear *qi* with its *yin* qualities resides below; murky *qi* is an attribute of the centre.

In the Mawangdui texts, 'murky' does not occur on its own but always as 'murky *yang*'. Thus, the Mawangdui 'Quegu' states: 'The murky *yang* blackens the four directions and clogs them up, it is the heavens' chaotic *qi*; when the sun rises, it becomes XY and misty' (*zhuo yang zhe, hei si sai, tian zhi luan qi ye, ji ri chu er X [wu] ye* 濁陽者 黑四塞 天之亂氣也 及日出而 x [霧] 也).[63] We note that the first clause *hei si sai* associates the 'murky

---

[59] *Shi jing*, '*Xiao ya*', 'Si yue' 四月, 13 (1), 462c. Translation based on Karlgren (1957:156). See also Roth (1991:616) and Graham (1986:22, 32) on *qing* and *zhuo* in Chinese cosmology.
[60] *Ling shu* 40, pp. 376–7.   [61] *Ling shu* 34, p. 365.   [62] *Ling shu* 1, p. 265.
[63] MWD 'Quegu' (1985:85). Compare and contrast with Harper (1998:308). In *Su wen* 5, p. 22, by contrast, 'being clear' is *yang*: 'The clear *yang* rises to heaven, the murky *yin* returns to the earth' (*qing yang shang tian, zhuo yin gui di* 清陽上天 濁陰歸地). See also *Su wen* 5, p. 19. On its p. 18, cold is associated with *zhuo*, and hot with *qing*! This inversion of *yin yang* qualities attributed to *zhuo* and *qing* parallels that mentioned in the introduction in *Su wen* 66, p. 182, and 5, p. 18, quoted on p. 34 and p. 37, n. 47. To understand why and how this inversion of *yin yang* occurred in medical history is beyond the scope of this study.

yang' with the colour black and the process of clogging up; the second speaks of the rising sun that makes it misty, presumably by heating it up.

In *Ling shu* 39, 'murky', in association with the colour black, describes a quality of blood: 'How is it that in small quantities blood becomes black and murky? ... *Yang qi* accumulates, and if after resting for a long time, it is not discharged, its blood becomes black and murky, hence it cannot spurt forth' (*xue shao hei er zhuo zhe, he ye? ... yang qi xu ji, jiu liu er bu xie zhe, qi xue hei er zhuo, gu bu neng she* 血少黑而濁者 何也... 陽氣畜積 久留 而不寫者 其血黑而濁 故不能射).[64] In *Ling shu* 38, 'murky' is an attribute of blood: 'If blood is murky and *qi* rough, and you swiftly discharge it, then the channels can connect' (*xue zhuo qi se, ji xie zhi, ze jing ke tong ye* 血濁 氣濇 疾寫之 則經可通也).[65] *Ling shu* 38 explicitly states 'blood is murky' (*xue zhuo*).

The Mawangdui 'Shiwen' furthermore mentions 'murky *yang*' in the context of speaking of the season spring: 'In spring avoid murky *yang*' (*chun bi zhuo yang* 春避濁陽).[66] It recommends avoiding the 'murky *yang*' then. Is it because the murky *yang* was thought 'to blacken and clog up the four directions', as in the Mawangdui 'Quegu', or because murky *yang* was associated with exuberance and rising heat? After all, the Mawangdui 'Quegu' speaks of it 'becoming misty' and case 1 mentions a 'rising heat' (lines 41–6). Whereas in canonical doctrine, blood has nutritive *yin*-qualities, perhaps the blood that rises in Yi's case 1 was conceived of as thick, hot and red? The rising murky *yang* blood thus would contrast with the water valued for its *yin*-qualities, i.e. its transparency, coolness, stillness and tendency to flow downward.[67]

Blood thus emerges as a key concept for explaining the pathological processes in case 1: it either clogs up, gets black and turns into a *ju*-abscess (lines 1–15) or, as it heats up, rises and is vomited, mixed with pus, triggers death (lines 33–46). When Yi says *qi* coming from the liver was 'murky', he probably had the 'murky *yang*' in mind, as known from the Mawangdui texts, not the 'murky *yin*' of medieval and later medicine. However, considering that in case 1 'being murky' is an attribute of liver *qi*, in cases 2 and 9 of heart *qi*, and in case 4 of kidney (or lung) *qi*, one starts wondering whether the 'murky' pulse was throughout thought to indicate disordered blood dynamics, since neither heart nor kidneys are as closely associated with them as the liver.[68] It therefore makes more sense to assume that in case 1 the pulse quality indicative of blood, which can coagulate to

---

[64] *Ling shu* 39, p. 374.   [65] *Ling shu* 38, p. 373.
[66] MWD 'Shiwen' (1985:147).   [67] e.g. *Laozi*, p. 316 and Lau (1963:128).
[68] The kidneys, which only arguably are mentioned in early texts (see case. 6, n. 100), certainly are not associated with blood in canonical doctrine (see case 4, line 35, and ch. 7, n. 29). The heart was in pre-dynastic China the seat of all emotion and cognition; in early medicine, accordingly, processes in the heart involved *qi* dynamics but in canonical and, particularly, contemporary medicine, they allude to blood dynamics.

form a *ju*-abscess, is '*qi* [coming] from the liver', a liver understood as blood depot.

The question then arises as to why 'being murky' qualifies the liver, heart and kidneys in cases 1, 2, 4 and 9. Interestingly, whenever 'murky' is mentioned, Xu Guang points out variant graphs in other editions: *meng* 眲 'clogged up' or *meng* 猛 'fierce, abrupt'. Perhaps *meng* was replaced by 'being murky'; perhaps due to a Han editor/commentator who conceived of it as 'murky *yang*' and considered the cases in question to concern *yang* and/or heat dynamics? Another possibility is that in contrast to the canonical body ecologic, where 'spleen and stomach' occupy the centre of the body, the architectural body accommodated within its internal/central space all viscera, 'murky' being indicative of any visceral disorder in the centre/interior of the body.

Several canonical passages suggest that 'murky' *qi* is produced by centrally located body parts, such as the above-quoted *Ling shu* 1, and also *Ling shu* 3: 'As to murky *qi* residing in the centre: one says that after all the water and grains have entered the stomach, their refined *qi* rises and pours into the lungs, while the murky *qi* flows downward into the intestines and stomach; one says that if the cold and warm are not adjusted, and one drinks and eats irregularly, the illness arises in the intestines and stomach, hence one calls it "murky *qi* resides in the centre"' (*zhuo qi zai zhong zhe, yan shui gu jie ru yu wei, qi jing qi shang zhu yu fei, zhuo liu yu chang wei, yan han wen bu shi, yin shi bu jie, er bing sheng yu chang wei, gu ming yue zhuo qi zai zhong ye* 濁氣在中者 言水穀皆入于胃 其精氣上注于肺 濁溜于腸胃 言寒溫不適 飲食不節 而病生于腸胃 故命曰 濁氣在中也).[69] *Ling shu* 3 locates 'murky *qi*' in the central region of the 'intestines and stomach'.

Incidentally, case 1 (line 6) mentions the region of the 'intestines and stomach' as the place where the *ju*-abscess erupts. However, according to text structure semantics not the centrally positioned 'intestines and stomach' but the stanza introduced by the phrase 'the means whereby I recognised that Cheng was ill were that ...' is expected to be indicative of it, namely '*qi* coming from the liver'. If 'murky' *qi* comes from a central body part, and liver *qi* is 'murky', the liver of case 1 presumably occupies the bodily 'interior/centre' (*zhong*). The minor *yang* seems to connect to it in lines 34–5. By contrast, the canonical liver is located in the 'abdomen' (*fu* 腹), often the 'small abdomen' (*xiao fu* 小腹) or 'minor abdomen' (*shao fu* 少腹), and connects to the 'dull *yin*' (*jue yin* 厥陰).[70] Thus, 'strung' rather than 'murky' is the canonical liver pulse, and while the canonical liver of the 'Mai fa' (lines 17–19), which is body ecologically comprehended, has

---

[69] *Ling shu* 3, p. 273. On stomach and *zhuo qi*, see furthermore *Ling shu* 4, p. 275. See also *Ling shu* 40, p. 376: 'In the case of receiving grains, it is murky, in the case of receiving *qi*, it is clear' (*shou gu zhe zhuo, shou qi zhe qing* 受穀者濁 受氣者清).

[70] *Ling shu* 10, p. 305.

as a main attribute its correlation with spring, the liver Yi refers to in his own vocabulary (lines 13–14) is centrally located and in charge of blood dynamics.

This points again in the direction of conceiving of *gan* 肝 as liver/womb, a reproductive organ in charge of blood dynamics. Due to its location in the innermost bodily sphere, the womb was considered *yin* (see case 5, line 3), and this may explain why in canonical doctrine the liver connects to the 'dull *yin*'.[71] But it also has *yang*-qualities. In *Ling shu* 41, 'the liver is the minor *yang* within the *yin*' (*gan wei yin zhong zhi shao yang* 肝為陰中之少陽),[72] in *Su wen* 34, 'the liver has one [degree of] *yang*-qualities' (*gan yi yang ye* 肝一陽也), while the heart 'has two [degrees of] *yang*-qualities' (*er yang* 二陽).[73] In *Su wen* 34, the liver's one *yang*-quality may have reflected its position in the lower *yin* sphere of the architectural body, as opposed to the heart with two *yang*-qualities in the upper one. Perhaps, therefore, the body architectural liver was associated with the minor *yang* and the body architectural heart, chest and stomach region with *yang* brightness. While one can easily understand why the hidden liver/womb would take on dull *yin*-qualities, one wonders whence its *yang*-qualities come. Perhaps from its association with blood, conceived of as 'murky *yang*'?

jing 靜 **– still (line 14)**   Since *qi* coming from the liver is 'still despite being murky' (*zhuo er jing*), one may be inclined to believe that 'still' was conceived of as opposite of 'murky'. However, in canonical texts, 'clear' (*qing*) is associated with the *yin*-qualities of water and considered the opposite of 'murky',[74] and 'still' is often given as the opposite of 'agitated' (*dong* 動).[75] 'Being still' is a *yin*-quality of earth, 'agitated' a *yang*-quality of heaven. Thus, *Su wen* 67 notes that 'in cases where one resonates with earth, there is stillness' (*ying di zhe jing* 應地者靜), and speaks of the 'agitation and stillness of heaven and earth' (*tian di dong jing* 天地動靜).[76] Heaven moves, earth is still.

Yi, however, uses the term 'still' to describe a person's behaviour, as in case 22, when he speaks of 'observing a person's stillness and activity' (*can qi ren dong jing*), and in case 21, when he says: 'This person liked to be quiet on his own, he was not hurried' (*qi ren xi zi jing bu zao* 其人喜自靜不躁). In a similar vein, 'still' refers in *Su wen* 25 to a state of mind: 'With still attentiveness look out for the appropriate' (*jing yi shi yi* 靜意視義),[77] as it

---

[71] The 'dull *yin*' is the last of the twelve *mai* in *Ling shu* 10 and the innermost 'warp' in the *Shang han lun*.
[72] *Ling shu* 41, p. 379.   [73] *Su wen* 34, p. 99.
[74] Xu Guang points out an edition with *jing* 靜 (still) as *qing* 清 'clear'/'cool' as opposite to 'murky'.
[75] *jing* 靜 means 'not moving' (*bu huo dong* 不活動) says Taki Mototane.
[76] *Su wen* 67, p. 186.   [77] *Su wen* 25, p. 80.

does in *Su wen* 54: 'With a still mind observe the patient, without looking left nor right' (*jing zhi guan bing ren, wu zuo you shi ye* 靜志觀病人 無左右 視也).[78] In *Su wen* 5, 'still' is opposed to 'hurried', and expresses a *yin yang* complementarity: '*yin* is still, *yang* is hurried' (*yin jing, yang zao* 陰靜陽躁).[79] *Su wen* 23 contrasts 'still' with 'angry' (*nu* 怒).[80] This is worth noting insofar as in many medical texts, anger, rising *qi*, and *yang* abundance are attributes of the liver.[81]

In case 1, *qi* coming from the liver is 'murky yet still': Yi considers this indicative of a 'disorder of the interior being closed off' (*nei guan zhi bing*). In light of the above, it appears correct to assume that 'being murky' indicates that there is a disorder in the centre of the body and 'being still' that this disorder has not become generally manifest.

nei guan zhi bing 內關之病 – 'disorder of the interior being closed off' (line 15)

The term *nei guan zhi bing* does not occur in canonical doctrine and poses great problems to the commentators. Zhang Shoujie quotes *Nan jing* 3,[82] with Lü Guang's comment on it, which is that the area between the 'gate' *guan* 關 (at the wrist) and the *chi ze* 尺澤 (acupuncture *locus* on the elbow) is called *nei guan*. But Taki Motokata points out that *nei guan* is the name of a disorder and not an acupuncture *locus*.

Nei guan zhi bing is also the name of the disorder in case 15, and *guan nei zhi bing* in case 12. As Wang Niansun points out, all three cases end in death. Despite their different names, cases 12 and 15, which arise from a 'damaged spleen' (*shang pi*), have more in common. Case 1 concerns an impairment of the liver, heat in the centre, an afflicted minor *yang*, and a *yang* brightness that is heated up. There are also continuities. The liver in case 1 clearly occupied the interior of the architectural body, and the spleen in cases 12 and 15, which stand out for their affinity with canonical doctrine,[83] is the most central of the five canonical viscera. Case 1 probably alludes to a body conception that pre-dated those of cases 12 and 15.

Wang Niansun glosses *nei guan* as *nei bi* 內閉: 'The interior is closed off.' He seems to read *nei* as a noun and *guan* (to close off) as a verb. One could, of course, argue that *nei bi* is a noun meaning 'internal closure' but it would then designate a condition accompanied by dysuria, as in *Ling shu* 22: 'If there is an internal closure and one cannot urinate . . .' (*nei bi bu de sou* 內閉 不得溲 . . .)[84] or in the *Zhu bing yuan hou lun*: 'Then the small intestine [abdomen] is painful and there is an internal closure, the urine and the

---

[78] *Su wen* 54, p. 146.
[79] *Su wen* 5, p. 18. See also *Su wen* 43, p. 122, quoted on p. 228, and *Ling shu* 23, p. 340, quoted on p. 322.
[80] *Su wen* 23, p. 75.   [81] e.g. *Su wen* 5, p. 21.
[82] *Nan jing* 3 (Unschuld 1986a:91, 96).   [83] See p. 23.
[84] *Ling shu* 22, p. 338. See also *Zhen jiu jia yi jing* 9.10, p. 1622.

faeces do not pass through [i.e. one cannot relieve oneself]' (*ze xiao chang [fu] tong nei bi, da xiao bian bu tong* 則小腸[腹]痛 內閉 大小便不通).[85] The idiom *nei bi* can also be an adverb-verb compound, as in *Su wen* 3: 'Internally it causes closure of the nine openings' (*nei bi jiu qiao* 內閉九竅).[86] Despite these examples, there is little doubt Wang Niansun means that *bi* in *nei bi*, and accordingly *guan* in *nei guan*, should be read as a verb.[87]

Nevertheless, *guan* is used as a noun in medical and meditation literature. In *Shen jian* 3, for instance, *guan* refers to a body part: 'Two *cun* [from] the navel is called *guan*' (*lin ji er cun wei zhi guan* 鄰隮二寸謂之關).[88] The noun *guan* designates the transverse bolt with which one locks a door, and may have alluded to a similarly transverse structure in the body. Finally, the noun *guan* also means '[mountain] pass' and accordingly it has been proposed that the landscape of the body drew on the geographical imagery of the region 'inside the passes' (*guan nei*) around the capital Chang'an.[89] This is a fanciful idea, and no evidence is given in its support. Moreover, why should the landscape of Qin have provided metaphorical imagery for a medical lineage in the culturally much more prestigious kingdom of Qi?

More importantly, various texts in the *Inner Canon* and *Mai jing*, which may have elaborated on the notion of *nei guan zhi bing* in case 1, invoke the same architectural imagery as *Shen jian* 3, and not a landscape metaphor. They allude to the conditions of the 'outside lock and inside trestle' (*wai guan nei ge* 外關內格) and the 'inside lock and outside trestle' (*nei guan wai ge* 內關外格),[90] where conditions of *guan* and *ge* are said to arise from an imbalance of *yin* and *yang*.[91] Taki Motokata suggests case 1 concerns such a *yin yang* imbalance. However, Yi does not appear to reason in *yin yang* complementarities in the first part of case 1, and in the end speaks only of a *yang* pathology, namely a rising heat that affected the *yang* brightness.

---

[85] *Zhu bing yuan hou lun* 14.4, p. 456. *Nei bi* is currently not used as a technical term, but *long bi* 癃閉 combines features attributed to *long* and *nei bi* in the *Nei jing*. See *Zhongyi neike* (Zhang 1985:239–44).

[86] *Su wen* 3, p. 12.

[87] Quoting line 34, Kaiho Gembi also considers *guan* 'to close' a verb like *guan* of *nei guan zhi bing*.

[88] *Shen jian* 3, p. 17 (Catherine Despeux 1995, p. c.).

[89] Watson (1961:1.23 nn. 7 and 25) mentions *guan nei* as a geographical term, and on the basis of this Lo (2000) claims that *nei guan zhi bing* in case 15 invokes a geographical imagery. This is flawed in more than one way. However, if *guan nei zhi bing* in case 12 is an interjection of a commentator, who had read other *Shi ji* chapters and was familiar with the geographical idiom *guan nei*, it would explain why he committed the mistake of interjecting *guan nei* instead of *nei guan zhi bing*. For early nosological terms as noun-verb complexes, see also *Zhi bing* case 2 (lines 3 and 15).

[90] e.g. *Mai jing* 1.4, p. 7. On *guan* and *ge* in the *Mai jing*, see Liao (1991:101–102).

[91] *Su wen* 9, p. 33; 17, p. 51; *Ling shu* 9, p. 294; 17, p. 323; 48, pp. 397–8; *Mai jing* 1.4, p. 7; *Zhu bing yuan hou lun* 14.4, p. 456.

Wang Niansun quotes *Ling shu* 9, which describes a similar condition of exuberance: 'If at the "opening of the *mai*" there is a fourfold abundance, once large, once frequent, you call it an "overflowing *yin*". The overflowing *yin* has as its characteristic that the interior is closed off. In cases where the interior is closed off, there is no connection. Death occurs, incurable' (*mai kou si sheng, qie da qie shuo zhe, ming yue yi yin, yi yin wei nei guan, nei guan bu tong, si bu zhi* 脈口四盛且大且數者 名曰溢陰 溢陰為內關 內關不通 死不治).[92] *Ling shu* 9, and also two other *Nei jing* texts,[93] culminate in a four-fold abundance, which is characterised by the pulse quality 'once large, once frequent' that comes close to Yi's description of the 'alternating' *mai* in case 6 (line 22), and ends in an overflowing *yin,* which triggers death. Perhaps the 'overflowing *yin*' in *Ling shu* 9 refers to overflowing blood? In case 1, rising heat which implicitly alludes to rising blood has been interpreted as 'murky *yang*'. Since *yin yang* attributions changed in medical history, and in canonical texts blood often is *yin* (while *qi* is *yang*), *Ling shu* 9 may well parallel case 1.[94] Not, however, cases 12 and 15.

Now, if the pulse quality 'being murky yet still' relates in an indexical and/or iconic way to the 'disorder of the interior being closed off', the terminally ill person would appear outwardly healthy with no complaints. Indeed, in cases 12 and 15 the patients did not feel ill before they died (*ren bu bing zi si* 人不病自死), but in case 1 the patient complains of a headache (line 1). This is odd. Furthermore, in contrast to Yi's otherwise medically fairly well-grounded account, it was difficult to find textual parallels for the idioms Yi used for explaining the headache (lines 45–6).

Summary   Text structure semantics postulates that the pulse qualities Yi mentions in his own vocabulary (lines 13–15) correlate with the name of the disorder (line 5). Accordingly, '*qi* coming from the liver' should indicate a '*ju*-abscess'. To someone familiar with canonical medical doctrine, this does not appear plausible. However, some of Yi's body conceptions and medical rationale pre-date canonical doctrine. It is possible that he considered the liver to be located in the interior if not the centre of the body, just like the womb. It appears that the pre-canonical, much like the canonical, liver stored blood and had reproductive functions. Yi states '*qi* coming from the liver' is 'murky yet still'. The 'still' may indicate the disorder has not yet broken out, the 'murky' and 'black' is an attribute of stagnating and coagulated blood, according to some canonical medical texts. Accordingly, the *ju*-abscess may have been thought to arise from a clogging up of blood. *Ling shu* 81 records this for *yong*-clogs.

---

[92] *Ling shu* 9, p. 294.
[93] See also *Ling shu* 48, p. 398, and a similar, but different, passage in *Su wen* 9, p. 33.
[94] Like Yi, *Ling shu* 48 and *Su wen* 9 mention only two locations for taking the pulse: the *mai kou* and *chi*.

Prognosticating the day of death (lines 33–40)

Yi clearly is interested in signs that allow him to prognosticate the time span before death in a quantified way. His reasoning appears to be derived from the same 'Fa' as that mentioned in case 6, which in case 8 is called 'Model for [Calculating] the Limits of one's Share' ('Fen jie fa' 分界法) and calculates the days before death in a numerology of five.[95]

In lines 33–5 and 36–40, Yi establishes a direct correlation between the number of *fen* and the progression of the disorder.[96] Thus, closure by one *fen* at the minor *yang* indicates that the *ju*-abscess is still intact (line 35), closure above two *fen* indicates the eruption of pus (line 38), reaching the 'boundary' (presumably a closure of five *fen*) correlates to the *yong*-clog swelling (line 39), which, as Yi stated earlier, happened after five days (line 7).[97] Strangely, death does not occur. In case 1, it takes three more days until, after eight days, death occurs as predicted (lines 8 and 40).[98]

A similar rationale of prognostication is recorded in *Su wen* 17: 'One recognises that that which divides the *mai* into allotments has time spans, hence one recognises the time of death' (*zhi mai suo fen fen zhi you qi, gu zhi si shi* 知脈所分分之有期 故知死時).[99] The idea that five *fen* make a whole is given in *Su wen* 19: 'A day and a night, divide them in five, this is the means by which one can prognosticate the time [lit. dawn and dusk] of life and death' (*yi ri yi ye wu fen zhi, ci suo yi zhan si sheng zhi zao mu ye* 日一夜 五分之 此所以占死生之早暮也).[100] In *Su wen* 19, the term *fen* is used as a verb, 'to divide a certain length of time', and not as a 'measure of length' or 'degree'.

In summary, Yi knows a method that allows him, in the manner of iatromantic diviners, to prognosticate the day of death. It is grounded in a numerology of five, as are the Shuihudi manuscripts. It consists of correlating the number of *fen* on the *mai* to the internal bodily processes and number of days before death occurs, and it has faint affinity with a few passages in the *Su wen*.

---

[95] Xu Guang points to an edition which renders *jie* 界 as *fen* 分. See parallel to *Su wen* 17, p. 51, on this page.

[96] *fen* 分 is a measure of length: a kernel of millet, equivalent to 0.1 *cun* 寸 (Dubs 1938:276, 279). *Kanseki kokujikai* 105, vol. 7, p. 31, also has *fen* as a measure of length: the three pulse diagnostic positions *cun guan chi* are each divided into five *fen*.

[97] The numerology of two and five (in lines 38, 36), but not of one (line 34), applies to the development of *yong*-clogs in *Zhu bing yuan hou lun* 32–3, p. 908. Consider comments on lines 34–5 in ch. 21, n. 16, in the light of this.

[98] Lines 8, 27 and 37 allude to a numerology of eight, i.e. five plus three. Grammatical and semantic incongruences before and after line 37 (e.g. change of subject) suggest line 37 was later interjected.

[99] *Su wen* 17, p. 51.   [100] *Su wen* 19, p. 60.

*Being exuberant (*you guo 有過*) and heat that rises (*re shang 熱上*) in tubular structures (lines 20–21, 22–5, 33–5, 41–4, 45–6)*

Based on text structure semantics, we have established that the pulse qualities given in Yi's own vocabulary (lines 11–15) provide an explanation for the diagnosis of the *ju*-abscess (line 5): *qi* that comes from the body architectural liver/womb, which stores blood, is indicative of the coagulation of blood which presumably gave rise to the *ju*-abscess. It has 'murky *yang*' qualities, but as the pulse quality 'being still' indicates, the illness has not yet broken out. The 'Mai fa' (lines 16–19) reinforces the idea that the liver is the host of the disorder, although its conception of liver as a viscus that correlates with the season spring is a body ecological one. Lines 20–21 and 22–5 speak of channels and linking vessels, and of the latter 'being exuberant', but they do not explicitly mention heat. Lines 26–9 explain the predictions of the *yong*-clog swelling and of death which Yi made in lines 6–8: the minor *yang* was alternating. This pulse quality, as lines 30–32 explain, indicates that the passageways are in disorder, which is a sign of death. Line 33, which states that the disorder in case 1 is governed by the linking vessels, is best taken as the opening line of the second part of case 1. Line 35 mentions heat for the first time but the following lines, 36–40, of that stanza relate prognosticatory calculations to the pathological processes which led to the *yong*-clog swelling, to the discharge of pus and to death, without making explicit reference to heat.[101] It is only at the very end of case 1, in lines 41–4 (and 45–6), that considerations of rising heat dominate medical reasoning. Lines 41–4 also mention tubular structures, such as 'linking vessels' (*luo mai*), the 'yang brightness' (*yang ming*), 'flowing links' (*liu luo*) and 'nodes of the *mai*' (*mai jie*).

To recapitulate, 'exuberance' (*you guo*), as given in the phrase the 'linking vessels are exuberant' (*luo mai you guo*; line 21), was visible to the onlooker according to Warring States medical rationale, which conceived of the body as a visible 'form' (*xing*) within which dwelt invisible *qi*.[102] As one would expect of an archaic term, the idiom causes problems to the commentators. 'Linking vessels that govern the disorder' (*luo mai zhu bing*; line 33), which pose no problems of comprehension to them, mention the term *zhu* 'to govern' in its body political sense, and show more affinity with canonical than Warring States rationale. This suggests line 33 was added to case 1 at a later stage than line 21, and perhaps the entire second part of case 1 (lines 33–46), even if additions may have been incremental. In what follows, the tubular structures are discussed: first, the 'linking vessels', which in canonical writings contain blood and can get hot and full.

---

[101] It is therefore possible that the *er*-phrase in line 35 *er zhong re* 'and the interior was hot' is a commentatorial interjection.

[102] See p. 32. Zhang Shoujie points to *tai guo* and *bu ji* in the *Su wen, passim*, quotes *Nan jing* 3 (Unschuld 1986a:91), and Lü Guang's comment on it.

Wine has the effect that 'linking vessels' become 'full' (*man* 滿) according to *Su wen* 45: 'When wine enters the stomach, then the linking vessels become full and the channels depleted' (*jiu ru yu wei, ze luo mai man er jing mai xu* 酒入於胃 則絡脈滿 而經脈虛). Their fullness is probably the same condition as their 'being exuberant'. The difference is that 'fullness' is felt – tangibly, subjectively, internally felt - and 'exuberance', first and foremost, is seen, at least in early medical contexts. Tangible and/or subjective internally felt heat is not mentioned in this *Su wen* 45 passage, but in another one (quoted on p. 146).

Ling shu 74 associates 'exuberance' with heat: 'For examining pain of a decaying tooth, press onto the coming of his *yang* [*mai*]. As to the one that is exuberant, if it alone is hot on the left, the left is hot; if [it alone is hot] on the right, the right is hot; if above, the above is hot; if below, the below is hot (*zhen qu chi tong, an qi yang zhi lai, you guo zhe, du re, zai zuo zuo re, zai you you re, zai shang shang re, zai xia xia re* 診齲齒痛 按其陽之來 有過者 獨熱在左 左熱 在右 右熱 在上 上熱 在下 下熱).[103] According to *Ling shu* 74, 'exuberance' in the *yang mai* manifests as heat.

Ling shu 22 does not explicitly mention 'linking vessels', but seems to allude to visibly bulging veins when it states that one can see 'those [places] that are exuberant': 'For treating those suffering from fits, live with them on a long-term basis, examine those places at which one must take [blood] from them. When the illness arrives, look out for those [places] that are exuberant, and discharge them. If you put their blood in the midst of a gourd bottle. When the time will come for it [the illness] to erupt, the blood will be agitated on its own' (*zhi dian ji zhe, chang yu zhi ju, cha qi suo dang qu zhi chu, bing zhi, shi zhi you guo zhe xie zhi, zhi qi xue yu hu hu zhi zhong, zhi qi fa shi, xue du dong yi* 治癲疾者 常與之居 察其所當取之處 病至 視之有過者寫之 置其血于瓠壺之中 至其發時 血獨動矣).[104] The recommendation of bloodletting for treating fits, presumably also epileptic fits, evidently assumes that 'linking vessels' were filled with blood.

Also in case 6 (lines 19–24) one cannot escape the impression that the 'linking vessels' (*luo mai*) were thought to contain 'blood' (*xue* 血). We have already encountered 'blood-links' (*xue luo* 血絡) in *Ling shu* 48 (on p. 131), and *Ling shu* 39 is even entitled 'Treatise on Blood-Links' (Xue luo lun 血絡論). Moreover, terms like 'blood vessels' (*xue mai* 血脈) and 'blood ways' (*xue dao* 血道) occur throughout the *Inner Canon*.

According to *Ling shu* 10, *yang* brightness 'governs disorders arising from blood' (*zhu xue suo sheng bing* 主血所生病).[105] This provides a further hint

---

[103] *Ling shu* 74, p. 455.
[104] *Ling shu* 22, p. 336. According to Epler (1980) and Kuriyama (1995b) bloodletting was common practice in early medicine but later discontinued. In *Ling shu* 39, p. 374, the Yellow Emperor asks: 'How is it that when making blood exit to large amounts, there is no agitation and shaking' (*duo chu xue er bu dong yao zhe, he ye* 多出血而不動搖者 何也)? Unfortunately, Qibo gives no response to this question.
[105] *Ling shu* 10, p. 301.

that the disorder Yi describes in case 1 relates to blood dynamics. Yi says rising heat 'heats up the *yang* brightness' (*xun yang ming* 熏陽明), an idiom not encountered in the *Inner Canon*. It probably denotes a process comparable to '*yang* becoming abundant' (*yang sheng* 陽盛).

The term 'flowing links' (*liu luo* 流絡) (lines 41–2) does not occur in the *Inner Canon* either. However, 'floating links' (*fu luo* 浮絡) are mentioned in the answer to the Yellow Emperor's question in *Su wen* 56: 'I hear the skin has divisions and parts, the *mai* have warps and threads, the sinews have knots and links, the bones have length and weight, the disorders to which they give rise are all different ...' (*yu wen pi you fen bu, mai you jing ji, jin you jie luo, gu you du liang, qi suo sheng bing ge yi* 余聞皮有分部 脈有經紀 筋有結絡 骨有度量 其所生病各異). Qibo thereupon explains that each of the six *mai* has visible 'floating links': 'In the cases where one sees in the midst of its [skin] parts that there are floating links, these all are the links of the A B vessel' (*shi qi bu zhong you fu luo zhe, jie A B zhi luo ye* 視其部中有浮絡者 皆 A B 之絡也).[106] Clearly, 'floating links' could be seen, but it is difficult to know whether the 'floating links' of *Su wen* 56 had any affinity with Yi's 'flowing links'.

The term *mai jie* 脈結 (line 43), which parallels the 'floating links' (*liu luo*), is here translated as a noun-noun compound word meaning 'nodes of the vessels'. However, *mai jie* in *Mai jing* 1.1 means 'the pulse is knotted', and *mai jie* in the *Nei jing* is generally a noun-verb phrase.[107] Thus, *Ling shu* 5 speaks of vessels that are knotted: 'If the pivot is broken, then the vessels have that which renders them knotted up and hinders passage through' (*shu zhe, ze mai you suo jie er bu tong* 樞折 則脈有所結而不通)[108] and *Ling shu* 9 mentions *mai* that are not knotted, in the sense of either vessels or pulses: 'If the *mai* of the six channels are neither knotted nor agitated ... this is called an even [i.e. healthy] person' (*liu jing zhi mai bu jie dong ye ... shi wei ping ren* 六經之脈不結動也 ... 是為平人).[109] *Su wen* 20 has *jie luo mai* meaning either 'knots, links and vessels' or 'knotted linking vessels': 'If above they are replete and below depleted, while pressing on them follow [their course], bind off their knotted linking vessels, needle them to make blood come out of them, and you will see them connect' (*shang shi xia xu, qie er cong zhi, suo qi jie luo mai, ci chu qi xue, yi xian tong zhi* 上實下虛 切而從之 索其結絡脈 刺出其血 以見通之).[110] *Ling shu* 64 has *jie luo* meaning 'knots and links' or, rather, 'knotted links' and also mentions *mai jie* meaning either 'nodes of vessels' or 'vessels that are knotted': 'In the case of knotted links, the blood in the nodes of vessels is not harmonious; breaking them open, brings them into motion' (*qi jie luo zhe, mai*

---

[106] *Su wen* 56, p. 151.
[107] *Mai jing* 1.1, p. 3. Note parallel to Yi's book title 'Qi luo jie', see ch. 6, n. 58. On *jie* as 'topknot of the hair', see Harper (1985:475).
[108] *Ling shu* 5, p. 281.　[109] *Ling shu* 9, p. 293.　[110] *Su wen* 20, p. 66.

*jie xue bu he, jue er nai xing*其結絡者 脈結血不和 決之乃行).[111] In *Ling shu* 64, *mai jie* could be read as the noun-verb phrase it is in other canonical texts, meaning either 'the vessel is knotted' or 'the pulse is knotted', to which is added the statement 'and the blood is not harmonious', but it is here rendered as a bisyllabic noun.

For reasons of rhythm, one is tempted to translate the sentence *liu luo dong, mai jie fa* (lines 41–2) as a noun-verb, noun-verb complex, with the nouns *liu luo* (flowing links) and *mai jie* (nodes of the vessels) as compound words. *Mai jie* as 'node of a vessel' would then occur in stanzas that speak of various tubular structures, and mention either the *yang* brightness or the dull *yin*, as do Yi's cases 1 (lines 41–4), 6 (lines 39–42) and 10 (lines 23–6).

The idiom the 'links intermingle' (*luo jiao* 絡交) (line 44) does not occur in the *Inner Canon* either.[112] It is mentioned in a clause which begins with the conjunction 'hence' (*gu* 故). Such 'hence' clauses usually reconfirm an earlier statement in the text.[113] If 'hence they intermingled' in line 44 follows this rule, 'they intermingled' must be interpreted as referring to the beginning of the second part of case 1, which states that 'the linking vessels govern the disorder' (line 33). This is a further hint that the last stanza (lines 45–6), which concerns the headache, is not intrinsic to case 1 and may have been added by a commentator.

A note on the cause of the disorder (line 9)

In case 1, the 'wine and women' (*jiu qie nei*) are, as in others, not crucial for the identification of the 'name of the disorder' (line 5),[114] and the parallels to *Su wen* 45 that Ando Koretora mentions are tenuous: 'This person must necessarily, after repeatedly drinking and simultaneously eating to his fill, have entered the bedchamber. *Qi* assembles in the midst of the spleen and cannot disperse' (*ci ren bi shu zui qie bao, yi ru fang, qi ju yu pi zhong, bu de san* 此人必數醉且飽 以入房 氣聚於脾中 不得散), 'alcoholic *qi* and cereal *qi* strike each other, and heat becomes abundant in the interior' (*jiu qi yu gu qi xiang bo, re sheng yu zhong* 酒氣與穀氣相薄 熱盛於中).[115] *Su wen* 45 suggests that social heat is turned into bodily heat.

---

[111] *Ling shu* 64, p. 433.
[112] Takigawa's punctuation 'the links intermingle with the hot' (*luo jiao re*) does not make sense.
[113] Hsu (1992:162–4; 1999:119–22) and Lloyd (1996:111–12).
[114] *nei* 內 means 'to ride on a woman' (*yu nü* 御女), says Cui Shi, who points to the parallel *jie nei* 接內 in case 6; Takigawa mentions *fang yu* 房慾 'to indulge in desires of the bedchamber' in case 7. For *nei*, see cases 3, 7, 23, 24, for *jie nei*, see cases 6, 10. In case 22, the term *jie nei* describes in a metaphoric sense a bodily process: *yang jie nei zhe* 'when *yang* joins inside'. On Confucius' use of *nei* and private sentiment, see case 8, n. 20.
[115] *Su wen* 45, p. 126.

Discussion

Text structure semantics postulates that the pulse quality is indicative of the name of the disorder, i.e. '*qi* [coming] from the liver' is indicative of the *ju*-abscess, a correlation that is not plausible from a canonical medical viewpoint. This correlation is given, as shown above, if one considers the liver to store blood, and *ju*-abscesses to arise from blood coagulations. '*Qi* [coming] from the liver' was 'murky yet still', which meant that the disorder was initially not outwardly manifest. Only the second part of case 1 reports on exuberance, rising heat, the vomiting of (blood with) pus, and death.

The first part of case 1 thus provides a rationale for diagnosing the name of the disorder (lines 1–15), the second for medicalising the cause of the disorder (lines 33–44): the social heat of 'wine and women' has turned into bodily heat. From the viewpoint of medical rationale, it is possible that these two parts date from different times, although there is only scant textual evidence to support this. Textual considerations suggest, in fact, that case 1 is a patchwork of mini-texts from more than two different periods. The text contains, for instance, blatant contradictions, which can be solved by suggesting that the same term may have been used in different senses in different passages. It contains phrases which reflect canonical medical rationale and idioms which may date to early medical rationale (but continued to be used later and therefore cannot be taken as unambiguous indices for dating a text). It is best taken as a collage with many layers.

Three pairs of tactile experiences are opposed to each other in case 1: being 'murky yet still' in Yi's vocabulary (line 14), being 'elongated yet strung' in the 'Mai fa' (line 17) and 'blending' versus 'alternating' in the following two stanzas (lines 20–1, 22–5). Among those, tactile descriptions could be found only for the pulses of the 'Mai fa' and for the 'alternating'. The latter will be discussed at more length in case 6.

Yi does not explicitly speak of blood in case 1.[116] But as noted above, *ju*-abscesses were known to arise from a coagulation of blood. The pulse quality 'being murky', if understood in the sense it has as 'murky *yang*' in the Mawangdui manuscripts rather than as the 'murky *yin*' of canonical medical texts, probably indicated both a clogging up and blackening of blood, on the one hand, and the rising hot blood mentioned in the end of case 1, on the other hand. In canonical texts the liver is known to have had functions of storing blood, the *yang* brightness to govern disorders that arise from blood, and linking vessels were thought to contain blood. Case 6, which compares in length and partially in contents with case 1, also alludes in some lines to blood dynamics, and case 2, which with certainty forms a contrasting pair with case 1, concerns a *qi* disorder.

---

[116] Yi mentions *xue* only when blood visibly streams out of the body (Hsu 1986:43).

12
Case 2

Translation (*Shiki kaichû kôshô* 105, pp. 27–8)

1. The youngest son of all the infants of the middle son of the King of Qi fell ill.
2. They summoned your servant, Yi. I examined him and pressed onto his *mai*.

Name:
3. I formally announced <u>saying</u>: 'It is a disorder of *qi* that is blocked.
4. The illness makes a person feel upset and oppressed.
5. Food does not go down.
6. At times, one vomits froth.'

Cause:
7. <u>The illness is contracted from</u> infantile irritability and [involves] frequently rejecting food and drink.
8. Your servant, Yi, immediately made for him a broth that causes *qi* to go downward and got him to drink it.
9. On the first day, the *qi* went downward.
10. On the second day, he was able to eat.
11. On the third day, the illness was cured.

Quality:
12. <u>The means whereby I recognised</u> the youngest son's illness were that
13. when I examined his *mai*, it was *qi* [coming] from the heart.
14. They were [or: it was] murky and hurried, yet [the condition was] transient.
15. This is a disorder of the links becoming *yang*.

1. 齊王中子諸嬰兒小子病

2. 召臣意診切其脈

3. 告曰氣鬲病

4. 病使人煩懣

5. 食不下
6. 時嘔沫

7. 病得之少憂 數忔食飲

8. 臣意即為之作下氣湯 以飲之

9. 一日氣下
10. 二日能食
11. 三日即病愈

12. 所以知小子之病者

13. 診其脈 心氣也

14. 濁躁而經也

15. 此絡陽病也

148

16. The 'Maifa' says:	16. 脈法曰
17. 'In cases where the *mai* come frequently and swiftly, and leave with difficulty, but are not one [in unison],	17. 脈來數疾 去難 而不一者
18. the host of the disorder resides in the heart.'	18. 病主在心
19. In cases where the entire body is hot and the *mai* are abundant,	19. 周身熱 脈盛者
20. it is a double *yang*.	20. 為重陽
21. As for the double *yang*, it overturns [the governor of] the heart.	21. 重陽者遏心主
22. <u>Hence</u> he was upset and oppressed.	22. 故煩懣
23. If the food had not gone down, then the linking vessels would have had excess.	23. 食不下 則絡脈有過
24. If the linking vessels had had excess, then the blood would have risen to get out.	24. 絡脈有過 則血上出
25. If the blood had risen to get out, he would have died.	25. 血上出者死
26. This is what a sad heart generates.	26. 此悲心所生也
27. The illness is contracted from being irritable.	27. 病得之憂也

Interpretation

An infant of the royal family gets ill (line 1), and Yi is summoned to examine him (line 2). He announces the name of the disorder (line 3), reports on signs and symptoms (lines 4–6), cause (line 7), treatment (line 8) and the course of recovery (lines 9–11). The remainder is medical speculation (lines 12–22), which ends with two additional statements on the cause of the disorder (lines 26–7).

Critical evaluation of retrospective biomedical diagnoses

Bridgman suggests an 'angina with a laryngitis that causes wheezing'.[1] Lu and Needham speak of 'difficulty in breathing, probably influenza or catarrh, perhaps acute laryngitis', and note that additionally 'some fever is implicit in the condition'.[2] They take the notion of *qi* very literally as 'breath', but as recent research on Chinese medicine has shown, *qi* has a much wider semantic stretch.[3]

---

[1] Bridgman (1955:70). [2] Lu and Needham (1967:231).
[3] e.g. Porkert (1974:166–76), Sivin (1987:46–54), Hsu (1999:67–87), Unschuld (2003:146–67). See also Lewis (1990) and Kuriyama (1999) on wind.

Infants often suffer from a viral gastritis or gastroenteritis, which makes them irritable; Yi gives an emotional disposition as illness cause. An irritable infant, who repeatedly refuses to eat and drink (*shuo yi shi yin* 數仡食飲), will suffer from a mild dehydration; all clinicians I consulted agreed on this. A dehydration can present with feelings of oppression, no appetite, froth at one's mouth (lines 4–6), and an elevated temperature (line 19), as also indicated by the 'hurried' *mai* (line 14) and 'frequent and swift' coming of the *mai* (line 17). Mild dehydrations are easily treated by consumption of a liquid (lines 8–11).

The name of the disorder

qi ge bing 氣鬲病 – disorder of *qi* that is blocked (line 3)   Yi's insistence on irritability as the cause of the illness (lines 7, 26, 27), his description of its signs and symptoms (lines 4–6), and the tender age of the patient (line 1) bring to mind the well-known children's disorder 'fright' (*jing* 驚).[4] However, 'fright' became a widely acknowledged medical disorder only by medieval times.

In the Warring States and Han, the term *jing* (fright) does not usually designate a disorder. Rather, it refers to a characteristic behaviour of horses, as in *Shuo wen* 10A: 'Fright is the startle of a horse' (*jing ma hai ye* 驚馬駭也).[5] Indeed, in case 4, the horses startled (*jing*), with the result that Xun fell into cold water and contracted a heat disorder, and in case 21, due to a horse being startled (*jing*), Shi Po fell onto a rock and injured his lungs. Likewise, *jing* is not mentioned as the name of a disorder but as a verb in the rubric on 'infants ailing from seizures' (*ying er bing xian* 嬰兒病癇) of the Mawangdui 'Recipes': 'In the case of a seizure, the body is [feverish] hot and frequently one is startled; while neck and spine get stiff, the abdomen is enlarged' (*xian zhe, shen re er shuo jing, jing ji qiang er fu da* 癇者 身熱而數驚 頸脊強而腹大).[6] Having said this, 'being frightened' is an aspect of a disorder of the agitated *yang* brightness in the Mawangdui 'Yinyang vessel text',[7] and the corresponding *Ling shu* 10,[8] and in the *Inner Canon*, it sometimes occurs in compound words like 'fright and shock' (*jing hai* 驚駭),[9] sometimes is associated with 'madness' (*kuang* 狂),[10] sometimes with a frightened awakening from one's sleep,[11] and occasionally with spasms.[12] *Su wen* 48 is an exception as it has *jing* as a disorder: 'If two *yang* are

---

[4] On fright, see Chen (2002:106–15). See also Cullen (2000) on *ke wu* 客忤.
[5] *Shuo wen* 10A, p. 14b; the graph *jing* 驚 has a horse radical.
[6] MWD 'Recipes' (1985:32). Harper (1998:233) has *shuo jing* 'constantly trembling'. Repeatedly startled' is grammatically also possible and medically more likely; it probably designates a series of minor fits.
[7] MWD YY (1985:10).   [8] *Ling shu* 10, p. 301.   [9] e.g. *Su wen* 3, p. 13.
[10] e.g. *Su wen* 63, p. 169.   [11] e.g. *Su wen* 48, p. 134.   [12] e.g. *Su wen* 74, p. 236.

intense, it is fright' (*er yang ji wei jing* 二陽急為驚),[13] which, incidentally, provides a rationale for the 'double *yang*' (*chong yang*) in case 2 (lines 20–21).

In compilations of the Sui and Tang dynasties 'fright' (*jing*) is described as a paediatric condition in its own right, such as in entries on 'fright syndrome' (*jing hou* 驚候), 'fright-seizure syndrome' (*jing xian hou* 驚癇候) and 'fright-crying syndrome' (*jing ti hou* 驚啼候) in the *Zhu bing yuan hou lun*.[14] By Song times, the assumption prevailed that the younger the child, the more dangerous the condition of fright (which explains the above choice of translation in line 1). There was a saying that 'among children's diseases, fright is the most serious one' (*xiao er zhi bing, zui zhong wei jing* 小兒之病最重惟驚).[15] Although the descriptions of 'fright', which multiply after the Song,[16] vary considerably, they nevertheless have striking similarities with case 2.

The signs and symptoms of *jing feng* 驚風 (wind of fright, convulsions due to fright), as the disorder is called in contemporary Chinese medicine, include 'high fever' (*zhuang re* 壯熱 or *gao re* 高熱), 'vomiting and spitting' (*ou tu* 嘔吐) and 'feelings of being upset and restless' (*fan zao* 煩躁).[17] They are reminiscent of some mentioned in case 2, namely: the entire body is hot (*zhou shen re*; line 19), one occasionally vomits (*shi ou*; line 6) and one feels upset and oppressed (*fan men*; line 4). There are also differences, as *jing feng* in contemporary medicine is marked by signs of 'shaking [with the head]' (*yao* [*tou*] 搖頭) or by 'stiffness [in the nape]' ([*xiang*] *qiang* 項強). These signs and symptoms, which invoke convulsions, are not mentioned in case 2. By contrast, case 2 mentions *ou mo* (line 6), which means either 'vomiting froth' or 'vomiting and foaming', and does not figure among the signs and symptoms of 'wind of fright'. This raises the question of why, in respect of a condition that otherwise is almost identical, convulsions are given as an aspect of the 'wind of fright' (*jing feng*) but foaming of the 'disorder of *qi* that is blocked' (*qi ge bing*)? In what follows, an explanation is sought by investigating the conception of body implied by the names of these disorders.

The name of the disorder 氣鬲病 is not attested elsewhere in the medical literature. The character 鬲 can be pronounced in at least two different ways, as *li* or *ge*. According to *Shuo wen* 3B: 'A *li*-cauldron belongs among the category of *ding* vessels' (*li ding shu ye* 鬲鼎屬也), and stood on three hollow feet.[18] It was a ritual utensil.[19] If the disorder 氣鬲病 is pronounced

---

[13] *Su wen* 48, p. 135; *er yang* could also be translated as the 'second *yang*', which designates the heart. See *Su wen* 34, p. 99, and case 1, n. 73.

[14] *Zhu bing yuan hou lun* 45–7, pp. 1288, 1291, 1348. *Zhu bing yuan hou lun* 1, pp. 37–9, lists *feng jing* 風驚 (wind-fright) syndromes that are associated with the heart, but not specified as paediatric conditions.

[15] *You ke shi mi*, p. 20. [16] e.g. Flohr (2000). [17] *Zhongyi erkexue* (Jiang 1985:63).

[18] *Shuo wen* 3B, p. 9a.

[19] On *li* bronze vessels, see Rawson (1990:311–33) and Loewe and Shaughnessy (1999:xxii).

qi li bing, it may have meant 'a disorder of *qi* [being trapped] in a *li*-cauldron'. In Zhou times (11th century–221 BCE), perhaps the body was understood as a pot and the disorder as *qi* trapped within it.[20]

If 鬲 is pronounced as *ge*, it means 'to separate, to cut off' (*ge* 隔) or may refer to the cognate 'diaphragm' (*ge* 膈).[21] The body is then perceived as bipartite, with an upper and lower space separated by the diaphragm. The character *ge* 鬲 is mentioned in two further case histories: in case 15 it possibly means diaphragm; in case 25 it certainly does. The *Yi shuo* of the twelfth century CE has *qi ge bing* 氣膈病, a 'disorder of the diaphragm of *qi*' or a 'disorder of *qi* and the diaphragm'.[22] However, this rendering of the name makes no sense. It appears more likely that case 2 refers to *ge* 隔, the verb. Thus, the name of the disorder 氣鬲病 is a 'disorder of *qi* that is separated' or 'blocked'.

The reading, in case 2, of *ge* 鬲 as verb *ge* 隔 'to separate' rather than as noun *ge* 膈 'diaphragm', as in cases 15 and 25, alludes to a body conception, according to which physicians attended to processes of specific body parts or in certain bodily regions without detailing their structures (see also case 3, line 4).[23] No doubt, the verb 'to separate' entailed the noun, 'diaphragm', that separates two spaces within a bipartite body. The diaphragm, like any gate, could be closed, as the phrase 'to close the gate' (*ge bi men hu* 鬲閉門戶) in *Han shu* 27 states, or, like 'the gate [that] is for opening and passing through' (*men wei kai tong* 門為開通),[24] could be conceived of as a connection between two separate spaces.

Yi treats the condition with a 'broth that causes *qi* to go downward' (*xia qi tang*).[25] The broth treats the complaints of 'feeling upset and oppressed', which affect the chest region (i.e. the upper bodily cavity above the diaphragm); the listlessness in eating, which is described very literally as 'food does not pass down' (i.e. from the upper to the lower bodily cavity); and 'vomiting froth', a sign of ascending instead of descending *qi* (due to a blockage between upper and lower bodily cavities). Upward movement is considered pathological, as in *Ling shu* 68, which opposes *qi* disorders above the diaphragm to 'bug' (*chong* 蟲) disorders below the diaphragm: '*Qi* [disorders] affect the area above the diaphragm, once food and drink

[20] No signs and symptoms affecting the parts below the diaphragm are mentioned, which may indicate that the disorder dates from a time when the body was conceived of as a pot with only one cavity.

[21] On *ge* 膈 'diaphragm', see *Huangdi nei jing*, pp. 1472–3. Not discussed in the *Shuo wen*.

[22] *Yi shuo* 5, p. 10b.

[23] The body conception in case 2, with *ge* the verb, certainly pre-dates that in cases 15 and 25, with *ge* as noun. See also the discussion of the *ju*-abscesses in cases 1 versus 22. It appears that cases 1–10 build on an earlier primary source than cases 11–25.

[24] *Han shu* 27, pp. 1413, 1425.

[25] Takigawa suggests to read it as *qi xia tang*, since *qi xia* is standard expression in canonical doctrine, e.g. *Su wen* 39, p. 113: 'If there is fear then the *qi* descends' (*kong ze qi xia* 恐 則氣 下). However, the broth *xia qi tang* treats chest problems also in *Bei ji qian jin yao fang* 13.7, p. 244.

have entered, they turn round to get out' (*qi wei shang ge zhe, shi yin ru er huan chu* 氣為上膈者 食飲入而還出).[26] Rising *qi* causes disorder; its downward movement reinstates health.

We established above that some signs and symptoms in case 2 (lines 4 first part, 5, 19) also figure in the description of *jing feng* (wind of fright), but others are not mentioned, like 'vomiting froth' (line 6). If *qi ge bing* were indeed to refer to a similar symptom complex as *jing feng*, Yi must have emphasised signs and symptoms that reinforced his bipartite body conception, and contemporary doctors attend to those they consider typical of wind. Thus, where contemporary doctors see in convulsions a manifestation of wind, Yi attends to vomiting froth and foaming as a sign of rising *qi*.[27]

If case 2 describes a condition later recognised as infantile 'fright' (*jing*), one could read the cause *shao you* (line 7), which is not attested elsewhere in the medical literature, as 'infantile irritability'. This is said in awareness that *shao* can mean 'to a lesser degree' and *shao you* may refer to 'minor indispositions'. It is also said in full awareness that commentator Zhang Wenhu suggests to read *shao you* as *xin you* (the heart is irritable), not least because of the similarity between the graphs *shao* 少 and *xin* 心. However, *Su wen* 28 mentions 'sudden anxiousness' (*bao you* 暴憂) which arises from a blocking off of *qi*: 'If separated and blocked, closed and severed, the upper and lower [parts] are not connected, then it is a disorder of sudden anxiousness' (*ge sai bi jue, shang xia bu tong, ze bao you zhi bing ye* 隔塞 閉絕 上下不通 則暴憂之病也).[28] The 'sudden anxiousness', *bao you*, with symptoms reminiscent of Yi's 'infantile irritability', *shao you*, semantically comes very close to the notion of sudden 'fright'.

In summary, the signs and symptoms (lines 4–6) and cause (line 7) of the infant's 'disorder of *qi* being blocked' (*qi ge bing*) are strikingly similar to those of the later disorder 'fright' (*jing*) and the contemporary 'wind of fright' (*jing feng*). Perhaps *qi ge bing*, *jing* and *jing feng* ultimately attend to a similar symptom complex, and different aspects of these illness events were noted in accordance with the physicians' body conceptions. Thus, Yi reported on foaming caused by rising *qi* where contemporary doctors see convulsions caused by wind. Yi furthermore emphasised age-sensitive epidemiological aspects (the illness affects infants), by saying the illness was contracted from 'infantile irritability', where canonical doctrine stressed phenomenological aspects (the sudden onset), when speaking of 'sudden anxiousness' and 'fright'.

---

[26] *Ling shu* 68, p. 442, continues: 'Bugs descend below the diaphragm . . .' (*chong wei xia ge* 蟲為下膈 . . .).

[27] Biomedically, convulsions and foaming belong among the concomitant signs of a mild dehydration.

[28] *Su wen* 28, p. 88. Consider also Wang Bing's comment on *bao you* 暴憂 on p. 164.

Text structure semantics

Text structure semantics causes one to expect that the qualities of *mai* (lines 12–18) correlate with constituents in the name of the disorder (line 3). However, to anyone familiar with canonical doctrine, there is no apparent correlation between the qualities of *mai* and the name of the disorder. The task of establishing one is complicated by the fact that Yi provides in two consecutive stanzas two different accounts of pulse qualities which invoke two entirely different body conceptions. The first relates pulse qualities in Yi's own vocabulary (lines 12–15); the second is the 'Mai fa' quote (lines 16–18). Since the *mai* in the 'Mai fa' are more familiar to us, I discuss them first.

lai 來, qu 去 – the coming and going of the 'Mai fa' pulses (lines 16–18)
The 'Mai fa', much in line with extant canonical writings, refers to both the 'coming' (*lai*) and 'going' (*qu*) of *mai*. By contrast, when Yi describes *mai* in his own terms, he does not speak of a coming *and* going. He only mentions the 'coming' of *mai*: in case 8 'its coming' (*qi lai*) is 'slippery' (*hua*), in case 10 'difficult' (*qi lai nan*), in case 18 'difficult and hard' (*qi lai nan jian*), and in case 21 'dispersed' (*qi lai san*). Therefore, he is in this study translated as speaking of *qi* 'coming' from a viscus after he examined *mai*.

In case 2 (line 17), the coming of the 'Mai fa' pulses is 'frequent' (*shuo*) and 'swift' (*ji*), and the going happens 'with difficulty' (*nan*); furthermore, they are not in unison (*bu yi*). The Japanese editor Takigawa provides a paraphrase: 'They arrived by coming swiftly and leaving retarded; they were numerous and simultaneously irregular' (*lai ji qu chi er zhi shu you bu tiao ye* 來疾去遲而至數又不調也). Since Yi provides comments on 'being frequent' in case 3 (line 17) and on 'coming with difficulty' in case 10 (lines 17–18), these terms will be discussed then.

'Swift', in contrast to 'frequent', is not a standard pulse in *Mai jing* 1.1, but it is in contemporary Chinese medicine, where it indicates a more life-threatening state.[29] In *Su wen* 33 (cited on pp. 189–90) it is also indicative of imminent death. Since the idiom *shuo ji* (frequent and swift) is not well documented in canonical medical texts, it is possible that either *shuo* or *ji* was later interjected. As *ji* (swift) qualifies the heart *mai* in early medical texts,[30] and *shuo* (frequent) was a well-known standard pulse, it was probably *shuo* that was interjected by a commentator.

The pulse quality 'and not being one' (*er bu yi*; line 17) causes problems. It occurs again in an and-phrase in case 21: 'They came dispersedly, arrived

---

[29] See *Zhongyi zhenduanxue* (Deng 1984:72). The 'frequent' is said to refer to five beats, or more, per inhalation, and 'swift' to seven, or more.

[30] e.g. ZJS 'Maishu' (2001:244). Zhang Wenhu notes that various editions wrongly render *ji* 疾 and *bing* 病; *ji* means 'swift' in case 2.

by several routes and were not one' (*qi lai san, shu dao zhi er bu yi ye* 其來散 數道至 而不一也). Since death is associated with dispersal,[31] also in pulse diagnosis,[32] one would expect 'not being one' to be indicative of death. Indeed, in case 21 the patient dies, but not in case 2. The People's Republic of China (PRC) editors, unaware of these semantic problems, punctuate the text by the rule of syntax: *mai lai shuo ji, qu nan er bu yi zhe*.[33] Takigawa's punctuation is more subtle: *mai lai shuo ji, qu nan, er bu yi zhe*. It has the effect that the *er*-phrase appears tagged on. Incidentally, there are medical parallels for the first part of the sentence (see below), while *bu yi* is not a pulse quality in the *Inner Canon*. Perhaps a commentator who was not a medic interjected *er bu yi* in cases 2 and 21 in an attempt to clarify the text.

Ando Koretora equates all qualities of *mai* mentioned in the 'Mai fa' quote with those of *Su wen* 19: 'The *mai* of summertime is the heart ... its *qi* comes abundantly and leaves weakened, hence it is called "hooked"' (*xia mai zhe, xin ye ... qi qi lai sheng qu shuai, gu yue gou* 夏脈者 心也 其氣 來盛 去衰 故曰鈎).[34] He proposes to equate coming 'frequently and swiftly' with 'abundantly' in *Su wen* 19 (a term given also in case 2, line 19), and going 'with difficulty' with leaving 'weakened'.[35] His comment reinforces Takigawa's punctuation and paraphrase *qi lai ji, qu chi*, and highlights its affinity with the canonical pulse quality 'hooked' (*gou* 鈎), earlier encountered in a Dunhuang quote (on p. 43). From the above it is evident that the 'hooked', which is indicative of a heart disorder, describes in an iconic way the hook-like movement of *qi*'s turning round inside the chest.

zhuo 濁, *zao* 躁, *jing* 經 – Yi's murky, hurried and transient (line 14)

Yi's discussion of *mai* in lines 12–15 bears little resemblance to canonical texts. The key to decoding this three-line stanza is that it parallels a three-line stanza in case 1 (lines 13–15): in both cases Yi first says that he examined *mai* and got *qi* [coming] from a viscus, he then describes the qualities of *qi* or *mai* with static verbs and, thirdly, maintains that these qualities are indicative of a certain disorder, *bing*. Thus, Yi says in case 1: 'When I, Yi, pressed onto his *mai*, I got the *qi* [coming] from the liver' (*qie qi mai, de gan qi*) and in case 2: 'When I, Yi, examined *mai*, it was the *qi* [coming] from the heart' (*zhen qi mai, xin qi ye*). In case 1, Yi then specifies that '*qi* [coming] from the liver was murky yet still' (*gan qi zhuo er jing*). In case

---

[31] Harper (1999).   [32] Hsu (2001d). See also discussion on *tuan* 'united' in case 7 (line 17).

[33] *Shi ji* 105, p. 2799.

[34] *Su wen* 19, p. 59. See slight variant in *Mai jing* 3.2, p. 72: 夏脈心也 ... 故其氣來盛去衰 故曰鈎. Note that the qualities attributed to *qi* in the *Su wen* and *Mai jing* are attributed to *mai* in the 'Mai fa' quote.

[35] Incidentally, Ando Koretora does not mention *er bu yi*. Does this mean that in his edition the commentator in question had not (yet) been at work, i.e. that it was interjected as recently as in the last three centuries?

2, the following sentence consists of a list of three static verbs: *zhuo zao er jing ye*,[36] but Yi does not specify whether these static verbs describe three qualities of the *qi* of three different *mai* or three qualities of one *mai*. The translation chosen, which in sentence structure parallels case 4 (line 30), mentions two qualities of the *qi* of two different *mai* and an assessment of the patient's overall condition: 'They were [or: it was] murky and hurried, yet [the condition was] transient.'[37]

luo yang bing 絡陽病 – **disorder of the links becoming *yang* (line 15)**   On the third line of the stanza (lines 12–15), which parallels case 1 (lines 13–15), Yi states that the above qualities of *mai* indicate 'disorder' (*bing*). Their names are of an entirely different order than those known to us from the extant medical literature. Yi says in case 1, *ci nei guan zhi bing ye* and in case 2, *ci luo yang bing ye*. If one treats *nei* and *luo* as nouns, and *guan* and *yang* as verbs, then case 1 reads: 'This is a disorder of the interior being closed off' and case 2: 'This is a disorder of the links becoming *yang*', i.e. taking on *yang*-qualities (and becoming hot). The translation of *nei guan zhi bing* and *luo yang bing* would then be modelled on the structure of the compound word *qi ge bing* (disorder of *qi* being separated/blocked), where *qi ge* is a noun-verb compound. Accordingly, *yang* 陽 would be a static verb.

It is also possible to treat *nei guan* and *luo yang* as noun-noun compound words. Taki Motohiro says the *Yi shuo* renders *luo yang* as *yang luo*, 'the link of the *yang*',[38] which he considers synonymous with what later became known as the 'pericard' (*xin bao luo* 心包絡). The noun *yang* is then perceived as designating the heart, and the noun *luo* as referring to a 'large tube within the body'.[39] Taki Motohiro's amendment of the text from *luo yang bing* to *yang luo bing* (line 15) tallies nicely with Zhang Shoujie's, who cites Yang Xuancao's (eighth-century) comment on *Nan jing* 18 in equating *xin zhu* (line 21) with *xin bao luo*, the 'pericard'.[40] However, these meaning-centred alterations of the text may well be anachronistic. In general, a grammatical analysis is more reliable than a meaning-oriented one, particularly if the latter is provided almost two thousand years later. The grammatical analysis above highlights the syntactic parallels between three names of disorders. In the late Warring States and early Han, names

[36] Taki Mototane suggests *er* 而 'and', 'yet' substitutes *zai* 在 'to reside in': 'It was murky and hurried in the channels' (*zhuo zao zai jing ye*), but this is unlikely.

[37] *jing* 經 is a static verb here, read in the fourth tone, meaning 'transient', synonymous with *jing* 徑. See HYDCD 9.860, entry 2, and 3.976, entry 4. Consider Kaiho Gembi on *jing* in case 6 (line 19): '*jing* means transient' (*jing zhe, li ye* 經者歷也). Osobe Yô (1994:66) suggests *jing* 'transient' is a pulse quality in case 2, but it may also qualify the patient's overall condition, much like *yu* 愈 'to recover' in case 4 (line 30).

[38] Not, however, in the edition of the *Yi shuo* 5, p. 10b, I consulted.

[39] *luo* 絡 does not always refer to tiny links on the body surface. See case 6 (lines 39–42).

[40] *Nan jing* 18 (Unschuld 1986a:248). However, *xin zhu* and (*xin*) *bao luo* can occur in the same text, with distinctive meanings. See *Ling shu* 10, p. 306; 12, p. 312; 71, p. 447.

of disorders seem to have assessed pathological processes in noun-verb phrases.

The above shows that the pulse qualities help elucidate the name of the disorder on the third line of the stanza (lines 12–15). In case 1, '*qi* [coming] from the liver' that is 'murky yet still' indicates a disorder of 'the interior being closed off' (*nei guan*), which suggests that the disorder initially was not outwardly manifest. In case 2, when *qi* or *mai* is/are said to be 'murky and hurried, but [the patient's overall condition] transient', the name of the disorder indicates that 'the links have become *yang*' (*luo yang*), i.e. have acquired *yang*-qualities. 'Murky' and 'hurried' both had *yang*-qualities (see pp. 136, 139). In the Mawangdui texts 'murky' is always juxtaposed to '*yang*' (*zhuo yang*) and in case 21 'still' (*jing*) contrasts with 'hurried' (*zao*), where context indicates that 'still' is *yin* and 'hurried' *yang*.[41] In what follows, we will discuss the implications of this finding.

chong yang 重陽 **– the double *yang* (lines 19–22)**   What may have been meant by calling an illness *luo yang bing* (disorder of the links becoming *yang*; line 15)? Lines 19–20 give an answer: 'If [first] the entire body is hot and [in addition] the *mai* are abundant, it is a double *yang*' (*zhou shen re, mai sheng zhe, wei chong yang*).[42] Body heat and abundant *mai* both are *yang*; if both are observed simultaneously, *yang* qualities are doubled. *Ling shu* 67 says of a 'person with a double *yang*' (*chong yang zhi ren* 重陽之人): 'He has an easily irritable spirit' (*qi shen yi dong* 其神易動), 'his *qi* easily errs about' (*qi qi yi wang ye* 其氣易往也) and 'there is a bounty of visceral *qi* of the heart and lungs' (*xin fei zhi zang qi you yu* 心肺之藏氣有餘).[43] Interestingly, *Ling shu* 67 speaks of *qi* dynamics and bounty within the 'sentimental body', not of heat. However, in the latter parts of case 2 heat and abundance emerge as central aspects of the 'double *yang*'.

When *yang* doubles, this affects the heart or, as the text puts it (lines 21–2): 'A double *yang* overturns the [governor of the] heart' (*chong yang zhe dang xin* [*zhu*]). There is some controversy among the commentators over whether the 'governor of the heart' (*xin zhu*) or the 'heart' (*xin*) is assaulted. Kaiho Gembi points out that Xu Guang from the fourth century says in his comment on *dang/tang*: 'the illness assaulted the "heart"' (*bing dang xin zhe* 病瘴心者), not 'the governor of the heart'. He deduces from this that early *Shi ji* editions referred to the 'heart'. Kaiho Gembi's and Xu Guang's observations could be used as further argument against Taki Motohiro's and Zhang Shoujie's above reading of *luo yang bing* as 'disorder of the pericard'.

---

[41] On *zao* 躁 (hurried), see case 5 (line 21) and *Su wen* 5 (quoted on p. 139).
[42] 重 *chong* is *zhong*, suggests Sima Zhen, but heat and abundance nicely add up to a double *yang*. See ch. 6, n. 61.
[43] *Ling shu* 67, p. 440.

The term *dang/tang* 盪 poses further problems to the commentators. Xu Guang pronounces it as *tang* and proposes to read it as *dang* 蕩 'to dash forth, to assault' (see quote above), which he suggests means 'to pierce the heart' (*ci qi xin* 刺其心).[44] Taki Motohiro cites *Mai jing* 6.3: 'The disorder of the heart [includes]: to be upset and have chest pressure, to have a short breath, to have great heat, the heat rises and dashes forth to the heart, to vomit, to cough slightly . . .' (*xin bing, fan men, shao qi, da re, re shang dang xin, ou tu, ke ni. . . .* 心病 煩懣 少氣 大熱 熱上盪心 嘔吐 咳逆).[45] Kaiho Gembi cites various texts which show that *dang* 盪 is used in military contexts in the sense of 'attack'. Researchers of the twentieth century, such as Bridgman and Yu Yunxiu, speak of palpitations, the latter in respect of *xin dang* 心蕩 'the heart is unsettled' in the *Zuo zhuan*.[46] However, 盪 read as *dang* 'to overturn', may be worth further exploration, as early medical rationale often framed bodily processes with reference to *yin yang* complementarities.

In this context *Su wen* 70 comes to mind: 'The heart aches, the stomach pit aches, there is an inversion and contravection, the diaphragm does not connect [i.e. allow passage through], this is governed by sudden velocity' (*xin tong wei wan tong, jue ni ge bu tong, qi zhu bao su* 心痛 胃脘痛 厥逆 鬲不痛 其主暴速).[47] *Su wen* 70 mentions a heart that is in pain, problems in the digestive system, and a diaphragm that does not allow passage through – aspects of discomfort contained also in Yi's case 2. *Su wen* 70 refers to an 'inversion' (*jue*), case 2 to an 'overturning' (*dang*); the former alludes to a process that in early Han medicine was framed in terms of *yin yang* inversions (see case 9, line 3), perhaps also the latter.

For understanding the relevance of the stanza comprising lines 19–22, it is important to know that Yi's medical speculation is generally geared towards explaining, in separate stanzas, first the name of the disorder, and then each of the concomitant signs and symptoms. Each of these stanzas ends in a summarising statement introduced by the conjunction *gu* 故 (therefore, hence). This stanza is an example par excellence of this recurrent feature in Yi's reasoning. The 'double *yang*' should explain a statement

[44] See also *Ling shu* 24, p. 342: 'If there is a fake heart pain, and the pain feels as though awls and needles were piercing the heart . . .' (*jue xin tong, tong ru yi zhui zhen ci qi xin . . .* 厥心痛 痛如以錐鍼刺其心). On *jue tong* as fake pain, see p. 318.

[45] *Mai jing* 6.3, p. 186.

[46] Yu (1953:123); *Zuo zhuan*, Duke Zhuang, fourth year, p. 1.163; Bridgman (1955:28, 70). See also MWD YY, in case 9, n. 31. HYDCD 10.1029 gives as pronunciation *dang* and *tang*; the latter for this *Shi ji* passage.

[47] *Su wen* 70, p. 206. *Wei wan* 'stomach pit' has been translated into English as 'gastric cavity' (*Hanying yixue dacidian* 1987) or 'stomach-duct' (Unschuld 1986a:741). See also *Shuo wen* 4B, p. 33b: '*wan* is the *fu* of the stomach' (*wan wei fu ye* 脘胃腑也), the definition of *fu* is given on the same page: '*fu* is dried meat' (*fu gan rou ye* 腑乾肉也). For *fu*, see also Karlgren (1957:101r, 46).

Yi made in line 4, namely why the infant had symptoms of 'feeling upset and oppressed' (*fan men*).

Counterfactual reasoning (for making sense of lines 23–5)   Lines 23–5 cause problems to the commentators. Taki Motokata considers these eighteen characters mistaken. He points out that the patient did not die. He also contests Ando Koretora's suggestion that they belong in case 25. Perhaps they belong in case 1? Another possibility is to consider this stanza a counterfactual, and disregard the anyway highly controversial claim of those psychologists and philosophers who maintain that the Chinese cannot reason in counterfactuals.[48] However, at least two objections instantly come to mind. First, this reading requires the stanza to begin with *shi bu xia*, 'If the food had not gone down . . .', and make a full stop after *fan men*, which is grammatically possible but not very rhythmical. Second, the name of the disorder *qi ge bing* alludes to movements of *qi*, but this stanza concerns blood.

The first objection can be countered by our analysis of the previous stanza (lines 19–22). The 'double *yang*' can explain why the person felt 'upset and oppressed' (*fan men*), but not why 'food was not going down' (*shi bu xia*). So, the punctuation is grammatically possible and semantically motivated. In response to the second objection, it has been suggested that the earlier rendering of a bodily process in terms of blood, by mistake, had not been translated into more recent medical jargon in terms of *qi*.[49] However, case 1 is about the liver and blood and case 2 about the heart and *qi*, which is in line with early medical rationale. So, perhaps, the graph for *qi* was later replaced by that for blood? In case 2, as opposed to *Ling shu* 67, the 'double *yang*' has features of heat. This makes anyone think of rising blood, probably also the commentator who presumably interjected this stanza. In case 4 (line 37), we will again encounter a counterfactual best interpreted as commentatorial interjection.

Movement certainly mattered over substance: irrespective of whether it was *qi* or blood, upward movement was considered pathological. Yi uses the same phrase with which *qi*-vapour from cooking is described, when it is trapped in a *li*-cauldron, as in *Shuo wen* 3B: 'The cooking vapours ascend to get out' (*chui qi shang chu ye* 炊氣上出也).[50] The phrase in line 25 'to ascend and get out' (*shang chu*) evidently also describes movements of *qi*.

In this context it is worth noting that the idea that it is good to have a cool head is in no way peculiar to early Chinese medical texts. It is a basic trait of common knowledge throughout South-east Asia. When Carol

---

[48] e.g. Bloom (1981), who already by the mid-1980s had been criticised for the inadequacy of the experimental setup, the samples taken and the leap he took from his experimental results to his conclusions.
[49] Paul Unschuld (2000 p.c.).   [50] *Shuo wen* 3B, p. 10b.

Laderman investigated cultural practices on the Malayan peninsula, which were shaped by competing ideas of local and Islamic medicines, she showed that the rituals and practices related to birth and postnatal care, despite the value that Islam attributed to heat, were framed in terms of the traditional local culture's high esteem for coolness.[51] Among the Orang Asli, 'a cool, spiritual liquid', *kahyek*, is infused into the head soul and heart soul of the ill'.[52] And in contemporary South Asia a patient of an Ayurvedic doctor was recorded to have said: 'The head must always be cool. Judgment (*putti*) must always be cool. The feet must always be hot. If the feet become cool it is very bad for the body.'[53] This ethnographic data shows that coolness in the head is today still highly valued in South and East Asia; it may well express encompassing values of cool water as the source of life.[54]

xin qi 心氣 – qi coming from the heart (line 13)   So far, the qualities of *mai* that Yi mentions (lines 14–15) and those in the 'Mai fa' (lines 16–18) have not provided us with a clue for the name of the disorder (line 3). The answer is found if one notes that both Yi and the 'Mai fa' mention pulse qualities indicative of a disorder in the heart. This would suggest that, according to text structure semantics, *xin qi* explains Yi's diagnosis of *qi ge bing*.

The correlation between '*qi* [coming] from the heart' (*xin qi*) and the 'disorder of *qi* being blocked' (*qi ge bing*) is not instantly obvious, because the two idioms allude to entirely different body conceptions and nosologies. The name of the disorder, *qi ge bing*, like *nei guan zhi bing* or *luo yang bing*, alludes to an understanding of illness arising from body parts affected by adverse changes. In these 'body part – subject to adverse change – disorders', the aspects of the body are given by a noun, '*qi*', 'the interior' – (*nei*) or 'the links' (*luo*), and those are modified by a verb, which shows that each is adversely affected: 'being separated' (*ge*), 'closed off' (*guan*) or 'becoming *yang*' (*yang*).

By contrast, the pulse quality *xin qi* alludes to a conception of illness based on the general idea that a disorder 'visits' (*ke*), is 'hosted by', is 'governed by' or 'governs' (*zhu*), or 'resides in' (*zai* 在, *yu* 於), a body part. If *xin* is understood primarily to refer to a space within the bodily architecture (rather than to the functions of the cardial system within the body ecologic), *xin qi* indicates that the illness resides in the upper bodily cavity. The pulse quality *xin qi*, which implies that *qi* is trapped within the body architectural heart, then correlates with the name of the disorder, *qi ge bing*, which speaks of *qi* being blocked. Text structure semantics thereby highlights a correlation not otherwise apparent.

---

[51] Laderman (1987).   [52] Roseman (1991:30–32).   [53] Trawick (1992:141).
[54] On water as the source of life, see Guodian *Laozi* in Jingmenshi Bowuguan (1998:125), Li Xueqin ([1999] 2001), Allan and Williams (2000:162–71, 228–31) and many more.

The cause of the disorder (lines 7 and 26–7)

The cause of the disorder is 'infantile irritability': 'The illness is contracted from infantile irritability and [involves] frequently rejecting food and drink' (*bing de zhi shao you, shuo yi shi yin*).[55] This is repeated in the last two lines of case 2: 'This is what a sad heart generates' (*ci bei xin suo sheng ye*), and 'The illness is contracted from grief' (*bing de zhi you ye*). Such repetition is puzzling.

xin 心 – the heart as seat of thought, morality and emotion (line 13) All three causes of the illness in case 2 (lines 7, 26 and 27) suggest that the 'heart' is not only understood as a body architectural space, the upper bodily sphere, but also as the seat of all emotions. The canonical 'heart', by contrast, is one of the five viscera, which each have separate functions of affect and cognition.[56] Case 2 seems to refer to an intermediate stage in medical history with the heart as an aspect of a bipartite bodily architecture and sentimental body. This bipartite body conception is also intrinsic to the idioms *xin gan* 心肝 (heart-liver) and *xin fu* 心腹 (heart-abdomen).

The 'heart-liver' (*xin gan*) can refer to one's overall feelings, as in a poem by Wang Can 王粲 (177–217 CE) of the Eastern Han: 'I was conscious of that man underneath the spring, the sighing hurts heart and liver' (*wu bi xia quan ren, kui ran shang xin gan* 悟彼下泉人 喟然傷心肝).[57] The Mawangdui vessel texts mention the 'heart' and 'liver/kidneys' (apart from the 'stomach') – and none of the other five viscera (see p. 42), but not *xin gan* as compound word. Nor does Yi. But he probably refers to the 'heart' (*xin*) as an aspect of the bipartite 'sentimental body', when he speaks of the cause of the illness.

The 'heart-abdomen' (*xin fu*), by contrast, does occur in the Mawangdui 'Recipes', and Ma Jixing explains that *xin* refers there to the 'upper bodily cavity', and not to the heart as seat of emotions; *xin* as upper bodily cavity complements *fu*, the lower bodily cavity, within the bipartite 'architectural body'.[58] Yi seems to have in mind this 'body architectural heart', when he speaks of the pulse quality *xin qi* (line 13).

In the *Dao de jing*, the term *xin* (heart) alludes to both the architectural space as well as the seat of thought and emotion that should be emptied for good government: 'Therefore, government for the sage person [consists

---

[55] 忆 *qi* 'to like' but *yi* 'to reject/detest'. HYDCD 7.412, Sima Zhen and Taki Motohiro read *yi*: '*yi* ... means the heart has no desire' (*yi ... xin bu yu* ... 忆 心不慾). For both interpretations, see Osobe Yô (1994:66, 68). Takigawa seems to suggest 'being forced to eat and drink' (*qiang shi yin ye* 強食飲也), although in early texts *qiang shi* means 'to eat heartily', see HYDCD 4.139 and Harper (1998:211), quoted on p. 257.

[56] For the *locus classicus*, see *Su wen* 4, p. 17, and 5, pp. 20–21.

[57] *Wen xuan* 23, p. 593. In standard modern Chinese *xin gan* refers to the character of a person, in colloquial speech it is the term by which one addresses one's beloved child or lover.

[58] Ma (1992:526). See also case 9, pp. 312–15.

of] emptying his heart-mind and filling his abdomen, weakening his will, and strengthening his bones' (*shi yi sheng ren zhi zhi, xu qi xin, shi qi fu, ruo qi zhi, qiang qi gu* 是以聖人之治 虛其心 實其腹 弱其志 強其骨).[59] Also Yi's use of the term alludes to both the architectural and sentimental body.

Another Han author, Wang Bao 王襃 (fl. 60–50 BCE), recommends that the entire *xin fu*, much like the *xin* in the *Dao de jing*, is emptied and opened up through self-cultivation: 'When one cleanses one's body and cultivates one's thought, while spitting out feelings, one opens up heart and abdomen' (*huo jie shen xiu si, tu qing su er ba xin fu* 或絜身修思 吐情素而拔心腹).[60] While Wang Can's 'heart-liver' (*xin gan*) refers to the feelings themselves, Wang Bao's 'heart and abdomen' (*xin fu*) is conceived as a receptacle for them.

Disorders of 'heart and abdomen' (*xin fu*) may also refer to troubles with digestion (see case 7, line 4), which in canonical writings is associated with 'spleen and stomach'. Although in early medicine the heart is mostly comprehended as an aspect of a bipartite body, it is also conceived of as the most central body part, as in *Shuo wen* 10B: 'The heart is the human heart. It is the viscus of earth. It resides in the midst of the body' (*xin ren xin, tu zang ye, zai shen zhi zhong* 心 人心 土臟也 在身之中).[61] The centrally located 'heart' is put in correlation with 'earth' (and presumably the earthbound function of digestion) as are spleen and stomach in canonical medical writings.[62]

In canonical doctrine, the feeling *xi*, 'happiness', generally correlates with the heart,[63] but in case 2, line 26, the feeling *bei* (sorrow) is explicitly attributed to the heart, and in line 27 *you* (grief), indirectly. The pentic correspondences between feelings and viscera vary greatly in the *Inner Canon*. This suggests that they were not yet standardised in Han times and that the pentic visceral system was promoted by physicians who had other preoccupations than attending to the psychology, i.e. the bipartite sentimental body, of an aristocratic clientele. The *Inner Canon* mentions *you* and *bei* as an aspect of the 'heart',[64] and also 'happiness' (*xi* 喜), 'fear' (*kong* 恐),[65]

---

[59] Translation based on *Laozi Daodejing He Shang gong zhangju* 1, p. 11. Compare and contrast with Lau (1963:59): 'Therefore, in governing people, the sage empties their minds but fills their bellies, weakens their wills but strengthens their bones'. See also *Laozi ... 3*, p. 71.

[60] *Wen xuan* 51, p. 1269.

[61] *Shuo wen* 10B, 23b. See also *Su wen* 79, p. 251, in case 1, n. 42.

[62] In contemporary clinical practice, students were exhorted to recognise heart conditions in patients who complained of stomach ache (fieldwork 1988–9). Rather than being given a biomedical explanation, we were told that historically the Chinese medical notions of 'heart' and 'stomach' were closely related.

[63] The *locus classicus* is *Su wen* 5, p. 21.

[64] e.g. *Su wen* 39, p. 113 and 62, p. 168, and *Ling shu* 8, p. 292, and 28, pp. 351–2, correlate 'sorrow' (*bei*) with the heart. E.g. *Su wen* 19, p. 61, *Ling shu* 4, p. 274, and 47, p. 391, correlate 'grief' (*you*) with the heart.

[65] e.g. *Ling shu* 4, p. 274.

'worry' (*si* 思)[66] and many more. Its rendering of many different feelings as correlates of the heart can be interpreted as testifying to the pre-dynastic heart as seat of all thinking and emotion.

bei 悲 – **sorrow (line 26)** The term *bei* (sorrow) generally has a narrower semantic stretch than *you* (grief) in medical contexts, although, as already stated, *bei* and *you* both are given as correlates of lungs or heart.[67] In the *Inner Canon*, *bei* is often mentioned in connection with 'sadness and mourning' (*ai* 哀). It is sometimes the emotion made responsible for tears.[68] Sometimes it is opposed to 'happiness' (*xi*), and while happiness tends to be associated with 'having bounty' (*you yu* 有餘) or 'repletion' (*shi* 實) of *qi* 氣 or *shen* 神 (spirits), 'sorrow' (*bei*) is related to conditions of 'insufficiency' (*bu zu* 不足) or 'depletion' (虛).[69]

Since case 2 concerns a state in which '*mai* are abundant', one wonders in which sense *bei* (sorrow) is used. It is unlikely that the infant is in a state of mourning, which would refer to *bei ai* and *bei* in the sense in which it is correlated with the lungs, autumn and the West (with its white deserts, associated with the land of the dead). In Yi's Memoir *bei* occurs only once more, in section one. After the document written by Yi's fifth daughter Tiying was given a hearing, 'the Emperor was saddened' (*di bei* 帝悲); he pitied her, and felt compassion.[70] It is most unlikely, however, that Yi considered the sentiment of the Emperor equivalent to that of a troubled infant. The issue remains unresolved.

you 憂 – **grief (line 27)** In the *Shi jing* of the first millennium BCE, there is a poem which relates the emotion *you* (grief) to the heart: 'While I do not see my husband, my heart cannot forget its grief . . . while I do not see my husband, my sad heart has no joy . . . while I do not see my husband, my heart is as if intoxicated with grief' (*wei jian jun zi, you xin qin qin . . . wei jian jun zi, you xin mi le. . . . wei jian jun zi, you xin ru zui* 未見君子 憂心欽欽 未見君子 憂心靡樂 未見君子 憂心如醉).[71] In the *Shi jing*, Legge translates *you* as deep-going 'grief'. In the *Mengzi* of the fourth century BCE, however, there is a phrase 'to be troubled by daily life problems' (*cai xin zhi you* 采薪之憂) with the word *you*, of which the commentator Zhao Qi (d. 201 CE) says: '*you* means to be in distress' (*you, bing ye* 憂病也).[72] In the *Mengzi*,

---

[66] e.g. *Su wen* 43, p. 122. *Ling shu* 28, p. 352; 66, p. 439, all refer to 'grief and worry' (*you si* 憂思).

[67] Consider in particular *bei* in *Su wen* 39, p. 113, and *you* in the same phrase in *Ling shu* 28, p. 352.

[68] e.g. *Su wen* 81, p. 254; *Ling shu* 28, p. 351, and 36, p. 369.

[69] e.g. *Su wen* 62, p. 168; *Ling shu* 8, p. 292. See also *Mai jing* 6.3 quoted on p. 164.

[70] *bei* 'to have compassion' as in Buddhist texts? A hint from semantics for dating the composition of the Memoir's section 1? Further evidence is necessary.

[71] *Mao shi, juan* 6.4, 'Chen feng' 晨風, p. 373b–c. Translation by Legge (1994:200–201).

[72] *Mengzi zhu shu* 4A, p. 2694a. See also Lau (1970:86).

you refers to 'minor daily worries'. This provides the basis for translating *you* as 'irritability' in case 2.

In the Warring States period, *you* certainly also had connotations of fear, as is evident from a phrase of the *Lü shi chun qiu* 20: 'I received my life from heaven and do my utmost in order to nurture the person. Life depends on nature, death on fate. What have I to fear from a dragon!' (*wu shou ming yu tian, jie li yi yang ren. sheng, xing ye. si ming ye, yu he you yu long ye* 吾受命於天 竭力以養人 生性也 死命也 余何憂於龍也).[73] It is possible that *you* also has connotations of anxiety and fear in case 2. In this context, it is interesting to note that the word *wei* 畏, which also means fear, arises from an imbalance in the heart in *Mai jing* 6.3: 'If the heart *qi* is depleted, then one continuously is sad, if repleted, then one constantly giggles ... if the heart *qi* is depleted, then ... if the heart *qi* is abundant, then in a state of confusion one is [simultaneously] cheery and apprehensive' (*xin qi xu ze bei bu yi, shi ze xiao bu xiu; xin qi xu, ze. . . . xin qi sheng, ze meng xi xiao ji kong wei* 心氣虛則悲不已 實則笑不休 心氣虛 則...心氣盛 則夢喜笑及恐畏).[74] In *Mai jing* 6.3 the feeling *kong wei*, which implies apprehensiveness and irritability, arises from abundant heart *qi*. Interestingly, *qi* coming from the heart that is 'hurried' or 'swift', and has been equated with 'being abundant', features also in case 2.

Relevant for the interpretation of case 2 is that *you* is considered to cause barriers in the body. Thus, *Ling shu* 8 states: 'In cases of worry and irritability, *qi* while being closed off and clogged up, does not move' (*chou you zhe, qi bi er sai bu xing* 愁憂者 氣閉塞而不行).[75] Wang Bing's gloss on 'disorders of sudden anxiousness' (*bao you zhi ji* 暴憂之疾) in *Su wen* 28 mentions a clogging up within a bipartite body, with upper and lower parts that are thereby separated one from the other: 'In cases of worry and anxiousness, *qi*, while being closed off and clogged up, does not move, hence there is a separation and clogging up, closing off and *pi*-clots. While *qi* and *mai* are cut off and severed, the above and below do not connect' (*ran chou you zhe, bi sai er bu xing, gu ge sai fou bi, qi mai duan jue er shang xia bu tong ye* 然愁憂者 閉塞而不行 故隔塞否閉 氣脈斷絕而上下不通也).[76] Wang Bing describes here bodily processes comparable to those in case 2, which corroborates the suggestion that the 'infantile irritability' (*shao you*) of case 2 refers to a condition comparable to the 'sudden anxiousness' (*bao you*) in *Su wen* 28 (see p. 159).

In support of this, *Mai jing* 6.3 relates 'anxiousness' (*you*) to 'fright': 'If one is troubled, anxious, worried and preoccupied, then this injures the heart. If the heart is injured, then one suffers from fright' (*chou you si lü, ze shang xin; xin shang, ze ku jing* 愁憂思慮 則傷心 心傷 則苦驚).[77] *Mai*

---

[73] *Lü shi chun qiu* 20.3, 'Zhi fen' 知分. Compare with Knoblock and Riegel (2000:519).
[74] See *Mai jing* 6.3, p. 180.   [75] *Ling shu* 8, p. 291.
[76] HDNJSW 28, p. 64.   [77] *Mai jing* 6.3, p. 182.

jing 6.3 does not fit the canonical five agents schema of the emotions, but it corroborates the analysis of case 2 insofar as it links 'irritability' and 'anxiousness' (*you*) to 'fright' (*jing*), and to the place in which the disorder resides, the 'heart' (*xin*). In summary, the *Mengzi*, *Mai jing* 6.3, *Ling shu* 8 and *Su wen* 28 all provide evidence in support of *you* 'minor daily worries' as cause of the disorder; the medical texts associate them with blockages and abundant *qi*.

We now may attempt to explain why line 26, with *bei* (sorrow), is followed by line 27, with its reference to *you* (grief, irritability). Probably, a commentator who had little understanding for Yi's rationale added line 26, but since sorrow (*bei*) typically arises in cases of feeling depleted, another commentator corrected him in line 27.

Discussion

Based on text structure semantics, one expects the pulse quality '*qi* [coming] from the heart' (*xin qi*) to correlate with the name, 'disorder of *qi* that is separated/blocked' (*qi ge bing*). It is difficult to see a correlation instantly. It is given if one considers the 'heart' to refer to the upper bodily cavity of a bipartite architectural body, and '*qi* [coming] from the heart' to indicate that *qi* is trapped in it. The 'Mai fa' reinforces this, but in a different language. It describes *mai* as 'coming frequently and swiftly, but leaving with difficulty; and not being one [in unison]', which incidentally is the movement of the 'hooked' (*gou*) pulse indicative of disorders in the heart.

The name 'disorder of *qi* that is separated/blocked' (*qi ge bing*) and the name of the remedy that treated it, 'broth that causes *qi* to go downward' (*xia qi tang*) refer to the same body conception: the body is bipartite, with an above and below, and the flow of *qi* matters. Its main axis is a vertical up–down movement, regardless of whether or not there was a bodily structure in the middle, the diaphragm, which could be opened or closed. This rationale is not only contained in the name (line 3), signs and symptoms (lines 4–6), treatment (lines 8–11), counterfactual statement (lines 23–5) and perhaps the term *dang* 'to overturn' (line 21) of case 2, but also in early medical manuscripts (quoted on p. 41) and several of Yi's case histories (e.g. case 1, 2, 3, 6, 9 and others).

Pulse qualities like *xin qi*, generally translated as 'heart *qi*', are in Yi's case histories translated as '*qi* coming from the heart', based on the observation that Yi only speaks of the coming of *mai* and *qi* (while the 'Mai fa' *mai* 'come' and 'go'). If the viscera were understood as seats of emotion and storage places for *qi*, it makes sense that once early Han physicians considered the *mai* to connect with the viscera, *qi* that came from the viscera started to flow in the vessels. Accordingly, palpation on the body surface made it possible to feel *qi* coming from the internal viscera.

The pulse qualities 'murky' (*zhuo*) and 'hurried' (*zao*), as Yi explicitly says, indicate that the 'links have taken on *yang*-qualities' (*luo yang bing*). 'Being murky and hurried', much like 'being frequent and swift', may have indicated that *yang*-qualities had doubled: the entire body felt hot and the *mai* were abundant. Such a 'double *yang*' resulted in overturning the heart and explains why the infant felt 'upset and oppressed'.

The tactile qualities of the pulses Yi mentions in his own vocabulary are difficult to know. 'Being hurried' primarily refers to an emotional disposition of the heart, rather than to a tactile perception. Yet the tactile experiences described by the 'Mai fa' reflect in an iconic and/or indexical way how the chest quickly fills up with *qi* as *qi* gets blocked and turns round in the upper bodily cavity, in a hook-like movement.

In this context, the Dunhuang text P3287 quoted on p. 43 comes to mind, for its striking parallels assure us that cases 1 and 2 form a pair. The Dunhuang text's first line parallels case 1, if one interprets *zhong bu* (middle part) as 'the interior' (*zhong*, where the pre-canonical liver resides), the pulse quality *zha shu zha shuo* as 'alternating' (*dai*, considering its definition in case 6, line 22), and *jing luan* (the passageways are in disarray) as 'the passageways are in disorder' (*jing bing*). Its second line parallels case 2, if one interprets *shang bu* (the upper part) as the 'heart', the pulse quality *gou* (hooked) as 'the *mai* come frequently and swiftly, leave with difficulty, yet are not one' (*mai lai shuo ji, qu nan, er bu yi*) and *bing zai luo mai* (the disorder resides in the linking vessels) as 'disorder of the links becoming *yang*' (*luo yang bing*). The Dunhuang text and Yi's cases 1 and 2 seem to elaborate on the same ancient source; it evidently was terse.

13
Case 3

Translation (*Shiki kaichû kôshô* **105, pp. 28–30**)

1. Xun, the Prefect of the Gentlemen of the Palace of Qi, fell ill.
2. All the many doctors considered it a numbness that had entered and struck the interior,
3. and needled him.

Name:

4. Your servant, Yi, examined him and <u>said</u>: 'It is a welling amassment.
5. It makes the person unable to urinate and defecate.'

6. Xun said: 'I have not been able to urinate and defecate for three days!'

7. Your servant, Yi, had him drink a broth [prepared by careful] regulation of fire.
8. After drinking the first [dose], he was able to urinate.
9. After drinking the second, he thoroughly relieved himself.
10. After drinking the third, the illness was cured.

Cause:

11. <u>The illness was contracted from</u> women.

Quality:

12. <u>The means whereby I recognised Xun's illness were that</u>
13. at the time when I pressed onto his *mai*,
14. at the right opening, *qi* was intense.
15. The *mai* did not have *qi* [coming] from the five viscera –

1. 齊郎中令循病
2. 眾醫皆以為蹶入中
3. 而刺之
4. 臣意診之曰 湧疝也
5. 令人不得前後溲
6. 循曰 不得前後溲三日矣
7. 臣意飲以火齊湯
8. 一飲得前溲
9. 再飲大溲
10. 三飲而疾愈
11. 病得之內
12. 所以知循病者
13. 切其脈時
14. 右口氣急
15. 脈無五藏氣

16. At the right opening, the *mai* were large, yet frequent.

16. 右口脈大而數

17. In cases of the frequent, the interior and lower parts are hot – yet welling.

17. 數者 中下熱而湧

18. The left is for [diagnosing] the lower parts, the right for the upper parts.

18. 左為下右為上

19. There was in all cases no response from the five viscera.

19. 皆無五藏應

20. <u>Hence</u> I said a welling amassment.

20. 故曰湧疝

21. The interior was hot,

21. 中熱

22. <u>Hence</u> the urine was dark.

22. 故溺赤也

Interpretation

Yi first accuses other unnamed doctors of misdiagnosis and mistaken treatment (lines 2–3), then provides his own diagnosis (line 4) and details its concomitant signs and symptoms (line 5). The patient affirms having suffered from those for three days,[1] and Yi treats him with a broth in three doses (lines 7–10). Yi then states the illness cause (line 11). The medical speculation that follows contains repetitions (lines 12–15 and 16–20), and ends with an explanation for a sign not previously mentioned (lines 21–2).

Critical evaluation of retrospective biomedical diagnoses

Bridgman considers this case an acute urinary retention, which he attributes either to kidney stones or to vesical complications due to schistosomiasis. Conditions caused by kidney stones used to be called 'pierre' in French, '*Steinleiden*' in German or 'the stone' in English (OED).[2] The common doctors may have shared this conception of urinary retentions, for Chinese lexicographers have glossed *jue* as 'stone'. However, Yi maintains *jue* 'the stone' is a misdiagnosis. From a biomedical viewpoint, this presumably means that he thought the urinary retention was not caused by kidney stones.

Lu and Needham state it 'was evidently vesical schistosomiasis, accompanied by haematuria, urinary retention, vesicular calculi, perhaps prostatorhoea'.[3] Their diagnosis elaborates, as in other cases, on Bridgman's. There is little doubt that the patient suffers from urinary retention, but their certainty about the vesical schistosomiasis is difficult to share and their claim that it involved haematuria outright mistaken. The idea of haematuria probably arose from translating *ni chi* as 'the urine is red' (line 22), and taking it as a sign of blood in the urine. However, recent scholarship has

---

[1] The patient verifies Yi's signs and symptoms, as otherwise only in cases 4 and 17.
[2] Bridgman (1955:72).   [3] Lu and Needham (1967:231).

made possible a more differentiated understanding: *ni chi* means the urine is dark yellow and indicates heat.[4]

The common doctors vainly attempt to treat *jue* with 'needling', which Yi applies successfully in cases 11 and 16, where *jue* is a heat condition (but not in case 9, marked by coldness). Yi's treatment takes place in three stages: the first dose restores the patient's 'urination' (*qian sou*). However, urinary retentions can hinder defecation as the pain they cause is all-encompassing, and after the second, the patient has a 'great relief' (*da sou*).[5] The disorder is cured only after the third dose, as though Yi distinguished between apparent complaints and an underlying disorder.[6]

The name of the disorder (lines 2 and 4)

Several terms in case 3 are known from canonical medicine, such as the names for the disorder, which all the many doctors call *jue* ('the stone', numbness, inversion) but Yi diagnoses as *shan* (tumour, hernia, amassment) and the qualities of *mai*. Nevertheless the case contains incongruencies.

jue 蹶/厥 – 'the stone'? (line 2)   In medical texts there are several graphs for *jue*, two of which are particularly frequent: 厥 and 蹶.[7] These graphs can have distinctive meanings but were often used interchangeably. Thus, *jue* in Takigawa's edition of *Shi ji* 105 only has *jue* 蹶, while Ren Yingqiu's *Nei jing* edition consistently has *jue* 厥. *Shuo wen* 9B defines *jue* 厥: "*jue* is an emitted/dug out stone" (*jue fa shi ye* 厥發石也).[8] This definition is given as basic meaning in all standard dictionaries on literary Chinese. All have as first entry for *jue* 厥 'the stone' (*shi* 石).[9]

The interpretation of *jue* as 'stone' is also given in Yang Liang's 楊倞 (ninth-century) gloss, "*jue* means stone" (*jue shi ye* 厥石也), on *Xunzi* 27:

---

[4] Although all clinicians I consulted emphasised no more can be said with certainty about this case than that it concerns a urinary retention, one is tempted to hazard the guess that dark urine hints at an infection, perhaps a prostatitis. This can be contracted through sexually transmitted pathogens (e.g. gonorrhoea) and can lead, if the prostate becomes very swollen, to urine retention, which, in turn, can manifest with central bloating, and often is so painful that it hinders defecation. It is quickly cured in its early stages.

[5] *da sou* 大溲 means 'to defecate', *xiao sou* 小溲 'to urinate', according to Zhang Shoujie. See also case 5. Wang Niansun suggests line 8 is corrupt and should read *qian hou sou* 前後溲 'to urinate and defecate', as it does in case 5 (line 6) and in the *Tai ping yu lan* 721. However, Wang Shumin (1983:2904) refutes this parallel between cases 3 and 5; the 'great discharge' (*da sou*) probably means 'discharge in the back' (*hou sou*).

[6] Zhang Wenhu points out three editions, and Takigawa yet another, that render *ji* 疾 (line 10) as *bing* 病 'disorder'. Alternative translation of line 10: "After drinking the third, he recovered swiftly" (*san yin er ji yu*).

[7] Wang Niansun notes *jue* 蹶 in case 3 should be read as *jue* 厥 and quotes the *Shi ming* on *jue* 厥. See also Yu (1953:233–5). On *jue*, see case 9.

[8] *Shuo wen* 9B, 20a. Duan Yucai comments "If one extends its [meaning] all that has been dug out is called *jue*" (*yin shen zhi fan you jue fa jie yue jue* 引伸之 凡有撅發皆曰厥). See also Karlgren (1957: 90–91).

[9] See HYDZD 1.76, HYDCD 1.936.

"Learning and culture are to men what polishing and grinding are to jade ... Bian He's *bi* disc was a stone from inside a well, but after the jade man carved it, it became the treasure of the son of heaven" (*ren zhi yu wen xue ye, you yu zhi yu zhuo mo ye ... He zhi bi, jing li zhi jue ye, yu ren zhuo zhi, wei tian zi bao* 人之於文學也 猶玉之於琢磨也 和之璧 井里之厥也 玉人琢之 為天子寶).[10] According to the translation of the *Xunzi* passage presented here, which differs from the usual one, *jue* would refer to a coarse stone taken out of the ground that one finds in the course of digging a well. Unlike stones from river beds, dug out *jue* stones were crude and coarse, and had to be subject to the work of culture, i.e. polished and carved by skilled craftsmen, before becoming highly treasured objects, such as *bi* discs.

The *Shuo wen* definition of *jue* as 'dug out stone' and *Xunzi*'s reference to *jue* as unpolished crude stone establish a stark contrast to the much valued *yu*-jade and *shi*-stones in early China, as is also evident from the name of Yi's book called 'Divinity of the Stone' (Shi shen). This is relevant in the medical context. Urinary retentions caused by kidney or bladder stones that cross-culturally were conceived of as 'the stone' could not have been called *shi*-stones and the common doctors may therefore have spoken of the *jue*-stone. 'Needling' may have been intended to cause an emission of stones. The washed out small 'stones' may have given the disorder its name. These small stones may or may not have been considered debris from one large 'stone' inside the characteristically protruding abdomen, which is caused by the accumulated waters of a urinary retention.[11]

In Late Imperial China, as in Europe, Santangelo notes, 'stones' (*shi* 石) had connotations of emotional coldness.[12] Among the four seasonal *mai* – where the *mai* of spring is likened to a 'bow-string' (*xian* 絃), that of summer to a 'hook' (*gou* 鈎), that of autumn to a 'hair' (*mao* 毛), and that of winter to a 'stone' (*shi* 石) – Majno translates the fourth as 'dead as a rock'.[13]

---

[10] *Xunzi* 27, p. 309. Translation based on Knoblock (1994:227–8), but modified. The usual reading is *Jingli zhi jue ye*: "The stone from Jingli". In *Han Feizi* 4.13, pp. 238–9, the stone is said to come from the Chu mountains 楚山, which a commentator glosses as Jing mountains 荆山. Jingli is generally considered a place name (Mark Lewis, 1995 p.c.). Since Jingli is unattested as a place name in the received literature, I give the above alternative translation. Perhaps it was unthinkable that an ordinary stone dug out of a well could become as treasured an object as Bian He's *bi* disc.

[11] Consider the ancient Greek author of *On Diseases* and his ideas about the formation of stones in the bladder:

> First he refers to the way in which a sediment forms when dirty water is left to stand in a cup or vessel, and he says that a sediment forms in the same way in the bladder when the urine is impure ... And then he suggests how a stone is formed from part of this sediment by referring to the smelting of iron from iron ore: while the stone remains and hardens in the bladder under the influence (he believes) of phlegm, the equivalent of the dross is passed out with the urine ... (Lloyd 1966:346–7)

> The Greek author considered stones in the urine debris of a large stone inside the body.

[12] Santangelo (1994:172 and unpubl. *Materials for an Anatomy of Personality in Late Imperial China*).

[13] Majno (1975:245) on the qualities of *gu* 鼓 'drum beating' in *Su wen* 7, p. 27. On *xian*, see case 1 (line 17); on *gou*, see case 2 (line 17); on *gu*, see case 6 (line 18).

However, in early China, not *shi*-stones but the unrefined *jue*-stones that had been dug out of the ground and were considered crude and coarse implied insensitivity, dullness and numbness. Duke Zhao was so completely lifeless that everyone considered him dead, when Bian Que diagnosed *bao jue* 暴厥 (sudden numbness) and *shi jue* 尸厥 (the corpse is numb/fake), and brought him back to life.[14] In Yi's case 25, the symptom *jue* is collocated with 'cold' (*han* 寒), which prompts its rendering as 'numb' in cases 3 and 23, and also parts of case 9. However, the *Shi ji* personage Yi has a more sophisticated concept of *jue* in cases 9, 11 and 16, and perceived it as an 'inversion' of *yin* and *yang* or heat and coldness.[15]

In summary, it is likely that the connotations of the dull, numb and cold apply to the many doctors' understanding of *jue* in cases 3 and 23. They certainly apply to the medical term *jue* in the third century BCE (see case 9, line 3). The commentators are wrestling with this early understanding of *jue*, and also with whether *zhong* in *jue ru zhong*, '*jue* entered and struck the interior', is a verb in a verb-verb complex or a deictic noun, designating a body part.[16]

shan 疝 – an amassment or, literally, a tumour (line 4)   The term *shan* 疝 with the phonetic part *shan* 山 'mountain' is in translation best approximated by 'tumour', which means 'hill' in Latin, but nowadays has unsuitable connotations. Likewise, *shan*'s rendering as 'hernia' is too specifically biomedical. Therefore, *shan* is here translated as 'amassment'. An 'amassment' designates an 'accumulation into mass' (OED). Although the word sounds unfamiliar, it accurately invokes a visible and tangible protrusion or swelling.

Shan are often given as the second constituent in compound words and function there as what lexical semanticists call a 'semantic categoriser'.[17] According to some authors there are five different kinds of *shan*, according to others seven, and only a cursory glance at the medical literature shows there are many more. 'Amassments' generally refer to men's disorders, and sometimes are contrasted with 'conglomerations' (*jia*) as women's disorders.[18] Such a gender-specific differentiation of *shan*, but not *jia*, is already given in the early medical manuscripts.[19] It is therefore not surprising that

[14] *Shi ji* 105.1, p. 2788 and p. 2790.

[15] Yi has 'wind-induced numbness/inversion' (*feng jue* 風厥) in case 9, 'heat inversion' (*re jue* 熱厥) in case 11, and an 'inversion above' (*jue shang* 厥上) in case 16. For Bian Que, *jue* too is a *yin yang* inversion.

[16] Takigawa points to an edition with *ru* 入 as *ren* 人, Wang Niansun to *feng ru zhong* 風入中 in case 10 (line 2). For *ru zhong* as verb-verb complex, see *shang chu* in case 2 (lines 24–5), *ru zhang* 入長 in case 9 (line 15) and *ru ru* 入濡 in case 17, see ch. 7, n. 29. See also MWD "Recipes" (1985:30, 31): "Wind enters and causes harm" (*feng ru shang* 風入傷). Alternative translation for *jue ru zhong* 'numbness entered the interior'.

[17] See ch. 10, n. 17.

[18] On *jia* (conglomerations), see case 7 (line 4). See also case 19 in ch. 7.

[19] MWD YY (1985:11). Quoted on p. 336.

in Yi's Memoir *jia* are not gender-specific disorders (as they tend to be in Late Imperial China), but it is strange that in case 10 a woman suffers from *shan*.

According to *Shuo wen* 7B, 'An amassment is abdominal pain' (*shan fu tong ye* 疝腹痛也).[20] Duan Yucai (1735–1815), the Qing commentator to the *Shuo wen*, relates *shan* to 'heart pain' (*xin tong* 心痛), correlated to ascending *qi*) and the 'swollen *yin*-parts, i.e. genitals' (*yin zhong* 陰腫, correlated to descending *qi*).[21] Yet in antiquity, as he points out, *shan* were marked by 'intense pain of the small abdomen' (*xiao fu ji tong* 小腹急痛). This is crucial to understanding *shan* in case 3.

Yi mentions *shan* three times in the name of the disorder (cases 3, 10, 25). The amassments in cases 3 and 10 present as urinary retentions that Yi can treat, but the 'male amassment' (*mu shan* 牡疝)[22] in case 25 is of a different order and ends in death.[23] The 'welling amassment' (*yong shan*) in case 3 and the 'amassment visiting the bladder' (*shan ke yu pang guang*) in case 10 have signs and symptoms that coincide with those in *Su wen* 55: 'If the disorder is in the minor abdomen, the abdomen is painful and one is not able to defecate and urinate, the name of the disorder is called an amassment' (*bing zai shao fu, fu tong bu de da xiao bian, bing ming yue shan* 病在少腹 腹痛不得大小便 病名曰疝).[24] *Su wen* 55 also notes that it "is contracted from the cold" (*de zhi han* 得之寒), but Yi speaks of sexual indulgence in all three cases. Nevertheless, we will return to the coldness mentioned in *Su wen* 55.

yong 湧 – welling (line 4)   The 'welling amassment' (*yong shan*) is not attested in canonical medical texts, this in contrast to 'welling' (*yong*). 'Welling' refers to upward movements of water, as in the canonical medical idioms 'welling water' (*yong shui* 涌水) or 'welling spring' (*yong quan* 涌泉).[25] As case 3 (line 17) currently reads, *yong* is mentioned in association with heat and means 'gushing' rather than 'welling'. However, textual anomalies point to serious problems in that passage. In early manuscripts

---

[20] *Shuo wen* 7B, p. 29b.
[21] e.g. Yu (1953:218–20 and 225–9) devotes a separate entry to 'heart pain' and 'swollen genitals'.
[22] Compare with the term 'male conglomeration' (*mu jia* 牡瘕) in ZJS (2001:235), discussed in case 7 (line 4). As suggested in Hsu (in press c), 'male' and 'female' disorders were named as such based on the experience of the reproductive organs. The former may have had a protuberant appearance; the latter caused bloody emissions. Compare with the gender-specific activities mentioned in case 7, n. 21.
[23] Note, again, the relative semantic consistency for *shan* in cases 1–10.
[24] *Su wen* 55, p. 149.
[25] e.g. *Su wen* 37, p. 108 and *Su wen* 17, p. 50. 'Yongquan' is also an acupuncture *locus*, e.g. *Su wen* 6, p. 25.

yong refers to the 'welling' of *yin* [waters][26] and in the canonical idioms as the above, it also alludes to water. Since water was and is generally classified as cool, *yong shan* meaning 'welling amassment' may also have implied coldness. This would align it with *Su wen* 55 that gives coldness as cause for any amassment.

Taki Motohiro considers the 'welling amassment' a 'transverse amassment' (*heng shan* 衝疝) and cites *Su wen* 60: 'When this one gives rise to a disorder, by following along the minor abdomen and rising to transverse to the heart region and when it is painful and one cannot urinate and defecate, it becomes a "transverse amassment"' (*ci sheng bing cong shao fu shang heng xin, er tong bu de qian hou, wei heng shan* 此生病從少腹上衝心 而痛不 得前後 為衝疝).[27] He identifies the 'transverse amassment' with '*qi* of a running piglet amassment' (*ben tun shan qi* 奔豚疝氣), a term that does not occur in the *Inner Canon*. The 'running piglet' (*ben tun*), however, does occur in *Ling shu* 4, and manifests with the same symptoms of 'being unable to urinate and defecate' that Yi mentions.[28]

Text structure semantics

According to text structure semantics, one would expect the quality of *qi* that Yi senses when he examines *mai* to correlate with the name of the disorder. Yi reports that at the 'right opening' *qi* is 'intense' (line 14) and that the *mai* were 'without *qi* [coming] from the five viscera' (line 15), and he calls the disorder a 'welling amassment' (line 4). No correlation is readily apparent.

Yi then describes qualities of *mai* in a different vocabulary (lines 16–20): they are 'large, yet frequent' (line 16). He then explains the implications of 'being frequent' (line 17), of *mai* examined on the 'right' and 'left' (line 18), repeats that none of the five viscera was affected (line 19), and ends by saying that hence he diagnosed a 'welling amassment' (line 20). Although Yi's reasoning appears coherent, it is difficult to correlate any pulse qualities with the name of the disorder. We will explore each in more detail.

ji 急 – **intense (line 14)**   All three static verbs qualifying pulses in case 3 are known from the received medical literature. 'Being frequent' is one of the standard pulses in *Mai jing* 1.1, 'intense' (*ji*) and 'large' (*da*) belong among the three well-known pairs of *mai* in the *Inner Canon*. Thus, 'relaxed or slack' is contrasted with '(in)tense', 'small' with 'large' in *Ling shu* 4: "I wish to ask what form the illness takes when the pulse is either slack or

---

[26] e.g. MWD YY (no. 2) in (Ma 1992:272) has *xin yong* (lit. 'the heart is welling'), see case 9, n. 28.

[27] *Su wen* 60, p. 161.   [28] *Ling shu* 4, p. 277.

intense, small or large, or slippery or rough" (*qing wen mai zhi huan ji xiao da hua se zhi bing xing he ru* 請問脈之緩急 小大 滑濇 之病形何如).[29] Qibo's answer mentions *ji* several times without, however, elucidating its meaning.

In the Mawangdui medical manuscripts, *ji* occurs in three different instances, with three distinct meanings: in one context, it refers to a time span and means 'instantly';[30] in another it refers to an inner state of mind, which Harper aptly translates as 'tense';[31] and third, it describes the sensation one has when touching the skin, which Harper translates as 'taut'.[32] This use of *ji*, for describing a 'taut skin', can also be found in *Ling shu* 4, where the quality of the skin at the *chi*-area correlates with that of the *mai*: "If the pulse is taut, then the skin at the *chi*-area is also taut" (*mai ji zhe, chi zhi pi fu yi ji* 脈急者 尺之皮膚亦急).[33] It resurfaces here and again in later texts, as for instance in the expression 'the skin is taut' (*pi ji* 皮急) in the *Zhu bing yuan hou lun*.[34]

The *Shi ji* case histories refer to *ji* in the above three senses too. In case 3, *ji* (approximated as 'taut' or 'intense') designates a tactually perceived quality. In case 7, *ji* modifies the length of a time span that is brief and intense insofar as it critically determines the outcome of the illness. In case 15, it modifies the heart and refers to a tense inner state of mind.[35] In cases 7 and 15, *ji* is an aspect of a condition that ends in death, and in the *Inner Canon*, *ji* belongs, together with others, among *mai* indicative of death. Thus, *Su wen* 28 states: 'If *mai*, in the case of being full and large, are slack/relaxed, then one will live, if they are taut/intense, then one dies' (*mai shi da ye, huan ze sheng, ji ze si* 脈實大也 緩則生 急則死).[36] In case 3, *ji* (taut, intense) also indicates urgency, but Yi says twice that the five viscera were not affected and he cures the patient.

A gloss not given by the commentators here but often cited elsewhere is: '*ji* means having difficulties' (*ji wei kun nan* 急謂困難).[37] With it Yin Zhizhang 尹知章 (d. 718) commented on *ji* in *Guanzi* 24: 'When initiating [military] ventures, if he understands the people's urgent needs, the masses will not become rebellious' (*ju zhi ren ji ze zhong bu luan* 舉知人急則眾不亂).[38] This meaning of *ji* that invokes a 'difficult' (*nan*) situation of crisis and urgency is variously given in medical contexts. Thus, amassments can present with 'difficulties in urination and defecation', as in case 10 (line 15), where incidentally Yi also senses *mai* 'coming with difficulty' (*qi lai nan* 其來難).

---

[29] *Ling shu* 4, p. 276. See also Hsu (in press e).   [30] MWD "Recipes" (1985:58).
[31] MWD "He yinyang" (1985:156), Harper (1998:419).
[32] MWD "Yangsheng fang" (1985:107), Harper (1998:342).
[33] *Ling shu* 4, p. 276.   [34] *Zhu bing yuan hou lun* 30.5, p. 852.
[35] There is some controversy over the graph *ji* in case 15. See ch. 7, n. 26.
[36] *Su wen* 28, p. 87.   [37] e.g. Ma (1992:998).
[38] *Guanzi* 3.24, "Wen" 問, p. 1b. Translation by Rickett (1985:369).

Furthermore, pain can be 'intense' (*ji*), as in *Su wen* 71: "When coldness arrives, then there are firm *pi*-clots, the abdomen is full, pain is intense, and the disorder of [urinary] inhibition arises (*han zhi, ze jian pi, fu man, tong ji, xia li zhi bing sheng yi* 寒至則堅否腹滿痛急下利之病生矣).[39] Applied to case 3, the 'intense' pain inside the body may well be reflected in the 'intense' quality of *qi* Yi sensed on the body surface. This is clearly stated in *Su wen* 18: 'When *mai* are intense, you call it an amassment or conglomeration, the minor abdomen is in pain' (*mai ji zhe, yue shan jia shao fu tong* 脈急者曰疝瘕少腹痛).[40] In *Su wen* 18, the pulse quality 'intense' reflects in an iconic/indexical way the 'intense' pain in the minor abdomen.

Also in *Su wen* 48 an 'intense' pulse indicates an amassment, although the intense pain is not mentioned: "When the kidney *mai* is large, intense, and sunken or when the liver *mai* is large, intense, and sunken, in all those cases it is an amassment" (*shen mai da ji chen, gan mai da ji chen, jie wei shan* 腎脈大急沈肝脈大急沈皆為疝).[41] *Su wen* 18 and 48 have *mai* rather than '*qi* that is intense' (*qi ji*), but all take 'being intense' as a sign of 'amassments' (*shan*). Text structure semantics can be applied to the second constituent of the name of the disorder in case 3: the 'amassment' correlates with 'being intense'.

shuo 數 – frequent (lines 16 and 17)

The stanza (lines 12–15) within which Yi mentions 'intense' as a quality of *qi* is followed by one where he describes *mai* as 'large, yet frequent' (*da er shuo*; lines 16–20). In contemporary Chinese medicine, *shuo* is recognised by its rapid pulse beat which, as in biomedicine, is taken as an indication of heat and fevers.[42] Interestingly, however, for defining the 'frequent pulse' (*shuo mai*), *Mai jing* 1.1 speaks of 'being intense': 'It goes and comes rapidly and intensely' (*qu lai cu ji* 去來促急).[43] And in the *Nei jing*, the graph 數 pronounced as *shuo*, does not primarily qualify *mai* nor imply heat. Rather, it is used for describing repetitive behaviour, such as 'urinating frequently' (*shuo xiao bian* 數小便), 'drinking frequently' (*shuo yin* 數飲) or 'frequently being drunk' (*shuo zui* 數醉).[44] *Ling shu* 3 mentions *shuo* in the context of needling techniques: 'The subtleties of needling reside in frequency and retardation' (*ci zhi wei*

---

[39] *Su wen* 71, p. 229. See also *Su wen* 74, p. 235: "Inside it is tense, there is violent pain" (*li ji bao tong* 裡急暴痛) (Paul Unschuld, 2000 p.c.).

[40] *Su wen* 18, p. 55. The translation 'conglomeration of an amassment' for *shan jia* is unlikely since each is an unambiguous name of a disorder in Yi's case histories. See also *Su wen* 19, p. 61, quoted on p. 276.

[41] *Su wen* 48, p. 135; *da* may also be an intensifier, meaning 'very'.

[42] *Zhongyi zhenduanxue* (Deng 1984:66).   [43] *Mai jing* 1.1, p. 1.

[44] *Huangdi nei jing*, pp. 1500–1501.

zai shuo chi zhe 刺之微在數遲者).[45] The needle's movement is described as *shuo*-frequent and *chi*-retarded.

In *Su wen* 7, 'being frequent' is again contrasted with 'being retarded' and now explicitly said to indicate a *yang* condition: 'Being retarded is *yin*, being frequent *yang*' (*chi zhe wei yin, shuo zhe wei yang* 遲者為陰 數者為陽).[46] In case 3, Yi states that 'being frequent' indicates heat. Heat clearly is an aspect of a *yang* condition in cases 1 and 2, and arguably also in case 5, where Yi states that 'hurried' (*zao*) rather than 'frequent' indicates heat in the interior. In summary, the 'frequent' pulse has traits of the 'intense' and is not always associated with heat in canonical medical texts.

da 大 – large (line 16)   The *mai* are not only 'frequent', but simultaneously 'large' (*da*). The 'large' is neither one of the twenty-four pulses in the *Mai jing* nor of the current twenty-eight, although it is one of the standard six in the *Nei jing* (quoted on pp. 173–4).[47] Yi mentions it three times in the case histories (cases 3, 5, 10).[48] In case 5 (line 20), Yi explains 'being large' indicates '*qi* [coming] from the bladder' (*pang guang qi*) and also in case 10 the bladder is affected. In case 3 (line 5), Yi says the patient cannot urinate and defecate. Since it is likely that urine was thought to accumulate in the region of the bladder, the 'large' pulse presumably indicates a disorder of the bladder also in this case.

It is strange that Yi does not explicate 'being large' in a topic-comment sentence after the one on 'being frequent' in line 17. Such topic-comment sentences are recurrently found in cases 1–10,[49] and despite considerable variation, they are an important rhetorical feature of these cases. There is a pattern to the case recordings of the *Shi ji* personage Yi. First, he reports on the 'name', 'cause' and 'quality' of the disorder (which can be singled out due to the recurrent phrases that introduce them), he then may quote the 'Mai fa', discuss it sometimes with yet another set of static verbs and, finally, elucidate these in topic-comment sentences. Since the terminology in the topic-comment sentences comes so close to the canonical writing style, these sentences were either added by the early first-century editor or represent commentatorial interjections.

Case 3 contains no 'Mai fa' quote but after Yi's statement in line 16 there is an elucidating topic-comment statement on 'being frequent' in line 17,

---

[45] *Ling shu* 3, p. 271. The following, *ji xu zhi yi* 疾徐之意, which contrasts *ji*-swift with *xu*-slow, can be read either as explanatory paraphrase or as detailing the mind set of the physician during the needling.

[46] *Su wen* 7, p. 26.

[47] *Huangdi nei jing*, p. 1580. See also case 10 (line 14).

[48] *da* 大 'being large' is also mentioned in case 5 (lines 15–16), arguably in the same sense as here, and case 6 (line 22), where it does not refer to a disorder in the bladder.

[49] In case 1 (line 30), case 2 (line 21), case 3 (line 17), case 4 (line 30), case 5 (lines 20–21), case 6 (lines 21–2), case 7 (lines 17–19), case 9 (lines 20–21), case 10 (line 17), but not in case 8.

which fits the above-outlined pattern. However, there is an *er*-phrase: 'yet welling' (*er yong*) which appears to be tagged on. While the first part of line 17, "In cases of the frequent, the interior/central and lower parts are hot", does not reflect early medical rationale, its second part may well do so. The 'frequent' pulse may indicate 'heat', but not a 'welling'. Nor is the 'welling' ever 'hot'. On the contrary, it is collocated with cool spring waters (see p. 172).

In the light of the Guodian manuscript that 'the Great One gives birth to water' (*da yi sheng shui* 大一生水),[50] it is likely that 'being large' was indicative of the 'welling' cool waters, in the bodily region of the bladder.[51] This would also be in line with *Su wen* 55 (quoted on p. 172), which states that amassments arise from the cold.

wu wu zang qi 無五藏氣 **– Without any *qi* coming from the five viscera (line 15)** If 'yet welling' (*er yong*), which evidently correlates with *yong*-welling in the name of the disorder, does not belong to line 17, may it once have been part of line 15 or line 16? If it had been part of line 16, the pulse qualities of being 'large, yet welling' both would have correlated with *yong* in the name of the disorder. Assuming that Yi reasons coherently, it is more likely that the quality of *mai* in line 15 was 'without any *qi* coming from the five viscera, while there was a welling'. The correlation between *yong* as pulse quality and as constituent in the name of the disorder would then be facile, comparable to that of 'wind *qi*' and 'wind' in cases 5 and 9. As we will see in case 9 (pp. 304–5), there is reason to assume that the first-century editor may have interpolated passages that establish such a facile correlation. Accordingly, lines 16 and 17, first part, may well be commentatorial interjections. We will return to this suggestion later.

Summary Text structure semantics postulates a correlation between the name of the disorder 'welling amassment' (*yong shan*) and Yi's pulse qualities. In case 3, the correlation is given twice. If one considers '*qi* that is intense' (*qi ji*) to reflect in an iconic or indexical way intense pain, it refers to the main characteristic of 'amassments' (*shan*), according to the *Shuo wen* and several *Su wen* texts (and also according to the general human experience of urinary retentions). 'Being intense' (line 14) indicates 'amassments' (line 4) also in canonical medical texts.

According to text structure semantics, the next pulse quality '*mai* did not have *qi* [coming] from the five viscera' (line 15) should correlate with the 'welling' (*yong*). This correlation is given, if one considers 'yet welling' (line

---

[50] Jingmenshi Bowuguan (1998:125). The graphs are here rendered as in the manuscript text as *da yi* 大一 rather than the usual *tai yi* 太一. The two graphs were often used interchangeably.

[51] See MWD YY graphs discussed in case 9, n. 28.

17) to have been part of line 15 at one stage in the textual history of case 3.

Furthermore, parallels to Yi's cases 1–10 and the Guodian *Laozi* point to an early correlation between 'being large' (*da*) and the cosmogonic waters of the bladder. So, with regard to the presumably commentatorial interjections in lines 16 and 17, text structure semantics also works but not as unambiguously as one would hope: 'being large' correlates with 'the welling' (*yong*) and 'frequent' with 'amassments', although no canonical parallels were found for the latter.

The concept of mai kou 脈口 – *opening of the* mai *(lines 14 and 16)*

you 右 – the right (lines 14, 16, 18)   Yi says first that he felt *qi* (on line 14), and then that he felt *mai* at the right opening (line 16). He speaks once of *qi* and once of *mai*, but this does not trouble most commentators.[52] They find it puzzling that he mentions twice the right opening. Xu Guang points to an edition which renders 'the right' (*you* 右) in line 14 as 'to have' (*you* 有): 'There was *qi* [coming] out of the opening, it was intense' (*you kou qi, ji*). Although this reading affects the rhythm of the phrase unfavourably and therefore is unlikely, it is conceivable that, as Yi presses onto the *mai*, he senses that there is much *qi* at the opening, and that this indicates that inside the body an amassment is blocking the opening for urination. If *you* 右 (the right) is read as *you* 有 (to have) in line 14, 'the right' would be mentioned only once, in line 16.

Ando Koretora, however, suggests that the 'right' should be read as 'left' (*zuo* 左) in line 16. He evidently assumes that *mai* can be examined on the left and right, as is implied by line 18, which states that pulses felt on the right and left are indicative of processes taking place in the upper or lower bodily spheres respectively. Line 18 parallels *Su wen* 5: 'Hence whenever one is affected by the noxious, if it is above, the right is very [much affected], if it is below, then the left is very [much affected]' (*gu ju gan yu xie, qi zai shang, ze you shen qi zai xia, ze zuo shen* 故俱感於邪 其在上則右甚 其在下則左甚).[53] Accordingly, sensing 'intense' *qi* on the right would indicate pain

---

[52] Taki Motokata notes that *qi* in *qi ji* (line 14) is used in the same sense as in *Su wen* 19, pp. 58–9, as *qi* of a *mai*. In line 14, Yi qualifies *qi*, in line 15 *mai*. Probably line 15 is an editorial interpolation. In line 15, the *mai* have qualities of *qi*, in line 19, which states there is no response/resonance (*wu ying*), they are expected to *ying* (to resonate). Perhaps line 19 is a commentatorial interjection?

[53] *Su wen* 5, p. 22. See also *Su wen* 74, pp. 231–2 (which dates to the same period). For a gender-specific differentiation between the left and right, see *Su wen* 15, p. 45: "The woman's right indicates the contravective, and the left indicates the smooth; the man's left indicates the contravective, and the right indicates the smooth, (*nü zi you wei ni, zuo wei cong, nan zi zuo wei ni, you wei cong* 女子右為逆 左為從 男子左為逆 右為從). In line with this rationale, *Su wen* 48, p. 135, reports on gender-specific 'one-sided withering' (*pian ku* 偏枯, in biomedical jargon inclusive, presumably, of hemiplegias) on the left in men and the right in women.

in the upper parts, and sensing the 'large yet frequent' *mai* on the left would indicate that the bladder in the lower parts was primarily affected. This alteration of the text makes perfect sense, but a caveat is necessary. Ando Koretora's emendation of the text may well derive from anachronistically imputing into the *Shi ji* the medical rationale from *Su wen* 5.[54] The rationale given in line 18, which obviously parallels that of *Su wen* 5, does not tally with that found otherwise throughout case 3. Rather than emending the graph for the 'right', there are reasons, presented in what follows, that a commentator of medieval times or later may have interjected line 18. Perhaps it was the same one who interjected the 'lower parts' (*xia*) in line 17.[55]

In the reading proposed here, which differs from Xu Guang's and Ando Koretora's, the text is divided into two stanzas (lines 12–15 and 16–20). These two stanzas report on the same condition in different vocabularies. Since they both report on the same condition, they both mention the 'right opening'.

Thus, the first stanza speaks of *qi* that is 'intense', and the second stanza of *mai* that 'are large, yet frequent'. The first stanza continues with speaking about *mai* that do not have the *qi* of the five viscera; the second stanza speaks of no response from the five viscera, or, more literally, a lack of *ying* 應 (resonance). Both stanzas describe the same diagnostic procedure: they both record the examination on the right (*you*). This suggests that contrary to the rationale in *Su wen* 5 and the perhaps interjected line 18, early Han physicians primarily investigated the right for detecting qualities of *qi*. There are hints for such a principle of diagnosis in Yi's cases 1–10.

kou 口 – **mouth, opening (line 14)**   Yi says that at the 'right opening' *qi* was intense, but it is difficult to know what exactly he meant by the 'right opening' (*you kou*). Literally, *kou* means 'mouth' but in Yi's case histories it generally designates a place on the body surface where Yi examines *mai*. In case 4 (line 33), Yi speaks of the 'opening of the major *yin mai*' (*tai yin mai kou*) and in case 5 (line 12) of the 'opening of the major *yin*' (*tai yin zhi kou*). In case 6 (line 31), as the text is punctuated in Takigawa's edition, Yi furthermore would mention the 'foot's minor *yang mai* opening' (*zu shao yang mai kou*); not, however, according to this study (see translation of case 6, lines 31 and 32, discussed on p. 257). The 'openings' evidently refer to a specific place on the *mai*. In the Mawangdui vessel texts, *mai* usually 'come out' (*chu* 出) near the tips of the extremities, and, accordingly,

---

[54] On the dating of *Su wen* 5, see ch. 3, n. 21, and case 1, n. 63.

[55] There are two reasons for postulating an interjection of *xia* in line 17: *zhong xia re* (the interior and lower parts are hot) is a strange idiom and *zhong re* (the interior is hot), which would have occurred first on line 17, is repeated on line 21.

Yi may have called these places, which were perhaps on the wrist and ankle, 'openings' (*kou*).

Yi's understanding of *kou* instantly brings to mind Wang Bing's comment on *Su wen* 11: '*Qi kou* then is *cun kou*, it is also called *mai kou*' (*qi kou ze cun kou ye, yi wei mai kou ye* 氣口則寸口也 亦謂脈口也),[56] which equates the 'opening of the *mai*' (*mai kou* 脈口) with the 'opening for *qi*' (*qi kou* 氣口) and the 'inch-opening' (*cun kou* 寸口). It would be wrong, however, to apply this medieval understanding unreflectedly to early medicine. There are important differences.

Case 7 mentions an 'opening of the *mai* on the right' (*you mai kou*; line 13), which probably is synonymous with the 'right opening' in case 3. Nowadays, it is located, as Takigawa says, one inch behind the thenar eminence. It is possible but not certain that this was its location in antiquity (a passage of *Su wen* 20 which parallels the Zhangjiashan "Maishu" suggests investigating the ankle). Although case 18 refers in its last paragraph to a 'left opening' when reporting on the viscus liver, which may or may not be a commentatorial interjection, we note that in cases 1–10, if specified (as in cases 3 and 7), the 'opening' Yi investigates is always on the right. His diagnosis consists of identifying qualities of *qi* indicative once of an amassment, once of a conglomeration, both of which are painful (e.g. *Su wen* 18, quoted on p. 175).

Canonical medical texts usually speak of the right and left simultaneously, but there are exceptions. One is *Su wen* 62: 'If while pain is on the left, the right vessel is in disorder, the big needle lances it' (*tong zai yu zuo er you mai bing zhe, ju ci zhi* 痛在於左 而右脈病者 巨刺之), which is repeated in *Su wen* 63: 'If pain on the left has not yet come to an end, and if the right vessel is the first to get into disorder, if it is such, one must [use] the big needle for lancing it' (*zuo tong wei yi er you mai xian bing, ru ci zhe bi ju ci zhi* 左痛未已 而右脈先病 如此者 必巨刺之).[57] *Su wen* 62 and 63 differ from all other *Nei jing* passages because they do not discuss left and right, and vice versa, but state that pain on the left manifests in *mai* on the right (no vice versa). They provide a rationale for the pulse diagnostic findings given in cases 3 (line 14) and 7 (line 13), which concern pain conditions diagnosed at the 'right opening'.

Another exception is a passage of the *Mai jing* that Zhang Shoujie cites: 'The right hand's inch-opening then is the opening for *qi*' (*you shou cun kou nai qi kou ye* 右手寸口乃氣口也). As so often, Zhang Shoujie's quote cannot be found in extant editions. It is mentioned here because it states *qi kou* is on the right. In *Su wen* 11, *qi kou* is indicative of the condition of the five viscera; in *Ling shu* 48, it indicates the overall state of the body's interior; and in *Su wen* 21, it is considered crucial for the prognosis of life and death. The canonical *qi kou* provides a rationale for Yi's findings

---

[56] HDNJSW 11, p. 30.   [57] *Su wen* 62, p. 171, and 63, p. 172.

recorded in case 3 (lines 15 and 19), insofar as those concern the overall state of the five viscera.

Su wen 11 begins with the Yellow Emperor asking: 'How is it that the "opening for *qi*" alone is the host of the five viscera?' (*qi kou he yi du wei wu zang zhu* 氣口何以獨為五藏主). Qibo answers: 'The flavours enter the mouth, are stored in the stomach and thereby nourish the *qi* of the five viscera – "the opening for *qi*" is the major *yin* – hence the flavours and *qi* of the five viscera and six bowels all come out from the stomach, and their anomalies are experienced at "the opening for *qi*"' (*wu wei ru kou, cang yu wei yi yang wu zang qi, qi kou yi tai yin ye, shi yi wu zang liu fu zhi qi wei, jie chu yu wei, bian jian yu qi kou* 五味入口 藏於胃以養五藏氣 氣口亦太陰也 是以五藏六腑之氣味 皆出於胃 變見於氣口).[58] Qibo emphasises that *qi kou* assesses the overall state of the five viscera.

In *Su wen* 11, Qibo also says '*qi kou* is the major *yin* [opening]'. We are reminded of *Su wen* 15 (quoted on p. 68), which stated the Model of 'Qi heng' investigates the 'major *yin*'. We established then that the term 'major *yin*' in its broadest sense refers to the interior of the body in general. In other words, when Yi says he investigates the 'opening on the right' and attempts to identify the state of the five viscera (lines 15 and 19), he follows the rationale given in the 'Qi heng' of the *Su wen*, or, rather, the 'Qi ke' received from his Master Yang Qing.

The above passage from *Su wen* 11, in which *qi kou* is equated with the major *yin* in a text about the stomach, brings to mind Takigawa's quote of Zheng Xuan's 鄭玄 (127–200) comment on the *Zhou li* which mentions the 'inch-opening of the *yang* brightness' (*yang ming cun kou* 陽明寸口) as the location at the body surface that indicates the overall condition of the viscera inside.[59] The 'inch-opening of the *yang* brightness' (*yang ming cun kou*), the 'beginning of the major *yin*' (*tai yin zhi shi*), 'the opening for *qi*' (*qi kou*), and Yi's 'right opening' (*you kou*) have in common that they all are investigated in order to know the general condition of body internal processes.

Su wen 21, much like *Su wen* 11, mentions *qi kou* in the context of discussing internal processes relating to the stomach, but it does so in order to decide whether the patient will live or die.[60] *Ling shu* 48 reinforces the idea that the 'opening' in question is used for investigating body internal processes when it states: "The inch-opening governs the interior, *ren ying* governs the exterior" (*cun kou zhu zhong, ren ying zhu wai* 寸口主中，人迎主外).[61] To appreciate this statement fully, it is important to know that the

---

[58] *Su wen* 11, p. 37.
[59] *Zhou li*, "Ji yi" 疾醫, p. 667c. In canonical medical doctrine, which is relevant here, the stomach correlates with the *yang* brightness; the stomach is the outer aspect of the spleen, which, in turn, correlates with the major *yin*.
[60] *Su wen* 21, p. 67.   [61] *Ling shu* 48, p. 397.

Ling shu mentions all three openings, *qi kou*, *cun kou* and *mai kou*,[62] and sometimes interchangeably pairs each of them with the position for taking the pulse that is called *ren ying*.[63] Whenever this happens, *ren ying* indicates *yang* excess, and *qi kou*, *cun kou* or *mai kou* all indicate *yin* excess. They thus are clearly known as places on the body surface where qualities of *mai* can be sensed that provide information about pathological processes of the body's interior *yin* sphere.

Yi is explicit that he examines 'openings' (*kou*) in cases 3, 4, 5 and 7 (not case 6). He mentions the 'left opening' (*zuo kou*) in case 18 and he strokes over the skin of the *chi* 尺 in case 19. He presses onto the *mai* (*qie mai*) at the 'opening', perhaps cutting through it vertically, and he strokes, presumably horizontally, over the skin of the *chi* (*xun qi chi*), which, as its name suggests, may have been one foot long.[64] Incidentally, *Su wen* 28 mentions a pulse diagnostic method which examines *mai* at two positions with exactly the same names: the *mai kou* and *chi*. *Su wen* 28 speaks of 'dearth' (*bu zu*) and 'bounty' (*you yu*) affecting 'channels' and 'links' in a framework of hot/cold pathologies.[65] Evidently, not only Yi but also other physicians in antiquity differentiated between two different locations for examining *mai*, and not, as one does today, between three.[66]

In summary, the idiom 'opening on the right' (*you kou*) in case 3 proba-bly refers to an 'opening', which in canonical medical texts is called 'vessel opening' (*mai kou*), 'inch-opening' (*cun kou*) and '*qi* opening' (*qi kou*).[67] *Qi kou* is in *Su wen* 11 and 21, and in *Ling shu* 48, indicative of a person's general condition of health based on knowledge of body internal processes, as is the 'right opening', which provides information on the overall state of the viscera, and by implication the person as a whole (lines 15 and 19). In Yi's cases 1–10, if specified as to whether the left or right is affected, as in cases 3 and 7, it is always the right opening. Cases 3 (lines 14, 16) and 7 (line 13) concern an 'amassment' (*shan*) and a 'conglomeration' (*jia*)

---

[62] *Ling shu* 3, p. 273; 5, p. 281; 9, pp. 293–4; 23, p. 339; 49, p. 400 mention *mai kou*. *Ling shu* 3, p. 271; 10, p. 306; 19, p. 331; 21, p. 335; 23, p. 339; 27, p. 371; 49, p. 400 mention *qi kou*. *Ling shu* 2, p. 267; 10, pp. 299–305; 13, p. 317; 35, p. 367; 48, pp. 397–8; 49, p. 400; 52, p. 407; 62, p. 424; 64, p. 433; 71, p. 447, and 74, p. 455 mention *cun kou*. The *Su wen* mentions *mai kou* once, in *Su wen* 28, and *qi kou* twice in *Su wen* 11 and 21 (all mentioned in main text). For *cun kou*, see *Su wen* 9, p. 33 (see case 3, n. 67); 18, p. 55; 27, p. 84; 74, pp. 231–2; 78, p. 249. Based on computer searches by Wang Zilan (2005 p.c.).

[63] *Ling shu* 9, pp. 293–4; 10, pp. 299–305; 19, p. 331 and *Ling shu* 48, pp. 397–8. See also *Su wen* 9, p. 33.

[64] See diagram in Unschuld (1986a:88), which elucidates *Nan jing* 2.

[65] *Su wen* 28, p. 86; *mai kou* and *chi* are mentioned nowhere else in the *Su wen* and *Mai jing*. On the two positions *chi cun*, see *Su wen* 5, p. 23; 67, p. 187; 78, p. 249; *Ling shu* 3, p. 273 (quoted on p. 298); 9, p. 293; 38, p. 372; and *cun* and *chi* in *Su wen* 74, p. 232.

[66] On the pulse diagnostic method *cun guan chi*, see e.g. *Nan jing* 18, Unschuld (1986a:243ff.) and Hsu (2008a).

[67] For the interchangeable *mai kou* and *cun kou*, compare *Ling shu* 49, p. 400, with *Ling shu* 9, pp. 293–4, and with *Su wen* 9, p. 33.

respectively, which do not affect the viscera but cause difficulties in urination and defecation. They are also marked by great pain, which, as in *Su wen* 62 and 63, Yi detects from the quality of *qi* on the right-hand side. By contrast, the *tai yin mai kou* and *tai yin zhi kou* are mentioned when the viscera are affected in cases 4 and 5 (i.e. bladder, kidneys/lungs), and the otherwise undocumented 'left opening' in case 18, when the viscus liver is affected.

A creative commentator's interjection? (lines 21–2)

ni chi 溺赤 – dark urine (lines 21–2)   In the last stanza, Yi states: 'The interior was hot, hence the urine was dark' (*zhong re, gu ni chi*). In this context, *chi* does not mean 'red'; rather it refers to the colour/quality of 'raw gold or copper' (*chi jin* 赤金).[68] Dark yellow urine is a well-known sign for heat in contemporary Chinese medical practice and indicates heat in chapters of the *Su wen* that presumably were interpolated by the medieval Wang Bing: 'The urine is yellow and dark' (*xiao bian huang chi* 小便黃赤).[69]

This last stanza is odd, as it makes use of the resumptive conjunction 'hence' (*gu*) in order to explain a sign not previously mentioned. The heat pathology is not given in the first part of case 3 (lines 1–14/15).[70] This is if one interprets *huo ji tang* as a broth that was prepared by simmering it over a carefully regulated fire (see case 5, line 5) rather than as 'fire regulatory broth',[71] and considers Yi's treatment to have been directed at dissolving an amassment rather than regulating heat. The main sign of heat in case 3 is the 'frequent' pulse, which is explicitly said to indicate heat in line 17. The last stanza in case 3, which also alludes to heat, reminds us of the incongruencies encountered in cases 1 (lines 45–6) and 2 (line 26). Perhaps it was added, like the others, by a commentator with little intimation of Yi's reasoning.

Discussion

Text structure semantics is not easily applied to case 3, which mentions four pulse qualities but has only two constituents in the name of the disorder. Repetitions in the text suggest that the same diagnostic process was described in two different vocabularies. Thus, Yi investigates the right opening, and reports on his findings first in terms of *qi* (lines 12–14/15), then in terms of *mai* (lines 16–20). He first says that *qi* is 'intense' (*ji*) and that the *mai* do 'not have *qi* coming from the five viscera' (*wu wu zang qi*)

---

[68] HYDCD 9.1163; *chi* means 'raw' in *chijiao yisheng* 赤腳醫生 (barefoot doctors, Ma Boying, 1987 p.c.).
[69] e.g. *Su wen* 71, p. 212, and *Su wen* 74, p. 234. In *Ling shu* 74, p. 455, it is not explicitly indicative of heat.
[70] On *gu* 'hence', see pp. 147 and 159.   [71] Harper (1998).

and then speaks of the *mai* 'being large and frequent' (*da er shuo*). Perhaps both pairs should correlate with both constituents in the name of the disorder?

The correlation between the pulse quality of *qi* 'being intense' (line 14) and the constituent 'amassment' (*shan*) in the name of the disorder (line 4) is straightforward, as the urinary retentions which amassments cause are notoriously painful, according to both medical and lexicographic texts, and because *ji*, which implies crises and difficulties, indicates pain. If *ji* is translated as 'taut', it assesses qualities of the skin and communicates a tactile experience, while *ji* 'intense' alludes to the feeling of acute pain. If translated as 'intense', the pulse quality reflects in an iconic way the feeling of 'intense' pain inside the body. If translated as 'taut', it relates in an indexical way contractions caused by pain. Yi may have implied both connotations.

The second constituent in the name of the disorder, *yong* meaning 'welling', brings to mind the cosmogonic waters of the Guodian *Laozi* and may point to an early conception of the bladder, which was associated with either the Great One (*tai yi*) or the large pulse (*da*). Accordingly, one would expect, as also text structure semantics posits, that in case 3 'being large' correlates with the 'welling'.

In line 17, 'being frequent' (*shuo*) is explicitly said to be indicative of heat and there is a textual anomaly *er yong*. However, no evidence in support of *shuo* as indicative of heat was found in the *Nei jing* and, perhaps, *er yong* may once have ended the sentence in line 15. In the reconstituted line 15, *mai* that do 'not have *qi* coming from the five viscera, while there is a welling' may well indicate that the viscera are not affected.

Case 3 becomes a heat condition only in the second part, due to the two idioms 'the interior has heat' (*zhong re*) and 'dark urine' (*ni chi*) (lines 17, 21–2). This invites the cautious guess that the idea that disorders arise from coldness, coagulations, blockages and amassments, and are treated by having them dissolved, was prominent in scholarly medical circles of eastern China during the early to mid-second century BCE (lines 1–14). By contrast, reasoning in terms of heat pathologies was fashionable elsewhere or it became so later, perhaps not exclusively among medical specialists but also among the non-medical intelligentsia. This is said in full awareness of their mutual interdependence and coexistence.

14

Case 4

Translation (*Shiki Kaichû Kôshô* **105, pp. 30–31**)

1. Xin, the Chief of the Palace Wardrobe of Qi, fell ill.
2. I entered [the palace] to examine his *mai* and formally announced <u>saying</u>:

Name:
3. 'It is the *qi* of a heat disorder.
4. So, you sweat [as one does] from summer heat.
5. The *mai* are barely weakened.
6. You will not die.'

Cause:
7a. I said: 'This illness is contracted when one formerly bathed in running water,
7b. while it was very cold, and once it was over, got hot.'

8. Xin said: 'Yes, so it is.
9. Last winter season, I was sent as the King's envoy to Chu.
10. When I got to the Yangzhou River in Ju county, the planks of the bridge were partly damaged.
11. I then seized the shaft of the carriage.
12. I did not yet intend to cross.
13. The horses became frightened and [I] promptly fell.
14. I was immersed in water, and almost died.
15. Some officers then came to save me and pulled me out of the water.
16. My clothes were completely soaked.
17. For a short time my body was cold.
18. And once it was over, it got hot like a fire.

1. 齊中御府長信病
2. 臣意入診其脈 告曰

3. 熱病氣也
4. 然暑汗
5. 脈少衰
6. 不死

7a. 曰 此病得之當浴流水
7b. 而寒甚已則熱

8. 信曰唯然
9. 往冬時 為王使於楚
10. 至莒縣陽周水而莒橋梁頗壞
11. 信則攣車轅
12. 未欲渡也
13. 馬驚即墮
14. 信身入水中幾死
15. 吏即來救信出之水中
16. 衣盡濡
17. 有閒而身寒
18. 已熱如火

19. Up to today, I cannot be exposed to the cold.'

20. Your servant, Yi, thereupon made for him a decoction [prepared by careful] regulation of fire, to drive away the heat.

21. After drinking the first dose, the sweating came to an end.

22. After drinking the second, the heat left.

23. After drinking the third, the illness ceased.

24. I then made him apply medicines.

25. After about twenty days, his body was without illness.

Quality:

26. The means whereby I recognised Xin's illness were that at the time when I pressed onto his *mai*, there was a paired *yin*.

27. The 'Mai fa' says:

28. 'In the case of a heat disorder, those whose *yin* and *yang* intermingle, die.'

29. When I pressed on them [the *mai*], there was no intermingling, but a paired *yin*.

30. In cases of the paired *yin*, the *mai* are smooth and clear, and [the patient] recovers.

31. Although his heat had not yet gone completely, he was still going to live.

32. *Qi* [coming] from the kidneys was sometimes for a moment murky,

33. at the opening of the major *yin mai*, however, it was thin.

34. This is a case of water *qi*.

35. The kidneys certainly govern water.

36. Hence by means of this I recognised it [the disorder].

37. If one neglects treating [such disorders] instantly, then they turn into chills and hot flushes.

19. 至今不可以見寒

20. 臣意即為之液湯火齊逐熱

21. 一飲汗盡

22. 再飲熱去

23. 三飲病已

24. 即使服藥

25. 出入二十日身無病者

26. 所以知信之病者切其脈時并陰

27. 脈法曰

28. 熱病陰陽交者死

29. 切之不交 并陰

30. 并陰者脈順清而愈

31. 其熱雖未盡猶活也

32. 腎氣有時間濁

33. 在太陰脈口而希

34. 是水氣也

35. 腎固主水

36. 故以此知之

37. 失治一時 即轉為寒熱

Interpretation

Yi discusses the condition with its signs and symptoms (lines 3–5), predicts recovery (line 6) and states the cause of the illness (line 7). The patient reconfirms it in an unusually long and personal account (lines 8–19). Yi then outlines his treatment in two stages (lines 20–23, 24–5). The remainder is medical speculation (lines 26–36), to which is added a statement on the progression of the illness, had it not been treated (line 37).[1]

Critical evaluation of retrospective biomedical diagnoses

Bridgman diagnoses malaria on the grounds of the names given in lines 3 and 37: a 'heat disorder' (*re bing*) is on the verge of becoming an 'intermittent coldness and heat' (*han re*). He argues that Xin contracted the malaria before the accident and considers Yi to have mistaken the true cause of the illness.[2] Indeed, *han re* can refer to the intermittent fevers of malaria.[3] However, rather than downgrade an ancient doctor's knowledge as erroneous, today's researchers are well advised to recognise the serious limitations of our own knowledge of ancient medicine: *han re* can refer to conditions other than malaria.

According to Lu and Needham, it is 'surely bronchitis or pneumonia'.[4] They do not search for a hidden cause when it is obvious that Xin caught a cold after being immersed in cold water. As we will see, theirs is an educated guess that takes account of canonical medical rationale.

It probably was pneumonia, because one would expect the patient to complain of a cough or chest pain in the case of bronchitis. The name 'heat disorder' points to a fever, as do the signs and symptoms of sweating (line 4) and fear of exposure to the cold (line 19). One would expect the pulse beat to be heightened, but Yi says it is 'barely weakened' (line 5); perhaps the temperature is only slightly elevated.

As the text reads now, the treatment has two stages. The first consists of three steps. In form it evidently is in line with other cases (e.g. cases 2 and 3), but in contents it is odd. Yi administers a liquid that stops the sweating, then lowers the temperature, and, third, cures the illness (lines 20–23). The procedure is odd, for one would expect the intake of liquid to increase the sweating and thereby lower the temperature. In fact, the entire stanza is odd, for if the illness ceased, why would Yi provide further treatment? The second stage involves 'externally applied medicines' (*fu yao*) for another

---

[1] This study of case 4 radically revises Hsu (2001b).   [2] Bridgman (1955:73).
[3] Yu (1953:235). On malaria treatment, see Miyasita (1979), Obringer (2001) and Hsu (2009).
[4] Lu and Needham (1967:231).

twenty days (lines 24–5).[5] This was the appropriate method for treating infections before the advent of antibiotics; European folk medicine, for instance, prescribed long-term hot fomentation (e.g. potato, onion or cabbage fomentation).

The final line, 37, concerns a general maxim of treatment (it is best read as a counterfactual, as lines 23–5 in case 2). It reads like a comment on the observation that patients, who have been weakened by repeated fevers, have insufficient energy to entertain their body temperature and therefore start shivering.

The names for the disorder

Yi speaks of *re bing qi* (heat disorder *qi*) in line 3, and in line 37 he remarks that if not treated, it would have turned into a *han re* (coldness and heat). He mentions *re bing* only in case 4, but *han re* also in cases 6, 18 and 19. Both terms frequently occur in the medical canons, but neither is mentioned in the Mawangdui medical manuscripts.

***re bing* 熱病 – heat disorder (line 3)**   The Mawangdui 'Zubi vessel text' does not have *re bing* but mentions 'hot sweat comes out' (*re han chu* 熱汗 出) among the disorders of the *yang* brightness *mai*.[6] Sweating is evidently a key characteristic of fevers. Likewise, *Su wen* 35 connects 'summer-heat' (*shu* 暑) and 'hot *qi* becoming abundant' (*re qi sheng* 熱氣盛) to 'sweating' (*han* 汗).[7] This is crucial for understanding case 4.

The *Inner Canon* often mentions 'heat disorders' (*re bing*), and some chapters discuss them extensively; *Su wen* 31, 33 and *Ling shu* 23 have 'heat disorder' in the chapter title.[8] Among the varied conditions described in those chapters, there is one in *Su wen* 31, 'If a person is harmed by the cold, then he will suffer from heat. Even if the heat is severe, he will not die' (*ren zhi shang yu han ye, ze wei bing re, re sui shen bu si* 人之傷於寒也 則為病熱 熱雖甚不死),[9] which provides a parallel in medical rationale to Yi's favourable prediction (line 6) as well as to the second cause of the disorder (line 7b).

***han re* 寒熱 – chills and hot flushes (line 37)**   *Han re* and *nüe* are often used interchangeably to mean 'intermittent coldness and heat', as in *Shuo wen* 7B: '*Nüe* is the disorder of an intermittent manifestation of the cold and

---

[5] *fu yao* 服藥 'to apply medicines' in early medical texts generally refers to external application, see Ma (1992:429, 432, 566, 568). For exceptions, see Harper (1982:407), Ma (1992:500) and Yi's cases 22 and 23.

[6] MWD ZB (1985:4).   [7] *Su wen* 35, p. 101.

[8] For extensive discussion of heat disorders (*re bing*), see *Su wen* 31–3, pp. 92–7; 61, p. 116; 71, p. 216, and *Ling shu* 23, pp. 339–41; 61, p. 423.

[9] *Su wen* 31, p. 92. See also *Su wen* 61, p. 166, last few sentences.

hot' (*nüe han re xiu zuo bing* 瘧 寒熱休作病).[10] They generally designate intermittent fevers, some of which may have been malarial, but not all. *Ling shu* 21 is entitled 'Disorders of Intermittent Coldness and Heat' (Han re bing) and *Ling shu* 70 'Intermittent Coldness and Heat' (Han re), but among the conditions they list none applies directly to case 4.

For elucidating *han re* in line 37, Taki Motohiro quotes *Su wen* 42: 'If it [the skin's pore pattern][11] is cold, one loses one's appetite for food and drink, if it is hot, it dissolves [i.e. causes a wasting of] the muscles and flesh, hence it makes that the person suddenly shivers and is unable to eat. Its name is called chills and hot flushes' (*qi han ye, [ze] shuai shi yin, qi re ye, [ze] xiao ji rou, gu shi ren tu li er bu neng shi, ming yue han re* 其寒也 [則]衰 食飲 其熱也 [則]消肌肉 故使人怢慄而不能食 名曰寒熱).[12] Evidently, *Su wen* 42 does not describe an intermittent fever. Taki Motohiro remarks that these 'chills and hot flushes' arise from 'depletion and overexertion' (*xu lao han re* 虛勞寒熱). He also cites *Su wen* 17, 'wind turns into chills and hot flushes' (*feng cheng wei han re* 風成為寒熱), to show that *han re* can refer to a progressed if not the end stage of an illness.[13] In Yi's Memoir, likewise, *han re* designates a serious (cases 4 and 18) if not terminal condition of utter exhaustion (cases 6 and 19).

In summary, *re bing* (heat disorders) and *han re* (intermittent coldness and heat) do not occur in the Mawangdui texts but are frequent in the *Inner Canon*, where they refer to many different disorders, of which only a few parallel case 4. While canonical texts on *re bing* tend to stress hot/cold complementarities, the disorder 'hot sweat comes out' (*re han chu*) in an early manuscript text highlights a connection between bodily heat and bodily waters: the former causes a loss of the latter. This leads to a state of utter exhaustion, the 'chills and hot flushes', as which Taki Motohiro proposes to interpret *han re* in line 37.

The 'Mai fa' quote

yin yang jiao 陰陽交 – *yin* and *yang* intermingle (line 28)   No canonical parallels were found for the 'Mai fa' quote in its entirety, but an 'intermingling of *yin* and *yang*' (*yin yang jiao*) as cause of death is commonplace in Chinese medicine.[14] For explaining *yin yang jiao*, Ando Koretora cites *Su wen* 33: 'The Yellow Emperor asked: if one is ill with warmth, and while one sweats and abruptly feels hot again, the pulses are hurried and swift, and it is impossible to effect that the sweating is lessened, and one speaks jibberish and cannot eat, what is the name of the disorder? Qibo answered:

---

[10] *Shuo wen* 7B, p. 31a.
[11] Harper (1998) has 'the skin's webbed pattern' for *cou li* 腠理.
[12] *Su wen* 42, p. 119.   [13] *Su wen* 17, p. 52.
[14] e.g. *Su wen* 33, p. 96; 67, p. 187. Fieldwork (1988–9).

the disorder is called an "intermingling of *yin* and *yang*". If they intermingle, one dies' (*Huangdi wen yue: you bing wen zhe, han chu zhe fu re, er mai zao ji, bu wei han shuai, kuang yan bu neng shi, bing ming wei he? Qibo dui yue: bing ming yin yang jiao, jiao zhe, si ye* 黃帝問曰 有病溫者 汗出輒復熱 而脈躁疾 不為汗衰 狂言不能食 病名為何 岐伯對曰 病名陰陽交 交者 死也).[15] In *Su wen* 33, which is a chapter on 'heat disorders', the 'intermingling of *yin* and *yang*' evidently delimits a state of delirium due to a high fever. In this state, *yin* and *yang* become blurred, if one follows Wang Bing's view: '*jiao* designates to intermingle and unite, the *qi* of *yin* and *yang* are not divided and separated' (*jiao wei jiao he, yin yang zhi qi bu fen bie ye* 交 謂交合 陰陽 之氣不分別也).[16] When *yin* and *yang* intermingle, one cannot distinguish them.

Since *yin* is cool and *yang* hot, one might have felt inclined to infer that Yi's final statement on *han re* provides a comment on 'intermingling *yin* and *yang*' in the 'Mai fa'. However, Wang Bing's gloss on *Su wen* 33 states that in the case of an 'intermingling *yin* and *yang*' the distinction between *yin yang* is blurred, whereas chills and hot flushes are marked by clearly demarcated, intermittently alternating states of *yin* and *yang*. So, *han re* (line 37) may be related to the illness cause of intermittently feeling hot and cold (lines 7b and 17–19), but not to the 'Mai fa'. In fact, the 'Mai fa' quote is not well integrated into case 4. Together with the observation of its surprisingly unaltered form from present-day maxims, the possibility of a late commentatorial interjection cannot be put aside entirely.

Text structure semantics

Text structure semantics postulates that the constituents in the name of the disorder correlate with the qualities of *mai*. Applied to case 4, this means that *re bing qi* (*qi* of a heat disorder) should be the name of the disorder, because it is mentioned after the recurrent phrase 'I said' (*yue*), and it should correlate with *bing yin* (paired *yin*) given after the recurrent phrase 'the means whereby I recognised the illness were' (line 26). However, in case 4 it is unlikely that the term *re bing qi* actually is a name of a disorder, nor that *bing yin* may be a pulse quality. Rather than naming the disorder Yi seems to be saying: 'It is the *qi* of a heat disorder'[17] which parallels his diagnosis in case 15 where he says: 'This one has the *qi* of having damaged the spleen' (*ci shang pi qi ye* 此傷脾氣也). Accordingly, text structure semantics cannot be made to apply to cases 4 and 15: *re bing qi* and *shang pi qi* are qualities of *qi* and not names of disorders. The *qi* in question qualifies a disorder rather than a viscus, whereas otherwise in cases 1–10 Yi examines

---

[15] *Su wen* 33, p. 96.   [16] HDNJSW 33, p. 70.

[17] Yamada (1998:117) renders *re bing qi* as: 'It is a fever of your *qi*', but this translates *qi zhi re bing*; it is grammatically incorrect and semantically nonsensical.

mai in order to elicit qualities of *qi* (of the liver in case 1, of the heart in case 2, of none of the five viscera in case 3; see table 5 on p. 349).

bing yin 并陰 – a paired *yin* (lines 26 and 30)   Probably the 'paired *yin*' (*bing yin*) designates a pathological condition, not a tactile experience. Ando Koretora speaks of processes inside the body, when he remarks: 'After the heat and the noxious has left, *yang* returns to *yin*, and unites inside, this is called a paired *yin*' (*re xie qu, yang gui yin, tuan zai li, wei zhi bing yin* 熱邪去 陽歸陰 專在裡 謂之并陰). In the *Inner Canon*, only one passage in *Su wen* 35 was found to mention *bing yin*: 'If the condition of intermittent coldness and heat has not yet broken out, [this is] if *yin* has not yet paired with *yang* and *yang* has not yet paired with *yin*, one can regulate it for this very reason. The true *qi* becomes peaceful and the noxious *qi* then takes flight' (*fu nüe zhi wei fa ye, yin wei bing yang, yang wei bing yin, yin er tiao zhi, zhen qi de an, xie qi nai wang* 夫瘧之未發也 陰未并陽 陽未并陰 因而調之 真氣得安 邪氣乃亡).[18] According to *Su wen* 35, the disorder *nüe*, i.e. an intermittent [*yin*-] coldness and [*yang*-] heat, breaks out when *yin* and *yang* pair up (although the idiom *yin bing yang* 陰并陽, or vice versa, is not attested). Thus, *bing*-pairing delimits a condition of intermittently alternating *yin*- and *yang*-qualities, where each retains its identity, in contrast to the *jiao*-intermingling that results in the loss of distinct *yin*- and *yang*-qualities. As technical terms, *jiao*-intermingling and *bing*-pairing describe very different processes.

In the Mawangdui medical manuscripts, *bing* generally means 'to mix' or 'blend'. It is used frequently in the Mawangdui 'Recipes', and for elucidating it, Ma Jixing quotes the *Ji yun* 集韻: '*bing* means to combine and blend' (*bing he he ye* 并合和也).[19] He also cites the *Yu pian* 玉篇: 'to pair, to combine, to follow each other, to be the same' (*jian ye, he ye, xiang cong ye, tong ye* 兼也 合也 相從也 同也), followed in the *Yu pian* by 'to unite' (*tuan ye* 專也). The *Yu pian* evidently reproduces definitions given in the *Guang ya* 廣雅, '*bing* means to pair' (*bing jian ye* 并兼也),[20] and the *Shuo wen*, '*bing* means to mutually follow each other' (*bing xiang cong ye* 并相從也), and mentions additional ones.[21] However, Ma Jixing omits the beginning of the *Yu pian* definition which is an entry on 竝. It states: '*bing* means to stand side by side, to mix' (*bing bing ye, za ye* 竝 併也 雜也).[22] Yet precisely the definition 'to stand side by side' highlights that *bing* designates a 'pairing' where both *yin* and *yang* retain their identity, and double it, if it is the same one.

In contrast to the above lexicographic works and early medical manuscripts, 'to pair' often has negative connotations in canonical medical texts.

[18] *Su wen* 35, p. 103.
[19] Emura (1987:131). Ma (1992:329). *Ji yun* 6.40, p. 25a.
[20] *Guang ya* 5B, p. 13a. *Bing* 并 is also used as a gloss to *hun* 捆 (to mix) and *jian* 兼 (to pair) in *Guang ya* 4A, p. 15b, and 5A, p. 11b.
[21] *Shuo wen* 8A, p. 43a.   [22] *Yu pian* C, p. 67b.

It is a desirable state that, as above in *Su wen* 35, *yin* and *yang* are not yet paired and that, as in *Su wen* 62, 'blood and *qi* are not yet paired' (*xue qi wei bing* 血氣未并).[23] In *Su wen* 23, the 'five modes of pairing' (*wu bing* 五并) bring forth strong emotions: 'When the essential *qi* pairs in the heart, then there is [private/selfish] love;[24] when it pairs in the lungs, there is sorrow; when it pairs in the liver, there is grief; when it pairs in the spleen, there is fear; when it pairs in the kidneys, there is apprehension' (*jing qi bing yu xin ze xi, bing yu fei ze bei, bing yu gan ze you, bing yu pi ze wei, bing yu shen ze kong* 精氣并於心則喜 并於肺則悲 并於肝則憂 并於脾則畏 并於腎則恐).[25] The five emotions, which in *Su wen* 23 correlate in unusual ways with the viscera, can be understood to arise either from an 'intermingling' of the 'essences' (*jing*) and *qi* or from a 'pairing' in the sense of a 'doubling' of the 'essential *qi*' (*jing qi*), as suggested above.

To summarise, *bing*-pairing probably designates the doubling of a quality rather than an intermingling of two. Yi contrasts the process of '*yin* and *yang* intermingling' (*yin yang jiao*), which is lethal (line 28), with that of a 'paired *yin*' (*bing yin*), which is not terminal (line 29). He explicates this in a topic-comment sentence (line 30): 'In cases of a paired *yin*, the *mai* are smooth and clear, and [the patient] recovers' (*bing yin zhe, mai shun qing er yu*). No canonical medical parallels for either of these statements (in lines 29 and 30) have been found. Perhaps the semantics of the static verbs provide a clue?

shun 順, *qing* 清, *yu* 愈 – smooth, clear and well (line 30)

The static verbs 'being smooth' (*shun*), 'clear' (*qing*) and 'well' (*yu*) all have positive connotations. They occur frequently in the medical canons but generally are not used for designating pulse qualities. This applies also to Yi's case histories: 'being smooth' (*shun*) modifies *mai* in case 15, 'person' (*ren* 人) in case 15, 'disorder' (*bing* 病) in case 20, and 'to die' (*si* 死) in case 21; 'being clear' (*qing*) modifies *mai* in case 15 and 'urine' (*sou* 溲) in case 10; and 'being well' (*yu*) modifies 'person' in case 15, 'illness' (*ji* 疾) in case 3, and 'disorder' in case 17. Evidently, all three verbs are used in a variety of contexts other than pulse diagnosis.

The three verbs occur in case 4 and also in case 15. 'Being smooth' and 'clear' qualify *mai* in both. The term *yu* (to get well), which consistently designates recovery in the *Inner Canon*,[26] is probably also used in this sense in cases 4 and 15. Yi speaks of a paired *yin*, which seems to imply that only two *mai* are affected; they are 'smooth' and 'clear'. This parallels case 2

[23] *Su wen* 62, p. 168.
[24] *xi* 喜 'happiness'/'love' goes against the socially approved and morally right *le* 樂 'joy' (Nylan 2001).
[25] *Su wen* 23, p. 74.
[26] Computer printout by Hermann Tessenow (2000 p.c.). See also *Huangdi nei jing*, pp. 1429–30. The few occurrences of *shun* are in *Su wen* 68, p. 191; 69, p. 200; 70, p. 204. On Wang Bing's interpolated chapters, see ch. 3, n. 21.

(line 14), where Yi speaks of a 'double *yang*' (*chong yang*), and, accordingly, mentions only two pulse qualities, namely 'being murky and hurried', indicative of a 'transient' condition (*zhuo zao er jing ye*).

The 'clear' and/or 'cool' (*qing*) as opposed to the 'murky' (*zhuo*) waters have been discussed in case 1 (line 14). *Shun* (smooth) is often given as the opposite of *ni* 逆 in the *Ling shu*, but it hardly occurs in the *Su wen*, where the opposite of *ni* is *cong* 從 (to follow).[27] While *shun* means 'to go with the stream', *ni* means 'to go against the stream'. Modelled on this imagery of the flow of water, *shun* and *ni* seem to invoke the imagery that there is a flow of *qi* inside the *mai*. There are other passages,[28] and some of those refer to a presumably tactually perceived pulse quality, like *shun mai*, which in *Ling shu* 23 is mentioned in the discussion of heat disorders and their treatment by induction of sweating.[29] The medical authors who used the terms *shun* and *ni* obviously were not troubled by the important distinction we make between postulated and perceived processes.

On its own, *shun* (to follow) often refers to appropriate conduct, such as living in accordance with the seasons, as in *Ling shu* 8: 'Hence those who have an understanding nurture [their] life. One must, by following the four seasons, accommodate to coldness and summer-heat; by harmonising happiness and anger, reside peacefully at one's place; by regulating *yin* and *yang*, harmonise the hard and soft' (*gu zhi zhe zhi yang sheng ye, bi shun si shi er shi han shu, he xi nu er an ju chu, jie yin yang er tiao gang rou* 故智者之養生也 必順四時而適寒暑 和喜怒而安居處 節陰陽而調剛柔).[30] In *Ling shu* 29, the Yellow Emperor asks: 'What does it mean to be *shun*?' (*shun zhi nai he* 順之奈何) and Qibo answers: 'When entering a country one asks about the customs; when entering a homestead, one asks about the taboos; when entering an ancestral hall, one asks about the rites; when attending to sick people, one asks about that which comforts them' (*ru guo wen su, ru jia wen wei, ru tang wen li, lin bing ren, wen suo bian* 入國問俗 入家問諱 入堂問禮 臨病人間所便).[31] In *Ling shu* 8 and 29, *shun* refers to an accommodating behaviour, and this is considered healthy.

In summary, the three static verbs 'to be smooth', 'clear' and 'well' (*shun, qing, yu*) do not exclusively assess tactile perception, neither in canonical texts nor in Yi's case histories. In case 4, they all indicate a favourable condition of *mai* and recovery of the patient. Insofar as *shun* describes a smooth flow of water, and *qing* its coolness, they allude to much-valued

---

[27] In Yi's Memoir, *ni* and *shun* are three times given as opposites (cases 21, 22, section four), but not in cases 1–10. In case 23, *ni* probably describes a symptom like 'burping'. Case 9, which describes similar processes to *ni qi*, does not mention the term; *ni qi* is not mentioned in cases 1–10.

[28] Note, however, *Ling shu* 3, p. 271: 'The small is contravective . . . the even is smooth' (*xiao zhe, ni ye* 小者逆也 . . . *ping zhe, shun ye* 平者順也).

[29] e.g. *Ling shu* 23, p. 340.   [30] *Ling shu* 8, p. 291.

[31] *Ling shu* 29, pp. 354–5.

qualities of water. Perhaps both *shun* and *qing* were thought to have the *yin* qualities of water, and together formed the 'paired *yin*'.

Interlude   So far, it has not been possible to apply text structure semantics to case 4. The '*qi* of a heat disorder' is not a name nor the 'paired *yin*' a pulse quality. However, apart from the two static verbs qualifying the 'paired *yin*' (line 30), Yi does mention two further pulse qualities, namely *qi* 'being murky' (*zhuo*) and 'yet being thin' (*er xi*) (lines 32–3). We instantly recognise Yi's peculiar vocabulary in the 'murky', which he idiosyncratically uses for assessing pulse qualities in cases 1, 2, 4 and 9.

Notably, 'being murky' qualifies *qi*, rather than *mai*, which as in case 3 (line 14) may hint at the possibility that lines 32–3 date, in part at least, from the presumed early second century document. Like the 'murky *yang*' of early manuscript texts that blackens and clogs up the four directions, 'murky' may have indicated that blood coagulated, became black and turned into a *ju*-abscess in the first part of case 1 (lines 1–15). Alternatively, it may have alluded to the harmful rising heat of, implicitly, hot blood in the tubular structures in the second part of case 1 (lines 41–4); or indicated *yang*-heat in the heart region in case 2; or pointed to a *yang*-wind in the heart region in case 9. In the light of this, 'being murky' (line 32) may well correlate with the constituent 'heat' (*re*) in the name of the disorder (line 3) in case 4. Yi says *qi* [coming] from the kidneys is murky, but not permanently, only 'sometimes' (*you shi*), and then only 'for a moment' (*jian*). This suggests the heat was not persistent.

xi 希 – **thin (line 33)**   In the Mawangdui texts, *xi* (thin, rare, scarce) once refers to a 'brief pause' (*xi xi* 希息) after cauterisation before recovery occurs, and once to 'few, rare' as opposed to 'frequent' (*shuo*) movements of the penis during sexual intercourse.[32] The term has not been located in the *Inner Canon*, *Nan jing* and other canonical medical texts but Yi appears to use it here in the sense of a pulse quality.

One could argue if 'being frequent' implies *yang* qualities, 'rare' indicates *yin* qualities. Indeed, 'being thin' indicates 'water *qi*' (*shui qi*), as Yi explains on line 34, and water is *yin*. 'Water *qi*' occurs fairly frequently in the *Su wen*, but not in the *Ling shu*,[33] and it often occurs in contexts that have no resemblance with case 4. However, *Su wen* 61, entitled 'Shui re xue lun' 水熱穴論 (Discourse on the *Loci* [for Treating] Water that has become Hot), is noteworthy. Although its contents do not exactly match case 4, in its description of various pathological conditions it mentions the kidneys, the lungs and water, as well as 'water *qi*' before ending in a discussion about the treatment of heat disorders. The parallels are tenuous, but they echo

[32] MWD YY (no. 2) and 'He yinyang' (1985:90, 156). See also Ma (1992:994).
[33] See *Su wen* 33, p. 97, and 34, p. 100; 35, p. 101; 37, p. 108; 49, p. 138; 61, p. 165; 68, p. 191; 76, p. 246. The term *shui qi* is not mentioned in the *Ling shu*.

Yi's account, which mentions the paired *yin*, the kidneys, water *qi* and a heat disorder.[34]

Text structure semantics postulates that the pulse quality 'thin', which is explicitly said to be indicative of 'water *qi*' (line 34), must in some way correlate with the name of the disorder. Consider the concomitant symptom: 'So, you sweat [as one does] from summer heat' (*ran shu han*) (line 4).[35] We are reminded of the disorder 'hot sweat comes out' (*re han chu*) in the Mawangdui 'Zubi vessel text' (quoted on p. 188). Sweating was a prime feature of fevers in early elite medical reasoning, and in case 4, rather than considering it a concomitant symptom, it could be considered part of a very long name. Without altering the text, 'sweating' (*han*) would then correlate with 'thin' (*xi*).

This means that, after all, text structure semantics also applies to case 4: the pulse quality 'being murky' correlates with the constituent 'heat' in the name of the disorder (line 3) and 'being thin' with the 'sweating' [and water] (line 4). One may now wish to proceed directly to the discussion on p. 201. The excursus that follows explores possibilities of engaging in the dangerous undertaking of making minor alterations to the extant text. It builds on the assumption that cases 1–10 are formulaic and their medical rationale consistent, this is, if one differentiates between the medical rationale of an early second-century medical document and that of a later editor, and if one allows for the possibility of numerous commentatorial interjections.

The first amendment consists of suggesting that in the medical document of the early second century the disorder was called *shui re* [*bing*], '[disorder of] water that has become hot'. This name, which parallels that in *Su wen* 61, fits into the schema of others in Yi's Memoir as it is a noun-verb phrase, like the 'disorder of the interior being closed off' (*nei guan zhi bing*) or the 'disorder of *qi* being blocked' (*qi ge bing*) in cases 1 and 2. The pulse quality 'being murky' would then correlate with the constituent 'becoming hot', and 'being thin' with 'water'. By altering the text only slightly and in ways that are given elsewhere in medical writings, the principle of text structure semantics can be made to apply elegantly to case 4.

Excursus: textual anomalies and the search for consistency in medical rationale

Interpolations and interjections (lines 26–31 and line 33)   To recapitulate, text structure semantics expects us to find Yi mentioning pulse qualities in

---

[34] *Su wen* 61, pp. 164–6.

[35] *ran* 然 means here *ru zhi* 如之 'like it', 'this so being', 'so' (Pulleyblank 1995:180); rather than as 'in spite of', a rendering of *ran* as in *sui ran* 雖然 'although'. Medical texts differentiate between types of perspiration, see case 9 (line 22); one such type may be *shu han* 暑汗 lit. 'it is a summer heat sweating'.

line 26, but 'being murky' (*zhuo*), which is indicative of heat, and 'yet being thin' (*er xi*), which correlates with sweating/water, occur in lines 32–3. In order to explain this textual anomaly, one could suggest that lines 26–31 were interpolated. This idea, motivated by a text structural concern, has already been suggested when discussing the semantics of the three static verbs mentioned in lines 26–31.

So far, we found that 'being smooth' and 'clear' (line 30), which may well qualify two *yin mai*, are used in many contexts other than pulse diagnosis both in Yi's case histories and in the *Nei jing*. Since these static verbs, together with 'being well', also occur in case 15, where Yi overtly reasons in terms of the five agents, they may be part of a text that has more affinity with canonical doctrine, and which dates from a later period than the early second century BCE. Since these three static verbs are frequently seen in canonical texts but are notoriously unspecific, the commentator/editor who interpolated them may have had superficial but not intricate knowledge of medicine. Notably, they qualify *mai*, as do the pulse qualities mentioned in lines 16–20 of case 3, which is a stanza that reflects ample workings of editor/s and commentator/s. By contrast, the pulse qualities Yi gives in his own vocabulary, like 'being intense' in case 3 (line 14) and 'murky' (respectively 'clogged up') in cases 1 and 2 (line 13), qualify *qi*. Based on the semantics of these technical terms, it appears reasonable to suggest that at least line 30, if not the entire passage of lines 26–31, is an editorial interpolation that has more affinity with canonical doctrine than do the two pulse diagnostic terms in lines 32 and 33.

Furthermore, the first part of line 33 appears to consist of a commentatorial interjection. Based on the observation that Yi tends to put two pulse qualities in relation with each other with the conjunction *er* 而, which indicates that they are aspects of the same phenomenon,[36] one expects 'being murky, yet thin' (*zhuo er xi*) to form a single clause. However, in the beginning of line 33, the phrase 'at the opening of the major *yin mai*' (*zai tai yin mai kou*) appears to have been interjected, which leads to the rather odd 'yet being thin' (*er xi*) at the end of the same line. This phrase *zai tai yin mai kou* could have been added by the same editor who interpolated lines 26–31. On grounds of grammar, however, it is more likely that this phrase was interjected, at a later stage, by a commentator.[37] The interjection in the beginning of line 33 and the interpolated passage in lines 26–31 appear to refer to the same medical rationale.

---

[36] See table 8 on p. 354: *zhuo er jing* in case 1, *da er shuo* in case 3, *bu ping er dai* in case 6, *da er shi* in case 10. On the particle *er* 而, see Pulleyblank (1995:44–5, 148–9).

[37] The clause *zai tai yin mai kou er xi* is grammatically problematic if not incorrect. An editor who elaborated on primary materials in his own prose is unlikely to have formed an ungrammatical sentence. It is more likely that *zai tai yin mai kou* is a brief interjection by a later commentator, who was unaware that he thereby transformed a syntactically well-formed clause, *zhuo er xi*, into a faulty construction.

The 'paired *yin*': the kidneys and lungs (lines 26–31, 32–5)   The 'paired *yin*' (lines 26 and 30) may well indicate that two *yin mai*, or *yin* viscera, are affected. Probably the commentator who interjected the beginning of line 33 considered the 'major *yin*' to have paired up with the 'kidneys' (*shen*), which in canonical doctrine correlate with the 'minor *yin*'. Bridgman, by contrast, believes that lines 32–3 describe the same condition,[38] and claims that in Yi's Memoir the 'major *yin*' correlates with the kidneys, which is indeed a correlation prevalent in inner alchemy.[39] However, if one considers the *Shi ji* personage Yi to be coherent in argumentation, it makes much more sense to interpret the two lines 32–3 as referring to two different tactile perceptions, namely 'being murky', which qualifies *qi* coming from the kidneys, and 'yet being thin', which qualifies what Yi felt at the 'opening of the major *yin*'s *mai*'. Accordingly, it is unlikely that the major *yin* designates the kidneys. So, which body part could the *Shi ji* personage Yi have meant? If 'at the opening of the major *yin*' is an interjection invoking canonical doctrine, he probably meant the lungs. According to *Ling shu* 10, the hand's major *yin* binds up with the lungs.[40] The *Shi ji* personage Yi must have thought that kidneys and lungs (lines 32–3) form a 'paired *yin*'.

Su wen 7 points to a disorder that wanders from the lungs to the kidneys, and anyone trained in Chinese medicine in China today instantly recognises this pattern.[41] *Su wen* 7 calls it a 'double *yin*' (*chong yin* 重陰),[42] which comes very close to Yi's notion of a 'paired *yin*'. There is only one problem with this interpretation, which is that it is at odds with the medical rationale found in other case histories of Yi's Memoir. In case 17, the kidneys correlate with the major *yang* and their condition is identified through the diagnostic method of inspecting *se* (colour), rather than palpating *mai*.[43] And in case 5 (line 3), the major *yin* will be shown to correlate with the bladder/womb.

One could point out that medical reasoning is more consistent across cases 1–10 than across cases 11–25, and that therefore a correlation given in case 4 need not coincide with one in case 17. Moreover, one could question the correlation postulated in case 5. We are here reminded that it is

---

[38] Bridgman (1955:142, 141–5). His hypothesis that the names of *mai* in Yi's case histories are wildly divergent from those of canonical doctrine builds on several such quick but mistaken readings. There are changes in attribution of *yin* and *yang* qualities to the viscera, but they happen in a patterned way, see pp. 360–63.

[39] Pregadio and Skar (2000).   [40] *Ling shu* 10, p. 299.

[41] Lu and Needham (1967), quoted on p. 187. *Su wen* 7 reminds one of the 'lung kidney *yin* depletion' (*feishen yinxu* 肺腎陰虛) in contemporary Chinese medicine, a 'distinguishing pattern' (*bianzheng* 辯証) with symptoms of heat and perspiration (Yin 1984:51), typically a slightly elevated temperature and night sweating (fieldwork 1988–9). Biomedically, it can describe pneumonia.

[42] *Su wen* 7, p. 27, quoted on p. 251.

[43] Perhaps Yi diagnoses *yang* disorders by inspecting colour, as he does in case 15, where the stomach may (or may not) correlate with the bright *yang*, and in case 17, where he diagnoses a disorder of the kidneys by examining the major *yang*.

important to differentiate between the rationale of the editor/commentator who interpolated lines 26–31 and of the later commentator who interjected the beginning of line 33, which both allude to canonical medical doctrine, and the rationale that the physician of presumably the early second century had, who spoke of *qi* 'being murky, yet thin'. Did this early physician consider *qi* to come from the kidneys or lungs?

In this context, we are reminded of the passage in *Ling shu* 66 (quoted on pp. 39–40) with its striking parallels to the aetiologies of Yi's cases 2, 4, 6, 15 and 17. A phrase in it states: 'A double coldness harms the lungs'. The passage in *Ling shu* 66 is a mini-compilation with patterned inconsistencies, as we established earlier when arguing that Warring States physicians alluded primarily to the 'sentimental body' rather than to the 'body ecologic' when framing disease. Thus, among the five viscera that it mentions, harmful emotions can arise only in heart and liver. We concluded that they alluded to a body conception that prevailed in the Warring States, although the two clauses that referred to heart and liver as seats of emotion occurred in a Han-Tang-Song canonical text.

Relevant to case 4 is the concluding sentence in this passage of *Ling shu* 66: 'These are the disorders that are generated by internal and external [aetiologies] and by the three parts'. The passage contains five clauses on five viscera yet refers to three parts in the concluding remark. It first mentions heart, lungs and liver, and in contrast to the aetiologies of spleen and kidneys given thereafter, the first three are written in three compact clauses with four characters each. There is little doubt that heart, lungs and liver are the 'three parts'. So, *Ling shu* 66 implicitly alludes not only to two but three body conceptions: the 'sentimental body' with heart and liver as seats of emotion, the canonical 'body ecologic' framed in five agents doctrine, and a body in 'three parts' affected by internal and external aetiologies. Within this body in three parts, feelings presumably harm heart and liver, and ecological factors, say, cold water in cold winter, affect the lungs. Perhaps the early second-century doctor who felt that *qi* was 'murky, yet thin' spoke of *qi* coming from the lungs rather than the kidneys? We will return to this question later.

The cause of the disorder: the cold and hot (lines 7b, 17–19)   The cause of the disorder mentions bathing in flowing water (line 7a), which is very cold, followed by an episode of subjectively felt heat (line 7b). Cases 4 and 2 are the only among the first ten not to blame wine and women. While case 2 located the 'infantile irritability' in the sentimental body, the cause in case 4 evidently affects the body ecologic. However, Yi's body ecological considerations do not invoke the five seasons but the hot and cold, which brings to mind the body ecological reasoning implied by the book title 'The Doubling of either Yin or Yang due to Resonances with the Four Seasons' that Yi mentions in section 4.3.

The cause of the disorder is introduced by the term 'I said' (*yue*). This is a textual anomaly that one would simply overlook if the cause of the disorder were not body ecological and showed discontinuities with other causes in other case histories. Keegan, in his text critical study of the *Inner Canon*, paid attention precisely to such rhetorical particles in order to detect the boundaries between different mini-texts of a compilation.[44] In full awareness that this one instance of a textual anomaly cannot be compared to the recurrent particles Keegan investigated, it nevertheless hints at line 7, or at least parts of it, as an interpolated text. If this were indeed so, the question is whether the narrative that follows, which is unusual in length and style, is also an interpolation (lines 8–19).

The patient on the cause of the disorder: water and winter (lines 7a, 8– 16)   The hot/cold complementarity that Yi gives as cause of the disorder (line 7b) is reconfirmed by the patient towards the end of his account (lines 17–19). It shows continuities with *Su wen* 31 (quoted on p. 188) that a person harmed by the cold will suffer from heat.[45] If pushed, one can also admit a faint affinity with the chills and hot flushes mentioned in line 37, although we established earlier that those typically arise from a state of utter exhaustion. More importantly, this hot/cold complementarity tallies with Yi's pulse qualities (lines 32–3), as 'being murky' correlates with heat, and 'being thin' with water, which has *yin* qualities. If this were so, lines 7b and 17–19 may well reflect early medical rationale intrinsic to case 4.

The patient's long narrative, which is most unusual in Yi's case histories, reports on an accident (lines 8–16): Xin fell in winter into the water. Although he does not once mention the word 'cold', Yi clearly alludes to a doubling of the cold. A 'double coldness' echoes the medical rationale of the 'paired *yin*' mentioned in lines 26–31. On the basis of this semantic continuity with lines 26–31, it is possible that the same commentator/editor interpolated also lines 8–16. Furthermore, as the above-mentioned textual anomaly 'I said' indicates, the cause of the illness in line 7a may also be an interpolation;[46] its semantics relate to the same kind of body ecological reasoning as lines 8–16: 'formerly bathing in running water' (*dang xi liu shui*). Since no parallels were found for this phrase in canonical medical texts, it may be testimony, once again, to a commentator/editor's familiarity with the basics of medicine but not its technical intricacies.

Winter is the season that correlates with the canonical kidneys; water is the agent of five agents doctrine that correlates with the canonical

---

[44] Keegan (1988).

[45] Kaiho Gembi notes '*xian* means to encounter' (*xian yu ye* 見遇也), also in cases 10 (line 8) and 24. See also case 15, quoted on pp. 118 and 213, and case 7 (line 14), where it is used in a slightly different sense. For the parallel *xian feng* 'being exposed to wind' in the MWD manuscripts, see case 5, n. 34.

[46] *dang* 'formerly' is used in a sense that is unusual in Yi's Memoir, see case 6, n. 9.

kidneys.[47] However, according to a mini-text in *Ling shu* 66, which alludes to an early body conception of a body in 'three parts', a 'double coldness' harms the lungs.

Further amendments and interjections   'The kidneys certainly govern water' (line 35) is no doubt an interjection by someone familiar with canonical doctrine, although the word 'certainly' makes one think that it may have been interjected by someone who was not a medical specialist.[48] It should explain that the water that escapes from the kidneys appears as sweat on the body surface. *Su wen* 33 likens sweat to refined essences: 'As for sweat, it is *qi* of refined essences' (*han zhe, jing qi ye* 汗者 精氣也).[49] In the Han, refined essences (*jing* 精) were thought to be stored in the viscera, the kidneys in particular, rather than in the brain.[50] Thus, *Su wen* 61 states: 'The sweat of the kidneys comes out' (*shen han chu* 腎汗出).[51] Sweating in *Su wen* 61 does not arise from a heat disorder but from overexertion and physical toil, as which sexual intercourse was understood in Han circles of the upper strata. Sweating causes and is indicative of an impairment of the kidneys.

Evidently, the kidneys control water/sweating in canonical doctrine, but did they do so already in the early second century BCE? If the pulse quality 'murky, yet thin' qualified *qi* in an early medical document, was it *qi* coming from the kidneys? The 'double coldness' in *Ling shu* 66 would suggest the lungs were harmed. Accordingly, the graph *shen* 腎 (kidneys) in line 32 would once have been *fei* 肺 (lungs). There is a precedent for substitution of a similar graph in case 10 (line 3), where Xu Guang mentions an edition that has the graph 肝 (liver) as variant to 肺 (lungs). However, a strict application of text structure semantics postulates that neither kidneys nor lungs should qualify *qi*, if the assumed early second-century case 4 was called 'Shui re' (the waters have become hot) and was recognised by the two pulse qualities '*qi* is murky, yet thin' (*zhuo er xi*). If yet another constituent of a pulse quality were added, say either kidneys or lungs, the name would be overdetermined!

Here, a comment on the kidneys is warranted. *Ling shu* 10 correlates them with the 'minor *yin*', *Su wen* 61 with the 'extreme *yin*' (*zhi yin* 至陰),[52] and inner alchemy with the major *yin*. However, case 17 associates the kidneys with the 'major *yang mai*', while case 5 suggests that the bladder correlates with the 'major *yin*', a finding that is corroborated by the verbs 'welling' and 'being large' in case 3, which make sense in the light of the Guodian *Laozi*'s cosmogony that 'The Great One gave birth to water'.

[47] e.g. *Su wen* 5, p. 21; 2, p. 10.
[48] *gu* 固 'certainly' in *shen gu zhu shui* case 4 (line 35), but contrast with the grammatical construction *gu se bian* 'the solid colour changed' in case 21, quoted on p. 30.
[49] *Su wen* 33, p. 96.   [50] Umekawa (2004: 165).
[51] *Su wen* 61, p. 164.   [52] *Su wen* 61, p. 164.

Incidentally, the bladder, as outer aspect of the kidneys, takes on their 'major *yang*' qualities in canonical doctrine. This swapping of the *yin*- and *yang*-qualities of kidneys and bladder parallels the swapping of the *yin*- and *yang*-qualities of spleen and stomach in pre-canonical texts and canonical doctrine. In the Mawangdui 'Yinyang vessel text', the major *yin mai* is that of the stomach, but in canonical doctrine, the spleen binds up with the major *yin mai* and the stomach with the bright *yang mai*.[53] A similar inversion of *yin yang* qualities has also been noted for the liver in Yi's case 1 (line 13) and its outer aspect in canonical doctrine, the gall bladder. Perhaps the canonical kidneys took on the function of governing water that in early medicine the bladder had and that it retains also in canonical doctrine albeit as the *yin*-kidney's subordinate, outer, major *yang* aspect.

Discussion

In case 4 correlations postulated by text structure semantics are not instantly evident. In the position where one would expect Yi to announce the name of the disorder, he speaks of '*qi* of a heat disorder' (*re bing qi*), which does not appear to be a name, and in the position where one would expect a pulse quality, he speaks of a 'paired *yin*' (*bing yin*), which in the canonical medical texts is not a pulse quality. The cause of the disorder in case 4 furthermore contains no hints of debauchery at the court of Qi, and records instead a body ecologically framed accident.

Case 4, as case 15, does not fit the formula of text structure semantics and is body ecologically framed. Case 4 alludes to two seasons, summer (line 4) and winter (line 9), where case 15 frames seasonal change in terms of the five agents. They both mention the static verbs 'being smooth' (*shun*), 'clear' (*qing*) and 'well' (*yu*), which in case 4 reinforces the idea that line 30, if not the entire stanza of lines 26–31, was interpolated by the same commentator/editor as the one at work in case 15.

Once the above commentatorial/editorial layer became apparent, others were spotted. The commentator/editor, who interpolated the stanza on the 'paired *yin*' (lines 26–31) and, in particular, the commentator who interjected the beginning of line 33, probably understood case 4 to report on a pairing of the canonical *yin*-kidneys and *yin*-lungs (lines 32–4). The 'paired *yin*' in the interpolated stanza is paralleled by the 'double coldness' of water and winter (lines 8–16), which therefore may also have been interpolated. 'Formerly bathing in running water' in line 7a and the statement that the 'kidneys certainly govern water' in line 35, which both allude to this rationale, may also represent later additions.

Once it became apparent that case 4 had been heavily edited, it was possible to apply text structure semantics and search for correlations between

---

[53] *Ling shu* 10, pp. 300–301.

constituents in a very long name of the disorder (lines 3–4) and static verbs that qualify *qi* (lines 32–3). Accordingly, 'being murky' (*zhuo*) is indicative of the constituent 'heat' (*re*) in the name of the disorder (line 3) and 'thin' (*xi*) probably of the 'sweating' (line 4). Since a fever is featured as 'hot sweat comes out' in an early manuscript text, and sweat was a sort of water, 'being thin' probably was indicative of 'water' (*shui*). Accordingly, the early medical name of the disorder may not have been '*re bing qi*' but rather '*shui re*', a name that is best read as a noun-verb complex: the waters got hot.

Case 4 emerges as a text with two major layers, each consistent in itself but alluding to a different medical rationale. The teasing out of the two layers was motivated by considerations of consistency in medical rationale, but syntax and semantics played a key role.[54] One alludes to a 'double cold-ness' or 'paired *yin*', the other to bodily waters that got hot. One alludes to body ecological knowledge communicated in a general vocabulary, the other reflects technical terminology of a medical document. We note that the cause given in line 7a alludes to general body ecological reasoning, which contrasts with the specifically medical reasoning partly paralleled by *Su wen* 31 in line 7b; that the narrative in lines 8–16 contrasts with the medical terminology in lines 17–19, which repeats contents of line 7b; that the medical treatment in lines 20–23 fits with the narrative formula of previous case histories, but that lines 24–5 actually make sense medically; and that the qualities in lines 26–31 are rendered with static verbs that are not specific to pulse diagnosis, but lines 32–3 report on pulse qualities that fit perfectly into the schema of text structure semantics. In summary, it appears that considerable textual material was interpolated into an early medical document. The commentator/editor who worked on case 4 differs from the one(s) in the previous three in that he consistently interpolated his text with his ideas first: line 3, line 7a, lines 8–16, lines 20–23, lines 26–31. The text contains furthermore a variety of interjections: the beginning of line 33, perhaps even lines 27–8, and furthermore lines 34, 35, 37, which each may have been added by a different later commentator. Perhaps the text of case 4 gradually incremented over the centuries?

Nevertheless, an overarching narrative theme emerges. Cases 3 and 4 form a pair, just like cases 1 and 2 (which concerned blood and *qi* dynamics in the liver and heart respectively). Case 3 concerns the welling up of cold waters that formed a mass, case 4 waters that became very hot; both are framed in terms of water dynamics.

---

[54] For lexical semantics, as applied to line 30, see pp. 192–4; as applied to line 19, see case 4, n. 45. For the textual anomaly in line 7a, see p. 213. For the syntactical problems that the interjection causes in the beginning of line 33, see case 4, n. 37; for variation in the use of the word *gu* meaning 'certainly' rather than 'solid' in the interjection of line 35, see case 4, n. 48; for the use of the word *dang* meaning 'formerly', see case 4, n. 46.

15
Case 5

Translation   (*Shiki kaichû Kôshô* 105, pp. 31–2)

1. The queen dowager of the King of Qi fell ill.
2. They summoned your servant, Yi. I entered [the palace] to examine *mai*.

Name:

3. I <u>said</u>: 'A wind-induced condition caused by overexertion is visiting the bladder.
4. One has difficulties with defecating and urinating, and the urine is dark.'
5. Your servant, Yi, had her drink the broth [prepared by careful] regulation of fire.
6. After drinking the first dose, she immediately could urinate and defecate.
7. After drinking the second, the illness ceased. She urinated as before.

Cause:

8. <u>The illness was contracted because</u>, while dripping with sweat, she went outside to dry up.
9. In cases of drying up, after having removed one's clothes, the sweat dries in the sunlight.

Quality:

10. <u>The means whereby I recognised the illness of the queen dowager of the King of Qi were that</u>
11. when your servant, Yi, examined her *mai*, and
12. when I pressed onto the opening of the major *yin*,
13. it was damp. In spite of this there was wind *qi*.

1. 齊王太后病
2. 召臣意入診脈

3. 曰 風癉客脬

4. 難於大小溲 溺赤

5. 臣意飲以火齊湯

6. 一飲 即前後溲

7. 再飲 病已 溺如故

8. 病得流汗出滫

9. 滫者 去衣而汗晞也

10. 所以智齊王太后病者

11. 臣意診其脈
12. 切其太陰之口

13. 淫然風氣也

203

14. The 'Mai fa' says:

14. 脈法曰

15. 'In cases when, as one sinks [into the *mai*?], it is very firm, and

15. 沈之而大堅

16. when, as one floats [on the surface of the *mai*?], it is very tight,

16. 浮之而大緊者

17. the host of the disorder resides in the kidneys.'

17. 病主在腎

18. When I pressed onto the kidneys, it was the opposite.

18. 腎切之而相反也

19. The *mai* was large, yet hurried.

19. 脈大而躁

20. In cases where it is large, it is *qi* [coming] from the bladder.

20. 大者 膀胱氣也

21. In cases where it is hurried, the interior has heat and the urine is dark.

21. 躁者 中有熱而溺赤

Interpretation

Yi announces the name of the disorder (line 3) and mentions concomitant signs and symptoms (line 4), similar to those in cases 3 and 10. He successfully treats the illness with *huo ji tang* (lines 5–7), as in cases 3 and 10. The cause of the disorder (lines 8–9) is not instantly evident – after all, Yi's client is the dowager queen herself – but basically the same as in cases 3 and 10. Yi's medical speculation that follows includes an explanation in his own vocabulary (lines 12–13), a 'Mai fa' quote (lines 14–17) and reports on his own findings (line 18). In the final stanza, Yi mentions qualities of *mai*, which he elucidates in two topic-comment sentences (lines 19–21). This case is one of the most transparent ones, once one knows how to follow Yi's line of argumentation.

Critical evaluation of retrospective biomedical diagnoses

Bridgman diagnoses 'acute cystitis'.[1] Lu and Needham consider the cystitis to be connected to nephritis, because the client suffered in their understanding from haematuria.[2] However, as in case 3 (line 22), *ni chi* means 'the urine is dark yellow'. Since blood is not always visible in urine, nephritis is nevertheless possible.

The retrospective diagnosis 'acute cystitis' was confirmed independently by the three clinicians I consulted; this case is the only one with unanimous agreement. The dark yellow urine is taken as a sign of heat, as is the accelerated pulse rate, into which Yi's 'hurried' *mai* is translated. Both are typical signs of dehydration and/or infection. The difficulties with urinating point to the bladder; the difficulties with defecating may come from the pain the cystitis causes. They disappear after drinking the

[1] Bridgman (1955:74).   [2] Lu and Needham (1967:231).

first dose, but Yi considers the illness to have ceased only after administering the second.

huo ji tang 火齊湯 – *broth [prepared by careful] regulation of fire (line 5)*

The remedy Yi repeatedly administers, *huo ji tang* (broth [prepared by careful] regulation of fire), is one of the few technical terms in Yi's Memoir about which modern scholarship has something to say, most importantly Yamada Keiji.³ In an entire chapter on this theme, Yamada first examines various terms for 'broths', or, more literally, 'hot liquids' (*tang* 湯) and 'decoctions' (*tang ye* 湯液 and *ye tang* 液湯), then explores the meaning of *ji* 齊 (regulation) and finally discusses all of Yi's case histories that mention *huo ji* 火齊 (regulation of fire). As he notes in a later chapter, *tang ye* (decoctions) are a basic trait of what is called 'Chinese medicine' and by the time of Zhang Zhongjing 張仲景 (ca 150–ca 219 CE) in the Eastern Han, they constituted the main treatment method for disorders identified through pulse diagnosis.⁴ With regard to Yi's Memoir, this means that the innovative diagnostic method of examining *mai* entailed an innovative therapeutic method: decoctions. Considering that Yi provides the first extensive account of pulse diagnosis in Chinese medical history, it may be no coincidence that he emphatically makes his patients drink their medicines (*yin* in the fourth tone, as Zhang Shoujie notes in case 3). They do so in ten out of the fifteen cases he treated,⁵ ingesting mostly *tang*.

What was a *tang*? Yamada explains in an earlier chapter that in the Mawangdui 'Recipes' nine out of 300 cases involve treatment with *tang*, and that *tang* is used there in at least three different senses: first, it refers to 'hot water'; second, to 'medicinal baths'; and, third, to a 'broth which dribbles out from steaming'.⁶ In this context, Yamada also mentions examples of prescriptions for treating disorders of the urinary tract, which he views as 'prototypes of decoction' insofar as 'the medicines are boiled in water for a comparatively long period of time'.⁷ He differentiates between three different 'prototypes': first, medicines boiled in water; second, medicines boiled in alcohol or alcohol and vinegar; and, third, a form of gruel made of the 'five grains'.⁸ 'Prototypes of decoction' were according to Yamada primarily

---

³ Yamada (1998:109–23).   ⁴ Yamada (1998:138).
⁵ External application was the common method of treatment. See case 4, n. 5.
⁶ Yamada (1998:95–8) uses 'broth' here in an unidiomatic way; a broth is the water within which meat is cooked. Literally, *tang* means 'hot liquid' and can refer to a tea, infusion, decoction or broth; it is here given as 'broth' for literary reasons (like *jiu* is given as 'wine' instead of the more accurate 'alcoholic beverage'). Cross-culturally, medicinal hot liquids often were/are broths (e.g. Zimmermann 1987). The simmering of plant materials in broths leads to the extraction of not only water- but also fat-soluble chemical compounds.
⁷ Yamada (1998:100).
⁸ Yamada (1998:101–6). The five grains are: setaria millet (*ji* 稷), panicum millet (*shu* 黍), rice (*dao* 稻), wheat and barley (*mai* 麥), legumes (*shu* 菽), according to Bray (1984:432). For a variant in medicine, see *Ling shu* 56, p. 413, detailed in a footnote to case 21 in Hsu and Nienhauser (in press).

used for treating urinary tract disorders, because like treats like: 'Fluids which closely resemble urine, and consequently were thought to belong to the same category [*tong lei* 同類], accelerated urination, and could be used as a diuretic.'[9] These prototypes of decoction, he argues, certainly had a prompt and drastically felt effect on the patient in that they enhanced the frequency of urination, regardless of their ultimate curative value. Yamada continues his argument, which is guided by considerations of their efficacy, by pointing out that warming medicines in alcohol probably led to a wider application because: 'Preparations boiled in alcoholic drink have the remarkable effect of inducing perspiration.'[10] Perspiration, like urination, is a prompt and drastically felt effect of any ingestion of fluids for any patient, regardless of its ultimate therapeutic value. According to Yamada, 'prototypes of decoction' were prepared by careful regulation of fire, over a small fire. The water-based ones enhanced urination, the alcohol-based ones perspiration.[11]

With the above in mind, let us turn to *Shi ji* 105. Yamada suggests, as already stated, that the medical knowledge in Bian Que's Memoir dates to the period of Sima Qian's life, while Yi's case histories date to the mid-second century, and that therefore the technical terminology in the two Memoirs has to be discussed separately.[12] Yi frequently refers to *huo ji*, but not Bian Que. This observation is the more interesting as *huo ji* is mentioned in the *Han Feizi* of the third century BCE but substituted in Bian Que's Memoir by the compound word *jiu lao* 酒醪, generally approximated as 'mixed alcohols'. This prompts Liao Yuqun to suggest that *tang ye* (decoctions) originally referred to fermented drinks,[13] but Yamada is more cautious: 'Undoubtedly, for Sima Qian to change *huo ji* into *jiu lao*, some sort of historical basis must have been contained within.'[14] It is not compelling that if a term, say *jiu lao*, substitutes another one, *huo ji*, the two terms have the same referential meaning. They may have designated related but different kinds of remedies. In the same passage, for instance, the 'flesh and fatty skin' (*ji fu* 肌膚) is substituted by 'blood vessels' (*xue mai* 血脈), and even though the two terms referred to the same layer within the skin, they certainly did not have exactly the same referential meaning.

The paragraph in question reads in the *Han Feizi*:[15]

> If the illness resides in the skin pore pattern,
> then hot compresses are that which reach it,
> if it resides in the flesh and fatty skin,
> then stone needles are that which reach it,

[9] Yamada (1998:101).   [10] Yamada (1998:101).
[11] See also case 9 (lines 5, 8, 22), on the 'drugged wine' (*yao jiu*).
[12] Yamada (1998:109). See also p. 61.
[13] Liao (1984).   [14] Yamada (1998:112).
[15] *Han Feizi* 7 (21), pp. 397, 399.

if it resides in the intestines and stomach,
then *huo ji* is that which reaches it,
if it resides in the bones and marrow,
then it belongs to fate, there is nothing you can do about it!

ji zai cou li, tang yun zhi suo ji ye 疾在腠理 湯熨之所及也
zai ji fu, zhen shi zhi suo ji ye 在肌膚 鍼石之所及也
zai chang wei, huo ji zhi suo ji ye 在腸胃 火齊之所及也
zai gu sui, si ming zhi suo shu wu nai he ye 在骨髓 司命之所屬無奈何也

In Bian Que's Memoir the wording of the passage is slightly modified:[16]

If the illness resides in the skin pore pattern,
then hot compresses are that which reach it,
if it resides in the blood vessels,
then stone needles are that which reach it,
if it resides in the intestines and stomach,
then mixed alcohols are that which reach it,
if it resides in the bones and marrow,
then it is a matter of fate, there is nothing you can do about it!

ji zhi ju cou li ye, tang yun zhi suo ji ye 疾之居腠理 湯熨之所及也
zai xue mai, zhen shi zhi suo ji ye 在血脈 鍼石之所及也
qi zai chang wei, jiu lao zhi suo ji ye 其在腸胃 酒醪之所及也
qi zai gu sui, si ming wu nai zhi he 其在骨髓 司命無奈之何

Both *huo ji* and 'mixed alcohols' were used for treating disorders in the 'intestines and stomach', which in some medical circles were thought to occupy the very centre of the body.[17] Perhaps Yi frequently administered *huo ji*, not least because he adhered to the teachings of 'Qi ke', which, as established earlier (pp. 67–8), was innovative in the importance it attributed to investigating body internal processes for correct diagnosis and treatment.

If one adopts Yamada's empiricist stance of analysis, which interprets *huo ji*'s characteristics on the grounds of its therapeutic use for treating conditions identified through retrospective biomedical diagnoses, and is interested in whether or not it was water-based or alcohol-based, so much can be said on Yi's Memoir: Yi administers *huo ji tang* in cases 3, 5 and 10, which all concern problems with urination. In those cases, as Yamada puts it, the broth is 'cathartic'.[18] In case 20, Yi administers a '*huo ji* rice porridge' (*huo ji mi zhi* 火齊米汁) for treating a condition on the verge of turning into a disorder called 'wind of the void' (*dong feng* 迵風), which in all likelihood designated a violent form of diarrhoea (see also case 8, line 4). And in case

---

[16] *Shiki kaichû kôshô* 105.1, p. 17.
[17] In *Su wen* 56, p. 152, disorders arise in the 'skin's body hair' (*pi mao* 皮毛), then proceed to the 'linking vessels' (*luo mai* 絡脈), 'channels' (*jing* 經), 'receptacles' (*fu* 府) and, finally, the 'intestines and stomach' (*chang wei*).
[18] See table 4 in Yamada (1998:122).

23, the '*huo ji* gruel' (*huo ji zhou* 火齊粥) is used for treating what Yi approximates as an 'obstruction' (*bi* 痺). There is little doubt that the broths Yi used for treating problems with urination in cases 3, 5 and 10 were water-based, and since a rice porridge or gruel generally are not considered fermented drinks, the '*huo ji* rice porridge' and 'gruel' in cases 20 and 23 were water-based too.[19] This would suggest, contrary to Liao Yuqun, that in Yi's Memoir, at least, *huo ji* was a water-based remedy rather than a fermented drink.

Once again case 4 (line 20) is an exception, this time in its use of *huo ji*. Yi administers a '*ye tang* [called] regulation of fire' (*ye tang huo ji* 液湯火齊). In Yamada's view, it is used in an 'antipyretic' way to treat an infection. Without calling into question the infection, we noted that Yi's account of its application was from a biomedical viewpoint slightly odd (lines 20–23); probably the externally applied medicines were antipyretic (lines 24–5). A further anomaly is that the term *ye tang* (lit. fluid liquid, i.e. decoction) is prefixed to *huo ji*. What does it mean and why is it *ye tang* rather than *tang ye* (decoction)? Taki Motokata cites *Han shu* 25B, 'In accordance with the winds he made a *ye tang*' (*shun feng zuo ye tang* 順風作液湯) and Ru Chun's (fl. 198–265) comment to that phrase, which is that a 'Canon of Ye Tang' (*ye tang jing* 液湯經) occurs in *Han shu* 30.[20] However, its title in the Zhonghua shuju edition of *Han shu* 30 is 'Model of the Canon of Decoctions' (*Tang ye jing fa* 湯液經法).[21] This would suggest that *ye tang* was later substituted by *tang ye*. Considering that several compound words in Yi's Memoir are inverted,[22] it is likely that *ye tang* in case 4 designates much the same kind of decoction as does *tang ye* (decoction) in other texts and in Bian Que's Memoir.[23] If *ye tang* meant 'decoction', *huo ji* is water-based also in case 4.

In the course of discussing *huo ji*, Yamada also explores the meaning of *ji*. He discusses passages from the *Zhou li* (Rites of Zhou), the *Li ji* (Record of Ceremony) and the *Han shu*, and comes to the conclusion that '*ji* means quantity or adjustment, or a preparation adjusted by the degree of quantity of medicines'.[24] Yamada later points to quotes from the *Li ji* and *Xunzi*,

---

[19] Note again consistency in treatment rationale across cases 1–10 (except case 4) versus cases 11–25.

[20] *Han shu* 25B, p. 1270. Translation based on Yamada (1998:117), but modified.

[21] *Han shu* 30, p. 1777. Yang and Yang (unpubl.) suggest 湯 does not mean 'hot liquid' but refers to the legendary Yi Yin 伊尹, famous cook of the Tang (period during the Shang dynasty ca sixteenth to eleventh century BCE), who invented the so-called 'Tang liquids' (Tang *ye*), i.e. 'decoctions'. The substitution of *tang ye* by *ye tang* is evidence to refute their claim. Yang Chengzu 楊承祖 and Yang Kai 楊凱 (unpubl.). 'Tangye de shizu – Yi Yin' 湯液的始祖 伊尹 (The First Ancestor of Decoctions – Yi Yin). Paper presented at the Shaanxi conference on pre-Qin medicine, 1985.

[22] For instance: *nei guan zhi bing* and *guan nei zhi bing* (in cases 1 and 15 vs case 12).

[23] *Shiki kaichû kôshô* 105.1, p. 9. See Yamada (1998:109ff.).

[24] Yamada (1998:114). See also Osobe Yô (1994:72–3), an interpretation I consider unlikely.

which make clear that the word *ji* in *huo ji* refers to a 'balance' between the raw and matured or between the raw and processed. Therefore *ji* is here rendered as 'regulation'.

The term *huo ji* (fire regulation) occurs both in the *Han Feizi*, which with certainty dates to the third century BCE,[25] and in Yi's case histories, which, as argued here, in places reflect medical knowledge from the early second century, but it is not mentioned in later medical texts. The question is what *huo ji* means. Harper emphasises the broth's effect of being 'fire regulatory'.[26] In the *Shi ji* text as it reads now, cases 3 and 5, and certainly case 4, involve heat, and *huo ji* may have been considered therapeutic by being 'fire regulatory'. Case 10 is more complex, the dark urine suggests heat but Yi also reports that the cold aggravates the condition, and he cauterises the patient first and only then administers *huo ji*. Nevertheless, it is difficult to construct an argument that in case 10 *huo ji* is 'fire regulatory'. Moreover, there is reason to question that heat was the prime pathological factor in the assumed early second-century document of cases 3, 5 and 10, on which Sima Qian elaborates (or whoever the editor/s was/were). So far, we noted that heat becomes an issue only towards the end of these three cases. Nor would the *huo ji* rice porridge and gruel of cases 20 and 23 respectively seem 'fire regulatory'.

Case 22, by contrast, which probably was composed at a more recent date than the primary source materials for cases 1 and 2 (and even all cases 1–10), definitely is framed in hot/cold complementarities. As in several later Han compilations, *huo ji* has become *shui huo zhi ji* 水火之齊 'regulation of water and fire'. This idiom occurs in *Han shu* 30 from the first century CE: 'As for the canonical recipes . . . they discuss the five bitter and six astringent [flavours], they enable the regulation of water and fire, in order to effect a passage through the closed and dissolve that which is knotted up' (*jing fang zhe . . . bian wu ku liu xin, zhi shui huo zhi ji, yi tong bi jie jie* 經方者 辯五苦 六辛 致水火之齊 以通閉解結), and also in the *Zhou li* (*ca* third century BCE to the first CE): 'The person in charge of boiling is responsible for offering the cauldron, and thereby provides the regulation of water and fire' (*peng ren zhang gong ding huo, yi ji shui huo zhi ji* 烹人掌共鼎鑊 以給水火之齊).[27] In case 22, Yi says of 'medicinal minerals' (or 'drugs and minerals', *yao shi* 藥石) that they are 'regulators of *yin* and *yang*, water and fire' (*yin yang shui huo zhi ji* 陰陽水火之齊).[28] There is little doubt that the term *huo ji* was then understood to effect a regulation between water and fire. As Yamada points out repeatedly, the meaning of the term changed over time. Accordingly, *huo ji* need not necessarily mean 'fire regulatory' in the late Warring States and early Han.

[25] Levi (1993) and Yamada (1998:112).   [26] Harper (1998).
[27] *Zhou li*, 'Tian Guan' 天官, p. 662. On its dating, see Boltz (1993:24–32).
[28] *Shiki kaichû kôshô* 105.2, p. 49.

Treatment rationale in the early second century may not have been guided, to an overriding degree as in many *Ling shu* texts, by the aim of balancing out the hot and cold. This is said in awareness that extreme coldness turned into extreme heat in case 4 and that oppositions of the dry and wet play a role in case 5. More often, however, treatment rationale appears to be focused on body internal processes of accumulation that were considered harmful: a coagulation of blood in case 1, a blockage of *qi* in case 2, and an amassment that hindered urination and defecation in case 3. All cases 1–10 were heavily edited, and as will become increasingly evident, cases 3, 5 and 10, where *huo ji tang* restored urination, became heat conditions primarily due to commentatorial interjections. There are indices that the water-based *huo ji tang* in cases 3, 5 and 10 dissolves amassments and dampness. It was a 'prototype I decoction', in Yamada's words, which like the later decoctions, presumably was prepared by simmering over a 'regulated fire'. It is unlikely that in texts of the third and early second centuries BCE the term *huo ji* refers to 'fire regulatory' therapeutic effects. Rather, its name reflects the procedure of its production as a broth 'prepared by means of a [careful] regulation of fire'.

What was so special about *huo ji*? *Su wen* 14 points out that *bi ji* 必齊 is used for treating the interior: 'Nowadays, the interior is treated by *bi ji* [i.e. *huo ji*?] and potent drugs, and the exterior is treated by using stone needles, acupuncture and moxibustion' (*dang jin zhi shi, bi ji du yao gong qi zhong, chan shi zhen ai zhi qi wai ye* 當今之世 必齊毒藥攻其中 鑱石鍼艾治其外也).[29] If Yamada is right that *bi ji* in *Su wen* 14 means *huo ji*,[30] and if *Su wen* 14 accurately reports on its usage, *huo ji* treated disorders of the 'interior'. *Su wen* 14 thus advocates the same use of *huo ji* as the *Han Feizi*, where the idiom 'stomach and intestines' stands for 'interior'. Notably, Yi did not treat disorders of the viscera with *huo ji*, although these occupied the bodily 'interior'; perhaps because they were conceived of primarily as storage places for *qi*, while drinking *huo ji* was meant to have body internal effects on fluids and regulate bodily waters.

In summary, the term *huo ji tang* has at least two different layers of meaning in Yi's Memoir. Accordingly, it may either be translated as 'fire regulatory broth' or as a 'broth [prepared by careful] regulation of fire'. The translation 'fire regulatory broth' emphasises its therapeutic effects within a medical rationale framed in hot/cold complementarities. The translation of *huo ji* as 'broth [prepared by careful] regulation of fire' points to the mode of preparation of being simmered over a regulated fire as the most characteristic feature of decoctions and 'prototype decoctions'. Commentators on Yi's case histories most likely considered *huo ji* 'fire regulatory', but the author of the early second-century medical document probably understood *huo ji* to refer to its mode of preparation over a 'regulated fire'.

---

[29] *Su wen* 14, p. 43; 15, p. 45.   [30] Yamada (1998:129).

The name of the disorder (line 3)

The name of the disorder, 'wind-induced condition caused by overexertion is visiting the bladder' (*feng dan ke pao* 風癉客脬) (line 3), is not recorded in canonical medical texts, but each of the constituents are. In what follows, the first constituent of the name, 'wind' (*feng*), is discussed in the light of other occurrences in Yi's Memoir; the second, *dan* (condition caused by overexertion), is explored by examining mostly non-medical texts; and the third, *pao* (bladder), by reading Chinese medical writings from a cross-cultural perspective.

feng 風 – **wind (line 3)**   'Wind' (*feng*) is one of the most central notions in Chinese medicine,[31] but it will be discussed in what follows only with respect to Yi's Memoir. 'Wind' occurs four times as a constituent of the name of the disorder: in the 'wind-induced condition caused by overexertion' (*feng dan*) of case 5, the 'wind of the void' (*dong feng*) of cases 8 and 20, the 'wind-induced numbness/inversion' (*feng jue*) of case 9, and the 'talkative wind' (*ta feng* 沓風) of case 24. In cases 5 and 9, the constituent 'wind' in the name of the disorder correlates with the pulse quality 'wind *qi*' (*feng qi*), which is what one would expect according to text structure semantics; case 8 (lines 4 and 12/13) is more complicated. In cases 20 and 24, Yi also reports on his examination of *mai*, but at this stage of the research it is difficult to see a connection between the qualities of *mai* and the name of the disorder, if ever there was meant to be one.

Whereas in cases 1–10 'wind' is mentioned among the pulse qualities, it figures as a cause of the disorder only in cases 13, 15 and 24. In case 24, where the patient contracted the illness 'By frequently drinking wine and by being exposed to great wind *qi*' (*shuo yin jiu yi xian da feng qi* 數飲酒以見大風氣), the constituent 'wind' in the name correlates with the cause of the disorder. Case 24 thus provides the most evident counterexample among all of Yi's twenty-five cases for challenging text structure semantics and its postulate that constituents in the name of the disorder correlate with the quality of the disorder rather than its cause. However, said correlation between cause and name of the disorder occurs only in case 24, and probably due to a commentator's interjection (see following paragraph). Wind is not once the cause of the disorder in cases 1–10.[32]

In cases 13, 15 and 24 wind is not the sole cause. The foul tooth in case 13 is not only 'contracted from wind' (*de zhi feng* 得之風), because of 'sleeping with an open mouth' (*wo kai kou* 臥開口), but also from 'eating and not rinsing the mouth' (*shi er bu sou* 食而不嗽). The slave in case 15 contracted

---

[31] On 'wind' (*feng*) in the Warring States and Han, see Lewis (1990:214–21). On wind in medicine, see Unschuld (1982), Kuriyama (1994, 1999), Hsu (2007c).

[32] We note again consistency in rationale, with regard to pulse qualities, across cases 1–10 and, in respect of illness causation, across cases 11–25; the exception is the 'wind of the void' (*dong feng*) in cases 8 and 20.

his illness from both 'profusely sweating' and 'frequently going outside', from 'having roasted by the fire' and 'being exposed to great winds when going outside' (*liu han shuo chu, jiu yu huo er yi chu xian da feng ye* 流汗 數出 灸於火 而 以出見大風也), and in case 24, cited in the previous paragraph, the patient not only indulged in frequent wine consumption but also exposed himself to great wind *qi*. In all three cases, wind is not the only cause of the disorder. It is thus possible, particularly in cases 15 and 24,[33] that wind as an illness cause was added to an already existent text that blamed bad habit. Bad habit put the patient into a vulnerable state before wind could cause harm.

In the above three cases, 'exposure to wind' (*xian feng* 見風) was considered detrimental to one's health. This idiom occurs in various Mawangdui medical manuscripts,[34] as does the notion 'taking precautions against wind' (*fang feng* 方[防]風),[35] but not in the Mawangdui vessel texts. In these early medical sources, 'wind' is not yet the all-encompassing concept it eventually becomes in canonical texts, like *Su wen* 60, which makes it the cause of all illness: 'Wind is the beginning of the hundred illnesses' (*feng zhe bai bing zhi shi ye* 風者百病之始也).[36] In case 10 (line 2), all the many doctors' concept of an intruding external 'wind' contrasts with Yi's notion of an internal *qi* (line 6). Neither 'wind' nor *qi* spans the wide semantic field they have in canonical doctrine.

By medieval times, wind gives rise to madness, seizures, fright and fits,[37] which from a biomedical viewpoint are dysfunctions in the neurological and neuro-muscular systems, but not in Yi's Memoir. In case 2 (line 3), Yi diagnosed a 'disorder of *qi* that is separated/blocked' (*qi ge bing*) and not 'wind of fright' (*jing feng*), although the symptom complex of these two nosological entities is strikingly similar. Again case 24 arguably is an exception, as its 'talkative wind' is predicted to end in dumbness, limpness and death.[38]

In Yi's Memoir, the queen dowager of the King of Qi in case 5 and the King of Jibei in case 9 both suffer from a disorder containing the prefix 'wind' in its name, that is, a 'wind-induced condition caused by overexertion' (*feng dan*) and a 'wind-induced numbness/inversion' (*feng jue*). In both cases, sweating belongs among the causes giving rise to their disorder.

---

[33] In support of this, note in case 15 the grammatically odd juxtaposition of the conjunctions *er* 'yet' and *yi* 'and'. Such textual anomalies are best interpreted as faultlines between two mini-texts. Note that also in case 24 the conjunction *yi* is used at the presumed faultline. See ch. 3, nn. 19 and 20.

[34] MWD 'Recipes' (1985:30) and MWD 'Yangsheng fang' (1985:116).

[35] MWD 'Recipes' (1985:56) and MWD 'Yangsheng fang' (1985:109, 110, 115).

[36] e.g. *Su wen* 60, p. 160.   [37] Chen (2002:124–50).

[38] The only early reference to wind-induced stiffness is in the MWD 'Recipes' (1985:30, S30), translation by Harper (1998:229): 'Rigidity occurs when there is a wound, wind enters the wound, and then the body becomes straight and cannot bend' (*jing zhe, shang, feng ru shang, shen xin* [*shen*] *er bu neng qu* [*qu*] 痙者 傷 風入傷 身信[伸] 而 不能詘[屈]).

According to *Su wen* 26, sweating was thought to open the skin's pore pattern,[39] and according to *Su wen* 33, this let the essences leak that, according to *Su wen* 61, came from the kidneys (quoted on p. 200). The *Shi ji* text is sufficiently vague that one can impute this canonical rationale into cases 5 and 9. However, a closer reading suggests that, overridden by a concern with 'sweating' and 'exposure to wind', cases 5 and 9 report on over-exposure to either *yang*-sunlight or *yin*-earthiness.

In case 5, the explicit cause of the disorder is that the queen dowager, when dripping with sweat, went outside, removed her clothes and let her sweat dry in the sunlight (lines 8–9). This sentence, which alludes to wet sweat and dry sunlight, is implicitly framed in *yin yang* complementarities and makes no allusion to wind. Perhaps it reflects early medical rationale. In case 9 (line 8), the cause of the King of Jibei's illness is not only sweating, but also lying prostrate on the ground, whence *yin* ascends, thereby causing numbness and an inversion of *yin* and *yang*. Finally, although one could put the cause of the disorder quite literally down to an exposure to either *yin* or *yang* and to sweating and wind, yet further connotations deserve consideration.

Shigehisa Kuriyama emphasises that wind alludes to the unregulated and irregular in medicine, epitomised in madness and seizures. These connotations of wind, which prevailed in Late Imperial China, are already given in the *Inner Canon*, which, however, also puts much emphasis on the regularity of the seasonal winds. Much like the songs and tunes, customs and local mores, which 'wind' connoted in the Zhou, the seasonal winds regulated people's conduct. The wind-induced disorder in Yi's case 5 may connote socially disapproved behaviour less with madness than with unrestrained wants and desires. Another aspect of wind is thereby brought to the fore, wind as 'breath of life', 'as generative agent that begets through transformation', as discussed mainly in non-medical pre-Han and Han texts.[40] The key to understanding why the queen dowager and the King of Jibei have disorders that are wind-induced, as we will see (discussion of case 9, line 3), is the notion *feng ma* 風馬 (lit. wind horse), the 'horse in heat',[41] which alludes to wind as a socially disruptive, unruly and wild, but ultimately life-engendering principle.

dan 癉 – **condition of overexertion (line 3)**   The term *dan* occurs in texts from the early Zhou, such as the *Shi jing*. It is ubiquitous in writings of the Warring States and Han, and appears also among disorders of the Mawangdui vessel texts, the Zhangjiashan 'Maishu' and Zhangjiashan

---

[39] *Su wen* 26, p. 82.   [40] Sterckx (2002:170).
[41] *feng ma* in this sense is given in *Matthews'* (Brandon Miller, 2005 p.c.), but not in other dictionaries.

'Yinshu'.[42] It has several pronunciations and many meanings, too many to be detailed here, and some connotations left out from discussion in case 5 will be addressed in case 6 (line 3). One of the reasons that makes the study of *dan* difficult is that *dan* 癉 and *dan* 疸 have the same pronunciation and therefore were used interchangeably in Han medical texts and later.[43] Thus, *dan* 癉 occurs in the sense of *dan* 疸 already in the Zhangjiashan 'Maishu'. Also non-medical texts use *dan* 癉 and *dan* 疸 interchangeably in the compound word *huang dan* 黃疸 (yellow disorder), which connotes what biomedicine calls 'jaundice'.[44]

In pre-Han texts, however, they have distinct meanings. These are still given in *Shuo wen* 7B, which lists the graphs side by side: '*dan* is a disorder of overexertion' (*dan, lao bing ye* 癉 勞病也) and '*dan* is the yellow disorder' (*dan, huang bing ye* 疸 黃病也).[45] However, as the Qing commentator to the *Shuo wen*, Duan Yucai, rightly points out, they are used interchangeably in the *Tai su* and the *Su wen*, where the colour yellow is an attribute of *dan* 癉 and overexertion of *dan* 疸.

Relevant for cases 5 and 6 is that *dan* can refer either to a 'state of over-exertion' or to 'heat-due-to-overexertion'. From a canonical medical view-point, these two conditions are interrelated: overexertion causes one to sweat and thereby lose internally stored cool waters, with the result that the state of overexertion is marked by subdued chronic heat. The graph *dan* is written either with the 61st radical as 憚 or the 104th as 癉. The former, which occurs in the *Shi jing*, is glossed as '*dan* means to be overex-erted' (*dan lao ye* 憚 勞也),[46] and the latter from the *Er ya* as '*dan* means to be overexerted' (*dan lao ye* 癉 勞也).[47] These definitions of *dan*, it is argued here, apply to case 5, certainly to its assumed primary source and probably also to its edited version of the early first century. By contrast, heat is an intrinsic aspect of *dan* in case 6, or rather, as will be argued then, of *xiao dan* 消癉 (wasting heat-due-to-overexertion). This crucial difference between *dan* in cases 5 and 6 was not noted by the commentators.

Taki Mototane cites *Han shu* 64A: *nan fang shu shi, jin xia dan re* 南方 署淫 近夏癉熱. This sentence is difficult to translate; Taki Mototane seems to have cited it because *dan* can here be interpreted as 'heat'.[48] If one con-siders the 'summer-heat and dampness' (*shu shi* 署濕) in the first phrase to

---

[42] e.g. MWD YY (1985:12, S65), Gao (1992:28–9), ZJS (2001:242, 289).

[43] Yu (1953:17). Phenomenologically, both designate a weakened constitution.

[44] Mathieu (1983:1.041–2).   [45] *Shuo wen* 7B, p. 33b.

[46] *Shi jing*, 'Xiao ya', 'Da dong 大東' (SBBY 13.3b). Ma (1992:264) cites this text passage as *dan lao ye* 癉勞也 but it actually reads: *dan lao ye* 憚勞也. See also the *Shi jing* edition called *Mao shi zheng yi* 13.1, p. 461a. In *Shi jing*, 'Da ya', 'Ban 板' (SBBY 17.15b), the gloss to *dan* is: '*dan* is a disorder' (*dan bing ye* 癉病也).

[47] *Er ya* 1, p. 4a.

[48] *Han shu* 64A, pp. 2781–2. By contrast, Yan Shigu (581–645) glosses *dan* as *huang dan* 'jaundice'.

contrast with '*dan* and heat' (*dan re* 癉熱) in the second, the heat of *dan* may have been marked by dryness.[49] Indeed, *dan* is clearly related to drought in the *Lun heng* 15.4: 'Hence, since heaven and earth have floods, how do we know it is not like man having water illnesses; since they have droughts, how do we know it is not like man having *dan* disorders?' (*gu fu tian di zhi you zhan ye, he yi zhi bu ru ren zhi you shui bing; qi you han ye, he yi zhi bu ru ren you dan ji ye* 故夫天地之有湛也 何以知不如人之有水病 其有 旱也 何以知不如人有癉疾).[50] If *dan* were indeed to designate a condition of dryness due to heat, it would come very close to the canonical 'heat-due-to-overexertion', after loss of one's cooling waters through perspiration.[51]

If, however, in *Han shu* 64A one considers 'summer-heat and dampness' to parallel the phrase '*dan* and heat', one could interpret *dan* as referring to a subtropical humid heat. In corroboration of this, Wang Bing's comment on *Su wen* 17, '*dan* turns into a wasting away of the centre' (*dan cheng wei xiao zhong* 癉成為消中), reads: '*dan* indicates dampness and heat' (*dan wei shi re ye* 癉謂溼熱也).[52]

To complicate the issue, Taki Mototane cites Wang Bing's comment on *Su wen* 17 in a variant edition: '*dan* indicates heat' (*dan wei re* 癉為熱). This comment parallels Wang Bing's on 'spleen *dan*' (*pi dan* 脾癉) and 'gall bladder *dan*' (*dan dan* 膽癉) in *Su wen* 47: '*dan* indicates heat' (*dan wei re ye* 癉為熱也). Taki Mototane also quotes Wang Bing on a 'heat-due-to-overexertion resulting in chills and hot flushes' (*dan nüe* 癉瘧) in *Su wen* 35: '*dan* is heat, extreme heat turns into it' (*dan re ye, ji re wei zhi ye* 癉熱 也 極熱為之也).[53] In Wang Bing's interpretation of the *Su wen*, *dan* designates 'dampness and heat', 'heat' and 'extreme heat'; Taki Mototane chooses to quote him for the '[dry] heat'.

Yu Yunxiu points out that the meanings of *dan* 癉 as overexertion (*Shuo wen*) and heat (Wang Bing) are interrelated;[54] it is common knowledge in Chinese medicine that 'depletion patterns' can give rise to internal 'fire' (*huo* 火).[55] Although the term 'depletion' does not figure in Yi's Memoir, the existence of a concept approximating it cannot be entirely excluded, as early manuscript texts also describe conditions that one could classify as such (quoted on p. 257).

---

[49] *dan re zhi bing* 癉熱之病 translated as 'consumption' (Forke 1962:183) occurs also in *Lun heng* 5.2, p. 330.

[50] *Lun heng* 15.4, p. 962. Forke (1962:344), based on the commentary, has *dan ji* 癉疾 as 'jaundice', but is mistaken.

[51] Biomedically, a dehydration; see retrospective diagnoses on p. 204.

[52] HDNJSW 17, p. 39.

[53] HDNJSW 47, p. 95; 35, p. 74. See also case 6 (line 4).

[54] Yu (1953:144).

[55] Yu (1953:349). One of the typical signs for such 'depletion patterns' is 'heat in the middle of the hands and feet' (*shouzu zhongre* 手足中熱), marked by 'the five hearts (the heart, and the hearts of hands and feet) being upset and hot' (*wu xin fan re* 五心煩熱). See *Zhongyi zhenduanxue* (Deng 1984:85).

In summary, in non-medical pre-Han and Han texts *dan* designates a 'condition of overexertion' and 'utter exhaustion'. Accordingly, as argued here, *dan* in case 5 refers to a condition caused by overexertion (without any reference being made to heat). In the Han and post-Han literature, *dan* generally refers to states of utter exhaustion marked by a subdued internal heat, either damp or extreme heat, or what in more recent times is referred to as internal dry 'depletion fire' (*xu huo* 虚火): in case 6, Yi speaks of *xiao dan* (wasting heat).

pao 脬 – bladder (line 3)   Closer examination of the term *pao* 脬 (bladder) instantly refers us to other words for 'bladder' and other bag-like structures of the body. For making sense of these in early China, our discussion will centre on body parts conceived of as bags from a cross-cultural perspective. This section may therefore be of particular interest to the anthropologist.

For elucidating the term *pao* 脬, Zhang Shoujie explains: '*pao*, also written as *pao*, is the bladder' (*pao, yi zuo pao, pang guang ye* 脬亦作胞膀胱也). He mentions in one sentence three different words meaning 'bladder'. Of these, only the first, *pao* 脬, has an entry in *Shuo wen* 4B: '*pao* is the bladder' (*pao pang guang ye* 脬旁光也).[56] The graph *pao* 脬 is also the only one of the three mentioned in the sense of 'bladder' in the Mawangdui medical manuscripts;[57] the graph for *pao* 胞, without semantic determinative and pronounced as *bao* 包, is there used in the sense of 'afterbirth'.[58] However, *pao* 脬 hardly occurs in the *Inner Canon*, while *pang guang* 膀胱 is very frequent; Ren Yingqiu's concordance contains no entry on *pao* 脬 but many on *pang guang* 膀胱.[59] This would suggest that in the late Warring States and early Han *pao* 脬 was the usual term for 'bladder'; that the graph 胞, pronounced as *bao* and *pao*, referred to the 'womb', the 'afterbirth' and other body parts inclusive of the 'bladder'; and that the two-syllabic term *pang guang* 膀胱 became the common term meaning 'bladder' in Han and post-Han medical doctrine.

The above observations raise several questions. Why should a graph, like 胞 meaning 'womb' and 'afterbirth' also refer to the 'bladder' and other body parts? Why was the word *pao* 脬 with the clearly demarcated meaning of urinary bladder replaced by another term? Was it that a new term had to be invented to suit the meaning of 'bladder' in canonical medical doctrine? Why did this new term *pang guang* 膀胱 have two syllables? The following explorations intend to throw some light on these questions.

[56] *Shuo wen* 4B, p. 22. Note that *pang guang* 旁光 is rendered there without semantic determinative.
[57] MWD 'Recipes' (1985:45, 46, 56), Harper (1998:253, 255, 274). See also annotations by Ma (1992:452, 458, 524).
[58] MWD 'Zaliao fang' and 'Tai chan shu' (1985:126; 137, 139), Harper (1998:367–8; 381, 384).
[59] *Huangdi nei jing*, pp. 1143, 1473.

In response to the first question about the graph 胞, the phonophoric part of the character gives some hints: *bao* 包 means 'to wrap'. Karlgren remarks that 'The graph [*bao* 包] was possibly the primary form of *bao* 胞... and may have been the drawing of a foetus in the womb'.[60] The womb is in many cultures likened to a bag. Thus, Gilbert Lewis notes that among the Gnau in New Guinea the term *gelugi*, which means both 'womb' and 'placenta', is derived from their word for 'stringbag'.[61] Or, Michèle Cros explains that among the Lobi in West Africa the word for womb, *kolor*, is best paraphrased as 'male wrapper' (*enveloppe mâle*).[62] And Geoffrey Lloyd points to an understanding of the bladder as a structure which is hollow inside when he says of the writer of *On Ancient Medicine* 22: 'He already knows that of the parts of the body the bladder, the head and the womb are of this shape, "tapering and hollow"', a shape which was thought to have the function of attracting fluids.[63]

One can easily imagine why *bao* 胞 in Chinese, or *gelugi* in Gnau, referred to both the 'womb' and 'afterbirth' since both are related to the process of generation.[64] One would, however, expect 'womb' and 'bladder' to be more clearly differentiated given their distinct physiological functions. But from an anatomical viewpoint their position in the body and also their form are quite similar: the womb and bladder are both bag-like and empty inside. Thus, the *Zhuangzi* says: 'The womb has double emptiness, the heart has the universe for roaming about' (*bao you chong lang, xin you tian you* 胞有 重閬 心有天游).[65] In the view of the *Zhuangzi*, the womb has emptiness as its main characteristic: it is the space which makes the accommodation of the foetus possible. This view of the uterus as a bag may explain why *bao* 胞, if pronounced as *pao*, was also used to refer to another bag-like structure in the body – the urinary bladder.

Bladder and womb metaphorically substitute one another, if they are not simply confused with each other. Thus, among the morris dancers in England, young women are hit on the head with a pig's bladder, which should effect

---

[60] Karlgren (1957:1113a, 285).   [61] Lewis (1974).

[62] Cros (1990:41).   [63] Lloyd (1966:355).

[64] Lewis (1974:65) notes gender-specific knowledge: only women call the afterbirth *gelugi*, men call it *gungi wolit* (lit. blood lake). He suggests that men know from their dealings with sows that the womb stays within the sow and that it is only the 'blood lake' that is lost at birth. By contrast, 'Women who may handle the human placenta while men may not, assert that the *gelugi* itself is what women lose at birth.'

[65] *Zhuangzi*, pp. 4.939, 4.941. This passage is difficult to interpret. I follow the commentators Guo Xiang 郭象 (d. 312) and Cheng Xuanying 成玄英 (fl. 630–60) that *lang* means empty; but the editors of the HYDCD 6.1236 cite Lu Deming's 陸德明 (556–627) comment that *lang* means 'foetus' in support of *bao* as 'afterbirth' (*tai yi* 胎衣). Cheng Xuanying understands *bao* to refer to the 'abdomen' (*fu* 服), but it is equally possible to read *bao* as 'uterus'. The double emptiness may have referred to the space in the uterus for both the foetus itself and the placenta. The placenta is in many cultures treated as a second self of the child and considered responsible for its well-being, also in early China (Harper 1998:367–8).

a pregnancy in the following year, and among the Na in south-west China, a pig's bladder hangs in the innermost storage rooms of the house.[66] In England and south-west China, the bladder takes on the role of the womb; not only its reproductive functions, but also its body architectural ones of occupying a central space.

The idea that the bladder is something flabby and bag-like becomes obvious in the following passage from *Ling shu* 63, in which *bao* 胞 probably designates the 'lining of the bag', rather than the bag itself: 'The *bao* 胞 of the bladder is thin and soft' (*pang guang zhi bao bo yi nuo* 膀胱之胞薄以 懦).[67] This aspect of the bladder, as a bag-like structure with a thin and soft membrane, which is elastic, is also emphasised in another context of the early medical texts. In the Mawangdui 'Recipes' there is a formula against haemorrhoids, which proposes to use the bladder as a balloon for therapeutic purposes: 'For when a nest obstructs the rectum. Kill a dog. Take its bladder, and use a bamboo tube for entering it into the centre of the rectum. Blow on it [the tube]. Draw it out. Slowly cut away the nest with a knife' (*chao sai zhi zhe, sha gou, qu qi pao, yi chuan yue, ru zhi zhong, chui zhi, yin chu, xu yi dao bao qu qi chao* 巢塞直者 殺狗 取其脬 以穿籥 入直中 炊之 引 出 徐以刀剝去其巢).[68] The procedure reflects that the bladder was understood as a hollow bag, which was soft and very elastic and could be filled with air like a balloon.

The above quotes mention all three terms for bladder – *pang guang* 膀 胱, *pao* 胞 and *pao* 脬; evidently, all three terms could be used for referring to the bladder as the epitome of elasticity. Among the three, *bao/pao* 胞 clearly has the largest semantic stretch, ranging from afterbirth to womb, from bladder to the membrane of the bladder. In *Su wen* 37, *bao* 胞 may denote yet another bag-like structure: the bag that envelops the heart, the pericardium.[69] It is mentioned as the first in a series that thereafter enumerates five of the six hollow organs of canonical doctrine: (namely *bao* 胞, *pang guang* bladder, small intestine, large intestine, stomach, gall bladder): 'If the womb shifts the heat to the *pang guang* bladder, then one suffers from a protrusion ailment and urinates blood' (*bao yi re yu pang guang ze long ni xue* 胞移熱於膀胱則癃溺血). While the meaning of *bao* 胞 as womb makes perfect sense in this context, it is also possible that *bao* 胞 designates the bag that is the pericardium, the *xin bao luo* 心包絡 (pericardium), which eventually became canonised as the sixth hollow organ. The enormous

---

[66] Thaxted in Essex, England, yearly outings with Carmen Blacker and Michael Loewe in the late 1990s; Yongning, Yunnan province, PRC, field trip in March 1996. See also He (1999:37).
[67] *Ling shu* 63, p. 426.
[68] MWD 'Recipes' (1985:56), Harper (1998:274), translation modified.
[69] *Su wen* 37, p. 108.

semantic stretch of the term *bao/pao* 胞, also written as 包, allows for the above ambiguities.[70]

The term *pao* 胕, by contrast, was more clearly defined, for it consistently refers to the bladder in the Mawangdui medical texts, the *Shuo wen* and the *Shi ji*. One wonders therefore why *pao* 胕 did not become integrated into canonical medical vocabulary and why it was replaced by the term *pang guang* 膀胱. I suggest this may have to do with the connotations of *pao* 胕: both Yi's Memoir and the Mawangdui 'Recipes' point out that the bladder *pao* 胕 was positioned in the 'interior/centre' (*zhong* 表) of the body, while canonical doctrine teaches that the *pang guang* 膀胱 bladder is the outer aspect of the kidneys (*shen* 腎).[71]

Indications that the *pao* 胕 bladder was considered to be located in the interior of the body if not its centre can be found both in Yi's case histories and the Mawangdui medical manuscripts. Thus, case 5 (line 21) states that the 'interior/centre has heat' (*zhong you re*). This statement only makes sense if one assumes that the *pao* 胕 bladder was considered to be located in the interior/centre. The Mawangdui 'Recipes' also point to proximity between the *pao* bladder and the interior: 'Protrusion [ailment]: there is pain in the bladder reaching the interior/centre, if the pain is aggravated, urinating x, if the pain is even more aggravated, x x x x' (*long, tong yu pao ji zhong, tong shen, ni x, tong yi shen, xxxx* 癃 痛於胕及表 痛甚 溺x 痛益甚x x x x).[72] These observations suggest that the notions of *pao* 胕 bladder and *bao/pao*胞 womb/bladder both referred to a bladder located in the interior/centre of the body. The *pao* 胕 bladder was positioned in the interior/centre of the architectural body and not considered an outer aspect of one of the viscera, as the *pang guang* bladder is in canonical medicine.

Interestingly, the *Shuo wen* definition of *pao* 胕 is given next to that of the 'stomach' (*wei* 胃). Just as food was central to Han Chinese culture,[73] so was the stomach to the canonical Chinese medical body: 'spleen and stomach' (*pi wei*) form a unity at the centre of the body. By the Eastern Han, when the extant version of the *Su wen* was first compiled (see ch. 1, n. 5), the this-wordly digestive functions of spleen and stomach enjoyed a central position, while in pre-Han China the womb/bladder with

---

[70] Lloyd (1983:162), in his discussion of the fluctuations in anatomical terminology, points to a similar semantic stretch of the word *stomachos*, which was used '1. of the oesophagus, 2. of the orifice of the stomach, 3. of the neck of the bladder, 4. of that of the womb and even, it seems, 5. of that of the vagina'.

[71] *Ling shu* 10, p. 303.

[72] MWD 'Recipes' (1985:45), Harper (1998:253), translation modified. Harper's footnote 7 on *zhong* reveals difficulties in understanding why the bladder should be proximate to the interior/centre; his understanding of the bladder is evidently informed by biomedicine or canonical Chinese medicine but not by early medicine.

[73] Sterckx (2005).

its reproductive functions occupied the bodily interior/centre (see also case 1, line 13).[74]

The urinary bladder of canonical doctrine, by contrast, is the outer aspect of one of the viscera, the kidneys. The constituent *pang* 膀 in the term *pang guang* 膀胱, which means 'side' or 'sideways' or 'by the side', unambiguously indicates that the *pang guang* bladder was not considered to be located in the centre. The definition of the *pang guang* bladder in *Su wen* 8 can be read in support of this: 'The *pang guang* bladder is the office of the capital of an [administrative] region, the fluids are stored within it; when there are *qi* transformations, then they can exit' (*pang guang zhe, zhou du zhi guan, jin ye cang yan, qi hua ze neng chu yi* 膀胱者 洲都之官 津液藏焉 氣化則能出 矣).[75] In *Su wen* 8, the '*pang guang* bladder' is mentioned last in the sequence heart, lungs, liver, gall bladder, chest centre, spleen and stomach, large intestine, small intestine, kidneys, triple burner, '*pang guang* bladder'. Furthermore, it is the only one likened to an office outside the central administration, which underlines its peripheral position.

The above explorations indicate that *bao/pao* 胞 referred to bag-like structures in the body, ranging from 'uterus' to 'bladder' and 'pericardium'. The main characteristic of these bags was that they were hollow and empty inside, and soft and elastic. One can easily see that these bag-like structures embodied *yin* characteristics: they were pliable and hidden inside, positioned in the interior of the body. The usual term for designating the bladder with these *yin* characteristics was *pao* 脬. Canonical doctrine, by contrast, had a clearly demarcated concept of the bladder as an outer aspect of the kidneys. In other words, the '*pang guang* bladder' had to have *yang* characteristics, and this may explain why the term *pang guang* 膀胱 replaced the term *pao* 脬.

With this in mind, let us return to case 5. We observe that both terms for bladder occur in case 5, *pao* 脬 (line 3) and *pang guang* 膀胱 (line 20). The *pao* bladder correlates with the innermost interior, and the *pang guang* bladder contrasts with the kidneys. How should one interpret Yi's use of two different terms with, in our minds, the same referential meaning? Here we are reminded of the observation in case 2 (line 2) with regard to the graph 鬲 (read either as *li* designating an ancient ritual vessel or as *ge* 'to separate, to block') which was brought into correlation with the body architectural space of the 'heart': names of the disorders may well contain constituents which allude to earlier conceptions of body and illness than the elaborate medical speculation of the *Shi ji* personage Yi. The *pao* 脬 bladder in the name alludes to an earlier understanding of the bladder than the *pang guang* 膀胱 bladder mentioned in the very end of case 5.

---

[74] In a similar vein, the concentric architectural layout of the Qin Imperial palace emphasises this-wordliness (Wu 1995: fig. 3.19) and contrasts with the linear alignment of Zhou ancestral halls (*ibid.* fig. 2.7), which celebrate lineage and continuity across generations, and, as argued here, reproduction.
[75] *Su wen* 8, p. 28.

Text structure semantics

According to text structure semantics, the qualities of *mai* explain why Yi called the disorder 'wind-induced condition of overexertion visiting the bladder' (*feng dan ke pao*). Yi's explanation has three parts: first, he describes the qualities of *mai* in his own vocabulary (lines 11–13); then, he quotes the 'Mai fa' (lines 14–17); and, last, he discusses ways in which his findings differ from those mentioned in the 'Mai fa' (lines 18–21). The pulse qualities given in Yi's own vocabulary are 'being damp' (*shi*) and 'wind *qi*' (*feng qi*) (line 13). Wind *qi* certainly correlates with the constituent 'wind' in the name of the disorder. This leaves us with two constituents in the name of the disorder, *dan* (condition of overexertion) and *pao* (bladder), but only one pulse quality.

Yi furthermore states that he pressed onto the 'opening of the major *yin*' (*tai yin zhi kou*). If one does not shy away from applying in this case the principle of text structure semantics which puts pulse qualities in correlation with constituents in the name of the disorder, there is little doubt that in case 5 the 'major *yin*' (line 12) correlates with the 'bladder' (*pao*; line 3). In case 5, it is unlikely that Yi considered the major *yin* to correlate with the lungs as it does in canonical doctrine (and in the interjected phrase of case 4; line 33) or with the Mawangdui stomach or the canonical spleen.

One could argue that the phrase in line 12, 'when I pressed onto the opening of the major *yin*' (*qie tai yin zhi kou*), might have been interjected by a commentator, as in case 4. Since it parallels Yi's statement in line 11, 'when I examined her *mai*' (*zhen qi mai*), it could be interpreted as redundant. In that case, Yi would have felt only two pulse qualities 'wind *qi*' and 'being damp', which interrelated either with *feng dan* and *pao*, or with *feng* and *dan*, but not with *pao*. However, there are no coercive linguistic or textual anomalies to suggest that the phrase was later interjected, this in contrast to case 4 (line 33; see n. 37). Moreover, the observation that Yi felt two pulse qualities at the position of the 'opening of the major *yin*' and that the disorder *feng dan* is positioned in the *pao* bladder invokes a parallelism of an elegance that is disarming.

shi 溼 – damp and *feng qi* 風氣 – wind *qi* (lines 11–13)   Yi says it was 'damp' (*shi*) at the 'major *yin*'. Although it is theoretically possible that 'being damp' designated, in a highly abstract fashion, a movement in the *mai*, it probably meant that the skin felt damp at the position of the major *yin*. Perhaps precisely because 'being damp' designated a quality of the skin rather than a movement of *mai*, it was not canonised and later fell into oblivion. 'Being damp' is not a pulse quality in canonical medicine.

Zhang Wenhu considers 'being damp' (*shi*) a scribal error. By the nineteenth century, pulse qualities had become so standardised that they invariably described movements in the *mai*. However, the twentieth-century

Li Li takes issue with him. The term *shi*, he says, is not a scribal error but indicates a disorder in the renal system: 'The kidneys are a water reservoir' (*shen, shui cang/zang* 腎水藏). Li Li's interpretation that correlates 'being damp' with the 'bladder' is based on the understanding that the canonical kidneys control water and the bladder is their outer aspect. However, based on text structure semantics, we have already established that the location at which Yi sensed two pulse qualities is the 'opening of the major *yin*', which correlates with the location affected by the disorder, namely the *pao* bladder. The correlation with 'being damp' is redundant.

'Being damp' could, of course, also correlate with the 'condition of overexertion' (*dan*). Accordingly, both commentators would be wrong: Zhang Wenhu to consider it a scribal error and Li Li to correlate it with the renal system. This is what is argued here. While *dan* in *Lun heng* 15 refers to drought, *dan* in case 5 probably is a 'humid heat', as it is according to Wang Bing's gloss on *Su wen* 17 and arguably in *Han shu* 64A (see p. 215).

The term *feng dan* is attested in the received literature, not as *feng dan* 風癉 but as *feng dan* 風疸, in *Qian jin yao fang* 10: 'In the case of *feng dan*, the urine is sometimes yellow and sometimes white, one shivers from chills and hot flushes, one has a craving to sleep and does not wish to move' (*feng dan, xiao bian huo huang huo bai, xian xian han re, hao wo bu yu dong* 風 疸 小便或黃或白 洒洒寒熱 好臥不欲動).[76] Although modern commentators emphasise the affinities of *feng dan* with a kind of 'jaundice' (*huang bing* 黃病),[77] the symptoms given could equally be attributed to a state of 'utter exhaustion' (*dan*), manifesting in 'chills and hot flushes' (*han re*).

In summary, the pulse quality *feng qi* (wind *qi*) correlates directly with the constituent *feng* (wind) in the name of the disorder, and the pulse quality *shi* (being damp) probably with *dan* (condition of utter exhaustion), in spite of commentators who correlated it with the bladder. Yi senses these two pulse qualities at the 'opening of the major *yin*', which in all likelihood correlates with the 'bladder' (*pao*). Since none of the three pulse qualities is prominent in canonical doctrine, there are barely any textual parallels for the above correlations. It has been possible to see them only due to a rigorous application of text structure semantics.

The 'Mai fa' quote (lines 14–17)

The 'Mai fa' quote is easier to interpret than Yi's explanations because it makes use of a vocabulary with which readers of canonical doctrine are familiar. Zhang Shoujie points to a parallel that comes close to *Mai jing* 1.13: 'If the pulse is large, yet firm, the illness is issued by the kidneys' (*mai*

---

[76] *Bei ji qian jin yao fang* 10.5, p. 196.   [77] *Zhongyi dacidian* (1995:304–5).

da er jian, bing chu yu shen 脈大而堅 病出於腎).[78] *Mai jing* 1.13 shows continuities with Yi's 'Mai fa' in that both consider the pulse quality 'firm' (*jian*) indicative of a disorder in the 'kidneys' (*shen*).

The 'Mai fa' quote is repeated almost verbatim in *Mai jing* 6.9.[79] The sentence itself is modified only slightly, but this alters its meaning sensitively.[80] More importantly, the context in which it is mentioned differs. In the *Mai jing*, the 'Mai fa' quote is preceded by the compound word *shen mai*: 'The pulse of the kidneys: if, when sinking deeply into it, it is large, yet firm and if, when floating on it, it is large, yet tight, then …' (*shen mai chen zhi da er jian, fu zhi da er jin* 腎脈沈之大而堅 浮之大而緊). The *Mai jing* unambiguously attributes the tactile qualities of being 'large, yet firm' and 'large, yet tight' to the kidney *mai*, whereas Yi's 'Mai fa' does not.

The 'Mai fa' does not explicitly attribute the above qualities to *mai*. Yi continues in line 18, saying: 'When I pressed onto the kidneys' (*shen qie zhi*), instead of 'the *mai* of the kidneys' (*shen mai qie zhi). One could call this a 'semantic anomaly' and explain it away by faulting a negligent copyist (as I myself did earlier). I had not noticed then that this sentence provides the striking evidence I needed for an argument put forth elsewhere, which is that before Confucian teachings were embraced by the Imperial bureaucracy, physicians did not hesitate to palpate the body on both extremities and body trunk.[81] The *Shi ji* text intimates Yi pressed onto the 'kidneys' themselves, as though physicians in antiquity had specific techniques of palpating body parts like the 'kidneys', and other viscera, perhaps by 'sinking deep' into the flesh or 'floating' on it in those areas on the body surface underneath which the viscera were thought to be located. The imagery of this technique becomes very vivid if one considers that early medical manuscript texts give the graph *tun* 臀 'buttocks' in place of a graph interpreted as *shen* 腎.[82] The 'Mai fa' quote in case 5 (lines 15–16), unlike others, details a pair of tactile qualities. While it is not impossible that at one stage in medical history a graph in place of *shen* 腎 referred to the pair of 'buttocks' in Yi's case 5, this is not the case in its extant version nor in case 17. In case 17, *shen* probably denotes the pair of the anatomical kidneys; it correlates with the 'major *yang*', is examined by inspection of the lower back, and its dysfunction causes dysuria.[83]

---

[78] *Mai jing* 1.13, p. 25 gives *chu yu* as *zai* 在. It records as comment on this quote: 'Bian Que said: it is small, yet firm' (*Bian Que yun: xiao er jian* 扁鵲云 小而堅).

[79] *Mai jing* 6.9, p. 209.

[80] The 'Mai fa' positions the particle *er* before the word *da*, but the *Mai jing* mentions it after it. The 'Mai fa' has *er da jian* 'very firm' and *er da jin* 'very tight', but *Mai jing* 1.13, p. 25 and 6.9, p. 209, have *da er jian* 'large yet firm' and *da er jin* 'large yet tight'.

[81] Hsu (2005a).   [82] See case 6, n. 100.

[83] Perhaps, paradoxically, the canonical *pang guang* [bladder] designated at one stage in medical history the pair of anatomical kidneys, located on either 'side' (*pang*) of the spine?

In case 5 (line 19), when Yi finally speaks of *mai*, he may imply that *mai* of the tactually explored body parts were investigated, i.e. those on the buttocks or on the lower back underneath which the canonical kidneys were thought to be located. Before letting our imagination run wild, however, let us consider the more likely scenario that line 19 mentions *mai* because it was added by a later commentator (see pp. 226–7).

***chen* 沈, *fu* 浮 – sinking and floating as body techniques (lines 15–16)**
'Sunken' (*chen*) and 'floating' (*fu*) belong among the twenty-four *mai* in *Mai jing* 1.1 and the twenty-eight contemporary pulse images. *Chen* is a pulse quality that can only be detected if one presses down deeply onto the *mai*,[84] and *fu* is detected by scarcely touching its surface. In case 5, however, *chen* and *fu* obviously refer to a body technique of tactile examination, and not to a pulse quality. Oka Hakku explains that *chen* means to press heavily, and *fu* means to press lightly. The 'Mai fa' advocates thus a procedure of pressing with two different strengths onto the body surface in order to detect the qualities 'firm' and 'tight'. This procedure has since been elaborated in the domain of pulse diagnosis. *Nan jing* 5 differentiates between five different levels of pressing onto *mai*, each correlating with one of the five viscera, and *Nan jing* 4 introduces the three different levels, which in *Nan jing* 18 are called 'indicators' (*hou* 候).[85] The method outlined in *Nan jing* 18 of examining the *mai* in three different sections of the wrist at three different pressure levels (*san bu jiu hou* 三部九候) is still practised today.[86] However, the 'Mai fa' quote in case 5 distinguishes between two levels only. Perhaps this method that opposes sinking to floating was developed in attendance to a body framed in *yin yang* complementarities?

***jin* 緊 – tight (line 16)**   The 'tight' (*jin*) pulse is one of the standard twenty-four in *Mai jing* 1.1, which says of its tactile quality: 'It is fast/sharp, and in appearance like a cutting cord' (*shuo ru qie sheng zhuang* 數如切繩狀).[87] It is also a standard contemporary pulse image: 'Its appearance is like a stretched out cord or a wound up rope' (*zhuang ru qian sheng zhuan suo* 狀如牽繩轉索).[88] For elucidating the word 'tight' (*jin*), Zhang Shoujie gives its pronunciation and cites a phrase from the *Su wen* (not located): 'If there is one like a cutting cord [a cord used for cutting], it is called tight' (*you si qie sheng, ming yue jin ye* 有似切繩 名曰緊也). Ando Koretora cites *Su wen* 18: 'If the pulse of sick kidneys comes like a stretched creeper and if, when you then palpate it, it becomes even firmer, you call it a disorder of the kidneys' (*bing shen mai lai ru yin ge, an zhi yi jian, yue shen bing* 病腎脈來

---

[84] *chen* 沈 is *shen* 深 in another edition, according to Zhang Shoujie.
[85] Unschuld (1986a:101–17, 243–58). See also Hsu (in press e).
[86] *Zhongyi zhenduanxue* (Deng 1984:63).
[87] *Mai jing* 1.1, p. 2. The commentary notes: 'Another [source] says: like the irregularity of a wound up rope' (*yi yue ru zhuan suo zhi wu chang* 一曰如轉索之無常).
[88] *Zhongyi zhenduanxue* (Deng 1984:68).

如引葛 按之益堅 曰腎病).[89] The commentators all focus on the tactile experience of 'being tight', which is likened to touching a stretched out cord. They do not speak of it as indicative of the cold and painful, as do other canonical texts (see case 7, line 13), and as it probably was understood by the commentator who may have interjected the final stanza (see below, lines 19–21).

jian 堅 – **firm (line 15)**   'Being firm' (*jian*) is neither one of the standard *Mai jing* pulses nor a current pulse image; but it is common in the *Inner Canon*. One would expect that 'firm' primarily designates a tactile experience, which sometimes is positively valued, sometimes not.[90] It describes the quality of the skin,[91] and more often the quality of 'flesh' (*rou* 肉) and 'callus' (*jun* 䐃).[92] Thus, when in *Ling shu* 53 the Yellow Emperor enquires about the pain that stone needles and fire-heated needles can effect (*zhen shi huo ruo zhi tong* 鍼石火 焫之痛), he qualifies the potentially affected body parts as follows: 'The strength and weakness of sinews and bones, the firmness and flabbiness of the flesh, the thickness and thinness of the skin, and the porosity and density of the skin pore pattern' (*jin gu zhi qiang ruo, ji rou zhi jian cui, pi fu zhi hou bo, cou li zhi shu mi* 筋骨之強弱 肌肉之堅脆 皮膚之厚薄 腠理之疏密).[93] In *Ling shu* 53, and elsewhere, being 'firm' has positive connotations when it describes the qualities of the skin or flesh. The flesh of a man in his prime is 'firm', that of a baby is 'flabby' (*cui*).[94] 'The flabby is easily harmed' (*cui zhe yi shang* 脆者易傷);[95] it is a sign of infirmity. This applies particularly to the 'firm' and 'flabby' quality of the viscera, as in *Ling shu* 47: 'If the lips are firm, the spleen is firm. If the lips are large, but not firm, then the spleen is flabby' (*chun jian zhe, pi jian, chun da er bu jian zhe, pi cui* 脣堅者 脾堅 脣大而不堅者 脾脆).[96] One could consider this diagnostic method to rely on iconicity: the firmness of the lips is an iconic sign of the spleen, i.e. both are marked by the feature of firmness, regardless of whether or not they are intrinsically related to one another. Alternatively, since the flourishing of the canonical spleen appears on the lips and the two are intrinsically related, as smoke is to fire, one could say the relation is indexical within the conceptual frame of Chinese medical theory.

---

[89] *Su wen* 18, p. 57. See also *Mai jing* 3.5, p. 92. Ando Koretora equates the phrase 'if, when one sinks, it is very firm' (*chen zhi er da jian*), with 'if you palpate it, it becomes even firmer' (*an zhi yi jian*), and the phrase 'if, when floating, it is very tight' (*fu zhi er da jin*) with 'it comes like a stretched creeper' (*lai ru yin ge*).

[90] On the positively valued 'form' in its firmed-up state, see pp. 29–33; on ambiguities surrounding the firm and hard, see case 6 (line 14).

[91] e.g. *Ling shu* 38, p. 372; 46, p. 387; 57, p. 414.

[92] e.g. *Ling shu* 6, p. 285; 38, p. 373; 47, p. 395; 53, p. 408.

[93] *Ling shu* 53, p. 408. The 'intestines and stomach' are assessed with the same static verbs as 'skin and flesh': being thin and thick, firm and flabby.

[94] *Ling shu* 38, p. 373.   [95] *Ling shu* 46, p. 387.

[96] *Ling shu* 47, p. 393.

In *Ling shu* 47, 'being firm' clearly has positive connotations, and 'flabby' has negative ones. Likewise, firmness of the flesh guarantees longevity in *Ling shu* 6: 'If the flesh is firm, then there is longevity' (*rou jian ze shou yi* 肉堅則壽矣).[97] In addition, firmness of the viscera ensures absence of illness according to *Ling shu* 47: 'If the five viscera are all firm, then there is no illness; if the five viscera all are flabby, then one is ridden by illness' (*wu zang jie jian zhe, wu bing; wu zang jie cui zhe, bu li yu bing* 五藏皆堅者無病 五藏皆脆者不離于病).[98] As in the above quote on lips and spleen, the firmness and flabbiness in this passage from *Ling shu* 47 can be interpreted to reflect in an iconic way the state of the viscera inside the body. Alternatively, it can be interpreted as describing the tactile perception of the viscera themselves underneath the palpated areas inside the body.

It would be wrong to assume that *jian* had only positive connotations. When *jian* qualifies *mai*, its connotations are often negative.[99] Thus, in *Ling shu* 75, where the congealing of *mai* is likened to water turned to ice, *mai* are 'firm and tight' (*mai ... jian jin zhe* 脈 ... 堅緊者) and 'by breaking them up, they are dissolved' (*po er san zhi* 破而散之).[100] Or in *Su wen* 48, where the '*mai* of the heart' (*xin mai* 心脈) is described as 'small, firm and taut' (*xiao jian ji* 小堅急), *jian* also has negative connotations.[101]

Finally, *Su wen* 48 outlines a body technique comparable to the 'Mai fa': 'If one floats on it [the *mai*], then it is slightly taut, if one palpates [presses] it, then it is firm and very taut' (*fu zhi xiao ji, an zhi jian da ji* 浮之小急 按之 堅大急).[102] The wealth of canonical medical excerpts which in some way elucidate Yi's 'Mai fa' quote suggests that conceptually the medical lineage that compiled the 'Mai fa' had much in common with the composers of the canonical texts. In contrast to the vocabulary Yi adheres to in the previous stanza (lines 11–13), the technical terminology in the 'Mai fa' has much affinity with the canonical one.

Yi's comments on the 'Mai fa' quote (lines 18 and 19–21)

Yi compares the dictum of the medical authority, the 'Mai fa' (lines 14–17), with his own findings (line 18 or lines 18–19). He states: 'When I pressed onto the kidneys, it was the opposite: the *mai* were large, yet hurried'. If one follows Kaiho Gembi in interpreting *ye* 也 as topic marker, the sentence is semantically and grammatically odd. Why does Yi speak of 'kidneys'

---

[97] *Ling shu* 6, p. 285.   [98] *Ling shu* 47, p. 394.
[99] An exception is *Su wen* 39, p. 113.
[100] *Ling shu* 75, p. 461.   [101] *Su wen* 48, p. 135.
[102] *Su wen* 48, p. 136. On *xiao*, see also case 7 (lines 10, 13); on *da*, see case 3 (line 16) and case 10 (line 14). They are interpreted adverbially here but could also mean 'small' and 'large', as in the previous quote. The same term is often used in a different sense in different paragraphs of an ancient medical text; sometimes this hints at a compilation of mini-texts from different sources (e.g. *dai* in case 1, lines 18 and 21), but not always.

rather than the 'kidney *mai*' in line 18? Or, if he first speaks of the kidneys themselves, does he thereafter refer to *mai* on the buttocks/kidneys in line 19? It makes more sense to read line 18 as one sentence, with *ye* in its usual grammatical function as end of sentence marker. This also makes much more sense semantically, as the following line and stanza can then be interpreted as a commentator's interjection (lines 19–21). It contains canonical medical terms and makes out of case 5 a heat pathology, which is incongruent with Yi's earlier statements.

***da* 大 – large (lines 19 and 20)**   If Yi says that he felt the opposite (line 18), full stop, he did not specify how it felt. If, due to commentatorial intervention, he is made to say the opposite felt 'large yet hurried', being 'large' is best interpreted as opposite of 'firm' and 'hurried' of 'tight'. There are textual parallels in support of this in canonical medical texts. Thus, 'large' is given as opposite of 'firm', in *Ling shu* 47 (quoted on p. 225) and 'being hurried', connoting heat, could be read as opposite of 'tight', which indicates coldness. Nevertheless, let us first explore whether 'large' (*da*) contrasted with both the 'very firm' and 'very tight'; and whether only 'yet hurried' (*er zao*), together with the final topic-comment sentence elucidating 'hurried' (line 21), was a commentatorial interjection.

The above explorations render the bladder as an epitome of the elastic and soft, which are *yin*-qualities that allow it to be enlarged and stretched beyond expectation, and the pulse quality *da* may have implied this. In other words, *da* may not primarily have connoted the 'big', hard and strong, but the 'large' and immense cosmogonic waters. Furthermore, 'being large' as an attribute of the bladder that contrasts with the 'tight' and 'firm' kidneys, may iconically have reflected the outer and inner aspects of the canonical renal system.

***zao* 躁 – hurried (lines 19 and 21)**   The term *zao* (being hurried), unlike *shuo* (frequent), is neither a standard *Mai jing* pulse nor a standard contemporary one, but it frequently occurs in the *Inner Canon*.[103] Neither *shuo* nor *zao* are primarily pulse qualities in the *Inner Canon* and, interestingly, the *Shi ji* text contains a line of explanation on each. Thus, Yi explains in case 3 (line 17) that the pulse quality 'frequent' (*shuo*) indicates that the interior and the lower parts are hot and, presumably, painful. And in case 5 (line 21), he says 'being hurried' (*zao*) is indicative of heat in the interior and of a dark urine.

In the *Inner Canon*, 'being hurried' generally designates a state of the heart-mind. It is mentioned in connection with the 'upset heart' (*fan xin* 煩心), the 'contravective' (*ni* 逆) and also 'bounty of *yin*' (*yin qi you yu* 陰氣

---

[103] *Huangdi nei jing*, p. 1580.

有餘), which in turn is associated with 'numbness' and 'inversions' (*jue* 厥).[104] In *Su wen* 69, it is furthermore related to heat: 'Disorders of the populace are that the body is hot, the upset heart hurried and anxious; while *yin* numbness rises, the lower parts and the interior get cold' (*min bing shen re fan xin zao ji, yin jue shang, xia zhong han* 民病身熱煩心躁悸 陰厥上 下中 寒).[105] Yet, even in *Su wen* 69, heat is linked to an upset heart that is hurried and anxious. Likewise, *Su wen* 43, which alludes to visceral states and spirits (*shen*), and to states of the heart, contrasts 'still' and 'hurried', when it states 'being still' indicates life, 'being hurried' death: 'As for *yin qi*, if it is still, then the spirits are stored within, if it is hurried, then there is disintegration and perishing' (*yin qi zhe, jing ze shen cang, zao ze xiao wang* 陰氣者 靜則 神藏 躁則消亡).[106] 'Being still', as opposed to 'hurried', has positive connotations also in *Ling shu* 23, where sweating can effect a change from one into the other, and thereby ensure the continuation of life (quoted on p. 322).

Based on text structure semantics, 'being damp', presumably from sweating, has been interpreted to be indicative of the 'condition-of-overexertion' (lines 1–15), and now Yi speaks of a 'hurried' pulse and heat, which make out of *dan* a 'heat-due-to-overexertion'. If one further accounts for the canonical medical terminology in the final stanza, it is best interpreted as commentatorial interjection.[107] Case 5 would then parallel cases 1, 2 and 3 insofar as it becomes a heat condition only towards the end of the case history, mostly, if not entirely, due to commentatorial interventions.

'Being hurried' (*zao*) indicates heat, much like 'being frequent' (*shuo*) in case 3 (line 17). The two different verbs hint at the hand of two commentators. One used the canonical pulse quality 'frequent' and was therefore medically *à jour*, the other not. Apart from defining 'being hurried' in a sense it does not usually have in early medicine, namely as indicative of heat in the bladder rather than anxiety in the heart, he also uses the unidiomatic *zhong you re* instead of *zhong re* for saying 'there is heat in the interior'. We are by now familiar with this rather confused commentator adding his remarks in the very end of almost every case history.

The cause of the disorder (lines 8–9)

The cause of the disorder contains a tentative answer for why the queen dowager became so utterly exhausted and why she was affected by wind. The four words *liu han chu xun* (flowing, sweat, to go out, *xun*) indicate the cause of the queen dowager's disorder (line 8). Among those, the first two

---

[104] For *fan xin*, see *Su wen* 69, p. 197; for *ni* and *yin qi you yu*, see *Su wen* 74, p. 234; *Ling shu* 1, p. 265; 3, p. 273; for *jue*, see also *Ling shu* 9, p. 297.

[105] *Su wen* 69, p. 197.

[106] *Su wen* 43, p. 122. See also *Ling shu* 1, p. 265; 3, p. 273. The meaning of *zao* is not straightforward in *Su wen* 70, p. 203, and *Ling shu* 72, p. 450.

[107] *ni chi* 'the urine is dark' (line 4) is best interpreted as commentatorial interjection, as in case 3 (lines 21–2) and case 10 (line 7).

certainly mean 'profuse sweating'. As comparison with other case histories shows, sweating as illness cause is given only in respect of the King of Jibei and the queen dowager of the King of Qi. It must speak in a coded way of a kind of social conduct Yi considers illness inducing (see pp. 117–18).

Yi may have used the word *xun* 㴞 in a similarly coded way. It solicits eloquence among the commentators, but leaves contemporary dictionaries laconic. Considering that Yi finds it necessary to explain what he means by *xun*, we may assume that the term was not entirely transparent to his readership. He may have used it in a rather specific sense. In an edition referred to as Mao's 毛 edition, *xun* 㴞 is given as *xiu* 潃. In contrast to other commentators,[108] Wang Yinzhi interprets *xiu* 脩 as *xiu* 脩, and glosses it as 'dried-up and dry' (*xiu qie gan ye* 脩且乾也). He considers the passage to say that heavily flowing sweat came out and dried up. However, one could go a step further. From the viewpoint of the case history's internal coherence, 'dried-up sweat' does not have much significance as a cause of the disorder.

Here Yi's own gloss on *xun* comes into play (line 9): 'In the case of *xun*, having discarded one's clothes, the sweat dries in the sunlight' (*xun zhe qu yi er han xi ye*). There is little doubt that what Yi describes here is sunbathing. The cause of the queen dowager's disorder is accordingly 'while sweating' (*liu han*), 'going outside to sunbathe' (*chu xun*). Indeed, wealthy elderly ladies on the shores of lake Zurich can spend hours lying in the sun, and elderly peasant women in rural China sometimes enjoy the afternoon sun, seated and dressed to the waist, in front of their houses.[109] The author of the early medical document may have been concerned primarily with the loss of *yin*-waters through sweating and exposure to *yang*-sunlight.[110] For the *Shi ji* personage Yi, however, the 'utter exhaustion' arose from activities that likened the queen dowager to a 'wind horse' (horse in heat), and discarding her clothes exposed her to 'wind'. Therefore the disorder was 'wind-induced'.

Discussion

Case 5 turns out to be one of the most transparent case histories, once one has clarified the meaning of terms such as *xun*, used in the sense of

---

[108] According to Xu Guang's gloss to *Shi ji* 61, p. 2120, *xiu* 潃 designates 'The juice after washing the rice' (*xi mi zhi ye* 淅米汁也), and, according to Gao You's gloss to *Huainanzi* 18, pp. 1915, 1917, 'dirty juice' (*chou zhi* 臭汁). According to the *Shuo wen* 11A, p. 32a, '*xiu* is old water of washed rice' (*xiu jiu gan ye* 脩久泔也). Ma's (1992:504, 571, 589) annotations to *xiu* in the MWD 'Recipes' point in the same direction. Such a reading of *xiu* would imply that the sweat is like that of rice water, say 'sticky' or 'viscous'. See Bridgman (1955:74). However, Harper (late 1990s p.c.) pointed to Wang Yinzhi.

[109] Personal observations; Charles Aylmer (late 1990s p.c.).

[110] From a biomedical viewpoint, the sweating, indicative of the queen dowager's excessive sexual life, may explain why she got cystitis; the subsequent sunbathing, why the cystitis was acute: due to a dehydration.

'sunbathing', or *feng*, which in not merely a medical sense explains why the condition is 'wind-induced'.

The name of the disorder, *feng dan ke pao*, has three nouns that can be put in correlation with the three pulse qualities that are given in Yi's own vocabulary in ways that text structure semantics postulates. Most apparent is the correlation between the first constituent 'wind' (*feng*) and 'wind *qi*' (*feng qi*). If the location the disorder is visiting, the *pao* bladder, correlates with the location at which Yi examines *mai*, which is the 'opening of the major *yin*', then *dan* correlates with the pulse quality 'damp' (*shi*). This points to a patient damp from sweat, and to an interpretation of *dan* as 'condition-of-overexertion'.

There are textual parallels for the correlations highlighted by text structure semantics but they are few. Thus, while *dan* no doubt designated a condition of overexertion in the Zhou (heat not being explicitly involved), I found no more than a possible reading of a passage in *Han shu* 64A and a comment by Wang Bing on *Su wen* 17 to mention dampness in the definition of *dan* disorders. Furthermore, while there is an early medical manuscript text that associates the *pao* bladder with the interior/centre of the body, and there are many indices that the *pao* bladder had *yin*-qualities, no text has been found that explicitly correlates it with the 'major *yin*'. Rather than dismissing the method of text structure semantics, I emphasise that textual parallels do exist, even if few in number, and I take this as a hint that the medical rationale of the lineage of learning Yi adhered to was later marginalised.

The 'Mai fa' pulses often are standard canonical ones, which are often defined in terms of tactile experiences. Two terms which later described pulse qualities, namely 'to sink' (*chen*) and 'float' (*fu*), outline here body techniques of a manual diagnostic procedure. The tactile experiences this palpation technique elicits are 'being firm' (*jian*), which often describes flesh in its healthy state, and 'tight' (*jin*). In canonical texts, the latter is often assessed by similes and tends to be compared to stroking a stretched out cord. The 'tight' pulse is also indicative of pain, as undoubtedly in case 7 (line 13), and of the cold.

Yi's comment on the 'Mai fa' is that he felt the opposite, without, however, specifying how exactly it felt (line 18). The final stanza (lines 19–21) discusses pulse qualities: the *mai* were 'large, yet hurried' (*da er zao*). Both are terms frequently encountered in canonical medical texts but not exclusively in the context of pulse diagnosis. The possibility of them both being added in a commentatorial interjection comprising lines 19–21 cannot be discarded entirely. Having said this, from the viewpoint of semantics, only 'yet hurried' (*er zao*) and the final line 21 pose problems. The 'large' pulse, which correlates with the outer aspect of the canonical renal system, the bladder, can be interpreted to contrast with the 'very firm' and 'very tight' that correlate with its inner aspect, the kidneys. Since the bladder and other bag-like structures were considered elastic and soft and, like a balloon, could easily be enlarged, the pulse quality 'large' may iconically have reflected this.

Alternatively, if the entire final stanza (lines 19–21) represents a commentatorial interjection, the 'large' pulse may have been understood as opposite of the 'firm', as it is in *Ling shu* 47, and the 'hurried', indicative of heat, as opposite of the 'very tight', indicative of coldness. The 'hurried pulse', together with *ni chi* (the urine is dark), makes case 5 unambiguously into a heat condition. However, as already noted, and as will become blatantly apparent in case 10, heat is in all these cases best interpreted to have arisen from commentatorial emendations.

The commentator/s in question probably understood *huo ji tang* in the sense of a 'fire regulatory broth'. However, word meaning is multilayered in Yi's cases 1–10. The same term in the assumed early second-century medical document, which the early first-century editor seems to have selectively embellished as he rewrote it, probably belonged among what Yamada called a 'prototype I decoction' that typically was prepared by simmering a liquid with medicinal ingredients over a carefully regulated fire. It therefore probably meant 'broth prepared by careful regulation of fire'. The broth may have been used in order to dissipate or drive out dampness.

16

Case 6

Translation (*Shiki kaichû kôshô* 105, pp. 32–4)

1. Cao Shanfu of the ward Zhangwu in Qi fell ill.
2. Your servant, Yi, examined his *mai* and <u>said</u>:

Name:

3. 'It is a lung consumption.
4. In addition there are chills and hot flushes.'
5. Forthwith, I informed the members of the household saying:
6. 'He will die. Incurable.
7. In accordance with what he needs, provide maintenance.
8. A doctor should not treat this one.'

9. The 'Model' says:
10. 'After three days, he will be in a state that matches madness.
11. In a frenzy, he will rise to walk about, desiring to run.
12. After five days, he will die.'

13. He then died at the end of the predicted time period.

Cause:

14. <u>Shanfu's illness was contracted from</u> being in great anger, and in this condition indulging in women.

Quality:

15. <u>The means whereby I recognised</u> Shanfu's illness were that
16. when your servant, Yi, pressed onto his *mai*, the *qi* [coming] from the lungs was hot.

1. 齊章武里曹山跗病
2. 臣意診其脈曰
3. 肺消癉也
4. 加以寒熱
5. 即告其人曰
6. 死 不治
7. 適其共養
8. 此不當醫治
9. 法曰
10. 後三日而當狂
11. 妄起行欲走
12. 後五日死
13. 即如期死
14. 山跗病得之盛怒而以接內
15. 所以知山跗之病者
16. 臣意切其脈 肺氣熱也

17.	The 'Mai fa' says:	17.	脈法曰
18.	'In cases of the uneven and not drumming, the body form is fading away.'	18.	不平不鼓 形獘
19a.	This one's [disorder in] the high one [among the five viscera] went the distant number.	19a.	此五藏高之遠數
19b.	And the passageways were in disorder.	19b.	以經病也
20.	<u>Hence</u> at the time when I pressed onto them [the vessels], they [the pulses] were not only uneven, but also alternating.	20.	故切之時 不平而代
21.	In cases when they are uneven, the blood does not reside in its proper place.	21.	不平者 血不居其處
22.	In cases when they alternate, from time to time three strokes arrive together, at once hurried, at once large.	22.	代者 時參擊並至 乍躁 乍大也
23.	This one's two linking vessels were severed.	23.	此兩絡脈絕
24.	<u>Hence</u> he died, and was incurable.	24.	故死 不治
25.	As for the reason why there were in addition chills and hot flushes,	25.	所以加寒熱者
26.	it was said that this person had fainted.	26.	言其人尸奪
27.	In cases of fainting, the body form has been fading away.	27.	尸奪者 形獘
28.	In cases where the body form has been fading away, it is not fitting to apply cauterisation and needle therapy, and to make [the patient] drink potent drugs.	28.	形獘者 不當關灸饞石 及飲毒藥也
29.	At the time when your servant, Yi, had not yet come to make an examination,	29.	臣意未往診時
30.	the Grand Physician of Qi had already examined Shanfu's illness.	30.	齊太醫先診山跗病
31.	He cauterised his foot's minor *yang* vessel, and	31.	灸其足少陽脈
32.	orally, he made him drink a bolus of *Pinellia*.	32.	口而飲之半夏丸
33.	The patient immediately discharged and got drained.	33.	病者即泄注
34.	The abdominal part of the interior was depleted.	34.	腹中虛
35.	Moreover, he [the Grand Physician] cauterised the minor *yin* vessel.	35.	又灸其少陰脈
36.	This harmed the hardness of the liver, causing a rupture deep inside.	36.	是壞肝剛絕深
37.	In this way, he [the Grand Physician] doubly diminished the *qi* of the patient.	37.	如是重損病者氣

38. <u>Hence</u> there were additionally chills and hot flushes.

38. 以故加寒熱

39. As for the reason why, after three days, he [Shanfu] was in a state that matches madness,

39. 所以後三日而當狂者

40. a link of the liver – the connecting and binding knot – was severed off from the *yang* brightness beneath the nipples.

40. 肝一絡連屬結絕乳下陽明

41. <u>Hence</u>, when the link was severed, it opened up the *yang* brightness *mai*.

41. 故絡絕 開陽明脈

42. When the *yang* brightness *mai* was damaged, then in a state that matches madness he [Shanfu] ran about.

42. 陽明脈傷 即當狂走

43. As for dying after five days,

43. 後五日死者

44. liver and heart are distant from each other by five degrees [*fen*]

44. 肝與心相去五分

45. <u>Hence</u> I said: 'After five days, it [the distance] is exhausted.

45. 故曰 五日盡

46. Being exhausted, he will thereupon die.'

46. 盡即死矣

Interpretation

This case concerns two disorders, and Yi names each (lines 3–4). He then declares the patient incurable, and advises the client's entourage to provide palliative care (lines 5–8).[1] His quote from the 'Model' (lines 9–12), which reads like a justification for his refusal to treat the client, prognosticates death in a numerology of three and five. This is verified (line 13), and the cause of the disorder stated (line 14). The remainder combines narrative on the course of the illness with medical speculation (lines 15–46). Yi explains the first disorder (lines 15–24), then discusses the second (lines 25–38), and ends with justifications for his two prognostications (lines 39–42, 43–6).

For explaining the first disorder (line 3), Yi follows the usual pattern of first reporting on the pulse qualities he sensed in his own vocabulary (lines 15–16) and then quotes the 'Mai fa' (lines 17–18). He thereafter provides an interpretation in highly abstract language (line 19a), mentions another set of pulse qualities (line 20) and explains their implications in two topic-comment sentences (lines 21–2). Another interpretation follows which explains why death occurred (lines 23–4).

The second disorder (line 4) is iatrogenic, and Yi details the incorrect treatment of the Grand Physician of Qi (lines 25–38). The last two stanzas

---

[1] Dong Fen reads *gong* 共 as *gong* 供 'to provide'.

provide the justification for the prognostication (given in lines 9–12), namely that the patient would be in a state matching madness after three days (lines 39–42) and die after five (lines 43–6).

Critical evaluation of retrospective biomedical diagnoses

Among medical historians in the PRC, case 6 is celebrated as the first medical account of diabetes. This is contested here. A more detailed analysis than usual is given in what follows, in full awareness that any retrospective diagnosis is laden with dangers of overinterpretation.

Before embarking on it, a caveat is necessary. Throughout this book, semantic, linguistic and rhetorical/textual analyses account for the cultural constructedness of any 'concept' or, rather, 'linguistic term', whether biomedical or Chinese medical. Nevertheless, inspired by recent research in 'holistic anthropology', which in natural scientifically informed and social scientifically sophisticated ways attempts to attend to continuities across cultures and biologies, the analysis that follows goes against the strong programme of relativism. As in the discussion of the names of the disorder in cases 2 and 5, it grants ancient physicians the ability to have been attracted to phenomena similar to those that attract the attention of practitioners today.[2]

Bridgman considers this case too complicated to hazard a diagnosis; he merely suggests the case involves a liver abscess that may have arisen from an amoebiasis.[3] Lu and Needham speak of a delirious fever due to 'acute hepatic cirrhosis, probably caused by liver and blood flukes'.[4] Wang Zhipu[5] and other PRC researchers consider this case of *fei xiao dan* (lit. lung wasting heat-due-to-overexertion) the first in the history of Chinese medicine that attests to *xiao ke* 消渴 (wasting thirst), which they equate, biomedically, with 'diabetes' (*tangniao bing* 糖尿病).[6]

The main argument for diabetes is that the constituents in the name of the disorder *fei xiao dan* are reminiscent of the names of other disorders that have been identified as diabetes. Chinese researchers list additional reasons. First, they point out that the client had a coma, and long-term diabetes in its final stages can indeed manifest in a diabetic coma. However,

---

[2] Naturally, one cannot speak of exactly the 'same phenomena' because different traditions of learning reach different consensus of what the phenomena are. See ch. 1, n. 20 and nn. 14–16. This study is undertaken in the spirit outlined by Parkin and Ulijaszek (2007), and builds heavily on the works in ch. 3, n. 24, which contain a reaction to Needham (1956) and any naïve programme of the writing history of science. For further examples that highlight the experiential validity of Yi's case material, see in case 2, n. 27, and case 5, n. 110.

[3] Bridgman (1955:78).   [4] Lu and Needham (1967:232).   [5] Wang (1980).

[6] *xiao ke* 消渴 that arises from 'a sweet and fatty diet' in *Su wen* 47 has affinities with type 2 diabetes mellitus, while polydipsia and polyuria attributed to *xiao ke* in Sui and Tang texts are typical of diabetes insipidus.

while hyperglycaemia can cause coma, it generally does not lead to delirium (as indicated by lines 10–11). They, secondly, have detected indirect evidence in case 6 for excessive thirst (polydipsia) and excessive urination (polyuria), which belong among the most conspicuous clinical manifestations of diabetes mellitus and diabetes insipidus.[7] However, Yi does not actually record these signs and symptoms.

One could argue that case 6 concerns a type 2 diabetes mellitus, which is acquired late in life and arises mostly in obese people. It often goes hand in hand with a deterioration of other basic functions resulting, for instance, in heart insufficiency, fat deposits in the liver, and deterioration of eyesight. However, in contrast to diabetes insipidus and type 1 diabetes mellitus, which can lead, as the illness progresses, to the person eventually becoming emaciated like someone suffering from consumption, type 2 diabetes mellitus generally improves with weight loss.[8]

Rather than imputing diabetes into case 6, the condition called *fei xiao dan* appears to approximate what in Europe was called 'consumption' (which has distinct connotations in European and early Chinese medical understandings). Yi says the 'lungs' (*fei*) are affected and treatment involves *Pinellia ternata* (*ban xia*), which was typically indicated in cases of coughing and a long-term deterioration of the lungs. It is therefore likely that case 6 concerns 'consumption' in the sense of long-term tuberculosis or another chronic condition of the lungs. Chronic lung conditions often cause a general degeneration of the right ventricle of the heart, which can lead to heart insufficiency. There are several indications for heart insufficiency: first, the quality of the pulse, which is 'not drumming' (*bu gu*), can be considered an arrhythmic pulse, which sometimes is a sign of heart insufficiency. Second, heart insufficiency can cause fainting. Third, heart insufficiency can trigger processes that eventually lead to so-called 'hepatic encephalopathy', which typically manifests in bouts of delirium after food intake.

Lu and Needham suggest delirium due to high fever. While damage of the *yang* brightness in the latter part of case 1 is related to 'heat' that rises, it typically results in madness in early and canonical medical texts. This appears to apply also to case 6. Yi speaks of a 'link' (*luo*) between the liver and the *yang* brightness (the canonical stomach), and says it was severed; this gave rise to a state 'matching madness',[9] perhaps a delirium. Incidentally, biomedicine also recognises an important link between the liver and the digestive tract: the portal vein. The portal vein transports nutritive blood from the intestines to the liver, where some of the substances are detoxified,

---

[7] *Harrison's* (1987:1725).   [8] *Harrison's* (1987:1782, table 327-3).
[9] *dang kuang* alternative reading: 'there will be madness'. Both translations are possible. The former is inspired by the retrospective diagnosis, and the latter by the meaning of *dang* in case 1 (line 7) and case 20; *dang* also means 'formerly' in case 4 (line 7a) and 'should' in case 6 (line 8) and section 4.4.

before they enter, through the liver veins, into the vena cava and the circulatory system. If due to heart insufficiency the liver is congested or, in the worst case, if there is liver cirrhosis (as suggested by Lu and Needham), this can lead to high pressure in the portal vein; as a consequence of this, the nutritive blood flows directly into the vena cava and the resorbed substances enter blood circulation without previously having been detoxified in the liver. If these substances cross the blood–brain tissue barrier, they can cause delirium.

The above suggests that what today is recognised as 'hepatic encephalopathy', which can arise due to liver disease secondary to heart insufficiency, was known to Yi; however, the stanza that details the processes may have been a commentatorial interjection (see p. 262). It makes the 'link' (*luo*) between the *yang* brightness and the liver responsible for the state of delirium. From the viewpoint of clinical observation, it is not impossible that physicians would observe a correlation between certain kinds of food intake and manifestations of delirium. From an anatomical viewpoint, the portal vein is very large and distinctive, a vessel as broad as a thumb, and if people in antiquity cut open corpses,[10] it is easy to imagine that they recognised in this structure a link between the intestines and the liver.[11] In fact, they need not even have cut open corpses, as the portal vein is also observed on a living body due to superficial vein dilation. Yi can thus be interpreted to describe a disruption of the usual functions of the portal vein that caused delirium.

In summary, case 1 involves not diabetes, as some Chinese researchers propose, but probably a chronic lung condition, such as tuberculosis, accompanied by a general deterioration of basic functions. We can be fairly certain that heart insufficiency belonged among these. Heart insufficiency may have been responsible, together with liver congestion/cirrhosis, for hepatic encephalopathy causing delirium. The patient was very weak, and apparently had had bouts of coma previously. He was additionally weakened through maltreatment, which probably triggered off another acute crisis of hepatic encephalopathy, and it seems that in this delirious state, when he was very agitated, he died of overexertion, probably due to heart failure. However, with the information at hand it was impossible to be certain about any one diagnosis to the exclusion of others.[12] Yi's terminology is vague

---

[10] Note *Ling shu* 12, p. 311: 'If he dies, it is possible to disentangle, cut open and inspect him' (*qi si ke jie pou er shi zhi* 其死可解剖而視之). A case of dissection? See also Hsu (2005a).

[11] Padel's (1992:15) quote from Euripides' (ca 480–406 BCE) *Electra* mentions the 'portal vein': 'Aegisthus gazed earnestly at the sacred parts taking them into his hands. There was no liver lobe to the *splanchna* [innards]! And the portal-vein [πύλαι] and gallbladder showed evil visitations near to the person looking at them.'

[12] Ritzmann in 1997 (p.c.) brought to paper the above diagnosis in German; Aronson in 2005 (p.c.) independently came to it. Flohr in 2000 (p.c.) did not dismiss it as impossible. But note concluding remarks in main text.

and indeterminate, the layers of meaning multiple, and the textual materials date probably from different time periods.

Text structure semantics

fei qi 肺氣 – qi coming from the lungs is re 熱 – hot (line 16)   According to text structure semantics, the name of the first disorder *fei xiao dan* (line 3) should correlate with the pulse qualities that Yi senses (line 16). However, the name of the disorder has three constituents and Yi senses only two pulse qualities: '*qi* [coming] from the lungs' (*fei qi*) and 'being hot' (*re*). To solve the problem, the middle constituent of the name, 'wasting' (*xiao*), is best viewed as part of a bisyllabic constituent of either *fei xiao*, which correlates with *fei qi*, or *xiao dan*, which correlates with *re*.

The meaning of *xiao* comes close to *dan*. In *Su wen* 17, *dan* in its protracted form is *xiao*: '*dan* turns into a wasting of the interior' (*dan cheng wei xiao zhong* 癉成為消中).[13] There is ample evidence in canonical medical texts that *xiao* and *dan* form a compound word, *xiao dan*, 'wasting [resulting in] heat-due-to-overexertion' or short: 'consumption' (but note caveat just mentioned). If *fei xiao* were the bisyllabic constituent, the rationale across cases 5 and 6 would be inconsistent: *dan* would in case 5 correlate with 'damp' and in case 6 with 'hot'. It is consistent if *xiao dan* is conceived of as a bisyllabic constituent of the name, with 'damp' (*shi*) in case 5 correlating with *dan* (condition of overexertion), and 'hot' (*re*) in case 6 correlating with *xiao dan* (consumption).

Neither '*qi* [coming] from the lungs' nor 'being hot' is one of the twenty-four *mai* in *Mai jing* 1.1. As with 'being damp', encountered in case 5, it is uncertain what felt 'hot': was it the temperature of the skin where Yi examined *mai*, or was it a quality that Yi imputed into a certain movement of *mai*, as, for instance, a rapid pulse beat? While it seems reasonable to suggest that in cases 5 and 6 Yi quite literally referred to the temperature and humidity of the skin when he spoke of the 'hot' and 'damp', we simply do not know.

In summary, the three constituents in the name of the disorder *fei xiao dan* correlate with only two pulse qualities. Medical rationale is consistent across cases 5 and 6 if in case 6 *fei* correlates with *fei qi* (lung *qi*) and *xiaodan* forms one bisyllabic constituent, which correlates with *re* (hot). The name of the disorder *fei xiaodan* is then best approximated as 'lung consumption'.

The name of the disorder (lines 3–4)

Two aspects of 'consumption' (*xiao dan*) are explored in what follows: first, its relation to body internal heat, and, second, to processes in the sentimen-

[13] *Su wen* 17, p. 52.

tal body, such as hard internal feelings and outward wasting of softened flesh. In case 6 the cause of the disorder is anger, which in *Ling shu* 47 is associated with emotional hardness that in turn gives rise to anger, heat and consumption. Case 6 has thus much affinity with *Ling shu* 47.

'Wasting thirst' (*xiao ke* 消渴) and 'wasting lungs' (*fei xiao* 肺消) are disorders today interpreted as diabetes, which contemporary Chinese research imputes into case 6. We will examine this claim by scrutinising canonical texts and show that, in contrast to case 6, they mostly concern imbalances in food intake, as does 'wasting grains' (*xiao gu* 消穀). Finally, striking parallels to the disorder *dan nüe* 癉瘧 (utter exhaustion resulting in chills and hot flushes) will be highlighted.

xiao dan 消癉 – consumption and heat (lines 3 and 16)

As remarked in case 5, *dan* (condition-of-overexertion) figures already in the *Shi jing* from the Zhou dynasty. In case 5 (lines 1–15), it correlates with the 'damp', but over time the condition increasingly took on features of 'heat'. In Wang Bing's comment to *Su wen* 17, it is still glossed as 'dampness and heat' (*shi re* 溼熱) (quoted on p. 215), but eventually it is no longer associated with the phenomenon of sweat pearls on the body surface, and refers to a body internal 'depletion fire' (*xu huo* 虛火).

The term *xiao* (wasting), much like *dan*, designates a state of utter exhaustion, in *Shuo wen* 11A: '*xiao* is to be exhausted' (*xiao jin ye* 消盡也).[14] It is frequently encountered in the canonical medical literature, and generally relates to a process marked by overheating.[15] Thus, in respect of *Su wen* 56, 'If heat augments, then the sinews become slack and the bones waste away' (*re duo ze jin chi gu xiao* 熱多則筋弛骨消), Wang Bing comments: '*xiao* means smelting' (*xiao shuo ye* 消爍也).[16] With regard to *xiao dan* (consumption) in *Su wen* 28, Wang Bing comments: '*xiao* means to waste away internally' (*xiao wei nei xiao* 消謂內消) and '*dan* means hidden heat' (*dan wei fu re* 癉謂伏熱).[17] The term *xiao* often but not always implies heat.

'Consumption' (*xiao dan*) occurs in many different contexts of the *Nei jing*. Sometimes it is collocated with *zhong re* 中熱 the 'interior is hot' or 'internal heat' as in *Ling shu* 29.[18] Sometimes it is found in the context of dysfunctions of one's outwardly visible bodily frame, such as 'sudden stroke' (*pu ji* 仆擊), 'one-sided withering' (*pian ku* 偏枯) and 'limpness and numbness' (*wei jue* 痿厥), as in *Su wen* 28.[19] Furthermore, as in *Ling shu* 46, it is mentioned in the following sequence: from *feng zhong* 風腫 (lit. wind swellings, or: wandering swellings) to *xiao dan* 消癉 (lit. wasting resulting in a

---

[14] *Shuo wen* 11A, 28b.

[15] e.g. *Su wen* 40, p. 115; 42, p. 119; 79, p. 206; 35, p. 104 (discussed on p. 243). See also *xiao gu* 消穀 (wasting grains) in the *Ling shu* discussed on p. 242.

[16] HDNJSW 56, p. 105. Consider also *Ling shu* 81, p. 481, 'brain smelting' (*nao shuo* 腦爍).

[17] HDNJSW 28, p. 64.   [18] *Ling shu* 29, p. 354.   [19] *Su wen* 28, p. 88.

heat-due-to-overexertion, or: consumption) to *han re* 寒熱 (intermittent coldness and heat, or: chills and hot flushes) to *liu dan* 留癉 (residual heat-due-to-overexertion) and *ji ju* 積聚 (gathering of accumulations).[20] In all these cases, *xiao dan* can be interpreted as 'consumption' insofar as it arises from an internal overheating and manifests in an emaciated bodily frame.[21]

gang 剛, *nu* 怒, *re* 熱, *xiao dan* 消癉 – emotional hardness, anger, heat and consumption (line 14)

Ling shu 46 corroborates much of what was said above: 'If the five viscera are all soft and weak, one is prone to ail from consumption' (*wu zang jie rou ruo zhe, shan bing xiao dan* 五藏皆柔弱者 善病消癉).[22] *Ling shu* 46 does not speak of internal heat but of soft and weak viscera.[23] It relates *xiao dan* to imbalances in the 'sentimental body', as it contrasts hard inner feelings, like anger, to a soft outer appearance, and wasting flesh. Thus, it elaborates, after the above phrase, on the softness of the flesh which is opposed to the hardness of the heart. A person with a thin skin and eyes that are firm, solid and deep-seated, is considered to have raised eyebrows and a heart that is hard (*qi xin gang* 其心剛), and such hardness implies that the person is frequently angry (*gang ze duo nu* 剛則多怒). It is important to note that in *Ling shu* 46 a 'heart that is hard' gives rise to illness, while in *Ling shu* 47, a 'heart that is firm' (*xin jian*) is a virtue.[24] The anger is considered to cause heat to rise into the chest, which, in turn, effects a wasting of the flesh and fat (*re ze xiao ji fu* 熱則消肌膚). The paragraph ends with the statement: 'This means that the person is [in character] violent and hard, but his skin and flesh is soft' (*ci yan qi ren bao gang er ji rou ruo zhe ye* 此言其人暴剛而肌肉弱者也). Interestingly, precisely this rationale seems to apply to case 6. Yi points out that the person was violent and hard in character, when he mentions that he was in anger even during sexual intercourse (line 14). Yet the account in *Ling shu* 46 is much more medicalised. Where Yi blames the patient for improper social conduct, *Ling shu* 46 details how the emotion anger is linked to a series of body-internal processes, and where Yi emphasises heat, *Ling shu* 46 elaborates on both, the hot and cold.

Ling shu 47 praises firmness of the viscera and claims their flabbiness results in consumption: 'If the heart is firm, then one stores tranquility and preserves the solid, if the heart is flabby, then one is prone to ail from con-

---

[20] *Ling shu* 46, p. 387.

[21] For *xiao dan* in this sense, see also *xiao dan* in *Lun heng* 3.1, p. 152.

[22] *Ling shu* 46, p. 388.

[23] Taki Mototane also points to visceral states, subtle and small ones, when quoting *Ling shu* 4, pp. 276–7: 'If the pulse of the heart, lung, liver, spleen, kidneys . . . is subtle and small, it is a consumption' (*xin, fei, gan, pi, shen mai . . . wei xiao wei xiao dan* 心 肺 肝脾 腎脈 . . . 微小為 消癉).

[24] *Ling shu* 47, pp. 391–2. Contrast with the early medical positive connotations of *gang* in case 6 (line 36), discussed on p. 260.

sumption and internal heat' (*xin jian ze cang an shou gu, xin cui ze shan bing xiao dan re zhong* 心堅則藏安守固 心脆則善病消癉熱中).[25] Consumption is here given as opposite to firmness and solidity; internal heat is tagged on at the very end. This suggests that implicit to the concept of *xiao dan* is the idea that the hard, solid and firm is healthy (see pp. 29–33); *xiao*-wasting implies dissolution and becoming soft in an unhealthy way.

***xiao ke* 消渴 (wasting thirst)**   Chinese researchers, by contrast, point out close affinities between *xiao dan* 消癉 (lit. wasting [resulting in] heat-due-to-overexertion) and *xiao ke* 消渴 (wasting [resulting in] thirst). For instance, *xiao ke* in the *Su wen* is given as *xiao dan* in the *Zhen jiu jia yi jing*. More precisely, a passage in *Su wen* 47 reports on *pi dan* 脾癉 (spleen heat-due-to-overexertion) turning into *xiao ke* (wasting thirst), and the very same passage in the *Zhen jiu jia yi jing* 11.6 records that *pi dan* turns into *xiao dan* (consumption).[26] Both centre on an imbalanced diet.

Su wen 47 contains in fact the only occurrence of *xiao ke* (wasting thirst) in the entire *Inner Canon*. The passage reappears under the heading 'All Syndromes of the Disorder of Wasting [resulting in] Thirst' (Xiao ke bing zhu hou 消渴病諸候) in *Zhu bing yuan hou lun* 5, which has as its opening sentence: 'In cases of wasting thirst, thirst does not cease and urination is plentiful. This is it' (*fu xiao ke zhe, ke bu zhi, xiao bian duo, shi ye* 夫消渴者 渴不止 小便多 是也).[27] However, while *xiao ke* in *Zhu bing yuan hou lun* 5 emphasises excessive thirst and frequent urination, *Su wen* 47 attributes the condition of *xiao ke* to people who have a sweet tooth: 'This condition is that which the fatty and sweet brings about; this person with certainty frequently eats not only the sweet, but also the very fatty. The fatty makes that the person has internal heat, the sweet makes the person full in the centre, hence the *qi* ascends and flows over, and the condition turns into a wasting thirst' (*ci fei mei zhi suo fa ye; ci ren bi shuo shi gan mei er duo fei ye, fei zhe ling ren nei re, gan zhe ling ren zhong man, gu qi qi shang yi, zhuan wei xiao ke* 此肥美之所發也 此人必數食甘美而多肥也 肥者令人內熱 甘者令人中滿 故 其氣上溢 轉為消渴). It is difficult to see any resemblance between case 6 and *xiao ke* in *Su wen* 47, let alone with *xiao ke* in the *Zhu bing yuan hou lun* and other works from the Eastern Han and Tang.[28] Furthermore, *xiao ke* in *Su wen* 47, which typically arises from obesity, has more in common with *xiao dan* in *Ling shu* 46, which consists of a wasting of soft flesh, than it has with the other forms of *xiao ke* recorded in the *Zhu bing yuan hou lun*, which centre on excessive thirst and frequent urination.

---

[25] *Ling shu* 47, pp. 391–2; applies also to the lungs, liver, spleen and kidneys, variations concern only details.

[26] *Su wen* 47, p. 132; *Zhen jiu jia yi jing* 11.6, p. 1750.

[27] *Zhu bing yuan hou lun* 5, p. 155.

[28] See also references to *xiao ke* 消渴 in *Mai jing* and *Jin gui yao lüe* in Yu (1953:214) and Wang (1980).

In summary, there is no textual evidence for interpreting Yi's *fei xiao dan* as the medieval *xiao ke* and the biomedical 'diabetes'. The condition of *fei xiao dan* in case 6 has more in common with *xiao dan* in *Ling shu* 46 than with *xiao ke* in *Su wen* 47 because it is caused by a hard emotion, namely anger, and does not allude to habits of food intake.

***xiao gu* 消穀 – wasting grains**   'Wasting grains' (*xiao gu* 消穀), described only in the *Ling shu*, must have resulted in emaciation, although none of the texts explicitly states it. 'Wasting grains' arises from 'stomach heat' (*wei re* 胃熱), which is eventually transformed into a coldness in the stomach that makes the patient uninterested in food, as outlined in *Ling shu* 80: 'The Yellow Emperor said: When a person with an inclination to hunger has no appetite, what kind of *qi* brings this about? Qibo said: If the essences and *qi* unite in the spleen, the hot *qi* stays in the stomach, and there is a stomach heat, then there is a wasting of the grains. The grains are wasted, hence the patient is prone to hunger. If the stomach *qi* inverts and rises, then the stomach pit gets cold, hence one has no appetite' (*Huangdi yue: ren zhi shan ji er bu shi shi zhe, he qi shi ran. Qibo yue: jing qi bing yu pi, re qi liu yu wei, wei re ze xiao gu. gu xiao gu shan ji. wei qi ni shang, ze wei wan han, gu bu shi shi ye* 黃帝曰 人之善饑而不嗜食者 何氣使然 歧伯曰 精氣并於脾 熱氣留於胃 胃熱則消穀 穀消故善饑 胃氣逆上 則胃脘寒 故不嗜食也).[29] *Ling shu* 10, 29, 36 and 80 all centre on attitudes to eating, such as loss of appetite and digestion.[30] The processes they describe characteristically involve a transition from heat to coldness. 'Wasting grains', like 'wasting thirst' in *Su wen* 47, centres on food intake. In this way, it differs fundamentally from states of 'consumption' (*xiao dan*) in the *Inner Canon* and the 'lung consumption' (*fei xiao dan*) in case 6.

***fei xiao* 肺消 – lung wasting (line 3)**   The *Su wen* disorder *fei xiao* (lung wasting) mentions some of the signs and symptoms of *xiao ke* (wasting thirst) in *Zhu bing yuan hou lun* 5. Taki Mototane cites *Su wen* 37: 'If the heart shifts coldness to the lungs, there is lung wasting. In cases of lung wasting, one urinates twice what one drinks. Death occurs, incurable' (*xin yi han yu fei, fei xiao, fei xiao zhe, yin yi sou er, si bu zhi* 心移寒於肺 肺消 肺消者飲一溲二 死不治).[31] On the grounds of these symptoms, Chinese researchers of the twentieth century, like Yu Yunxiu, suggest *fei xiao* is a form of *xiao ke* (wasting thirst). Wang Zhipu even goes so far as to suggest that not only *fei xiao* in the *Su wen* but also Yi's *fei xiao dan* designates a condition

---

[29] *Ling shu* 80, p. 478. See also *Ling shu* 10, p. 301; 29, p. 354; 36, p. 369.
[30] This brings to mind anorexia nervosa, but retrospective diagnoses are always highly problematic.
[31] *Su wen* 37, p. 108. The text continues on the lungs affected by heat: 'If the heart shifts heat to the lungs, it turns into a wasting of the diaphragm' (*xin yi re yu fei, zhuan wei ge xiao* 心移熱於肺 傳為鬲消).

of *xiao ke* (wasting thirst).[32] The *Shi ji* text has accordingly been 'corrected'. Thus, based on the *fan qie* 反切 method, Zhang Shoujie outlines the pronunciation of *dan* in Takigawa's and other *Shi ji* editions: '*dan*, pronounced as *d-an h-an*, exchanged [i.e. *d-an*]' (*dan, yin dan han fan* 癉 音單旱反).[33] But in the PRC *Zhonghua shuju* edition his comment reads: '*dan*, pronounced as *dan*, is drought' (*dan, yin dan, han ⟨ye⟩ [fan]* 癉 音單旱⟨也⟩[反]).[34] So, *dan* means drought! A comment on pronunciation has forcefully been changed into a gloss on meaning. Readers are probably meant to infer that *dan*, like 'wasting thirst', is marked by drought.

The attempt to explain *fei xiao dan* in case 6 in terms of *fei xiao* (lung wasting) in *Su wen* 37 is flawed for at least three reasons. First, Yi does not mention thirst and frequent urination as concomitant signs and symptoms. Second, *fei xiao* arises if the lungs are affected by the cold, but *fei xiao dan* is indicated by a hot pulse. Third, text structure semantics in combination with considerations of consistency in medical rationale across cases 1–10 has demonstrated that *xiao dan* rather than *fei xiao* should be taken as a bisyllabic constituent in the name of the disorder. Furthermore, *xiao dan* is in canonical writings much more frequent than *fei xiao*.[35] It is therefore much more likely that the early medical document, on which this *Shi ji* text elaborates, had *xiao* or *xiao dan* as name of the disorder, to which the early first-century editor prefixed *fei* (the lungs).

dan nüe 癉瘧 – utter exhaustion resulting in chills and hot flushes

Considering that in case 6 the lungs are primarily affected, *Su wen* 35 contains an interesting parallel: 'In cases of *dan nüe*, the lungs alone have heat…it causes the person to waste and smelt away and makes the flesh drop off, hence it is called *dan nüe*' (*dan nüe zhe, fei su you re…ling ren xiao shuo tuo rou, gu ming yue dan nüe* 癉瘧者 肺素有熱 令人消爍脫肉 故命曰癉瘧).[36] In *Su wen* 35, the 'heat-due-to-overexertion' (*dan*), which arises from heat in the lungs, leads to the patient's emaciation and eventually turns into an 'intermittent coldness and heat' (*nüe*), which, as established in case 4 (line 37), probably designates 'chills and hot flushes' that arise in a condition of utter weakness. Clearly, *dan nüe* (heat-due-to-overexertion ending in chills and hot flushes) comes much closer to the 'lung consumption' (*fei xiaodan*) and 'chills and hot flushes' (*han re*) that Yi diagnoses (lines 3 and 4) than do *xiao ke* (wasting thirst) and *fei xiao* (lung wasting).

In summary, *xiao dan* (consumption) is a disorder of either an overheating that smelts the flesh or a dissolution of softened flesh. Canonical medical

---

[32] Yu (1953:213–14), Wang (1980).   [33] *Shiki kaichû kôshô* 105.2, p. 31.
[34] *Shi ji* 105.2, p. 2801. See also Wang (1980:79).
[35] HYDCD 5.1209 discusses *fei xiao dan* in the rubric on *xiao dan*.
[36] *Su wen* 35, p. 104.

descriptions of *xiao dan*, *xiao ke* (wasting thirst) and *xiao gu* (wasting grains) centre on eating habits and on the stomach as locus of the disorder. Coldness in the lungs gives rise to *fei xiao* (wasting lungs), with signs and symptoms reminiscent of diabetes, but case 6 is not a form of *fei xiao*, for the three reasons detailed above. Heat in the lungs leads to *dan nüe* (heat-due-to-overexertion ending in chills and hot flushes), so far completely ignored by the secondary literature. It comes closest to Yi's 'lung consumption' (*fei xiao dan*) ending in 'chills and hot flushes' (*han re*).

The 'Mai fa' quote (lines 17–18)

xing bi 形獘 – fading (lines 18 and 27)   The 'Mai fa' is often illuminating as it explains in a, to the contemporary Chinese medical researcher, more familiar language what Yi states earlier in his own vocabulary. However, in contrast to all other cases, the 'Mai fa' quote in case 6 has no canonical medical parallel and Yi's subsequent comments on it pose difficulties of comprehension (lines 19–24). For elucidating *xing bi* neither dictionaries nor the concordance of the thirteen classics provided further leads.

The term *bi* 弊, which apparently is synonymous with *bi* 獘 in *xing bi*, can refer to both a sudden event or a gradual process: it can mean both 'to fall forward' or 'to be [gradually] exhausted'. Thus, the gloss of the commentator Zheng Xuan 鄭玄 (127–200) on the *Zhou li* reads: '*bi* means to fall forward' (*bi pu ye* 弊 仆也), while the commentator Yin Zhizhang 尹知章 provides the gloss '*bi* means to be exhausted' (*bi jie ye* 弊 竭也) in respect of *Guanzi* 35 (quoted on p. 245). Accordingly, *xing bi* can refer to either a body form that suddenly collapses or a body form that gradually fades away.

Su wen 14 defines *xing bi* as follows: 'The Emperor said: If the body form fades away and blood is exhausted, yet every effort [for effecting a cure] is unsuccessful, why is this so? Qibo said: The spirits do not cause things to happen [i.e. they are not effective]. The Emperor said: What does it mean to say: "the spirits are not effective"? Qibo said: In cases when needles and stones provide a way [for treatment], but the essences and spirits do not advance, and impulse and intent are not controlled, there will hence be no recovery. Now, if the essences have been spoilt and the spirits have left, the constructive and defensive *qi* cannot be retrieved. Why is this so? If one while ridden by endless desire, worries incessantly, the essences and *qi* are spreading and spoilt, the constructive drips out and the defensive is eliminated, hence once the spirits have left it [the body form], there is no recovery' (*Di yue: xing bi xue jin er gong bu li zhe he? Qibo yue: shen bu shi ye. Di yue: he wei shen bu shi? Qibo yue: zhen shi dao ye. jing shen bu jin, zhi yi bu zhi, gu bing bu ke yu. jin jing huai shen qu, ying wei bu ke fu shou. He zhe? Shi yu wu qiong, er you huan bu zhi, jing qi shi huai, ying qi wei chu, gu shen qu zhi er bing bu yu ye* 帝曰 形幣血盡而功不立者何 歧伯曰 神不使也

帝曰 何謂神不使 歧伯曰 鍼灸石道也 精神不進 志意不治 故病不可愈 今精壞神去 榮
衛不可復收 何者 嗜欲無窮 而憂患不止 精氣弛壞 榮泣衛除 故神去之而病不愈也).[37]

Su wen 14 provides a definition of *xing bi* that Yi could not have had; Yi
does not speak of 'essences and spirits' (*jing shen* 精神), nor of the 'constructive and defensive' (*ying wei* 榮衛). Of interest here is, however, that the
Yellow Emperor mentions *xing bi* in juxtaposition with *xue jin* 血盡, an
exhaustion of the blood. This reminds us of Yi's comment on the 'Mai fa',
which states that the 'uneven' (*bu ping*), together with 'not drumming' (*bu
gu*), indicates *xing bi*. The 'uneven', as Yi explains, points to blood outside
its place (line 21). This would suggest that both Yi and the authors of *Su
wen* 14 considered 'blood' (*xue* 血) an aspect of the 'body form' (*xing* 形),
and that they viewed 'blood outside its place' or 'blood that is exhausted'
as a characteristic feature of *xing bi*.

Not only blood but also bodily fats and lubricants can be 'exhausted' (*bi*).
Notably, in *Guanzi* 35, 'since the marshes had not been drained, there was
sufficient nourishment' (*ze bu bi er yang zu* 澤不弊而養足),[38] the verb *bi*
modifies 'marshlands' (*ze* 澤). Incidentally, *ze* is the landscape metaphor
with which medical authors refer to a shiny and lubricated bodily surface.[39]
Thus, *Ling shu* 10 mentions a 'bodily structure without fats and lubricants'
(*ti wu gao ze* 體無膏澤).[40] By analogy, the verb *bi* may well describe the
gradual drying up and drainage of the body's 'fats and lubricants' (*gao ze*).
Accordingly, *xing bi* means 'the body form fades away' in a gradual
process.

shi duo 尸奪 – fainting (line 27)   The term *xing bi* occurs twice in case 6,
once in the above 'Mai fa' quote (line 18) and once in the course of discussing the second disorder, the chills and hot flushes, where it is meant to elucidate the term *shi duo* (line 27): 'In cases of *shi duo*, there is *xing bi*' (*shi
duo zhe, xing bi*). The grammar of the sentence is such that *shi duo* can be
interpreted as the synonym of *xing bi*, and this is how some Chinese
researchers read it, likening *shi duo* to 'consumption'.[41] However, another
interpretation is also possible.

The graph 脫, read as *duo* or *tuo*, can mean 'to suddenly drop off' or 'to
gradually drop off'. It probably reads *tuo* in *Ling shu* 12: 'In cases where,
while one wastes away and becomes emaciated, the flesh of the body
form drops off . . .' (*xiao shou er xing rou tuo zhe* 痟瘦而形肉脫者 . . .).[42] But
in case 6 (line 26), it is more likely that it reads *duo*, and *shi duo* means

[37] *Su wen* 14, p. 44. Translation based on Nanjing zhongyi xueyuan (1991:107).
[38] *Guanzi* 4.35, 'Chi mi' 侈靡, p. 1a. Translation based on Rickett (1998:305), with
modifications.
[39] On *ze* 澤, see Bodde (1981).
[40] *Ling shu* 10, p. 304. Compare with MWD YY (1985:9) on p. 257.
[41] e.g. Wang (1980:79).
[42] *Ling shu* 12, p. 313. The characters *xiao* 痟 and *xiao* 消 can be used interchangeably, see
HYDCD 8.320. For other substitutions, see Ma (1992:540, 724, 963).

'fainting'. Taki Motohiro comments: 'As the flesh of the body form drops off, one becomes like a corpse, hence you call it "the corpse is falling"' (*xing rou tuo er ru shi, gu yue shi duo* 形肉脫而如尸 故曰尸奪). 'The corpse is falling' (*shi duo*) is like 'the body form is fading away' (*xing bi*), a noun-verb phrase, as we noted of other early medical names of disorders in cases 1, 2 and 4. The interpretation of *shi duo* as 'fainting' is reinforced by the word *yan* (line 26): 'It was said' (*yan*).[43] Yi had been told that his patient had previously fainted. If *shi tuo* referred to 'a gradual dropping off', Yi would have been able to observe it himself, instead of relying on hearsay; the term *yan* would be redundant. So, *shi duo* means 'fainting' in line 26.

shi jue 尸厥 – going numb (*Shi ji* 105.1)

Taki Motohiro adds: 'The *Tong ya* takes it for a *shi jue*, but this is wrong' (*Tong ya wei shi jue, fei ye* 通雅為尸厥 非也).[44] The term *shi jue* (lit. the corpse is numb/fake), which occurs in Bian Que's Memoir, arises from a *yin yang* inversion that ends in a corpse-like state: 'Hence the body form is still and the appearance is as if [the person] were dead' (*gu xing jing ru si zhuang* 故形靜如死狀).[45] Bian Que cures 'the corpse that is numb' with needling and various other therapies. Likewise, *Su wen* 63 recommends needling 'the corpse that is numb': 'When the five links are all exhausted, this effects in a person that all the vessels on the body [surface] are agitated, while, simultaneously, the bodily form is without consciousness. Its appearance is like that of a corpse. Some call it 'the corpse is numb'. Needle the inner side of the big toe, on top of the nail' (*wu luo ju jie, ling ren shen mai jie dong, er xing wu zhi ye; qi zhuang ruo shi, huo yue shi jue; ci qi zu da zhi nei ce zhua jia shang* 五絡俱竭 令人身脈皆動 而形無知也 其狀若尸 或曰尸厥 刺其足大指內側爪甲上).[46] *Su wen* 63 lists a sequence of locations for treating 'the corpse that is numb' (*shi jue*) with needle therapy. By contrast, Yi maintains, 'the corpse that fell' (*shi duo*) should not be treated with cauterisation, needle therapy and potent medicines (line 28).[47]

In summary, *xing bi* (the body is fading away) in the 'Mai fa' quote, like Yi's *fei xiao dan* (lung consumption), designates a gradual process of emaciation. However, where consumption (*xiao dan*) tends to be understood as a process where inner heat smelts the flesh, *xing bi* makes no allusion to heat. Rather, *bi* invokes the landscape metaphor of draining the marshlands, i.e. the lubricating fats and fluids. Furthermore, blood is men-

---

[43] *yan* 言 'there is a word/saying' in case 8 (line 23); 'it is said' in cases 6 (line 26) and 10 (line 20).

[44] *Tong ya* 18, p. 18b (SKQS 857:399).

[45] *Shiki kaichû kôshô* 105.1, pp. 14–15.   [46] *Su wen* 63, p. 177.

[47] Perhaps *shi duo* and *shi jue* referred to different kinds of fainting. Biomedicine differentiates between a variety of comas. An apoplectic coma can be accompanied by rigor and partial paralyses. In such a case, acupuncture and moxibustion are indicated (Ma Kanwen, 1990s p.c.).

tioned: *Su wen* 14 says that it is 'exhausted' (*jin*) and Yi that 'it is out of its place' (*bu ju qi chu*).

Considering that both terms *tuo* and *bi* can be used either in the sense of a sudden collapse or a gradual fading away, one wonders whether the distinction between a gradual fading and sudden dropping worried Chinese physicians. From an experiential viewpoint, one would have expected that a sudden collapse and a gradual wasting were distinctive. It is odd that the vocabulary used for referring to these processes is not unambiguous.

The pulses of the 'Mai fa' (line 18)

The 'Mai fa' mentions two pulse qualities, 'uneven' (*bu ping*) and 'not drumming' (*bu gu*). Both occur in canonical medical texts, but neither belongs among the twenty-four in *Mai jing* 1.1. Xu Guang points to yet a third one, mentioned in another edition, which has 'uneven' and 'dispersing' (*san* 散). We will attend to this one first.

san 散 – dispersing (line 18)   'Wasting' (*xiao* 消) is often likened to 'smelting' (*shuo* 爍) in canonical medical texts, but mostly conceived of as a kind of 'dispersal' (*san*) in Warring States and early Han texts, where not infrequently one encounters the compound word *xiao san* 消散 (to dissolve).[48] This compound word occurs, in my reading, also in the Mawangdui 'Shiwen': 'Sleep causes the disintegration of food, dissolves medicines and makes them [the food and medicines] flow through the body form' (*fu wo shi shi mi, xiao san yao, yi liu xing zhe ye* 夫臥使食靡 宵散藥 以流刑者也).[49] Its meaning 'to dissolve' is still contained in Wang Bing's gloss to *Su wen* 17: 'Wasting means to dissolve' (*xiao wei xiao san* 消謂消散).[50] The sentence in *Su wen* 17 that Wang Bing elucidates correlates the 'dispersed' (*san*) pulse with the condition of 'wasting' (*xiao*): 'If the heart pulse beats/strokes ... are soft, yet dispersed, there will be [or: it matches, it corresponds to] a wasting of the waist [lit. the ring], it gets better on its own (*xin mai bo ... ruan er san zhe, dang xiao huan, zi yi* 心脈搏 ... 耎而散者 當消環 自已).[51] Evidently,

---

[48] HYDCD 5.1205.

[49] MWD 'Shiwen' (1985:151). The graphs *xiao*宵and *xiao* 消, *xing* 刑 and *xing* 形 are interchangeable. This translation takes *xiao san* as a compound word and differs both from Ma (1992:963) and Harper (1998:409). *Su wen* 62, p. 169, has *xiao* in this sense, precisely, of dissolving in order to make it flow: 'If you warm it [blood *qi*], then by dissolving it, you make it go' (*wen ze xiao er qu zhi* 溫則消而去之).

[50] HDNJSW 17. p. 38.

[51] *Su wen* 17, p. 52. Modern editions tend to give *xiao huan* 消環 as *xiao ke* 消渴, thereby amending the text in accordance with the *Zhen jiu jia yi jing*, *Mai jing* and *Tai su*. Wang Bing in HDNJSW 17, p. 38, interprets *huan* as cycle, unaware that *huan* 環 (ring) was a body part in early Chinese medicine – the 'waist'. See MWD 'Maifa' (1985:17) and ZJS (2001:144): 'When the vapor [*qi*] ascends and does not descend, discern which *mai* has excess and cauterize it at the ring [i.e. the waist].' Harper's (1998:214) translation, as so often, is based on Ma (1992:282).

a 'dispersed' (*san*) pulse indicated 'wasting' (*xiao*). In this context we are reminded that *Su wen* 1 mentions the verb 'to disperse' (*san*) in the same sentence as a body form in danger of collapsing or fading (quoted on p. 35). 'Becoming dispersed' is thus characteristic of both a 'body form fading away' (*xing bi*) and 'wasting' (*xiao*), and highlights their semantic closeness. The pulse quality *san* (dispersed) would thus appear central to the medical rationale of the presumed early second-century document on which case 6 in *Shi ji* 105 elaborates.

bu ping 不平 – **uneven (lines 18 and 21)**   In *Su wen* 18, the 'even pulse' (*ping mai* 平脈) is contrasted with the 'pulse indicative of disorders' (*bing mai* 病脈) and the 'pulse indicative of death' (*si mai* 死脈).[52] Here, the even pulse clearly refers to a normal if not normative state, or what one nowadays calls 'health'; it varies seasonally and in respect of the state of each of the five viscera.[53] In *Mai jing* 5.3, the 'even pulse' is defined by the rhythm of breathing: 'If a person inhales once and the pulse arrives twice, you call it an even pulse' (*ren yi xi mai er zhi wei ping mai* 人一吸 脈二至 謂平脈).[54] Earlier, in *Su wen* 18, exactly the same state is attributed not to the 'even pulse' but to the 'even person' (*ping ren* 平人): 'If a person exhales once and the pulse moves twice, and if he inhales once and the pulse moves twice again, you call it an even person' (*ren yi hu mai zai dong, yi xi mai yi zai dong ... ming yue ping ren* 人一呼脈再動 一吸脈亦再動 命曰平人).[55] *Su wen* 18 continues by saying: 'The even person does not get ill' (*ping ren zhe, bu bing ye* 平人者 不病也). Such a definition of the 'even person' is also given in *Ling shu* 9: 'The so-called even person does not get ill' (*suo wei ping ren zhe bu bing* 所謂平人者不病).[56] The 'even' is indicative of health, and the 'uneven', accordingly, of illness.

The above definitions of the 'even pulse' and 'even person' from the medical canons do not contradict Yi's understanding of 'even' (*ping*). Yet, importantly, in his comment on the 'Mai fa', he defines the 'even' in respect of whether blood resides in its place or not (line 21). Although Zhang Shoujie cites a very similar *Su wen* passage (not located),[57] only *Ling shu* 81 has been found to mention *ping* as a verb that qualifies blood, when it speaks of 'the evenness and unevenness of the blood *qi*' (*xue qi zhi ping yu bu ping* 血氣之平與不平).[58] Yi does not specify which bodily processes cause blood, as he says in a rather unusual idiom, 'to be out of its place'. Perhaps

---

[52] *Su wen* 18, p. 57.

[53] Zhang Shoujie cites the 'even' pulses of the seasons according to *Mai jing* 3 (see p. 68 in spring; p. 73 in summer; p. 81 with noticeable variation in the sixth month; p. 87 with slight variation in autumn; p. 93 with slight variation in winter).

[54] *Mai jing* 5.3, p. 151.   [55] *Su wen* 18, p. 54.   [56] *Ling shu* 9, p. 293.

[57] 'If blood *qi* changes its place, you call it uneven. If the vessel indicator is agitated but not steady, you call it "alternating"' (*xue qi yi chu yue bu ping, mai hou dong bu ding yue dai* 血氣易處 曰不平 脈候動不定曰代). Taki Motohiro notes this *Su wen* text no longer exists, but *dai* is defined as such in *Lei jing* 5.4, p. 117.

[58] *Ling shu* 81, p. 480.

in the light of *Su wen* 17, 'as to the *mai*, they are the receptacle of the blood' (*fu mai zhe, xue zhi fu ye* 夫脈者 血之府也),[59] blood out of its place is blood that is not in the *mai*? Yi is vague.

In summary, the 'even pulse' (*ping mai*) and 'even person' (*ping ren*) refer to what we would call a 'healthy' state and to a certain extent invoke a normative concept of 'health'. In the *Inner Canon* and in medieval medical manuscripts, they are usually defined in respect of a normative number of pulse beats or instances of breathing (exhalations and inhalations),[60] while the 'Mai fa' indirectly and Yi explicitly point to blood dynamics, where blood either is 'exhausted' or 'out of place'.

bu gu 不鼓 – not drumming (line 18)   The idiom 'not drumming' (*bu gu*) occurs four times in the *Su wen*, where it always designates a pulse quality,[61] but it is not mentioned in the *Ling shu*. The term *gu* 鼓 occurs more frequently and is used in several different senses. It is used for qualifying *mai*,[62] for describing a movement of trembling[63] or for designating the sound of drumming.[64] In some passages drumming is likened to the echo, and perceived as a form of resonance or vibration, as in *Ling shu* 45: 'The inner and outer mutually duplicate one another, like the drumming responds to the drumstick, the echo responds to the sound, and the shadow resembles the form' (*nei wai xiang xi, ru gu zhi ying fu, xiang zhi ying sheng, ying zhi si xing* 內外相襲 如鼓之應枹 響之應聲 影之似形).[65]

In *Su wen* 7, *gu* (drumming) seems to designate an intensified form of beating, perhaps a heavy or loud pounding: 'If the three *yang* all beat together and if, moreover, they are drumming, one dies in three days' (*san yang ju bo qie gu, san ri si* 三陽俱搏且鼓 三日死).[66] In this sentence, *gu* is indicative of death. Elsewhere in *Su wen* 7 (see p. 170), *gu* (drumming) is used for qualifying the *yin* and *yang* in ways that result in the pulse qualities which are hook-like, body hair-like, bowstring-like and stone-like. In those sentences, *gu* seems to mean 'beating/drumming' in a general sense. Evidently, the term *gu* qualifies *mai* in rather different ways, i.e. it is not a highly standardised term in the *Inner Canon*.

Osobe Yô interprets *bu gu* as *bu gu dong*: 'If the pulse is not drumming and moving, then it does not have strength' (*mai bu gu dong, ze wu li* 脈不鼓動 則無力).[67] In Osobe Yô's view, 'to have no strength' reflects that the

---

[59] *Su wen* 17, p. 50.   [60] Hsu (In press b).

[61] *Su wen* 48, p. 134, quoted on p. 282; 74, p. 239; and twice in *Su wen* 79, p. 250 (based on computer printout by Hermann Tessenow, 2000).

[62] e.g *Su wen* 7, p. 27; *Su wen* 48, p. 136.

[63] e.g. *Su wen* 35, p. 101; *Su wen* 70, p. 206; *Su wen* 74, pp. 236 and 241; *Ling shu* 21, p. 335.

[64] e.g. *Su wen* 74, p. 241.

[65] *Ling shu* 45, p. 386. See also *Su wen* 66, p. 183.

[66] *Su wen* 7, p. 27. Note parallel to MWD ZB (1985:5). For reading 俱搏 as *ju tuan*, see case 7 (line 17).

[67] Osobe Yô (1994:82).

'body form is gradually fading away' (*xing bi*). Taki Motokata suggests a different reading of *bu gu*: 'Rhythmically drumming must have regular intervals' (*zou gu bi you jie* 奏鼓必有節). Accordingly, *bu gu* is 'arrhythmic'. This would make the pulse quality *gu* (drumming) a very desirable one, much like *ping* (even), but it would render the meaning of *gu* as diametrically opposed to that of *gu* (drumming loudly) in *Su wen* 7, which, as seen above, is indicative of death.

Since the 'Mai fa' says the pulses are 'uneven and not drumming' (*bu ping bu gu*) and Yi, in his comments on the 'Mai fa', that 'while being uneven, they are alternating' (*bu ping er dai*), Ando Koretora suggests: '*bu gu* means the pulse is *dai*, i.e. "alternating" or in this particular context, given the weakness of the patient, "intermittent"' (*bu gu yan mai dai ye* 不鼓言脈代也). However, considering that Yi's comments on the 'Mai fa' often concern observations that come close to it but are not exactly identical, one could argue that *bu gu* (line 18) and *dai* (line 20) designate two distinct pulse qualities. Accordingly, *bu gu* would describe either an 'irregularly drumming' pulse or one 'without strength', characteristic of a condition of wasting, while *dai* 'alternating' would indicate a progressed stage that is terminal.

In summary, for the 'Mai fa' quote of case 6 there is no parallel in the canonical medical literature, although for each of the three idioms – *bu ping*, *bu gu*, *xing bi* – at least one could be found. Canonical medical texts variously mention 'even' (*ping*) and 'drumming' (*gu*), but not exclusively in the context of pulse diagnosis. They also speak of the 'uneven' and 'not drumming', but not necessarily in Yi's sense. The two terms are used in different contexts, interpreted often in opposite ways, and no one standard definition was found to apply to all their occurrences, yet they appear intuitively intelligible and appear meaningful even to the uninitiated. In the light of this, one wonders whether the 'Mai fa' reflects medical knowledge at the interface between popular and scholarly medical knowledge.

Yi's comments on the 'Mai fa' (lines 19–24)

gao zhi yuan shu 高之遠數 – the 'high' one went to the 'distant' number (line 19a)   Yi's comments on the 'Mai fa' are difficult to decode. Comparison with case 5 has us expect that Yi cites the 'Mai fa' first, and then announces that his findings are slightly different. According to this pattern we expect to read the 'Mai fa' (line 18) as declaring that the pulse qualities *bu ping* and *bu gu* are indicative of a 'body form that fades away' (*xing bi*); meanwhile Yi states that he felt slightly different pulse qualities (line 20), namely *bu ping* and *dai*, which he then each explains (lines 21–2).

Before and after this statement are two sentences that begin with the conjunction *ci* 此 'this one' (lines 19a and 24). They are so technical that extended research was necessary to make sense of them. Due to the re-

sumptive pronoun with which they begin and the existence of parallel
canonical medical passages, one's first hunch is to view them as commentatorial interjections. However, they allude to an early medical bipartite
body.

For elucidating the first of these two sentences (line 19a), Kaiho Gembi
points to Wang Bing's comment on *Su wen* 74: 'The heart and the lungs are
the proximate ones, the liver and the kidneys the distant ones' (*xin fei wei
jin, shen gan wei yuan* 心肺為近 腎肝為遠).[68] In *Su wen* 74, the liver is the
'distant' (*yuan*), the lungs the 'proximate' one (*jin*). In case 6, accordingly,
the 'distant' (*yuan*) one among the five viscera is the liver, and the 'high'
(*gao*) one the lungs. Kaiho Gembi points out that in the first part of this
case history the disorder affects the lungs (lines 3, 16) and only in the second
part the liver (line 36). It is more likely, however, that the high one referred
not to the canonical lungs (line 3) but to the heart/lungs in the upper bodily
sphere of the early medical body (line 44), as opposite of the liver/womb/
bladder in the lower sphere. Yi's 'Model' also invokes this body conception
(line 44).

Kaiho Gembi does not comment on *zhi* 之, probably because he did not
consider it a problem. There is little doubt that it is a verb and Yi speaks
of the disorder 'going' from one viscus to another, as in *Su wen* 7: 'When
the liver [disorder] goes to the heart, you call it "giving birth to *yang*"; when
the heart [disorder] goes to the lungs, you call it "causing the death of *yin*";
when the lung [disorder] goes to the kidneys, you call it "doubling the *yin*";
when the kidney [disorder] goes to the spleen, you call it "opening up the
yin"; death occurs, incurable' (*gan zhi xin, wei zhi sheng yang, xin zhi fei,
wei zhi si yin, fei zhi shen, wei zhi chong yin, shen zhi pi, wei zhi pi yin, si
bu zhi* 肝之心 謂之生陽 心之肺 謂之死陰 肺之腎 謂之重陰 腎之脾 謂之辟陰 死不
治).[69] Although the text explicitly mentions the 'five viscera', the movement
from lungs to liver is not actually recorded in *Su wen* 7, nor elsewhere in
the medical canons.[70] This reinforces the above suggestion that Yi refers to
the early medical heart/lungs that went to the liver/womb.

Kaiho Gembi reads *shu* 數 (number) as adverbial, referring to a gradual
process, but it is here best read as a noun. One variously encounters it in
canonical medical writings, with meanings known only to the initiated. In
Ling shu 81, it is collocated with *jing* 經 (channels): 'Now the constructive
and defensive in the blood vessels circulate without pausing, above they
resonate with the lodges of the stars, below with the numbers of the channels' (*fu xue mai ying wei, zhou liu bu xiu, shang ying xing xiu, xia ying jing*

---

[68] HDNJSW 74, p. 187.
[69] *Su wen* 7, p. 27; *zhi* 之 'to go'. See also *Ling shu* 42, pp. 380–81, quoted on p. 288.
[70] Osobe Yô (1994:82), in line with canonical doctrine, says the disorder wandered from the
lungs to the kidneys but considers it odd and medically unfounded. On *chong yin* 'double
yin' and *bing yin* 'paired *yin*', see case 4 (lines 26, 29).

shu 夫血脈榮衛 周流不休 上應星宿 下應經數).[71] Since *Ling shu* 81 has the 'number of the channels', Yi may here speak of 'number'.

liang luo mai jue 兩絡脈絕 – two linking vessels are severed (line 23) The second sentence beginning with the resumptive pronoun *ci* (line 23) alludes to lungs and liver, according to Ando Koretora, i.e. the two 'numbers' in line 19a. It also is written in a fairly abstract language. Given that 'number' is an aspect of the system of *jing* (passageways, channels), as are 'links' or 'linking vessels', the same body conception appears to be implied by both lines 19a and 23.

The two links that are severed bring to mind *Su wen* 7: 'If two *yang* get knotted up, you call it wasting' (*er yang jie, wei zhi xiao* 二陽結 謂之消).[72] Admittedly, the alternative translation of *Su wen* 7, 'if the second *yang* [i.e. the heart-lungs] gets knotted, you call it wasting', precludes a possible parallel. Regardless of whether *er* 二 is interpreted as a cardinal or ordinal number, *Su wen* 7 provides a textual parallel to the 'wasting' heat in the 'lungs' of case 6.

jing bing 經病 – the passageways are in disorder (line 19b) The statement 'And the passageways were in disorder' (*yi jing bing ye*) in line 19b reads like an emendation tagged onto line 19a or, if it was interjected, line 18.[73] In that case, it is either an editorial interpolation or a later commentatorial interjection.

Kaiho Gembi comments: '*jing* means transitory' (*jing zhe, li ye* 經者 歷也), but it is not likely that he meant *jing bing* was a 'transitory illness' because it ends in death.[74] Rather, he took *jing bing* as a 'disorder of transition', from the heart/lungs to the liver or from life to death. The concept of *jing*, much like that of *mai*, is marked by meronymy: *mai* and *jing* designate a movement (the pulse or transition) and the thing in which it takes place (the vessel or passageway).[75] Transitions take place in passageways.

Whereas Yi refers to 'passageways' (*jing*) in cases 1 and 6, the canonical medical literature has 'channel-vessels' (*jing mai* 經脈).[76] The *locus classicus* is *Ling shu* 10: 'There are twelve channel-vessels, they travel in a hidden way between the divided flesh (i.e. bundles of muscles?), since they are located deeply [inside the flesh], one does not see them' (*jing mai shi er zhe, fu xing fen rou zhi jian, shen er bu xian* 經脈十二者 伏行分肉之間 深而不見).[77]

---

[71] *Ling shu* 81, p. 480. See also Wang Bing on HDNJSW 7, p. 23, quoted in case 7, n. 98.
[72] *Su wen* 7, p. 27.
[73] *yi . . . ye* 以 . . . 也 alternative reading: 'because' (Pulleyblank 1995:161–2; example 596), suggested by Mark Lewis (1995 p.c.).
[74] *jing* 經 'transitory' probably applies to case 2 (line 14).
[75] For meronymy, see Cruse (1986:160–80): for *mai* as a meronym, see Hsu (1986:46).
[76] Yi does not speak of *jing mai*, except in the book titles of section 4.7, discussed on p. 66.
[77] *Ling shu* 10, p. 306.

in *Ling shu* 10, *jing mai* are deeper-lying structures than the 'links' (*luo*) that, like bulging veins, can be seen.

Su wen 20 mentions a 'disorder of the channels' (*jing bing*) as opposed to a 'disorder of the second-generation, tiny links' (*sun luo bing* 孫絡病): 'In the case of a disorder of the channels, one treats the channels; in the case of a disorder in the tiny links, one treats the tiny links and makes them bleed' (*jing bing zhe, zhi qi jing, sun luo bing zhe, zhi qi sun luo xue* 經病 者 治其經 孫絡病者 治其孫絡血). The 'tiny links' are located on the body surface, the 'channels' in deeper-lying structures. In *Su wen* 20, *jing bing* refers in all likelihood to a 'disorder of the channels'.[78]

In *Su wen* 20, *jing bing* is a noun-noun compound word, but in cases 1 (line 30) and 6 (line 19b), it probably is a noun-verb phrase. In early Chinese medicine, as repeatedly shown, the names of the disorders often were noun-verb phrases. In cases 1 and 6, the term *jing bing* meaning 'the passageways are in disorder' and the pulse quality *dai* (alternating) occur in a context where Yi states that the disorder is lethal.

In summary, *jing bing* can be read in two different ways, depending on how the pulse quality *dai* is interpreted. According to the first reading, following Ando Koretora, *dai* would be a synonym of *bu gu*. Yi would then consider the 'passageways that are in disorder' (*jing bing*) more or less synonymous with the condition of 'the body form that is fading away' (*xing bi*). This is possible if the passageways were indeed considered part of the body form (*xing*), which is, however, debatable.[79]

The second reading is that the patient suffered not only from a body fading away (*xing bi*), but, even worse, from 'passageways that are in disorder' (*jing bing*). Yi explains that the passageways were in disorder, 'hence' he sensed slightly different pulse qualities (line 20): they were not only uneven, but also alternating (*dai*). This second reading presents Yi as engaging in a coherent argument when commenting on the 'Mai fa'.

***dai* 代 – alternating (lines 20 and 22)**   The 'alternating' (*dai*) has been discussed in case 1 (line 30). In case 6 (line 22), Yi describes the tactile perception of the 'alternating' in two different ways. Both have canonical medical parallels. In respect of Yi's first characterisation of *dai*, 'from time to time three strokes arrive together' (*shi san ji bing zhi*), Ando Koretora cites *Su wen* 20: 'If the upper, lower, right and left pulse mutually resonate like three pestles [simultaneously] pounding grain, the disorder is grave' (*shang xia zuo you zhi mai, xiang ying ru san chong zhe, bing shen* 上下左右之脈 相應 如參舂者 病甚).[80] The threefold pounding of grain is likened to the simultaneous arrival of three strokes.

---

[78] *Su wen* 20, p. 66.
[79] In case 1 (lines 22–3), the term *jing* in the narrow sense of 'channels' was put in connection with sinews and bone marrow, which certainly were not part of *xing*, the outwardly visible body form.
[80] *Su wen* 20, p. 65. See also MWD ZB (1985:5).

Yi's second characterisation of *dai* as alternating between being 'at once hurried, at once large' (*zha cao zha da*) is reminiscent of its description in *Ling shu* 48 as 'at once it is much, at once it is remittent' (*zha shen zha jian* 乍甚乍間).[81] Elsewhere in *Ling shu* 48 this passage reoccurs, but with interesting modifications. Here *dai* is a sign of pain that comes and goes: 'If it [the pulse] is intermittent, then at once there is pain, and at once it ceases' (*dai ze zha tong zha zhi* 代則乍痛乍止). We are reminded of *Su wen* 23 (quoted on p. 131), where *dai* is indicative of pain in the central part, namely the spleen and stomach. Perhaps the quality given there, 'briefly rare and briefly frequent' (*zha shu zha shuo*), does not only describe tactile qualities of *mai* but also reflects in an iconic way processes inside the body, such as intermittent pain.

In Yi's case histories, *dai* is always mentioned at the end of a list of pulse qualities and indicates the end stage.[82] In cases 1 and 6, this final stage of the illness is marked by exuberance in the links, and *dai* seems to be indicative not of a depletion pattern (as it is today), but of an alternation of presumably two pulse qualities.

Summary of case 6, part one (lines 1–24)

In line with text structure semantics the two qualities of *mai* that Yi senses can be made to correlate with the three constituents in the name of the disorder by suggesting one is bisyllabic: 'consumption' (*xiao dan*) correlates with 'being hot' (*re*), the 'lungs' (*fei*) with '*qi* coming from the lungs' (*fei qi*). The reading of *fei xiaodan* as 'lung consumption' highlights that case 6 has no affinity with *fei xiao* (lung wasting) and *xiao ke* (wasting thirst), nor with diabetes.

The main problem of comprehension in case 6 concerns the 'Mai fa' (lines 17–18) and Yi's subsequent comments on it (lines 19–24). According to the usual pattern, Yi first speaks of his own pulse qualities, which explain his diagnosis. He then quotes the 'Mai fa' and in a comment on it compares his own findings with those of the 'Mai fa'.

At first glance, it is difficult to see a connection between *fei xiao dan* and the *xing bi* of the 'Mai fa'. Detailed investigations of *xiao* (wasting), *xing bi* (the body form is fading away), *shi duo* (the corpse is falling) and *shi jue* (the corpse is numb) show that *xing bi* interpreted as 'gradual fading' comes close to 'wasting' (*xiao*). The main difference is that *xing bi* refers to a fading of the bodily frame during which fats and bodily lubricants are drained and blood is out of place, but *xiao* implies wasting from either a process of dissolution or from internal heat and smelting.

---

[81] *Ling shu* 48, pp. 397–8.
[82] See case 1 (lines 21, 30), case 6 (line 22), case 7 (line 19).

The 'Mai fa' pulses indicative of the 'body form that is fading away' (*xing bi*) are the 'uneven' (*bu ping*) and 'not drumming' (*bu gu*). However, because the passageways became disordered, Yi reports he felt they were 'uneven, yet alternating' (*bu ping er dai*). Yi finds it necessary to explain the implications of being 'uneven' (*bu ping*) and 'alternating' (*dai*) in two topic-comment sentences. In both cases the topic is marked by the same particle *zhe*, but despite the identical grammatical structure of the two sentences (lines 21 and 22), Yi provides very different information on these terms. He outlines for the 'uneven' (*bu ping*) the pathological processes it indicates, and for the 'alternating' (*dai*) the tactile experiences by which it is identified.

The reasons for the deterioration of the condition and the ensuing death are given in two sentences that both begin with the resumptive pronoun *ci* 此 (lines 19a and 23). The first explains that the disorder in the heart/lungs went to the liver and the second that two linking vessels were severed. Death is inevitable. Since *Su wen* 7 proves particularly useful for elucidating the meaning of several terms in these two sentences[83] and highlights an intricate affinity in technical terminology between lines 19a and 23, these two *ci*-sentences appear to be an interjection by a later, medically trained commentator. On the other hand they do allude to an early medical bipartite body.

Case 6, part two (lines 25–46)

The second disorder, *han re*, probably designates 'chills and hot flushes' in an end stage of exhaustion (see also case 4, line 37). Yi was told that the patient had fainted earlier (line 26) and explains that fainting belongs among the various manifestations of a 'body form fading away' (*xing bi*) (line 27). He declares one ought not treat persons whose form is fading with cauterisation, needle therapy and potent medicines (line 28). However, the Grand Physician at the court of Qi, who had earlier treated the patient, first cauterised the foot's minor *yang mai* and made the patient drink *Pinellia* (lines 29–32). This depleted the patient's abdominal part of the interior (lines 33–4). He then cauterised the minor *yin mai* (line 35). This harmed the liver (line 36). He thereby doubly diminished the patient's *qi* (line 37), and added 'chills and hot flushes' (*han re*) to the 'lung consumption' (line 38). From the viewpoint of medical history, Yi's account is remarkable because it reports, first, on an interdiction of treatment and, second, on an iatrogenic illness.

---

[83] *Su wen* 7, p. 27, mentions *zhi* 'to go' (see case 6, n. 69) and *er yang* 'the second *yang*' or 'two *yang*', *xiao* 'wasting' (case 6, n. 72), and Wang Bing mentions in a comment on it *shu* 'number' (quoted in case 7, n. 98). It also has *gu* 'drumming', which perhaps replaced an earlier *san* 'dispersed'.

The treatment interdiction (line 28) Both the manuscript and canonical medical literature contain interesting parallels to the treatment interdiction mentioned in case 6 (line 28).[84] Thus, *Su wen* 40 notes: 'The Masters are numerous who say that if there is heat in the interior and wasting of the interior, one cannot administer fats and grains,[85] aromatic herbs[86] and mineral drugs. The mineral drugs make one break out in [epileptic] fits, and the aromatic herbs make one break out in madness' (*fu zi shu yan re zhong xiao zhong, bu ke fu gao liang fang cao shi yao, shi yao fa dian, fang cao fa kuang* 夫子數言熱中消中 不可服高粱芳草石藥 石藥發瘨 芳草發狂).[87] *Su wen* 40 prohibits 'mineral drugs', reminiscent of Yi's 'potent drugs' (*du yao*), but not 'cautery and needling' (*guan jiu bian shi*), as does Yi in line 28.[88] It also states that the use of 'aromatic herbs' will cause madness, which shows striking parallels to Yi's state that matches 'madness', inter alia, after ingestion of the aromatic herb *Pinellia*.[89]

Su wen 40, unlike Yi, also includes the interdiction not to indulge in a diet rich in fats and grains: 'Those with heat in the interior and wasting of the interior all are rich and noble people, now if one prohibits fats and grains, this does not accommodate with their minds, and if one prohibits aromatic herbs and mineral drugs, this has the effect that the disorder is not cured, I'd like to hear elucidations on this' (*fu re zhong xiao zhong zhe, jie fu gui ren ye, jin jin gao liang, shi bu he qi xin, jin fang cao shi yao, shi bing bu yu, yuan wen qi shuo* 夫熱中消中者 皆富貴人也 今禁高粱 是不合其心 禁芳草石藥 是病不愈 願聞其說). This question suggests that the Yellow Emperor speaks from experience with a rather demanding genteel clientele who are unwilling to change their diet. In his answer, Qibo does not insist on the dietary regime, but stresses that one is prohibited to administer aromatic herbs and mineral drugs. *Su wen* 40, which links wasting to the lavish lifestyle of the good and rich, reveals that its medical authorship was well aware that

---

[84] See MWD 'Tai chan shu' (1985:136ff.), for food prescriptions and interdictions during pregnancy. For interdictions of cauterisation, and dietary and sexual restrictions, see Wuwei medical manuscripts (Gansusheng bowuguan and Wuweixian wenhuaguan 1975:18, S90A and 90B, and also: 6).

[85] *gao liang* 高粱 is *gao liang* 膏粱 in *Zhen jiu jia yi jing* 11.6, p. 1753; p. 1752.

[86] *fang cao* 芳草 *Asclepias curassavica* L. See ZYDCD (1995:1807, no. 3699). This term is frequently used for referring to aromatic herbs in general (Georges Métailié, late 1990s p.c.).

[87] *Su wen* 40, p. 115.

[88] Yamada (1998:44) translates *guan jiu bian shi* as 'moxibustion and acupuncture'. Vivienne Lo (1998 p.c.) suggests 'cauterisation at the joints and stone needles'; *guan jiu* comes close to *guan ci* 關刺 'needling at the joints' in *Ling shu* 7, p. 289. Taki Motohiro suspects *guan* is mistaken, but this is unlikely; a phrase of four words is more common than one of three. The term *shi* 石 could also designate minerals, as *wu shi* 五石 'five minerals' in case 22 or *shi yao* 石藥 'mineral drugs' in *Su wen* 40.

[89] If *shi* 石 in line 28 were translated as minerals, it is worth noting that the patient fainted, and *Su wen* 40 says that the minerals cause fits. Although fainting and fits may not present in exactly the same way, both present in a sudden collapse of the body frame.

certain disorders are caused by lifestyle and that their epidemiology is restricted to sociologically distinct groups.[90]

Interdictions of needling and cautery are too numerous to follow up here. The Grand Physician cauterised the minor *yin mai* and, incidentally, the Mawangdui 'Yinyang vessel text' contains a treatment recommendation – in fact, the only one in the vessel texts – in respect of the minor *yin*: 'When you cauterise it, force [the patient] to eat raw meat, loosen the belt, leave the hair unbound, and for walking have him use a large stick and wear heavy shoes; cauterise for a few moments, and the disorder will desist' (*jiu ze qiang shi chan rou, huan dai, bei fa, da zhang, zhong lü er bu, jiu ji xi ze bing yi yi* 久則強食產肉 緩帶 皮髮 大丈 重履而步 久幾息則病已矣).[91] In the translation offered here, the patient is recommended to take a protein-rich diet (eat raw meat), relax (by untying belt and hair), and exercise arm and leg muscles (by holding a large stick and wearing heavy shoes when walking). In Harper's translation, however, it is the doctor who ought to take these precautions: 'When cauterizing the Minor Yin vessel, eat raw meat heartily, leave the belt loose, and the hair unbound, and walk with a large stick wearing heavy shoes.'[92] Harper stresses the irrational and magical in early texts, but he cannot explain why the doctor ought to do this when cauterising the minor *yin mai*. The above translation, guided by daily life experiences, emphasises the therapeutically relevant in cases where a patient's body form has been fading away.

The iatrogenic illness (lines 29–38)   As the text reads now, three treatment interventions cause the iatrogenic illness: cauterising the foot's minor *yang mai* (line 31), making the patient ingest orally a bolus of *Pinellia* (line 32), and cauterising the minor *yin mai* (line 35).

For explaining what may have motivated the Grand Physician of Qi to cauterise the foot's minor *yang mai*, the Mawangdui 'Yinyang vessel text' provides a hint: 'To be without fatty tissue' (*wu gao* 無膏), it states, arises if the vessel is agitated and it accordingly recommends treating the condition with cauterisation.[93] According to Takigawa's punctuation, the Grand Physician cauterised the 'opening' of the foot's minor *yang mai*, but since there are no parallels for such an 'opening' in the medical literature, I suggest altering the punctuation.

The second treatment intervention accordingly reads: 'Orally, he made him drink a bolus of *ban xia* 半夏.' Contemporary dictionaries say that *ban xia* is *Rhizoma pinellia*, dried tuber of *Pinellia ternata* (Thunb.) Breit. Its

---

[90] See also *Su wen* 28, p. 88, on 'consumption' (*xiao dan* 消癉) and a whole range of other disorders in 'fat noble men' (*fei gui ren* 肥貴人), known as 'illnesses of the fats and grains' (*gao liang zhi ji* 高粱之疾).

[91] MWD YY (1985:12); based on comments to *Ling shu* 10 (Nanjing zhongyi xueyuan zhongyixi 1986:108).

[92] Harper (1998:211); see also Ma (1992:265–7).

[93] MWD YY (1985:9). Compare with *Ling shu* 10, p. 304, quoted on p. 245.

flavours are 'pungent and bitter' (*xin, ku* 辛苦), its *qi* is 'warming' (*wen* 溫) and it 'contains toxicity' (*you du* 有毒). It enters the spleen and stomach channels (as Yi notes in line 34). Its main indication is that 'it dries up the damp and transforms phlegm' (*zao shi hua tan* 燥濕化痰). It is therefore used for treating 'wind- and cold-induced cough' (*feng han ke sou* 風寒咳嗽), 'phlegm- and damp-induced cough' (*tan shi ke sou* 痰濕咳嗽), 'wheezing due to phlegm that obstructs the lungs' (*tan chuan bi fei* 痰喘閉肺) and 'depleted *qi* of the lungs and spleen' (*fei pi qi xu* 肺脾氣虛).[94] Interestingly, most of the above-listed 'distinguishing patterns' concern the lungs and one even lung depletion. It is of course unacceptable to the medical historian to elucidate the use of *ban xia* in the early Han on the grounds of contemporary Chinese medical knowledge. Needless to say that a physician of the Western Han did not conceive of disorders as 'distinguishing patterns' and had no concept of 'phlegm' (*tan* 痰), and that ideas about the therapeutic use of *Pinellia ternata*, and for that matter the identification of the referent itself, may have changed over time.

Incidentally, *ban xia* is already mentioned in the early medical manuscripts.[95] It is mostly externally applied, as in the Mawangdui 'Recipes', where it treats chin abscesses.[96] This may explain why Yi emphasises that the Grand Physician applied it orally and made the patient drink a bolus. The Grand Physician probably administered *ban xia* with the intention to treat the lungs,[97] because the earliest *materia medica*, the *Shennong ben cao jing* of presumably the first century CE, in its reconstructed edition, mentions among the many disorders that *ban xia* treats 'slight coughing' (*ke ni* 咳逆),[98] a complaint characteristic of any long-term deterioration of the lungs. Yi, however, may have conceived of *ban xia* as a 'potent/poisonous drug' (*du yao*), as it later became classified among the 'inferior drugs' (*xia pin* 下品), which 'have potency/toxicity' (*you du* 有毒).[99] In lines 33–4, he reports that this harmed the interior (*zhong*), which is in line with the above canonical medical understanding that *ban xia* enters the spleen and stomach channels. However, Yi also mentions the abdomen (*fu*) in line 34. This poses problems unless one considers *fu* an interjection by a commentator who was not familiar with medical rationale.

[94] ZHYH (1993:1300–1304). See also ZYDCD (1986:775, no. 1550). Not to be confused with *Arisaema consanguineum* Schott (ZYDCD 1986:329, no. 0656), as does Bridgman (1955:76–8).

[95] For *ban xia* in the early manuscript literature, see Zhang (1997:18). See Gansusheng wenwu kaogu yanjiusuo (1991:563A), Gansusheng bowuguan and Wuweixian wenhuaguan (1975:9, 12–13; S55, S8A, S80B), Fuyang Hanjian zhenglizu (1988:37, 39; W016, W064).

[96] MWD 'Recipes' (1985:68, S378–9), Ma (1992:599), Harper (1998:293).

[97] Taki Motokata claims *ban xia wan* is a 'draining and purging recipe' (*xie xia ji* 瀉下劑), but today it is mainly used for treating 'cold *qi* in the upper *jiao*' (*shang jiao leng qi* 上焦冷氣). Today, the bolus of *ban xia* contains additionally *Syzygium aromaticum* (L.) Merr. and Perry (*ding xiang* 丁香) and a processed form of *Zingiber officinale* Rosc. (*bao jiang* or *pao jiang* 泡姜). See ZHYH (1993:1303).

[98] *Shennong ben cao jing* 4, no. 244, p. 335.

[99] On potency/toxicity of drugs, see Unschuld (1986b) and Obringer (1997).

Thirdly, the Grand Physician cauterised the minor *yin mai*. The Mawangdui 'Yinyang vessel text' provides again a possible explanation. Among the disorders that the minor *yin mai* produces is *dan* 'overexertion', and in case 6 the patient suffered from *fei xiao dan*: cauterisation of the minor *yin* is recommended for treating weakened, and presumably emaciated, patients. We are reminded of the above treatment recommendation (quoted on p. 257). There is no need to impute the irrational into it merely because it is ancient and other.

In Yi's view, the adverse effect of the Grand Physician's treatment was that 'the hardness of the liver was harmed' (*shi huai gan gang*; line 36). According to the Mawangdui 'Yinyang vessel text', the foot's minor *yin* vessel is attached to the kidneys or, perhaps rather, the buttocks,[100] but according to the 'Zubi vessel text', it 'comes out at the liver' (*chu gan* 出 肝).[101] This may explain why, according to Yi, cauterising the minor *yin mai* harmed the hardness of the liver. The Grand Physician and Yi seem to have adhered to medical rationale of different lineages.

Yi then says the Grand Physician 'doubly diminished' (*chong sun*) the *qi* of the patient (line 37), an idiom which brings to mind 'doubling the exhaustion' (*chong jie*) in *Ling shu* 1: 'If, although the *qi* of the five viscera is already severed/exhausted inside the body, one uses needles and repletes its outer parts, this is called "doubling the exhaustion"; a doubling of the exhaustion necessarily leads to death' (*wu zang zhi qi, yi jue yu nei, er yong zhen zhe, fan shi qi wai, shi wei chong jie, chong jie bi si* 五藏之氣 已絕於內 而用鍼者 反實其外 是謂重竭 重竭必死).[102] 'Doubling the exhaustion' in *Ling shu* 1 arises when a doctor needles a patient and thereby increases *qi* in the superficial body parts, which in a patient whose visceral *qi* is already exhausted, doubles the exhaustion. This rationale does not apply to case 6. However, it also is an iatrogenic condition.

It is not clear what 'doubly' diminished the patient's *qi*. The Grand Physician's treatment has three steps, but effected a double diminishment of *qi*. One could object that any number of therapeutic steps can doubly diminish *qi*, or if one insists that there must have been two, that the first two were conceived of as one, as they both harmed only one body part: the abdominal part of the interior (*fu zhong*). Or one could suggest line 37 was later

---

[100] MWD YY (1985:12), Ma (1992:258) and Harper (1998:210) follow *Ling shu* 10, p. 303, where the foot's minor *yin mai* is attached to the kidneys and read the graph in question as *shen* 'kidneys'. Ma (1992:259) specifies that it is only given in one out of the three versions of the MWD YY, the *jia ben* 甲本 (no. 1). Rudolf Pfister (2000 p.c.) examined the graph on the published photographs available and found that only the lower part of the graph is legible, but not the upper one. In other words, there is no graph 'kidneys' (*shen* 腎) in any of the three versions of MWD YY! ZJS 'Maishu' (2001:78, S39; 241) has *tun* 臀 'buttocks' on the photo of the strip, according to Pfister (2000 p.c.), but kidneys in transcription.

[101] The connection to the liver is also mentioned in the paragraph on the minor *yin* in *Ling shu* 10, p. 303, in the section 'As to its main axis' (*qi zhi zhe* 其直者), which often contains parallels to the MWD ZB. On the liver, see also ch. 4, n. 63 and n. 65.

[102] *Ling shu* 1, p. 265.

interjected. The noted slight incongruence is reinforced by another one: the minor *yang* vessel is closely connected to the interior/centre in case 1 (lines 34–5), which was found to arise from a coagulation of blood in the centrally located pre-canonical liver/womb, but in case 6, the cauterising of the minor *yin* is said to harm the hardness of the liver. This slight inconsistency in medical rationale prompts text critical investigations, first, of line 36, then of lines 33–4 and finally of lines 31 and 35.

Line 36 contains two idioms that deserve closer scrutiny. The first is *gan gang* 'hardness of the liver', which poses problems to the commentators. Ando Koretora quotes *Su wen* 8, where the liver is the office of the military general and accordingly, he says, the liver is hard. Taki Motohiro cites *Ling shu* 10: 'The sinews are for hardness' (*jin wei gang* 筋為剛).[103] We are here reminded that *Ling shu* 46 mentions hardness as an attribute of anger (quoted on p. 240), although the anger there arises not in the liver, but in the heart as seat of all emotion and cognition, as it was in pre-dynastic times (and continued to be in some contexts). Anger has negative connotations in that context, as it generally does in canonical medical doctrine, but not every anger is negative.[104] The 'hardness of the liver' in line 36 reminds us of the positively valued 'firmness' of the 'form' (*xing*) in the *Guanzi* (quoted on p. 30) and of the flesh and viscera in several canonical medical texts.[105]

The two words *jue shen* 絕甚 in line 36 are not usually found in this combination in medical writings, but *jue* 絕 is frequent.[106] It is used in different senses, too many to discuss here. In canonical medical texts it sometimes means, quite literally, to cut apart (as, for instance, 'to cut the skin' *jue pi* 絕皮),[107] but it usually describes the severing of a string-like structure, such as a vessel or a link (as in lines 40–1). Thus, *Ling shu* 7, after prohibiting needling *mai* close to the body surface, recommends severing these string-like structures by pressing onto them: 'By pressing, sever these vessels, and needle them only then' (*an jue qi mai, nai ci zhi* 按絕其脈 乃刺之).[108] Or, in *Ling shu* 19, it is the string-like structure of the duct to the eye that is said to be severed: 'If the ducts to the eyes are severed, after one and a half days, then one will die' (*mu xi jue, yi ri ban ze si yi* 目系絕 一日半則死矣).[109] In case 1 (line 24), we encountered *jue* as a quality of *mai*,[110] i.e. a string-like

---

[103] *Su wen* 8, p. 28; *Ling shu* 10, p. 299.
[104] On 'anger' as a morally justified emotion, see Rosaldo (1980). On the therapeutic use of anger, see Sivin (1995e). On anger in contemporary Chinese medicine, see Ots (1990b).
[105] *Su wen* 3, p. 14. See also case 5 (line 15), case 6 (line 3), case 7 (line 13).
[106] Taki Motohiro points to a variant *niu* 紐 'to be knotted'. According to Harper (1985:475ff.), *niu* is a 'knot which can be untied', while *jie* is a 'knot which cannot be untied'.
[107] For *jue pi* 絕皮, see *Su wen* 25, p. 79; *Ling shu* 7, pp. 288–9. For *jue pi fu* 絕皮膚, see *Ling shu* 19, p. 328. For *jue fu* 絕膚, see *Su wen* 61, p. 165.
[108] *Ling shu* 7, p. 288.   [109] *Ling shu* 19, p. 298.
[110] See also e.g. *Su wen* 18, p. 55, or *Ling shu* 10, p. 305. On *jue* 絕 as *xuan* 懸, see Ma (1992:261).

mai. In *Su wen* 27 *jue* means 'to terminate a person's long life' (*jue ren chang ming* 絕人長命),[111] the implication being, perhaps, that life is like a string? In addition, '*jue* means to be exhausted' (*jue jin ye* 絕盡也), according to the commentator Gao You 高誘 (ca 168–212), in a gloss on the phrase in the *Huainanzi*: 'the Yangtze and the Yellow river and the three tributaries were exhausted and did not flow' (*jiang he san chuan jue er bu liu* 江河 三川 絕而不流).[112] Even in the sense of 'being exhausted', *jue* invokes a string-like structure: the river bed, within which the flow of water ceases – yet another landscape metaphor implicit to a medical term.

Relevant for *jue* in case 6 is the Mawangdui 'Zubi vessel text', which uses *jue* to refer to the string-like structure of a 'torn sinew/tendon' (*jue jin*): 'In cases of a *yang* [vessel] disorder, a broken bone or a torn sinew, but no *yin* [vessel] disorder, death does not occur' (*yang bing zhe gu jue jin er wu yin bing, bu si* 陽病折骨絕筋而無陰病 不死).[113] Considering that in canonical doctrine, the sinews are an aspect of the liver, and Yi speaks of the liver being *jue* (ruptured, torn), we note a second and direct parallel to the rationale in the Mawangdui 'Zubi vessel text'.

Evidently, line 36 with idioms like 'hardness of the liver' (*gan gang*) and its 'rupturing' (*jue*) shows striking continuities to the early medical manuscripts; it probably testifies to second-century medical rationale. By contrast, the bisyllabic word forms *bing zhe* 病者 (patient), *xie zhu* 泄注 (to leak) and, arguably *fu zhong* 腹中 (abdominal part of the interior) in lines 33–4, which speak of the harm of *Pinellia* in line with canonical medical rationale, probably were interjected.[114] Since early medical manuscripts report on *Pinellia* treatment, the cauterisation of the major *yang* and of the minor *yin*, it is difficult to make a strong case that reference to any represents a later addition to the text. From a grammatical viewpoint, however, lines 32–3 which report on the *Pinellia* treatment are probably an interjection.

In summary, it was possible to find parallels in medical rationale for every step leading to the aggravation of the patient's condition. Thus, the Mawangdui 'Yinyang vessel text' provides a possible rationale for the Grand Physician's cauterisations: that of the minor *yang* is indicated if the patient is 'without fatty tissue' (*wu gao*) and that of the minor *yin* for treating 'utter exhaustion' (*dan*). Yi's rationale for the adverse effects on the abdominal part of the interior (line 34) or liver (line 36) after cautery of the minor *yang* can be interpreted to show continuity with case 1. The

---

[111] *Su wen* 27, p. 85. See also *Su wen* 70, p. 208.

[112] *Huainanzi* 8, p. 802, p. 815.

[113] MWD ZB (1985:5, S23). See also S22 and MWD 'Recipes' (1985:30, S32; 31, S38; 53, S239). In MWD 'Tianxia zhi dao tan' (1985:164, S32;165, S38), *jue* is the sixth of the seven detriments (Harper 1998:431): 'To force it when desire is lacking is "curtailment"' (*fu yu qiang zhi yue jue* 弗欲強之 曰絕).

[114] The phrases beginning with (*bing* [*zhe*]) 'the patient' in case 6 (lines 33–4) and case 10 (line 8) cause slight medical incongruencies (see also p. 338–9).

harm to the liver after cautery of the minor *yin* is in line with the Mawang-dui 'Zubi vessel text', where the minor *yin* connects to the liver.

Prognosticatory calculations (lines 39–46)   The last two stanzas both begin with Yi stating his intention to explain the numerical aspect of the prediction contained in the 'Model' (lines 10–12).[115] In cases 6, 7, 8, 12, 15 and 24 Yi cites a 'Model' for making quantified prognostications on the course of the illness and the time span before death. The prognosticatory calculations are grounded in a numerology of five in cases 1, 6 and 8.

yang brightness and madness (lines 39–42)   The first of the two stanzas on prognostication (lines 39–42) does not actually explain why it was after three days that the client went into a state matching madness, although it purports to do so in its opening statement. This is somewhat odd (and indicative of a late commentatorial interjection?). It reports instead on a sequence of the postulated processes inside the body which affect the *yang* brightness and lead to a state that matches 'madness' (*kuang*). The stanza is rife with references to tubular structures, reminiscent of case 1 (lines 41–4) and case 10 (lines 19–22). Based on textual anomalies, the stanza in case 10 can be shown to be a commentatorial interjection. By analogy, as is argued here, this may also be the case for the corresponding stanzas in cases 1 and 6.

The architectural structures the text reports on are 'links' (*luo*), not viscera. In particular, Yi mentions a link between the liver and the *yang* brightness (line 40). This link differs from the 'links' in the medical canons, which often are 'linking vessels' (*luo mai*) or 'second-generation, tiny links' (*sun luo* 孫絡) on the body surface.[116] It reminds one of the manifold internal tubular structures mentioned in the *Inner Canon*. Among them was a 'large link of the stomach', as in *Su wen* 18: 'The large link of the stomach is called "the empty place", it pierces through the diaphragm, links to the lungs, and exits underneath the left breast, its movements resonate with one's clothes' (*wei zhi da luo, ming yue xu li, guan ge luo fei, chu yu zuo ru xia, qi dong ying yi* 胃之大絡 名曰虛里 貫鬲絡肺 出於左乳下 其動應衣).[117] Large links were bag-like. *Ling shu* 10 says the 'large link of the spleen' (*pi zhi da luo* 脾之大絡) is called 'large bag' (*da bao* 大包).[118] Elsewhere, it mentions the 'pericard', generally translated as 'heart-bag link', which could

---

[115] If one alters the punctuation, as Ando Koretora notes, Yi refers to a 'Model for Treatment' (Zhi fa 治法). But this is unlikely, since line 8, 'A doctor should not treat this one' (*bu dang yi zhi*), reoccurs in section 4.4.

[116] In *Su wen* 63, p. 172, *sun luo* contrast with *da luo* (large links) as part of the *jing luo* system. The 'large links' of *Su wen* 18, *Ling shu* 10 and 18 by contrast are large structures inside the body trunk.

[117] *Su wen* 18, p. 55; *xu li* 虛里 'the empty place', following Hermann Tessenow (2000 p.c.), but see Unschuld (2003:126).

[118] *Ling shu* 10, p. 307.

also be conceived of as a 'bag-link' or 'baggy link of the heart' (*xin bao luo* 心包絡).[119] *Ling shu* 60 mentions another 'large link' (*da luo*) attached to the stomach: 'That through which *qi* and blood exit the stomach is the channel-tunnel. The channel-tunnel is the large link of the five viscera and the six bowels' (*wei zhi suo chu qi xue zhe, jing sui ye; jing sui zhe, wu zang liu fu zhi da luo ye* 胃之所出氣血者 經隧也, 經隧者 五臟六府之大絡也).[120] The 'channel-tunnel' (*jing sui*), issued by the stomach, is a link between the viscera and bowels, which reminds us of the one Yi mentions between liver and *yang* brightness.

The *Ling shu* mentions many more large tubular structures inside the body and on its surface that were considered 'links' (*luo*). Thus, *Ling shu* 4 refers to a 'large link' visible on the body surface and *Ling shu* 19, 27 and 75 to 'large links' close to the body surface, some apparently filled with blood.[121] By contrast, *Ling shu* 62 has 'large links of *qi*': 'The four extremities are the gathering [place] of *yin* and *yang*, these are the large links of *qi*' (*fu si mo yin yang zhi hui zhe, ci qi zhi da luo ye* 夫四末陰陽之會者 此氣之大絡也).[122] *Ling shu* 38 and 62 refer to a 'large link of the minor *yin*' (*shao yin da luo* 少陰大絡).[123] In the light of these different links, it is not surprising Yi speaks of a link between the liver and *yang* brightness, although no textual parallel was found for it.[124]

The relation between the area 'beneath the nipples' (*ru xia* 乳下) and the *yang* brightness vessel (line 40) is well established in both the Mawangdui vessel texts[125] and in *Ling shu* 10.[126] Zhang Shoujie cites the *Su wen* (not in extant version): 'The *yang* brightness underneath the nipples is the stomach link' (*ru xia yang ming wei luo ye* 乳下陽明胃絡也). The term 'stomach link' (*wei luo* 胃絡), to which Zhang Shoujie refers, is probably the same as the 'large link of the stomach' (*wei zhi da luo*), mentioned in the above-quoted *Su wen* 18.

A damaged *yang* brightness gives rise to madness (lines 41–2). This is well-known. The Mawangdui 'Yinyang vessel text' contains, among the disorders that an agitated *yang* brightness *mai* produces, detailed descriptions approximating what people feel and do in a psychotic state. The corresponding *Ling shu* 10 uses the same circumscriptions, and mentions also the word *kuang* 狂 (madness). *Su wen* 30, the chapter on the *yang* brightness to which Ando Koretora refers, contains statements of much the same kind: 'The heat becomes abundant in the body, hence one throws off one's clothes and intends to run' (*re sheng yu shen, gu qi yi yu zou ye* 熱盛於身 故

---

[119] e.g. *Ling shu* 10, p. 303.   [120] *Ling shu* 60, p. 420.
[121] *Ling shu* 4, p. 278; 19, p. 331; 27, p. 384; 75, p. 462.
[122] *Ling shu* 62, p. 425.   [123] *Ling shu* 38, p. 373; 62, p. 425.
[124] *yun shu jie* 運屬結 'connecting and binding knot' (line 40), based on *shu jie* 屬結 'colon vessel' in Hübotter (1927:12); no textual parallels for either have been found in the *Inner Canon*.
[125] MWD ZB and YY (1985:4, 10).   [126] *Ling shu* 10, p. 300.

棄衣欲走也).[127] So, when 'heat becomes abundant' (*re sheng* 熱盛), one throws off one's clothes; but, as stated elsewhere in *Su wen* 30, when '*yang* becomes abundant' (*yang sheng* 陽盛), one 'runs about in a delirium' (*wang zou* 妄走). Yi speaks of the '*yang* brightness *mai* getting damaged' (*yang ming mai shang*), rather than of an 'abundance of *yang*', and of *dang kuang zou* 'running about in a state matching madness' rather than of *wang zou* 'running about in a delirium'. However, notions of 'delirium', 'madness' and 'states matching madness' are not well defined and refer to a similar experiential realm.

According to contemporary Chinese medical textbooks, 'delirium' and 'madness' (*zhan kuang* 譫狂) is a heart disorder, and not mentioned among the stomach disorders.[128] In contemporary medical practice, however, not only the heart but also the stomach are taken into account in a case of delirium and madness.[129] This is one of many instances, where practice, as opposed to written theory, retains knowledge of former times.

In summary, instead of providing prognosticatory calculations, this stanza details processes in tubular structures leading to the delirium. It first refers to a link, not attested elsewhere in the canonical medical literature, between the liver and the *yang* brightness (the canonical stomach). The link got severed, the *yang* brightness *mai* damaged and the patient became delirious. Parallels for this process of damage to the *yang* brightness causing madness are in Mawangdui 'Yinyang vessel text', *Ling shu* 10 and *Su wen* 30.

The prognostication of death (lines 43–6)   Lines 43–6 provide a rationale for the pentic numerology of the 'Model' (lines 10–12). The prognosticatory calculation consists of equating the distance between two viscera, in terms of *fen*, with the time span until death occurs. For expressing the distance between the viscera, Yi uses the expression *xiang qu* 'to be distant from each other'. It is unclear which distance Yi refers to, whether it is one that can be measured on the body surface at the wrist, as some later Japanese commentators suggest,[130] or whether he refers to the distance of the two viscera inside the body.

The 'Model' (line 45) may have been based on a less sophisticated conception of the body than the *Shi ji* personage Yi had. It may have built on the conception of a bipartite body, with 'heart' and 'liver' referring to the upper and lower body spheres respectively. In that case, the 'heart' to which the 'Model' alludes is probably an older and definitely more general term than the lungs mentioned in the name of the disorder.

[127] *Su wen* 30, p. 91.   [128] *Zhongyi jichu lilun* (Yin 1984:30, 44–5).
[129] Fieldwork (1988–9).   [130] e.g. *Kanseki kokujikai*, vol. 7, p. 31.

Note on the cause of the disorder (line 14)

The cause of the disorder is an emotion. Anger is in canonical doctrine located in the liver, and in case 6 the liver was harmed. Notably, not by anger, but by the Grand Physician of Qi's incorrect treatment. In canonical texts, anger gets medicalised and becomes framed in hot/cold complementarities, as in *Ling shu* 46, where the imbalance between a hard inner emotion, anger, and the soft flesh of the bodily frame is given as cause for 'consumption' (quoted on p. 240).[131]

Discussion

Cases 6 and 1 stand out for their length and composite character of disorders which end with the patient's death after five plus three days. In both cases, Yi is concerned with providing an accurate prognostication of the day of death, although his calculations are minimal and given at the very end of a very long narrative. Both involve 'passageways in disarray' (*jing bing*) and an 'alternating' (*dai*) pulse. While case 1 is concerned with two consecutive stages of one disorder, case 6 discusses two named disorders. The first relates to medical rationale presented in the usual formulaic way; the second is an iatrogenic illness caused by a disregard for treatment interdictions.

Some Chinese researchers are adamant that case 6 contains the first recording of diabetes in Chinese medical history, but this is contested here. Instead, a 'link of the liver', mentioned in a presumably interjected passage (lines 40–1), is interpreted to refer to the portal vein. Given its distinctive thumb-thick appearance, it is not impossible that Chinese medical doctors, like the ancient Greeks, recognised it and linked its dysfunction to the striking clinical observations that can be made between a patient's food intake and subsequent delirium-like strange behaviour.

The iatrogenic illness in the second part is caused by a court physician. Yi's statements on treatment interdiction and therapeutic intervention can all be elucidated with textual parallels: the former, mostly with canonical texts, the latter, with the Mawangdui vessel texts. Interestingly, the rationale of both the Grand Physician of Qi and Yi tally well with knowledge recorded in the vessel texts from distinct medical lineages. Historians agree that the Mawangdui 'Yinyang vessel text' became canonised in large parts.[132] No wonder the court physician adhered to its rationale, while Yi's medical rationale echoes the Mawangdui 'Zubi vessel text'.

Text structure semantics can be applied to elucidating the trisyllabic name, *fei xiao dan,* although Yi mentions only two pulse qualities, namely 'qi [coming] from the lungs' (*fei qi*), which is 'hot' (*re*). The correlation

---

[131] *Ling shu* 46, p. 388.   [132] Keegan (1988), Han (1999).

between *fei qi* and *fei* is straightforward, and for that between being 'hot' and *xiao dan* (wasting heat-from-overexertion) many textual parallels were found; *xiao dan* is a frequently encountered compound word in the medical canons. Case 6 thus concerns a 'lung consumption'.

Three further pulse qualities are mentioned in case 6, two in the 'Mai fa', namely 'uneven' (*bu ping*) and 'not drumming' (*bu gu*), and one in Yi's comments on the 'Mai fa', 'alternating' (*dai*). Yi describes the tactile experience of 'alternating', but not of the two other pulses, which have notoriously variable meanings. Yi appears to use them in a sense that differs from that in the most representative scholarly medical texts. This could be taken as a hint that he quotes a saying at the interface of popular and scholarly medical knowledge. No parallels have been found in the extant medical literature for the entire 'Mai fa' quote, but each of its three terms occurs at least once in the *Inner Canon*.

17

Case 7

Translation (*Shiki kaichû kôshô* 105, pp. 35–6)

1. Pan Manru, the Commandant of the Capital of Qi, fell ill
2. with pain in the minor abdomen.
3. Your servant, Yi, examined his *mai* and <u>said</u>:

Name:
4. 'It is a conglomeration of remanent accumulations.'
5. Your servant, Yi, then said to the Grand Coachman Rao and to the Clerk of the Capital Yao:
6a. 'If the Commandant does not any further restrain himself from an indulgence in women,
6b. then he will die in thirty days.'

7. After twenty-odd days, he passed blood and died.

Cause:
8. <u>The illness was contracted from</u> wine and women.

Quality:
9. <u>The means whereby I recognised</u> Pan Manru's illness were that
10. when I, your servant, Yi, pressed onto his *mai*, they were deep, small and soft,
11. abruptly they were confused,
12. this is *qi* [coming] from the spleen.
13. At the right *mai*'s opening, *qi* arrived tight and small,
14. it manifested as *qi* [coming] from conglomerations.

1. 齊中尉潘滿如病
2. 少腹痛
3. 臣意診其脈曰

4. 遺積瘕也
5. 臣意即謂齊太僕臣饒內史臣繇曰

6. 中尉不復自止於內則三十日死

7. 後二十餘日 溲血死

8. 病得之酒且內

9. 所以知潘滿如病者

10. 臣意切其脈 深小弱
11. 其卒然合合也
12. 是脾氣也
13. 右脈口氣至緊小

14. 見瘕氣也

15. They [the *mai*] took turns in mutually riding on each other,

15. 以次相乘

16. <u>hence</u> [I said] he would die after thirty days.

16. 故三十日死

17. In cases where the three *yin* are entirely united, it is according to the 'Model'.

17. 三陰俱搏者 如法

18. In cases where they are not entirely united, the decision resides within the 'intensive time span'.

18. 不俱搏者 決在急期

19. In cases where they once are united and once are alternating, [death] is near.

19. 一搏一代者 近也

20. <u>Hence</u> when the three *yin* struck, he passed blood and died as [said] above.

20. 故其三陰搏 溲血如前止

Interpretation

After specifying the pain that the disorder involves (line 2), Yi names it (line 4). He then addresses Pan Manru's entourage, prognosticating death unless he changes his behaviour (line 6). His prognostication is basically verified, although death occurs sooner than predicted (line 7). Yi then states the cause of the disorder (line 8). The remainder is medical speculation (lines 9–20).

Critical evaluation of retrospective biomedical diagnoses

Bridgman diagnoses a cancer of the bladder on the assumption that *sou xue* 溲血 means 'to urinate blood'.[1] Lu & Needham do not discuss this case. It abounds in medical speculation and mentions only two complaints that can be used for biomedical diagnosis: pain in the minor abdomen (line 2) and *sou xue* (lines 7, 20), which can also mean 'to defecate blood' or 'to have a haemorrhage'. It triggered the patient's death.

Although the wise option is not to hazard a guess, further possible diagnoses that come to mind are septicaemia, which tends to be lethal, and subacute diverticulitis, which typically arises when undigested food residues are retained and form into a hard mass, known as *fecalith*.[2] The latter often presents with lower abdominal pain and fever, and may lead to an abscess of the colon. If the abscess ruptures, there can be a haemorrhage. Simultaneously, the pus and blood of the abscess can break through internally and invade the abdomen causing peritonitis that results in death.

The name of the disorder (line 4)

Introductory remarks   Cases 7 and 19 both concern a *jia* disorder. Interestingly, for explaining each, different medical texts prove useful. Thus, for

---

[1] Bridgman (1955:80).   [2] *Harrison's* (1987:1293).

elucidating case 7, the *Su wen* is useful, and for elucidating *jia* in case 19, the *Zhu bing yuan hou lun* entry on *rao jia* 蟯瘕 (and other infestations classified as *jia*) provides parallels, but not the *Su wen*. This in itself is noteworthy. *Jia* was a condition sufficiently undifferentiated to have already been elaborated in early medicine in rather different ways.[3] It highlights again a difference in nosological understandings between cases 1–10 and 11–25.

The name of the disorder, *yi ji jia*, could be either a '*yiji* conglomeration' (*yiji jia*) or '*yi* accumulations and conglomerations' (*yi jijia*). Taki Motokata treats *jia* as a superordinate term, as do other commentators, but text structure semantics will provide evidence in favour of the second reading. The texts with most parallels to case 7 are in *Su wen* 48,[4] but the parallels are tenuous. *Su wen* 48 mentions the 'minor abdomen' (*shao fu*) in the first paragraph, relates the pulse quality 'small' (*xiao*) to 'conglomerations' (*jia*) in the second, and correlates the three *yang* with 'conglomerations' in the third.[5] Instead of dwelling on these few parallels, *jia* is explored throughout the early and canonical medical literature in what follows.

***jia* 瘕 – conglomerations in the Mawangdui and Zhangjiashan medical manuscripts** The term *jia* is mentioned both in the Mawangdui and Zhangjiashan manuscripts. In the Mawangdui 'Yinyang vessel text', *jia* is mentioned once as one of the five disorders to which the arm's major *yin mai* gives rise,[6] and possibly among the ten lethal disorders of the major *yin mai* of the stomach, in the context of discussing 'pond-water diarrhoea' (*tang xie* 溏泄). However, the text is corrupt in the position that may have been occupied by *jia*: 'If there is a pond-water diarrhoea, one dies; if there is x x blockage together, then one dies' (*tang xie, si; x x bi tong ze si* 溏泄死 x x 閉同則死).[7] The corresponding text in *Ling shu* 10 has a modified word sequence: *tang jia xie, shui bi* 溏瘕泄 水閉; but *Su wen* 74 gives one that could be faithfully replicating the Mawangdui text: *tang xie jia shui bi* 溏泄瘕水閉.[8] Terms like *tang xie* and *tang jia* also occur elsewhere in canonical medical texts[9] and contemporary Chinese medicine.[10]

The Zhangjiashan 'Maishu' differentiates between seven types of *jia*. Six of them concern troubles in the intestines:

---

[3] Yu (1953:129–30) shows despair because texts on *jia* diverge enormously.
[4] *Su wen* 48, pp. 134–5.
[5] Bridgman (1955:209) notes the parallel, suggesting Yi's source book 'Qi ke shu' 奇咳術 is the 'Da qi lun' 大奇論, the chapter title of *Su wen* 48.
[6] MWD YY (1985:12).
[7] MWD YY (1985:11); *tang* 溏 refers to fine mud or silt. See HYDCD 6.34.
[8] *Ling shu* 10, p. 301, and *Su wen* 74, p. 233.
[9] e.g. *Zhen jiu jia yi jing* 11.5, p. 1746.
[10] *tang xie* is diarrhoea with visible undigested pieces in the faeces (fieldwork 1988–9).

[The disorder] ...

if it resides in the midst of the intestines and if, when small, it is like a large wart,[11] and if, when large like a cup, it due to its hardness is painful, and if it oscillates,[12] it is a male conglomeration.

If [the disorder] resides in the midst of the intestines, and if there is pain, it is a blood conglomeration.

If there is a [parasitic] infestation,[13] and it arises from the spine and the chest, causing the abdomen to become inflated, and if, while one has the urge to fart,[14] one can only rarely do so, it is a *qi* conglomeration.

[If there is an infestation],[15] and the abdomen swells and it is in appearance like the skin when it expands,[16] and there is a croaking like a concert of frogs, it is a fat conglomeration.[17]

[If there is an infestation], and the [intestine's] interior gets wound up and causes a narrowing [stenosis],[18] and the upper and lower body parts do not connect, it is a faeces conglomeration.[19]

If [the disorder] resides in the midst of the intestines, and to the left and to the right there are no transformations, and one has diarrhoea, it is a pond-water conglomeration.[20]

[*bing* ... 病 ...]

zai chang zhong, xiao zhe ru ma hou, da zhe ru bei er jian tong, yao, wei pin jia
在腸中 小者如馬侯 大者如盃而堅痛 榣 為牡叚

zai chang zhong, tong, wei xue jia 在腸中 痛 為血叚

---

[11] ZJS 'Maishu' (2001:235); *ma* 馬 means 'large' (*da* 大), *hou* 侯 means 'wart' (*hou* 瘊), according to Gao (1992:16). He cites *Yu pian* B, p. 10a: '*hou* is a wart disorder' (*hou you bing ye* 瘊疣病也).

[12] '*yao* 榣 is the movement of trees' (*yao shu dong ye* 榣 樹動也; *Shuo wen* 6A, p. 25).

[13] *zhou* 肘 means *zhou* 疛, a so-called 'abdominal disorder' (Gao 1992:17).

[14] *de qi* 得氣 (lit. 'to obtain *qi*') is 'farting' (*da pi* 打屁) (Gao 1992:17).

[15] The following two clauses begin with 'it' (*qi* 其), which I understand to refer to the infestation *zhou*.

[16] *zhen* 胗 means 'to swell' (*zhong* 腫), *zhang* 張 means 'to expand' (*zhang* 脹; Gao 1992:17). In corroboration of this reading, see *Shuo wen* 4B, p. 28: "*zhen* is a blister on the lips" (*zhen chun yang ye* 胗唇瘍也) and HYDCD 6.1235: 胗, read as *zhun*, refers to the bulging stomach of a bird.

[17] '*gao* means slippery and lubricant' (*gao hua ze ye* 膏 滑澤也; *Guang ya*, 5A, p. 27a). The inflated skin is glossy and shiny (Gao 1992:17).

[18] I follow Gao (1992:18) in interpreting *yue* 約 as 'to wind' (*chan fu* 纏縛); I do not follow Gao when I interpret *qi* 其 as referring to the '[parasitic] infestation' (*zhou*), *zhong* 裹 as 'interior garment' and *tuo* 隋 as *tuo* 橢, as given in HYDCD 11.1057; *tuo* 橢 means 'narrow and long' (*xia er chang ye* 狹而長也), according to Zhu Xi's (1130–1200) gloss on the phrase in the *Chu ci* 3, p. 66: 'From the north to the south the earth is longer and narrower' (*nan bei shun tuo* 南北順橢). Translation by Hawkes (1959:49).

[19] 柣 is 'socle' (*zhi* 楮; Gao 1992:18) or 'faeces' (*shi* 矢; ZJS 2001:235).

[20] The text continues: 'If [the disorder] resides in the intestines, and to the left and right there are no transformations, it is a blocked interior' (*zai chang, zuo you bu hua, wei sai zhong* 在腸 左右不化 為塞中).

zhou, qi cong ji xiong qi, shi fu zhang, de qi er shao ke, qi jia ye.
肘 其從脊胸起 使腹張 得氣而少可 氣叚也

qi fu zhen zhen ru fu zhang zhuang, wu ru xia yin, gao jia ye.
其腹胗胗如膚張狀 嗚如蝦音 膏叚也

qi zhong yue tuo, shang xia bu tong, shi jia ye.
其裹約隋 上下不通 柣叚也

zai chang zhong, zuo you bu hua, xie, wei tang jia 在腸中 左右不化 泄
為唐叚

The most striking aspect in the above text is the almost identical structure of the sentences describing the 'male conglomeration' (*mu jia*), the 'blood conglomeration' (*xue jia*) and the 'pond-water conglomeration' (*tang jia*). In each case, the sentence begins with the phrase 'If [the disorder] resides in the intestinal parts of the interior' (*zai chang zhong*), and sometime thereafter a one-word statement is made 'If it oscillates' (*yao*) or 'If it is painful' (*tong*) or 'If it leaks out [i.e. if one has diarrhoea]' (*xie*), followed by the statement 'It is an AB conglomeration'. In the above reading, which is based on recent text critical studies that view even early manuscript texts as compilations, the three clauses on the 'infestation' (*zhou*) are taken as a mini-text that was interpolated after the first two on the 'male' and 'blood conglomeration'.[21]

The term *zhou* generally is given as 'abdominal disorder'. As argued here, it refers more specifically to a '[parasitic] infestation'. The conglomerations arising from an infestation are called '*qi* conglomeration' (*qi jia*), 'fat conglomeration' (*gao jia*) and 'faeces conglomeration' (*shi jia*), names closely linked to their appearance: airy like farts and *qi*, slippery and shiny like frog-skins and fat, and bulging like the socle of a pillar or faeces. These three conglomerations differ from the other three not only in their naming. The text contains no indication that the 'male conglomeration', the 'blood conglomeration' and the 'pond-water conglomeration' are [parasitic] infestations. This suggests already a mid-second-century manuscript outlines two different types of 'conglomerations'.

The common definition of *zhou* is 'abdominal disorder', most prominently in *Shuo wen* 7B: '*zhou* is an illness of the small abdomen' (*zhou xiao fu bing* 疛 小腹病).[22] However, as argued here, this 'abdominal disorder' may have been considered to arise primarily because of a 'parasitic infestation'. With regard to the above *Shuo wen* entry, Duan Yucai insists that *xiao fu*

---

[21] The male conglomeration 'oscillates', the blood conglomeration is 'painful'; their name and determining feature allude to gender-specific activity and experience of the male and female reproductive organs.

[22] *Shuo wen* 7B, p. 29a–b.

should read *xin fu* 心腹, which makes out of *zhou* an 'illness of the heart and abdomen' (*xin fu bing* 心腹病).[23] This raises the question of what a *xin fu bing* is. Although the term *xin fu bing* does occur in the *Zhu bing yuan hou lun* and other medical works as a superordinate syndrome, contemporary dictionaries have hardly anything to say on it.[24]

In the non-medical literature of particularly Han times and later, 'illnesses of heart and abdomen' were contrasted with 'illnesses of the feet and hands' or of the 'four limbs'. This suggests that they were understood to refer to internal problems as opposed to superficial and external ones. Thus, *Hou Han shu* 66 relates 'sufferings in heart and abdomen' (*xin fu zhi huan* 心腹之患) to serious problems of 'internal government affairs' (*nei zheng* 內政) and opposes them to the outer 'illnesses of the four limbs' (*si zhi zhi ji* 四支之疾), problems at the periphery of the state.[25]

However, in the *Zhan guo ce* of the Warring States, the troubles in heart and abdomen are compared to a parasitic infestation in wood: 'The state of Qin had the state of Han, much like wood has parasites and people are troubled in heart and abdomen' (*Qin zhi you Han, ruo mu zhi you du, ren zhi you bing xin fu* 秦之有韓 若木之有蠹 人之有病心腹).[26] In the Warring States, 'being troubled in heart and abdomen' invokes a chronic condition, which typically cannot be eradicated and has become an intrinsic part of one's very existence. This persistent malaise in wood is caused by parasites, but in man by the daily worries of heart and abdomen. Such was my initial reading of the text. Now, if this sentence were to describe a parasitic relationship three times – of the state of Han towards the state of Qin, of parasites to wood and of 'being troubled in heart and abdomen' to man – *bing xin fu* may not primarily refer to emotional worries (associated with the heart as seat of emotion) as much as to those caused by parasitic infestations (in the body architectural upper and particularly lower abdominal spheres). This is said in awareness that emotional and digestive troubles are often interrelated and from an experiential point of view are difficult to disentangle.

In corroboration of the idea that troubles in the heart/stomach and abdomen may primarily have been considered to be caused by parasites, a phrase in a manuscript from Wuwei comes to mind: 'In order to treat the heart-and-abdomen's large accumulations that go up and down and have an appearance as if they were bugs...' (*zhi xin fu da ji shang xia xing ru chong zhuang* 治心腹大積上下行如蟲狀).[27] Admittedly, this quote could be used as counterevidence against the idea that *xin fu bing* refers to infestations by bugs: it concerns large accumulations in heart and abdomen that

---

[23] *xin* 心 is the body architectural sphere above the diaphragm, see cases 2 (line 13), 9 (line 11).
[24] *Zhu bing yuan hou lun* 16, pp. 513–20. The nine entries are in content so diverse that it is difficult to find commonalities between them.
[25] *Hou Han shu* 66, p. 2164, quoted in Rosner (1991:28).
[26] *Zhan guo ce* 5, 'Qin san' 秦三, p. 192. Translation by Crump (1970:106).
[27] Gansusheng bowuguan & Wuweixian wenhuaguan (1975:7, S45).

are not parasitic infestations, but have an appearance as if they were bugs. However, one could read into the simile 'as if there were bugs' that it implies that parasitic infestations typically were considered to move up and down in heart and abdomen and, accordingly, that disorders in heart and abdomen typically ,were considered to be caused by parasitic infestation.

Further evidence in favour of reading *zhou* in the Zhangjiashan 'Maishu' as a '[parasitic] infestation' is found when, in respect of the above *Shuo wen* quote, one follows up Gao You's definition of *zhou*, of which Duan Yucai gives an abbreviated version: '*zhou* is an abdominal illness' (*zhou fu bing ye* 疛 腹病也). In fact, Gao You's comment to *Lü shi chun qiu* 3 reads: '*fu* [*zhou*]:[28] there is a jumping and moving, this all belongs among the abdominal illnesses' (*fu [zhou], tiao dong, jie fu bing* 府 [疛] 跳動皆腹病).[29] Here *fu*, which should be read as *zhou*, is collocated with the jumping and moving. What jumps and moves? Surely, bugs, worms and other parasites. In this way, Gao You's comment provides additional evidence that *zhou* refers to a '[parasitic] infestation'.

The above should make clear that in some contexts *zhou* designated a '[parasitic] infestation', which in consideration of the history of hygiene may well have been implied even by those Chinese authors who defined *zhou* in more general terms as an 'abdominal disorder'. If at an early stage in medical history, to which the Zhangjiashan 'Maishu' testifies, *zhou* in the sense of '[parasitic] infestations' are mentioned among *jia* disorders, it may come as no surprise that in later texts *jia* were defined as 'disorders caused by bugs'. This interpretation of *jia* as referring to bug infestations, and the like, is unambiguously given by Guo Pu's 郭璞 (276–324) comment on *Shan hai jing* 1: '*jia* are bug disorders' (*jia chong bing ye* 瘕 蟲病也).[30]

To complicate the issue, the Zhangjiashan 'Maishu' also mentions a conglomeration located outside the digestive tract: 'If the urine comes out white like foam, it is a white conglomeration' (*ruo [ni] chu bai ru mu [mo], wei bai jia* 弱[溺]出白如沐[沬]為白瘕). Modern commentators equate the 'white conglomeration' (*bai jia*) to 'white mucus' (*bai dai* 白帶), and consider the above to describe a gynaecological disorder.[31] They cite *Shuo wen* 7B from the second century CE: '*jia* is a women's disorder' (*jia nü bing ye* 瘕 女病

---

[28] *fu* 府, should here be read as *zhou* 疛 according to Pi Yuan 畢沅 (1730–97).
[29] Gao You (ca 168–212) comments on the sentence in *Lü shi chun qiu* 3.2, p. 4b. 'Flowing water does not become foul ... If the essences do not flow, then the *qi* becomes clogged up. If, when it clogs up ... it resides in the abdomen, then there is an expansion and a [parasitic] infestation' (*liu shui bu fu ... jing bu liu ze qi yu, yu ... chu fu ze wei zhang wei fu [zhou]* 流水不腐 精不流則氣鬱 鬱 處腹則為張為府[疛]). Compare with Knoblock & Riegel (2000:100).
[30] *Shan hai jing* 1, p. 2. For *chong jia* 蟲瘕, see *Ling shu* 24, p. 343. On *chong*, see Fèvre (1993).
[31] e.g. Gao (1992:22–3). Note absence of gender-specificity also in *Su wen* 19, p. 61, quoted on p. 276.

也).[32] Indeed, in later medical texts many types of *jia* are female disorders. However, there is no textual indication in the Zhangjiashan 'Maishu' from the second century BCE that *jia* is a gender-specific disorder.

It is noteworthy that in the Zhangjiashan 'Maishu' conglomerations can be detected through the urine or faeces, and that in Yi's case 7, *sou xue*, apart from referring to a haemorrhage, can mean both to defecate and/or to urinate blood. For a canonical Chinese medical diagnosis, troubles with defecating would be considered indicative of a disorder in the splenetic system, and troubles with urinating of one in the renal system; in a biomedical diagnosis one would distinguish between the digestive tract and the urogenital system. The notion of *jia* does not allude to conceptions of a body known by functions of a splenetic and renal system. It is a disorder that physicians recognised in a body that pre-dates canonical body conceptions.

In summary, the Zhangjiashan 'Maishu' contains a long list of *jia* (conglomerations), which are, however, rather heterogeneous. In the above interpretation of the text, it records three kinds of *jia* 'residing in the midst of the intestines' (*zai chang zhong*), three '[parasitic] infestations' (*zhou*) and one sort of *jia* that affects urination. Yi also mentions both a non-parasitic *jia* conglomeration in the digestive tract (case 7) and *jia* as a parasitic infestation (case 19). From a body architectural viewpoint, *jia* have in common that they occupy the interior bodily sphere. From a canonical medical viewpoint, six *jia* are located in the splenetic tract, and one in the renal tract. Considering that the six *jia* are mentioned in a sequence, the compiler of the Zhangjaishan 'Maishu' already thought along the lines of medical rationale that later became canonised. Although *jia* is in the *Shuo wen* of the second century CE defined as a women's disorder, there is no textual evidence in the Zhangjiashan 'Maishu' that any of the seven *jia* are gender-specific.

jia 瘕 – conglomerations as chronic disorders (line 4)   Taki Motokata considers *yi ji jia* a type of *jia* and enumerates various others: for 'conglomerations' (*jia* 瘕) as opposed to 'amassments' (*shan* 疝) he points to *Su wen* 48,[33] for *shan* [*xian*] *jia* 疝[仙]瘕 he points to *Su wen* 18 and 19,[34] for 'hidden conglomerations' (*mi* [*fu*] *jia* 密[虑]瘕) to *Su wen* 37,[35] for 'women's [discharge] conglomerations and assemblages' (*nü zi* [*dai xia*] *jia ju* 女子[帶下]瘕聚) to *Su wen* 60[36] and *Nan jing* 29,[37] for 'stone conglomerations' (*shi jia* 石瘕) to *Ling shu* 57,[38] for 'diarrhoea of great conglomerations' (*da jia*

---

[32] *Shuo wen* 7B, p. 30b.   [33] *Su wen* 48, p. 135.
[34] *Su wen* 18, p. 55; 19, p. 61.   [35] *Su wen* 37, p. 108.
[36] *Su wen* 60, p. 161, quoted on p. 276.
[37] *Nan jing* 29 (Unschuld 1986a:333) replaces 帶下 with 為.
[38] *Ling shu* 57, p. 414.

xie 大瘕泄) to *Nan jing* 57,[39] for 'solid conglomerations' (*gu jia* 固瘕) to a certain 'Yang ming pian' 陽明篇,[40] for 'conglomerations due to *rao*-worms' (*rao jia* 蟯瘕) to case 19, and one could enumerate many more.[41] Taki Motokata explains that in all those cases there were originally no 'things' (*wu* 物) inside the abdomen, but that due to the illness something took on 'form' (*xing* 形).

In canonical medicine *jia* and *ji* and other related terms take on many meanings. In some canonical texts one finds the idioms *zheng jia*[42] and *ji ju*,[43] in others *zheng* and *jia*, and *ji* and *ju*.[44] Yan Shigu glosses *jia* in the *Ji jiu pian* 急就篇 (Quick Reference Book in Case of Need) as: 'A conglomeration is a [kind of] concretion' (*jia zheng ye* 瘕 癥也).[45] The Song work *Sheng ji zong lu* 聖濟宗籙 states: 'So, there are also *zheng jia* [concretions and conglomerations] and *pi jie* [bits and knots], they are alternative names for *ji ju* [accumulations and assemblages], their manifestations are not uniform, but if you investigate the roots of these disorders, they are generally much alike' (*ran you you zheng jia pi jie zhe, ji ju zhi yi ming ye, zheng zhuang bu yi, yuan qi bing ben da lüe xiang lei* 然又有癥瘕癖結者 積聚之異名也 証狀不一 原其病本大略相類).[46] In contemporary medical practice, one speaks of body internal 'congealments' (*zheng ji* 癥積) and 'coagulates' (*jia ju* 瘕聚), and most practitioners maintain that the latter are more likely to 'have form' (*you xing* 有形). In some cases, this means that they are tangible when the abdomen is palpated, but not always: some processes inside the body are known to have form, even if they are not tangible.[47] From the wealth of information on *jia*, it is difficult to decide which aspects are relevant to the interpretation of case 7.

Perhaps the idea that *jia* 'has form' arises from that of *jia* as a persistent if not chronic condition, as defined in the *Yu pian*: '*jia* is a long-lasting disorder' (*jia jiu bing ye* 瘕 久病也).[48] It is well known that over time soft lumps were considered to harden,[49] and this correlated with their taking on form.

[39] *Nan jing* 57 (Unschuld 1986a:510).

[40] *gu jia* cannot be located in modern editions of the *Inner Canon*. See also computer printout by Hermann Tessenow (2000 p.c.). The 'Yang ming pian' is discussed at length in Keegan (1988).

[41] Several more are enumerated in *Zhongyi dacidian* (1995:1670).

[42] See *Jin gui yao lüe* 4.2, p. 106, and *Zhu bing yuan hou lun* 19, pp. 577–89.

[43] See *Ling shu* 46, p. 389; *Nan jing* 55 (Unschuld 1986a:495); *Jin gui yao lüe* 11.20, p. 314. See also *Zhu bing yuan hou lun* 19, pp. 564–76.

[44] e.g. *Zhongyi dacidian* (1995:1255 on *ji* and *ji ju*; p. 1649 on *ju*; p. 1670 on *jia*; p. 1742 on *zheng* and *zheng jia*). Today, dictionaries differentiate whether or not the pain or lump is moving; an immobile lump is classified as *yin* and a mobile one as *yang*. However, distinctions of this kind need not apply to canonical texts, let alone pre-canonical ones.

[45] *Ji jiu pian* 4, p. 268. The entry on which Yan Shigu glosses reads: 'Amassments and conglomerations, seizures, madness, muteness' (*shan jia dian ji kuang shi xiang* 疝瘕癲疾狂失響).

[46] *Sheng ji zong lu* 71, p. 1263.

[47] Fieldwork (1988–9), clinic notes 17.5.89, Hsu (1992:130).

[48] *Yu pian* B, p. 8b.

[49] e.g. commentary to *Jin gui yao lüe* 4, p. 106.

In case 7, a contrast between soft 'accumulations' (*ji*) and hard 'conglomerations' (*jia*) may be implied, as hinted at by the pulse qualities of the soft versus tight (lines 10 and 13).

For understanding case 7, it is important to know that conglomerations can be very painful. This is not given in the name but clearly stated in line 2: 'The minor abdomen is painful' (*shao fu tong*).[50] The Zhangjiashan 'Maishu' also mentions pain as an attribute of the first two conglomerations, the male *jia* and the blood *jia*.[51] Zhang Shoujie quotes the *Long yu he tu* 龍魚河圖 as cited in the *Gu wei shu* 古微書: '*quan*-dogs, *gou*-dogs, fish and birds, if one eats them when they are undone, they turn into conglomerations, it is painful' (*quan gou yu niao, bu shu shi zhi, cheng wei jia tong* 犬狗魚鳥 不熟食之 成為瘕痛).[52] Pain as an aspect of *jia* is also given in *Su wen* 19: 'If the spleen transmits it [the disorder] to the kidneys, the name of the disorder is 'amassments and conglomerations', the minor abdomen, while oppressed and hot, is painful and expels white [mucus]' (*pi zhuan zhi shen, bing ming yue shan jia, shao fu yuan re er tong, chu bai* 脾傳之腎 病名曰疝瘕 少腹冤熱而痛 出白).[53] In *Su wen* 19, the pain from amassments and conglomerations is located in the minor abdomen. These different textual sources all indicate that 'conglomeration' disorders are not only long-lasting but also painful.

jia 瘕 – a gender-specific disorder   Over time certain types of *jia* became gender-specific, and were classified as women's disorders. We quoted the *Shuo wen* above. As *locus classicus* Chinese scholar-physicians usually cite *Su wen* 60: 'If the conception vessel develops disorders, in men it leads to internal knots and the seven amassments and in women to discharge and conglomerations and assemblages' (*ren mai wei bing, nan zi nei jie qi shan, nü zi dai xia jia ju* 任脈為病 男子內結七疝 女子帶下瘕聚).[54] Indeed, *shan* amassments and *jia* conglomerations are often opposed to each other as male and female disorders. However, only *shan*, but not *jia*, has gender-specificity in the Mawangdui vessel texts.[55]

By Song times, the notion of 'blood' (*xue* 血) had become a very sophisticated concept, not least as a gender-specific classifier of bodily processes.[56] Conglomerations were often associated with 'blood': 'As to concretions,

---

[50] The commentators ponder as to whether it is *shao fu* or *xiao fu*, see case 10 (lines 9 and 22).

[51] See also ZJS 'Maishu', quoted on pp. 270–71.

[52] *Gu wei shu*, p. 670.

[53] *Su wen* 19, p. 61. Note the parallel to the white conglomeration of the ZJS 'Maishu', cited on p. 273.

[54] *Su wen* 60, p. 161; slightly modified in *Nan jing* 29 (Unschuld 1986a:333). See also *Ling shu* 10, quoted on p. 336.

[55] See also discussion of *fu, xiao fu* and *shao fu* in case 10 on pp. 335ff.

[56] Furth (1999).

they are bound up with *qi* [disorders], as to conglomerations, they are bound up with blood [disorders]' (*zheng zhe, xi yu qi ye; jia zhe, xi yu xue ye* 癥者 系於氣也 瘕者 系於血也).[57] Their association with blood certainly put them into the realm of women's disorders.

In case 7, the patient dies after 'passing blood' (*sou xue*) and in this way the conglomeration in question could be considered to be associated with 'blood'. While it is the case that already in Han times, *qi* and blood became complementary concepts, they were rarely used for a gendered account of illness. Even though the compiler of the Zhangjiashan 'Maishu' lists the 'blood' and '*qi* conglomeration' in a sequence,[58] it would be absurd to take that as early evidence for classificatory gender schemas which became predominant during the Song.

Having said this, the *Nei jing* mentions gender-specific conglomerations, but they are not distinguished from each other in respect of *qi* or 'blood'. In *Ling shu* 57, the 'stone conglomeration' is a gender-specific disorder: 'When a stone conglomeration arises in the midst of the womb, and cold *qi* lodges at the gate of the womb, the gate of the womb closes and becomes blocked, the *qi* cannot pass through and the ugly blood ought to leak out but does not leak out, and becoming congealed it remains at a halt. By the day it becomes bigger, the appearance is like that of being pregnant, the menses do not descend in time. All this arises in women, one can by [the gymnastics of] guiding make it descend' (*shi jia sheng yu bao zhong, han qi ke yu zi men, zi men bi sai, qi bu de tong, e xue dang xie bu xie, pei yi liu zhi, ri yi yi da, zhuang ru huai zi, yue shi bu yi shi xia, jie sheng yu nü zi, ke dao er xia* 石瘕生于胞中 寒氣客于子門 子門閉塞 氣不得通 惡血當寫不寫 衃以留止 日以益大 狀如懷子 月事不以時下 皆生于女子 可導而下).[59] *Ling shu* 57, which reminds one of pseudopregnancy, mentions *qi* within the very same passage as 'blood' (*xue*); evidently, blood is not the gender-specific concept it is in many medical texts from the Song onward.

Text structure semantics

There is no parallel for the trisyllabic name *yi ji jia* 遺積瘕 (line 4), but there are many for each constituent. Text structure semantics postulates that the pulse qualities correlate with these constituents. Yi first speaks of '*qi* [coming] from the spleen' (*pi qi*; lines 9–12), and then of '*qi* [coming] from conglomerations' (*jia qi*; lines 13–14). The match between *jia qi* and *jia*, i.e. the pulse

---

[57] *Zhong zang jing* 18, p. 1.1047. The *Zhong zang jing*, attributed to Hua Tuo, was compiled in the Song (Ma 1990:156–8), in 1064. See Sivin (unpubl.) *An Index of References to Classical Chinese Medical Books*. Draft No. 2 (1990), 221 p.

[58] The ZJS 'Maishu' 'male' and 'blood conglomeration' are not gender-specific disorders, but named in respect of their appearance that brings to mind male and female reproductive organs. See case 7, n. 21. The '*qi* conglomeration', associated with farting, is of a different order and part of a more recent textual layer.

[59] *Ling shu* 57, p. 415. Notably, not mentioned by Taki Motokata.

quality '*qi* [coming] from conglomerations' and the 'conglomerations' in the name is instantly evident, but it is unclear whether '*qi* [coming] from the spleen' correlates with *yi* (leaking, remaining) or *ji* (accumulation).

Since the constituent in the name of the disorder *ji* 積 (accumulations) occurs in many different contexts of the *Inner Canon*, it is impossible to investigate its meaning in any comprehensive way. However, only a cursory glance shows that one of the most coherent accounts on 'accumulations' (*ji*), given in *Ling shu* 66, correlates them with the 'splenetic system' (*pi*).[60] *Ling shu* 66, which begins with the Yellow Emperor asking how accumulations arise and reach their completion, discusses problems of mostly the 'intestines and stomach' (*chang wei*). It ends with an answer to a question about 'accumulations' that arise in the *yin* sphere. This reply, which refers to the spleen, contains a phrase reminiscent of the cause of the disorder (line 8): 'Being drunken and entering the bedchamber ... harms the spleen' (*zui yi ru fang ... shang pi* 醉以入房 ... 傷脾). The similarities between this paragraph in *Ling shu* 66 and case 7 are striking: accumulations in the digestive tract, indulgence in wine and women as cause of the disorder, and in particular the correlation of 'accumulations' (*ji*) with the 'spleen' (*pi*).

This means the third constituent in the name, *yi* 遺, which in medicine generally means 'to lose', 'to leak', 'to excrete', does not correlate with a pulse quality. Now, if the method of text structure semantics, which postulates correlations between each pulse quality and each constituent in the name, is to work in this case, two possibilities arise. First, one correlates 'spleen *qi*' with *yi*, and 'conglomeration *qi*' with the bisyllabic *ji jia* (conglomerations and accumulations). However, although *ji jia* is an idiom found in the non-medical literature of the Tang,[61] it is most unlikely that in case 7 *jia qi* correlates with *ji jia*, for reasons emerging from the discussion of the qualities of *mai*. The second possibility is that one correlates 'spleen *qi*' with a bisyllabic constituent, meaning 'remanent accumulation' (*yi ji*). This reminds us of case 6, where the pulse quality 'hot' (*re*) correlates with the bisyllabic constituent *xiao dan* (consumption). However, in contrast to case 6, where the compound word *xiao dan* is widely attested in the medical literature, the term *yi ji* is found neither in medical texts nor dictionaries.

Notably, *yi* also means 'stools'.[62] Accordingly, *yi ji* would designate an 'accumulation of stools' and *yi ji jia* a 'conglomeration disorder from an accumulation of stools'. However, *yi ji* in case 7 has a striking parallel in the idiom *yi ni* 遺溺 in case 10 (line 8). As a technical medical term, *yi ni* means 'enuresis', but in case 10 it leads to a swelling of the small abdomen.

---

[60] *Ling shu* 66, pp. 438–9, is the *locus classicus* for *ji* (accumulations). See Xie (1954:4145).

[61] See HYDCD 8.144.

[62] *yi* 遺 'stools', see HYDCD 10.1186, no. 15, as noted by the reading group of Robert Chard (2005 p.c.).

It therefore is best translated as 'remanent urine'; elsewhere in the *Shi ji yi* is used in the sense of "to remain",[63] and here in case 7, Sima Zhen comments: '*yi* means "to remain" ' (*yi you liu ye* 遺猶留也). Accordingly, *yi ji* could mean 'remanent stools'. This idiom is not discussed in medical dictionaries and is probably a colloquialism, but later commentators seem to have understood it precisely in this sense.[64]

In summary, considering that case 7 reports on two pulse qualities, '*qi* [coming] from the spleen' and '*qi* [coming] from conglomerations', which each can be shown to correlate with a constituent in the name, that is, *ji* and *jia*, one could say that the term *yi*, which elsewhere in the *Shi ji* is used in the sense of 'remanent', must be viewed as a constituent in the name of the disorder that has no correlate. It may well have been a later commentator's emendation, the same one who interjected *yi ni* in a non-technical sense in case 10 (line 8). The name, as given in the *Shi ji* editions consulted, is therefore best translated as 'conglomeration disorder of remanent accumulations' or, implicitly, 'conglomerations of remanent stools'. However, text structure semantics postulates that the name of the disorder in the early first century, as composed by the editor who structured the case histories formulaically, probably was 'accumulations and conglomerations' (*ji jia*).

The pulse qualities given in Yi's own vocabulary (lines 9–14)   In the interpretation of the name given here, the first stanza on medical speculation explains why Yi diagnosed 'accumulations' (lines 9–12), and the second why he diagnosed 'conglomerations' (lines 13–14). The third stanza (lines 15–16) provides a justification for the prognostication of the day of death in thirty days (line 6b), as does the fourth (lines 17–19 or 17 and 19). The fourth stanza also explains why initially there was a chance of survival (line 18 for line 6a), but death occurred earlier than predicted (line 7). The last line, 20, appears to have been added by a commentator who misinterpreted the text.

With regard to the first two stanzas, except for *jin* (tight), none of the static verbs belongs among the twenty-four pulses of *Mai jing* 1.1, nor the twenty-eight pulse images, but all occur in the medical canons, although not exclusively in the context of pulse diagnosis.

The first question that arises when investigating the static verbs that describe the qualities of *mai* is whether the three terms *shen xiao ruo* (line 10) and *zhi jin xiao* (line 13) are to be interpreted as three static verbs that describe the qualities of the three *mai* or whether they comprise two static verbs for describing the qualities of two *mai*, modified by the first as an

---

[63] e.g. *Shi ji* 9, p. 422. See also case 10, n. 32.
[64] Ando Koretora's comment on line 18 is that case 7 involves spleen and lungs. The spleen is obviously affected by the conglomerations and stools are formed in the large intestine, i.e. the outer aspect of the canonical lungs.

adverb. If the latter were the case, *shen* would translate as 'very' and *shen xiao ruo* as 'very small and soft' (line 10) and *zhi* would mean 'extremely' and *zhi jin xiao* 'extremely tight and small' (line 13). In cases 1 (line 14) and 2 (line 14), in particular, Yi speaks of only two pulse qualities, such as 'murky, yet still' or 'murky and hurried'. If he felt these qualities at the wrist, his possible implicit allusion to two *mai* may parallel the Mawangdui vessel texts, which have only two *yin mai* of the arm. The canonical literature, by contrast, generally refers to three *yin* vessels on the inner side of the arm.[65]

Since, in line 17 the 'Model' speaks of 'three *yin*', presumably the three *yin mai*, one is inclined to assume that three static verbs describe three *mai* in line 10, namely 'deep' (*shen*), 'small' (*xiao*) and 'soft' (*ruo*). However, a parallel with *Su wen* 7 hints at the possibility that line 17 once only referred to two *mai* (see p. 289) and, accordingly, the *Shi ji* editor, in contrast to how the text reads now, may have implied two qualities of *mai* in line 10 and two of *qi* in line 13.

Yi refers to two pulse qualities in terms of *qi* when saying it is 'murky, yet still' in case 1 (line 14), 'murky and hurried, yet [the condition] is transient' in case 2 (line 14), and 'murky, yet thin' in case 4 (lines 32–3). Notably, even when the *Shi ji* personage Yi speaks in terms of *mai*, he often alludes to two qualities, for example 'being large, yet frequent' in case 3 (line 16), 'large, yet hurried' in case 5 (line 19), 'large, yet replete' in case 10 (line 14) and 'smooth and clear, and [the patient] recovers' in case 4 (line 30), 'uneven and not drumming' in the 'Mai fa' quote of case 6 (line 18).

In case 7, the *Shi ji* personage Yi differentiates between qualifications of *mai* (line 10) and *qi* (line 13). In the medical canons this can be put down to *variatio* since the static verbs describing pulses indiscriminately qualify *mai* or *qi*, but in Yi's Memoir the difference is telling. In cases 1 and 2, Yi examines *mai* but communicates his findings with two static verbs qualifying *qi*. In case 4, Yi uses static verbs qualifying *qi* and *mai*, and those qualifying *mai* were found to have more parallels in canonical medical texts than those qualifying *qi*. Accordingly, it seemed reasonable to suggest that stanzas with static verbs qualifying *mai* do not reflect early second-century medical rationale (case 4, lines 26–31). In case 3 (lines 14–15) and case 7 (lines 13–14), Yi also reports on qualities of *qi*, however, after having pressed onto the 'right [*mai*] opening' (*you* [*mai*] *kou*). So, in contrast to cases 1, 2, 4 and 9, the qualities of *qi* he reports on may or may not reflect knowledge of the assumed early second-century medical document. As we will see, both stanzas in cases 3 and 7 can be read in ways for which canonical medical texts provide many parallels. However, the various possibilities need to be explored before drawing any conclusions.

[65] MWD ZB and YY (1985:3–13) and *Ling shu* 10, pp. 299ff.

zhi 至 – **congested, to arrive or extremely (line 13)**   If one translates *zhi* 至 (line 13) as 'congested', the quality of *qi* at the 'right vessel opening' (*you mai kou*) would correlate in an iconic or indexical way with the body internal process that leads to the formation of 'conglomerations' (*jia*). There are non-medical texts from the Warring States in which commentators have argued on grounds of the context in which *zhi* is mentioned that *zhi* 至 means *zhi* 窒 'congested'.[66] Perhaps *zhi* 'congested' was the pulse quality given in the assumed early second-century document, which has since fallen into oblivion?

However, *zhi* is also a verb as in *qi zhi* 氣至 '*qi* arrives' or an adverb, 'extremely', as in *zhi yin* 至陰 (extreme *yin*). Zhang Shoujie reads *zhi* as 'to arrive', when he proposes to change the word order to '*qi* arrives slightly tightened' (*qi zhi xiao jin*). It is, however, possible to translate line 13 without altering the word sequence '*qi* arrives tight and small' (*qi zhi jin xiao*), although *xiao* does indeed appear misplaced.

To account for Zhang Shoujie's concern, let us consider the following very hypothetical scenario: the early second-century document only had *qi zhi* '*qi* is congested', indicative of the 'conglomerations', the early first-century editor did not understand *zhi* in this sense and altered the phrase to *qi zhi jin* '*qi* arrives tightly', which correlated with the pain of conglomerations, and a commentator, who pre-dated the eighth-century Zhang Shoujie, by adding *xiao* changed it to *qi zhi jin xiao* '*qi* is extremely tight and small'. In canonical doctrine, 'small' but not 'tight' is indicative of conglomerations (see below).

The following line 14 reports on an overt correlation between 'conglomeration *qi*' and 'conglomerations', like 'lung *qi*' and 'lungs' in case 6, 'wind *qi*' and 'wind' in cases 5 and 9 (and seemingly in case 8). Since correlations dating from the presumed early second century document are more covert, line 14 probably is an editorial interpolation. It is introduced by the verb 'to manifest' (*xian*), which prompted commentatorial attention in case 4 (line 19), rather than by a resumptive term like *shi* (this) or *ci* (this one), which would allow one to argue that in line 14 the text continues in manner 1 (see table 4). Is this minute textual anomaly sufficient to call into question the above suggestion that the assumed early second-century document centred on *jia* (conglomeration) and to point instead to *ji* (accumulations) as the core disorder of case 7? It is difficult to know.

---

[66] HYDZD 2.2814 refers to a comment of Yin Tongyang 尹桐陽 (nineteenth to twentieth century) of whom there is little good to say (Loewe 1993:121, 373); the comment appears indeed irrelevant for the respective *Guanzi* passage. HYDCD 8.784, however, refers to a text passage in the *Han Feizi* 20 (55), p. 1142: 'Hence in reality when there is that which is blocked, then the principle is deprived of its measure' (*shi gu you suo zhi, er li shi qi liang* 實故有所至 而理失其量), and Yu Xingwu's 于省吾 (1897–1984) gloss on it that *zhi* 至 should be read as *zhi* 窒. See Yu Xingwu (1962:310–11).

***jin* 緊 – tight (line 13)**   In the *Inner Canon*, 'being tight' (*jin*) occurs three times in juxtaposition with 'being firm' (*jian* 堅), namely in *Su wen* 62 for describing the quality of the 'skin and flesh' (*ji rou* 肌肉),[67] in *Ling shu* 73 for describing the quality of 'knots and links' (*jie luo* 結絡),[68] and in *Ling shu* 75 for describing a pulse quality indicative of knots.[69] Evidently, 'tight' is indicative of the tactile experience of hardened aspects of the body, like knots, and one surmises, by implication, also conglomerations.

In *Su wen* 46, 'being tight', together with 'sunken' (*chen* 沈), is given as the *mai* of the season winter: 'If one examines them [the *mai*] in winter and if the pulse on the right-hand side is solid, matching the sunken and tight [or: certainly it should be sunken and tight], this [person] resonates with the four seasons' (*dong zhen zhi, you mai gu, dang chen jin, ci ying si shi* 冬診之 右脈固 當沈緊 此應四時).[70] *Su wen* 46 explains that 'being tight and sunken' (*chen jin*) are indicative of winter, which is the time when everything hardens and congeals due to coldness.[71] If *gu* is translated as 'solid', rather than as 'certainly', then *Su wen* 46 clearly states that the 'tight and sunken' is 'solid'. The phrase *dang chen jin*, 'matching the sunken and tight', is then to be read as a comment by a later Han, Tang or Song scribe on the then poorly understood idiom *mai gu*, 'the vessels are solid'. As demonstrated in chapter 4 (p. 30), *mai gu* alludes to the body conception of the Warring States that opposes the outwardly seen solid form (*xing*) to the invisible inner *qi* and feelings. Notably, *Su wen* 46 records this in respect of the right *mai*, and Yi speaks of tightness at the right *mai*'s opening in line 13.

Ling shu 9 says noxious *qi* is 'tight': 'If noxious *qi* comes, it is tight and swift; if grain *qi* comes, it is slow and harmonious' (*xie qi lai ye, jin er ji; gu qi lai ye, xu er he* 邪氣來也 緊而疾 穀氣來也 徐而和).[72] *Ling shu* 48 explains 'being tight' is a sign of pain: 'If it is tight, then there is a painful obstruction' (*jin ze wei tong bi* 緊則為痛痹).[73] *Ling shu* 48 also contains the idiom 'tight pain' (*jin tong* 緊痛). Evidently, 'being tight' (*jin*) indicates the pain mentioned in line 2, but it does not actually correlate with the 'conglomerations' in line 4.

***xiao* 小 – small (line 13)**   'Being small' (*xiao*), as opposite of 'large', belongs among the six standard *mai* of *Ling shu* 4 (quoted on p. 174). This opposi-

---

[67] *Su wen* 62, p. 170. The three were found through the computer printout by Hermann Tessenow (2000 p.c.).

[68] *Ling shu* 73, p. 452.   [69] *Ling shu* 75, p. 461.

[70] *Su wen* 46, p. 129.

[71] *Su wen* 47, p. 133. 'Tight' co-occurs here with 'large' (*da* 大). It is associated with 'abundant' (*sheng* 盛) in *Su wen* 18, p. 55, and with 'floating' (*fu* 浮) in *Su wen* 76, p. 246, and *Ling shu* 49, p. 400. See also *Su wen* 69, p. 199.

[72] *Ling shu* 9, p. 295.   [73] *Ling shu* 48, p. 397.

tion is also given in *Su wen* 28, when Qibo comments on the prognosis for 'seizures' (*dian ji* 癲疾): 'If the pulse is throbbing, large, and slippery, they [the seizures] will eventually cease by themselves. If the pulse is small, firm and intense, death occurs, incurable' (*mai bo da hua, jiu zi yi, mai xiao jian ji, si bu zhi* 脈搏大滑 久自已 脈小堅急 死不治).[74] 'Small', in combination with other pulse qualities, indicates death.

In *Su wen* 48, *xiao ji* could mean both 'slightly intense' or 'small and intense': 'When the pulse of the kidneys is small and intense, when the pulse of the liver is small and intense, when the pulse of the heart is small and intense, and when there is no drumming, it is a case of conglomerations' (*shen mai xiao ji, gan mai xiao ji, xin mai xiao ji, bu gu, jie wei jia* 腎脈小急 肝脈小急 心脈小急 不鼓 皆為瘕).[75] Together with the 'intense' pulse, it indicates conglomerations. *Su wen* 48 thus provides a parallel for case 7.

In summary, of the qualities of *qi* at the right *mai* opening (line 13), 'being tight' (*jin*) is indicative of the hardened knots that conglomerations are and of the pain they cause, although no passage was found where *jin* is indicative of conglomerations. The term *xiao* is in some contexts adverbially used, meaning 'slightly'; in others it clearly means 'small'. In canonical writings, it occurs mostly in combination with other pulse qualities, as in *Su wen* 48 or 28. In *Su wen* 48 these pulses indicate conglomerations, in *Su wen* 28 they indicate hardness, presumably from dryness, and death. In the extant *Shi ji* text, the term *zhi* means either 'extremely' or 'to arrive'; and line 13 probably refers to two pulse qualities. Let us now turn to line 10.

shen 深 – deep or very (line 10)   In canonical texts, 'being deep' (*shen*) generally does not describe tactile qualities of *mai*. Instead, it is used for locating a disorder 'deeply' inside the body.[76] Or, in the context of needling, it refers to a 'deep' insertion of the needle.[77] In *Ling shu* 78, the disorder that is called 'deep obstruction' (*shen bi* 深痺) can be reached with long needles,[78] although, generally, disorders 'deep' inside the body cannot be reached from the outside. If Yi took *shen* (deep) as a sign that in an iconic and indexical way indicates a body internal process, he considered, in line with canonical doctrine, the spleen the most central of the five viscera, located 'deep' within the body.

Ando Koretora reads *shen* (deep) as *chen* 沈 (sunken), which is a standard pulse, still today, and according to *Ling shu* 49, can also be used for assessing the quality of colour: 'The five colours each appear in their own parts [of the face]; investigate whether or not they are floating or sunken, in order

---

[74] *Su wen* 28, p. 87.
[75] *Su wen* 48, pp. 134–5. On *xiao*, see also case 5, n. 102. On *bu gu* 'not drumming', see case 6 (line 18).
[76] e.g. *Ling shu* 75, p. 463.   [77] e.g. *Ling shu* 45, p. 386.   [78] *Ling shu* 78, p. 471.

to know the shallowness and depth [of the disorder]' (*wu se ge xian qi bu, cha qi fu chen, yi zhi qian shen* 五色各見其部 察其浮沈 以知淺深).[79] *Ling shu* 49 correlates 'floating' (*fu*) and 'sunken' (*chen*), as perceived on the body surface, with 'shallowness' (*qian*) and 'depth' (*shen*) of the disorder within the body.

In *Su wen* 48, the 'sunken' pulse, in combination with others, is indicative of 'amassments' (*shan* 疝), 'intestinal *pi*-fluids' (*chang pi* 腸澼) and a 'lopsidedly withered diaphragm' (*ge pian ku* 鬲偏枯).[80] In *Su wen* 18, it indicates 'accumulations' (*ji* 積): 'If the pulse at the inch-opening is sunken, yet presents itself transversely, you call it "having accumulations beneath one's flanks [ribs]". If in the abdominal parts of the interior there are transverse accumulations, it is painful' (*cun kou mai chen er heng, yue xie xia you ji, fu zhong you heng ji tong* 寸口脈沈而橫 曰脅下有積 腹中有橫積痛).[81] *Su wen* 18 establishes for case 7 a striking correlation between 'being sunken' (*chen*), 'the interior' (*zhong*) and 'accumulations' (*ji*).

xiao 小 – small (line 10) 'Being small' (*xiao*), as shown above, is indicative of conglomerations (p. 283), but there is no parallel in the *Inner Canon* to consider it indicative of accumulations and/or spleen disorders. In some contexts it is considered protective against bad influences, as in *Su wen* 27: 'If it is large, then noxiousness arrives, if it is small, then there is evenness' (*da ze xie zhi, xiao ze ping* 大則邪至 小則平).[82] This parallels *Ling shu* 47, where, however, an additional phrase attributes it with negative qualities: 'If the five viscera are all small, one has few illnesses, but suffers from a worrisome heart, great anxiety and worry; if the five viscera are all large, then one is lax in one's affairs and only with difficulty can be made to worry' (*wu zang jie xiao zhe, shao bing, ku jiao xin, da chou you, wu zang jie da zhe, huan yu shi, nan shi yi you* 五藏皆小者 少病 苦燋心 大愁憂 五藏皆大者 緩 于事 難使以憂).[83] Elsewhere in *Ling shu* 47 'being small' indicates an infirmity of the stomach, which is the outer aspect of the spleen: 'In cases where the flesh and callus are not only small, but also thin, the stomach is not firm' (*rou jun xiao er mo zhe, wei bu jian* 肉䐃 小而麼者 胃不堅). However, since 'small' also indicates problems in the 'small intestines' (*xiao chang*), which are the outer aspect of the canonical heart, it is difficult to derive from *Ling shu* 47 a generally valid correlation between 'being small' and 'spleen' disorders.

---

[79] *Ling shu* 49, p. 401. For identical technical terms in *mai* and *se* diagnosis, see case 5 (lines 14–17) and case 7, n. 106.   [80] *Su wen* 48, p. 135.

[81] *Su wen* 18, p. 55. The translation of *zhong* as noun rather than adverb assumes that this *Su wen* passage on the nosological term *ji*, which, like *jia*, may pre-date canonical doctrine, was additively edited over time. See also case 6 (line 34) and its discussion on p. 258.

[82] *Su wen* 27, p. 84.   [83] *Ling shu* 47, p. 394. See also case 5, pp. 225–6.

ruo 弱 – **soft (line 10)**   The static verb *ruo* often means 'being weak', but in case 7 is probably best read as 'soft'. 'Being soft' can have connotations of 'weak', for instance, when it qualifies the flesh, which is an aspect of the splenetic system in canonical doctrine. Thus, *Ling shu* 50 refers to a 'thin skin and soft flesh' (*bo pi ruo rou* 薄皮弱肉), which is afterwards opposed to a 'skin that is thick and flesh that is firm' (*pi hou rou jian* 皮厚肉堅).[84] The pulse quality 'soft' (*ruo*) clearly correlates with the spleen, as becomes evident from two passages in *Su wen* 18 and 19 (quoted on p. 287) and *Ling shu* 77, which says of the 'great soft wind' (*da ruo feng* 大弱風) that 'when it harms the person, internally it lodges in the spleen and externally it resides in the flesh [close to the skin]' (*qi shang ren ye, nei she yu pi, wai zai yu ji* 其傷人也 內舍於脾 外在於肌) and that 'its *qi* governs intrinsic characteristics of being soft' (*qi qi zhu wei ruo* 其氣主為弱).[85] *Ling shu* 50 and 77 highlight the close correlation between the 'spleen', the 'flesh' and being 'soft'.

Comparison of the pulse qualities (lines 10 and 13)   The question as to whether lines 10 and 13 speak of two or three pulse qualities has to take account of their textual history. If both lines referred to three, 'being deep' (*shen*) in line 10 would correlate with the canonical 'spleen' located deep inside the body and 'congested' (*zhi*) in line 13 with 'conglomerations', but since neither is a canonical pulse quality, it is more likely that lines 10 and 13 were understood to refer to two pulse qualities each. The text would then contrast the 'very small and soft' with the 'extremely tight and small'. Indeed, the contrast between 'soft' accumulations and 'tight', hard and painful conglomerations is noticeable, but one wonders why 'small' is mentioned twice. Moreover, in the context of pulse diagnosis *zhi* usually means 'to arrive'.

Comparison with canonical texts shows that 'soft' (*ruo*) is generally a negative characteristic of the flesh, which is a correlate of the spleen, and 'small' (*xiao*), in combination with other pulse qualities, indicates death and conglomerations. So, the received text should be read as opposing the 'soft' and 'small'.

The comparison of cases 3 and 7 shows interesting parallels: Yi examines in both cases the 'right opening', diagnoses thereafter either a 'conglomeration' or an 'amassment' and mentions qualities of *qi* indicative of pain: 'it arrives tightly' (*qi zhi jin*) in case 7 and is 'intense' (*qi ji*) in case 3. In case 3, where Yi senses *qi* that is 'intense' but no *qi* from the five viscera, the patient recovers, but in case 7, where he feels that *qi* is coming from a viscus, the spleen, and is 'confused' (*qia qia*), the patient dies. Perhaps cases 3 (line 14) and 7 (line 13) speak of *qi*, because Yi investigates the 'right opening' and the 'right *mai*'s opening' respectively, which in canonical medicine was

---

[84] *Ling shu* 50, p. 403.   [85] *Ling shu* 77, pp. 468–9.

the 'opening for *qi*' (*qi kou*). Perhaps Yi speaks here of *qi*, not necessarily because the phrase dates from the early second century but because these 'right openings', like *qi kou*, in canonical medicine, were understood to inform on the dynamics of *qi*. Accordingly, contrary to the suggestion made earlier in this study, one could also argue that case 3 (lines 14–15) and case 7 (lines 13–14) could have been added by either the early first-century editor or a later commentator.

qia qia 合合 – **confused (line 11)**   Yi's wording 其卒然合合也是脾氣也 (lines 11–12) causes considerable debate among the commentators. First, the graph *zu* 卒 causes problems; Xu Guang, Zhang Shoujie and Takigawa point to other editions which have *lai* 來 (to come) in place of *zu*. However, there is no need to emend the text; *zu* 卒 can be read as *cu* 猝, and *cu ran* 猝然 as 'abruptly'. This is a common reading of *zu ran* 卒然 'abruptly' in the *Su wen*.[86]

Secondly, the commentators debate over whether the pulse quality consists of the monosyllabic verb *he* 合 (mixed) in the phrase: *qi zu ran he* 其卒然合, followed by the explanation that *he* indicates spleen *qi*: *he ye, shi pi qi ye* 合也是脾氣也, or whether it is described by a reduplication: *qia qia* 合合 (confused) or *ta ta* (rapid) 沓沓. Zhang Shoujie quotes a *Su wen* passage in favour of *he*. Kaiho Gembi considers it irrelevant and points, inter alia, to the gloss in *Guang ya* 2B: . . . 沓 . . . 合也, and takes 合合 to mean *ta ta* 沓沓. He quotes Yan Shigu's comment: '*ta ta* means to run rapidly' (*ta ta ji xing ye* 沓沓 疾行也) on the passage in *Han shu* 22, which says of the 'movement of the spirit' (*shen zhi xing* 神之行) that 'it gallops rapidly' (*qi ta ta* 騎沓沓). In his reading, *ta ta* describes an irregularity of the pulses that parallels that of being 'at once united, at once alternating' (*yi tuan yi dai*) mentioned in line 19 (see pp. 290–2).[87]

A systematic investigation of all Yi's glosses on pulse qualities shows that he is consistent in saying either '*XYZ. Z zhe*, *AB ye*' or '*XYZ ye. shi AB ye*', but not '*XYZ. Z ye, shi AB ye*'. According to the schema '*XYZ. Z ye, shi AB ye*', line 11 would read as: *qi zu ran he. He ye, shi pi qi ye* (It was suddenly mixed. The mixed is [indicative] of the spleen).[88] Although the presentation of the text in Takigawa's edition may insinuate this reading, this is precisely a schema Yi does not adhere to. This means that the above phrase should read as '*XYZ ye. shi AB ye*', i.e. 'It was abruptly *qia qia*' (*qi zu ran qia qia ye*). 'This is *qi* coming from the spleen' (*shi pi qi ye*). This is

---

[86] See *Huangdi nei jing*, p. 1045, and e.g. *Ling shu* 50, p. 403. See also Yan Shigu's comment: '*zu* reads as *cu*, *cu* means suddenly' (*zu du yue cu, cu bao ye* 卒讀曰猝 猝 暴也) on *Han shu* 27B(2), pp. 1412–13: 'Out of the Catalpa pillar at the grave gate suddenly grew branches and leaves' (*mu men zi zhu zu sheng zhi ye* 墓門梓柱卒生枝葉).

[87] *Guang ya* 2B, p. 10a–b. *Han shu* 22, p. 1066.

[88] See table 4, manners 1 and 2, on p. 115.

also the reading proposed by Taki Motohiro, who remarks, however, that the sentence must be corrupt.

There is no need to consider the clause 'it was suddenly confused' (*qi zu ran qia qia ye*) faulty, nor to replace the term *qia qia* with *ta ta*, since digestive problems, which according to canonical doctrine are associated primarily with the splenetic system, are often assessed with reduplicated terms. For instance, *Ling shu* 26 has 'the abdomen is echo-echo-like' (*fu xiang xiang ran* 腹嚮嚮然) or 'in the abdominal part of the interior it gu-gurgitates' (*fu zhong gu gu* 腹中穀穀).[89] It is conceivable that *qia qia* has an onomatopoetic meaning aspect, just like the pulse quality *cu cu ran* or *qi qi ran* 戚戚然 in case 19, which incidentally also concerns a conglomeration disorder. Apparently, *qia qia* can mean either 'in a united fashion' (*xiehe mao* 協和貌) or 'in a confused fashion' (*fencuo mao* 紛錯貌).[90] The second reading in particular appears to capture the descriptions of *mai* found in *Su wen* 18 and 19, discussed in what follows, where a soft pulse, in combination with an irregular one, indicates a lethal condition.

Thus, *Su wen* 19 states: 'If as the true pulse of the spleen arrives, it is soft, yet at once dense, at once dispersed,[91] and if the colour is yellow and blue-green and not shiny, and if the body hair is brittle, then death occurs' (*zhen pi mai zhi, ruo er zha cu zha shu, se huang qing bu ze, mao zhe, nai si* 真脾脈至 弱而乍數乍疏 色黃青不澤 毛折 乃死). *Su wen* 18 likewise associates 'soft' with the splenetic system and also states that if additionally the pulse is irregular, death is certain: 'If the long-summer stomach [pulses] are subtle, tender and soft, you call it even. If the soft ones are numerous and those of the stomach few, you call it a disorder of the spleen. However, if they are alternating and there are none of the stomach, it means that death occurs' (*chang xia wei wei ruan ruo yue ping, ruo duo wei shao yue pi bing, dan dai wu wei yue si* 長夏胃微耎弱曰平 弱多胃少曰脾病 但代無胃曰死).[92] If 'at once dense, at once dispersed' (*zha cu zha shu*) in *Su wen* 19 and 'alternating' (*dai*) in *Su wen* 18 are viewed as equivalent to 'abruptly confused' (*qi zu ran qia qia ye*) in case 7, the conditions described in *Su wen* 18 and 19 would be similar to those in case 7, insofar as the 'soft' pulse correlates in all these cases with the 'splenetic system' and the pulses of 'being confused',

[89] *Ling shu* 26, p. 345. For *xiang xiang*, see HYDCD 3.537 where *xiang* 嚮 is used as an alternative graph for *xiang* 響 (echo). For *gu gu*, see Nanjing zhongyi xueyuan (1986:205).

[90] HYDCD 3.147.

[91] *Su wen* 19, p. 62. I follow Mark Lewis (1995 p.c.) in reading *shu* 疏 as 'dispersed' and 數 as *cu* 'tightly knit', 'dense'. Alternative translation: 'at once retarded, at once swift', as in *Lü shi chun qiu* 26.5 (Knoblock & Riegel 2000:660): 'He takes care of what he planted, without causing it to accelerate, and also without causing it to slow down' (*shen qi zhong, wu shi shuo, yi wu shi shu* 慎其種 勿使數 亦勿使疏). See also *Huainanzi* 17, p. 1821, ending with the phrase: 'The correct is between the slow and frequent' (*zheng zai shu shuo zhi jian* 正在疏數之間), on which Gao You comments: '*shu* also means slow [or delayed]' (*shu you chi ye* 疏猶遲也) and '*shuo* also means swift' (*shuo you ji ye* 數猶疾也).

[92] *Su wen* 18, pp. 54–5.

'alternating' or 'at once dense, at once dispersed' indicate death. In particular the pulse of the spleen in *Su wen* 19, 'it is soft, yet at once dense, at once dispersed' (*ruo er zha cu zha shu*), shows some affinity with Yi's pulse qualities attributed to the spleen in case 7: 'Deep, small and soft; abruptly they were confused' (*shen, xiao, ruo, qi zu ran qia qia ye*).

In summary, the pulse quality *qia qia* is best interpreted as an onomatopoetic term for describing digestive problems within the splenetic system, which means 'to be confused'. Kaiho Gembi suggests that *qia qia* in line 11 describes the same state as 'not entirely united' *mai* in line 18. Like the 'alternating' in *Su wen* 18 and being 'at once dense, at once dispersed' in *Su wen* 19, if felt in combination with the 'soft' pulse, the quality *qia qia* indicates death.

The prognostication of death (lines 15–20)

yi ci xiang cheng 以次相乘 – they took turns in riding on each other (line 15)   Line 15 contains two terms used in the context of five agents doctrine. The idiom *yi ci* 以次 (to take turns), which is mentioned twice in the *Su wen* and four times in the *Ling shu*,[93] means 'in accordance with the usual sequence [of transmission]'. In *Ling shu* 42, it describes the transmission of an illness from one viscus to another, following a known sequence, a process that ends in death: 'If the disorder first breaks out in the heart, after one day it goes to the lungs, after three days to the liver, after five days to the spleen; if it then does not come to an end within three days, death occurs; in winter at midnight, in summer at midday' (*bing xian fa yu xin, yi ri er zhi fei, san ri er zhi gan, wu ri er zhi pi, san ri bu yi, si, dong ye ban, xia ri zhong* 病先發于心 一日而之肺 三日而之肝 五日而之脾 三日不已 死 冬夜半 夏日中). *Ling shu* 42 prognosticates death also in the case of disorders arising first in the lungs, liver, spleen, stomach, kidneys and bladder. The paragraph ends by stating: 'As to all disorders: if they are mutually transmitted to each other according to a sequence, in those cases, they all have a set time of death, and it is not permitted to apply needling' (*zhu bing yi ci xiang zhuan, ru shi zhe, jie you si qi, bu ke ci ye* 諸病以次相傳 如是者 皆有死期 不可刺也).[94] In *Ling shu* 42, the expression *yi ci xiang zhuan* means that the disorders follow a set course of transmission from one viscus to the other.

The term *cheng* 乘 literally means 'to ride on', and the term *xiang* 相 'mutual' presupposes that two parties are involved. In canonical doctrine, *xiang cheng* is used in the sense of 'to multiply'.[95] Apart from the two well-known cycles of five agents doctrine, those of 'giving rise to each other'

---

[93] *Su wen* 19, p. 61; 65, p. 181. *Ling shu* 37, p. 371; 41, p. 379; 42, p. 380; 56, p. 512. Based on computer printout by Hermann Tessenow (2000 p.c.).

[94] *Ling shu* 42, pp. 380–81. See also *Su wen* 65, p. 181.

[95] *cheng* 乘 'to multiply' in mathematics (Needham 1959:63).

(*xiang sheng* 相生) and of 'overcoming each other' (*xiang sheng* 相勝, also known as *xiang ke* 相克), there are two lesser-known ones: 'to mutually insult each other' (*xiang wu* 相侮) and 'to multiply each other' (*xiang cheng* 相乘).[96] Perhaps Yi meant that *mai* coming from the spleen and *qi* coming from conglomerations were mutually taking turns in riding on each other, and he therefore predicted the patient would die in thirty days?

san yin 三陰? – the three yin? (line 17)   In line 17, Yi explains that in cases where the three *yin* are entirely united, it is *ru fa*, which could mean 'normal', but Taki Motokata says *ru fa* refers to what Yi had predicted, namely that the patient would die in thirty days. One expects that Yi's prediction was 'according to the "Model"' (*ru* 'Fa'). However, none was mentioned so far. This 'Model' differs from those encountered in cases 1 and 6 in that it evidently is framed in a numerology of three rather than five. Rather than equating *fen* (degrees) with days for calculating the time span before death, it appears to pay attention to interrelations between the three *yin mai*.

Such a numerology of three is given in the Mawangdui 'Yinyangmai sihou' where the three *yin* are *mai* of death: 'All three *yin* are [indicative of] *qi* [coming] from the earth; they are the *mai* of death. When [x] is not only ailing, but also chaotic, death occurs within ten days (*fan san yin, di qi yi [ye], si mai [mai] yi [ye], [x] bing er luan, ze [bu] guo shi ri er si* 凡三陰 地氣殹[也] 死脈[脈] 殹[也] [x] 病而亂 則[不]過十日而死).[97] Yi may have had such a maxim in mind when he spoke of the 'Model'.

Taki Motokata cites *Su wen* 7: 'In cases where three *yin* are united in their entirety, one dies after twenty days at midnight' (*san yin ju tuan, er shi ri ye ban si* 三陰俱搏 二十日夜半死),[98] but does not quote *Su wen* 7, which elsewhere reports that if one *yin* is united in its entirety, then one dies in ten days and if two *yin* are united in their entirety, one dies in thirty days.[99] Interestingly, *Su wen* 7 and Yi both predict death in thirty days. Now, if the character for three 三 in line 17 is read as two 二, we would not only have found a textual parallel in *Su wen* 7 for the prognostication of death in thirty days, but also have established coherence in argumentation across lines 10, 15–16, 17 and 19, insofar as all would speak of two pulse qualities. Yi can be interpreted to refer to two rather than three pulse qualities in lines 10

---

[96] Porkert (1974:51–4), Sivin (1987:77), Hsu (1999:210–12).

[97] MWD 'Yinyangmai sihou' (1985:21), with variant in MWD ZB (1985:5): 'If there is disorder and chaos among the three *yin*, death occurs within ten days' (*san yin zhi bing luan, bu guo shi ri si* 三陰之病亂 不過十日死). Translation based on Harper (1998:219 and 199–200), with modifications.

[98] Note *Su wen* 7, p. 27. Taki Motokata adds Wang Bing's comment. See HDNJSW 7, p. 23: 'This is the excess of the complete number of spleen and lungs' (*pi fei cheng shu zhi yu* 脾肺成數之餘).

[99] *Su wen* 7, p. 27; *ju* means here 'entirely' rather than 'together' (Mark Lewis, 1995 p.c.). On 搏 as *bo* or *tuan*, see pp. 290–2.

and 13; a reader trained in canonical medicine may even have considered them to be *yin* in line 10 insofar as they come from a viscus, the spleen, and *yang* in line 13, where they come from conglomerations.[100] Line 17 would explain the prediction (line 6b), line 18 a state of uncertainty (line 6a) and line 19 why the patient died sooner (line 7). However minimal such amendments to however plausible 'mistakes', they are always dangerous. All that can be said with certainty is that the Mawangdui 'Yinyangmai sihou', *Su wen* 7 and the *Shi ji* personage Yi investigate *yin mai* for calculating the time span before death. This would emphasise that at the core of case 7 are pulse qualities that relate to the pre-canonical 'interior' (lines 10–11 rather than line 13).

bo 搏 or *tuan* 搏 – to strike or to be united (lines 17, 18 and 19)   According to Ru Chun, the graph which in Takigawa's edition is given as *bo* 搏 should be pronounced as *tuan*.[101] The graph 搏, if read as *tuan*, means 'to unite' or 'to bundle', and if read as *zhuan* it means 'to link up to form a circle'.[102] Perhaps *ju tuan* in line 17 and *xiang cheng* in line 15 delineate a similar process?

The term *bo* 搏 (to strike) takes on various shades of meaning in the *Inner Canon*. Perhaps this wide semantic stretch of the term *bo* comes from its graph being confused with the graph *tuan* 搏. Ren Yingqiu's edition of the *Inner Canon*, for instance, makes no distinction between the two graphs. The term *bo* is well known as a constituent in the idiom 'mutual resonance' (*xiang bo* 相搏) between, for instance, the hot and the cold, as in *Ling shu* 75.[103] Taki Motokata notes it is not a regular pulse and glosses it as 'suppressed drumming' (*fu gu* 伏鼓). In a more literal sense, it is likened to tapping, as in *Su wen* 19: 'If when the true pulse of the kidneys arrives, and as it strikes, is severed, like a finger tapping onto a stone, *bi bi*-like ...' (*zhen shen mai zhi, bo er jue, ru zhi tan shi bi bi ran* ... 真腎脈至 搏而絕 如指彈石辟辟然).[104] This notion of 'striking' as 'tapping' appears to be implied also by *Su wen* 23: 'If the noxious enters *yang*, then one becomes mad, if it enters *yin*, then one develops obstructions; if it [superficially] strikes *yang*, then it makes that one has a fit, and if it strikes [superficially] *yin*, then it makes that one [suddenly] becomes mute' (*xie ru yu yang ze kuang, xie ru*

---

[100] The canonical spleen correlates with the 'major *yin*'. Conglomerations are indicated by *yang mai* in *Su wen* 48, p. 135: 'If the three/third *yang* are/is intense, it is a conglomeration; if the three/third *yin* are/is intense, it is an amassment' (*san yang ji wei jia, san yin ji wei shan* 三陽急為瘕 三陰急為疝).

[101] *tuan* 搏 in *Shi ji* 105, p. 2803.   [102] HYDCD 6.827.

[103] *Ling shu* 75, p. 463.

[104] *Su wen* 19, p. 62. Note the parallel between 'striking, yet severed' (*bo er jue* 搏而絕) in *Su wen* 19, p. 62, and 'striking, yet immobile' (*bo er bu xing* 搏而不行) in *Ling shu* 56, p. 412. See also *Su wen* 48, p. 135: 'If the pulse upon its arrival strikes ... one dies' (*mai zhi er bo ... si* 脈至而搏 死).

yu yin ze bi, bo yang ze wei dian ji, bo yin ze wei yin 邪入於陽則狂 邪入於陰則痺 搏陽則為巔疾 搏陰則為瘖). In *Su wen* 23, 'striking' or 'tapping' of the body surface (*bo*) is opposed to 'entering' (*ru*) inside the body.

In other contexts when it is used in the sense of 'bundled' which is opposed to 'dispersed' (*san* 散), the graph *bo* in Ren Yingqiu's *Nei jing* edition probably should be replaced with that for *tuan*.[105] The above-cited passage of *Ling shu* 49 (on pp. 283–4), which refers to diagnosis by investigating colour, continues by stating: 'Investigate whether it [the colour part (of the face)] is lubricant or short-lived, in order to see whether one will be successful or fail [in treating the disorder], and investigate whether it is scattered or bundled in order to know whether [death] is far away or nearby' (*cha qi ze yao, yi guan cheng bai, cha qi san tuan, yi zhi yuan jin* 察其澤夭 以觀成敗 察其散搏 以知遠近).[106] The 'bundled' (*tuan*) and 'dispersed' (*san*), which elsewhere describe pulse qualities, refer here to colour, perhaps to its intensity. Interestingly, if the graph is read as *tuan,* it is, as in this case history (lines 17–20), mentioned in the context of prognosticating whether death is 'near' (*jin*) or 'far' (*yuan*).

The question is whether the graphs 搏 given in lines 19 and 20 should be read as *tuan* 搏 as well. Ando Koretora, as above already Kaiho Gembi, suggests the pulse quality given in line 19 refers to that of *qia qia* in line 11. This reading is possible regardless of whether one reads the graph in question as *bo* or *tuan*. Line 20, 'hence when the three *yin bo/tuan*, he passed blood and died as said before', would mean the patient died when the three *yin* 'united' (*tuan*). The idea that *mai* that are united, rather than dispersed, should indicate death blatantly contradicts the understanding of death arising from 'disintegration' (*san*) or 'chaos' (*luan*). In line 20, it makes more sense to read the graph 搏 as *bo*. This would suggest, however, that lines 17–19 and line 20 (or lines 17–18 and lines 19–20) form two different stanzas. The last line (or two lines) would then represent a comment added by a late commentator that builds on a misunderstanding of the previous text: he misread 搏 *tuan* as *bo* and creatively added a comment on *bo*.[107]

To summarise: following Ru Chun, *bo* 搏 should read *tuan*, 'to be united', *ju tuan* should be rendered as 'to be entirely united' and *bu ju tuan* as 'not to be entirely united' in lines 17 and 18. Thereby a semantic continuity is established between 'To ride on each other' in lines 15–16 and 'to be united' in lines 17–19 (or 17–18). If, however, the graph 搏 is read as *tuan* in line

[105] See *Su wen* 17, p. 52; *Ling shu* 49, pp. 401–2.

[106] *Ling shu* 49, p. 401. On further terms shared by *mai* and *se* diagnosis, see ch. 4, n. 28, and case 7, n. 79.

[107] In cases 1–4, the final and/or penultimate line appears odd because it is irrelevant (case 1), is in its approximation of what was already stated so wrong that it was later corrected (case 2), alludes to an observation not previously mentioned (case 3), is from the viewpoint of what is biomedically possible a reasonable comment but framed in an entirely different Chinese medical rationale (case 4).

20, the text would be contradictory and say that death occurs 'in thirty days' if the three *yin* are 'united in their entirety' (*ju tuan*) in line 17, and 'instantly' if they are 'united' (*tuan*) in line 20. Moreover, the rationale that *mai* that are united should instantly lead to death is difficult to comprehend to someone familiar with early and canonical medical texts. Accordingly, the graph 搏 is best read as *tuan* in lines 17–19 (or 17–18) and as *bo* in line 20 (or 19–20). The different readings of the graph 搏 suggest that these two stanzas form separate textual units.

Questions of timing (lines 17–20)   Two terms refer to the time span before death, *zai ji qi* 在急期 'to reside in an intense time span' and *jin* 近 'near'. With regard to *jin*, we can be fairly certain that, as in *Ling shu* 49 (on p. 291), the pair 'far and near' (*yuan jin*) refers to the length and brevity of the time span before death in *Ling shu* 81: 'Among the time spans of life and death, there are the far and the near, how can one gauge them?' (*si sheng zhi qi, you yuan jin, he yi du zhi* 死生之期 有遠近 何以度之).[108] Both in *Ling shu* 49 and 81,[109] 'near' (*jin*) indicates that death is near. In all likelihood this applies also to line 19.[110]

The idiom *zai ji qi*, meaning literally 'within the intense time span', may refer to a time span before death occurs (line 18). One could consider *zai ji qi* and *jin* hierarchically ordered, indicating shorter and shorter time intervals. However, no parallels have been found for this. Rather, *zai ji qi* may well refer to a period of crisis, within which the decision (*jue*) of whether or not the patient will die is made. This would explain why Yi seems to imply hope for recovery if the patient changes his behaviour (line 6a). However, although there is evidence for a concept in early China reminiscent of what we know today of the Greek crisis days,[111] the idiom *ji qi* has not been located in the *Inner Canon*.

Given the remarkable parallels for line 17 in *Su wen* 7 (see p. 289) and line 19 in *Ling shu* 41, which mentions *tuan* (to unite) and *jin* (near) in the same passage, it is also conceivable that line 18, with the rather unusual term *zai ji qi*, was interjected by a non-medical commentator. Considering that lines 15–16 already provide an explanation for Yi's prognosis that the patient would die in thirty days, line 17 itself may have been added, evidently, by someone who was well-versed in medicine. Like case 6 (lines 19a,

---

[108] *Ling shu* 81, p. 480. Note identical usage in *Ling shu* 49, p. 401.
[109] *jin* 近 refers to temporal proximity also in *Mai jing* 5.5, p. 162.
[110] Ando Koretora notes *jin* 近 is *ni* 逆 'counter-flowing' in *Yi shuo* 3, p. 33a, but this solves nothing.
[111] There are other texts, which point to a concept akin to 'critical days' in Chinese medicine. See *Su wen* 32, p. 94 and *Ling shu* 23, p. 340, quoted on p. 322. Early iatromantic manuscript texts have days of 'slight curing' (*shao chou* 少瘳), of 'great curing' (*da chou* 大瘳) and of 'death and life' or, rather: 'of death *or* life' (*si sheng* 死生) (Harper 2001:109). On Greek crisis days, see Lloyd (1987:264–70).

23), line 17 shows striking parallels to *Su wen* 7. Can this be taken as a hint that the same person was at work? Lines 17, 18 and 19 probably all speak of *tuan* 'to be united', although each may have been added by another commentator. At a later stage, yet another commentator may have added line 20, which uses *bo* 'to strike' in a medically idiomatic way, but out of context. It is best interpreted as a confused comment on a misread graph.

Discussion

Is case 7 a pun for fun? It stands out for its wealth of medical speculation. Making sense of it has therefore been a rather impossible task, particularly due to the many terms for which there are no clear referents outside the linguistic system.

By means of text structure semantics it was possible to correlate two qualities of *mai* with two constituents in the name of the disorder, approximated here as a 'Conglomeration of remanent accumulations' (*yi ji jia*). It is evident that '*qi* [coming] from a conglomeration' is indicative of a 'conglomeration' (*jia*). The correlation between '*qi* [coming] from the spleen' and 'accumulations' (*ji*) could be established because, incidentally, the *locus classicus* for defining 'accumulations' in *Ling shu* 66 attributes them to the 'splenetic system'. This leaves the constituent *yi* meaning 'remanent' with no correlate, and suggests that it was added later, perhaps by a commentator who was unaware of the formulaic structure that the presumed early first-century editor had given to cases 1–10. Indeed, *yi ji* meaning 'remanent stools' parallels the colloquial *yi ni*, the 'remanent urine' in case 10 (line 8), which will be shown to be an interjected phrase.

Yi mentions various static verbs for describing *mai* and *qi*. They are 'small' (*xiao*) and 'soft' (*ruo*), which correlate with the conglomerations and splenetic accumulations; and 'confused' (*qia qia*), an onomatopoetic word indicative of disorders of the digestive system. Furthermore, Yi mentions *zhi* meaning either 'being congested' or 'extremely', or 'to arrive'; *jin* 'tight', which certainly is here indicative of pain; and *shen* meaning either 'very' or 'deep'. Possible readings of Yi referring to twice three or twice two or once three and once two pulse qualities have been explored. The assumed early second-century document may have had only one, either *qi* 'being congested' at the opening of the right *mai*, indicative of 'conglomerations' or, perhaps more likely, the onomatopoetic *qia qia*, which indicated 'accumulations'.

The end of case 7, concerned with the prognostication of death (lines 15–20), is riddled with incongruencies, and best explained as the result of additive amendments by perhaps as many as two, three or four commentators.

18
Case 8

Translation (*Shiki kaichû kôshô* 105, pp. 36–7)

1. Zhao Zhang, the Chancellor of the Noble of Yangxu, got ill.
2. They summoned me, Yi.
3. All the many doctors took it for a coldness striking the centre.

Name:

4. Your servant, Yi, examined his *mai* and <u>said</u>: 'It is the wind of the void.'
5. In cases of the wind of the void,
6. drink and food go down the throat, are immediately evacuated and not retained.
7. The 'Model' says: 'Death occurs after five days.'
8. However, it was after ten days that he eventually died.

Cause:

9. <u>The illness was contracted</u> from an indulgence in wine.

Quality:

10. <u>The means whereby I recognised</u> Zhao Zhang's illness were that
11. when your servant, Yi, pressed onto his *mai*,
12. the *mai* came slippery.
13. This is *qi* [coming] from the wind of the within.
14. In cases where drink and food go down the throat, are immediately evacuated and not retained,
15. according to the 'Model', death occurs after five days.

1. 陽虛侯相趙章病
2. 召臣意
3. 眾醫皆以為寒中

4. 臣意診其脈曰 迥風
5. 迥風者
6. 飲食下嗌 而輒出 不留

7. 法曰 五日死
8. 而後十日乃死

9. 病得之酒

10. 所以知趙章之病者
11. 臣意切其脈
12. 脈來滑
13. 是內風氣也

14. 飲食下嗌 而輒出 不留者

15. 法 五日死

16. All this concerns the above-mentioned 'Model for [Calculating] the Limits of one's Share'.

17. [Zhao Zhang] eventually died after ten days.
18. As for the reason whereby he exceeded the predicted time:
19. this person liked to eat gruel,
20. <u>hence</u> the viscera in the interior were replete.

21. The viscera in the interior were replete,
22. <u>hence</u> he exceeded the predicted time.

23. A word of the Master says:
24. 'Those who accommodate with ease to cereals will live beyond the appointed time.
25. Those who reject cereals will not reach it.'

16. 皆為前分界法

17. 後十日乃死
18. 所以過期者

19. 其人嗜粥
20. 故中藏實

21. 中藏實
22. 故過期

23. 師言曰
24. 安穀者 過期

25. 不安穀者 不及期

Interpretation

Yi is summoned to examine a client of high rank (lines 1–2). He claims the common doctors made a mistaken diagnosis (line 3), provides the correct one (line 4) and finds it necessary to spell out its signs and symptoms (line 5). He cites a 'Model', and prognosticates death (line 6). The prognosis is verified (line 7), but the patient lives longer than predicted (line 8). The cause of the disorder (line 9) and the qualities of *mai* Yi felt (lines 10–13) follow. Yi then gives a justification for the prognosis by alluding to said 'Model' (lines 14–16) and explains why the client outlived the predicted span (lines 17–22) by quoting a 'Saying' of a certain Master (lines 23–5).

Critical evaluation of retrospective biomedical diagnoses

Bridgman considers this case reminiscent of an intestinal stoppage, accompanied by unrestrained vomiting.[1] He evidently takes seriously *Ling shu* 4 (quoted on p. 297). Lu and Needham note: 'The description ... suggests total failure of digestion, intense diarrhoea, possibly due to enteric fever, perhaps to cholera.'[2] Since the patient dies within less than a fortnight and cannot retain any liquids, it is likely that the diarrhoea was caused by an infection. The infection may have become worse after excessive alcohol intake, which can reduce the functions of the immune system.

The name of the disorder

dong feng 迵風 – the wind of the void (line 4)   The term *dong feng* is not attested in the medical literature but is mentioned again in case 20, where

---

[1] Bridgman (1955:80–81).   [2] Lu and Needham (1967:232).

a patient, who suffers from symptoms that are said to be on the verge of becoming *dong feng*, is cured with 'rice porridge [prepared by careful] regulation of fire'.

The graph *dong* 迵, in contrast to *dong* 洞, is rare. In the Mawangdui 'Daoyuan' 道原 of the early second century BCE, it is a noun: 'At the beginning of the eternal primordial, the void was the same as the great emptiness, and the emptiness was the same as the one' (*heng xian zhi chu, dong tong da xu, xu tong wei yi* 恆先之初,迵同大[太]虛,虛同為一).[3] It means 'the void': 'Hence it has no form, the great void is without name' (*gu wu you xing, da dong wu ming* 古[故]無有刑[形]大迵無名).[4] In *Huainanzi* 21 of the mid-second century BCE, it is a verb, collocated twice with *tong* 通, which means 'to pass through'.[5] The *Yu pian* also has it as a verb: '*dong* means to pass through and reach' (*dong tong da ye* 迵通達也).[6] The above meanings of *dong* are semantically related, and can be characterised by meronymy: *dong* designates both the 'void' as a place and the movement that takes place in it, 'to pass through'.[7]

The commentators take *dong* 迵 as a verb, in the sense of *dong* 洞 in *Shuo wen* 11A: '*dong* means to flow swiftly' (*dong ji liu ye* 洞疾流也).[8] Pei Yin of the fifth century says it means 'to penetrate and enter the four limbs' (*dong che ru si zhi* 洞徹入四支). In his view, wind affects the four limbs. However, in Yi's case histories with the exception of case 24, wind does not affect the limbs. Nor is exposure to the invading outdoor winds, which is given as cause of the disorder in cases 13 and 15, very explicit in cases 1–10, where 'wind' occurs as a semantic categoriser in the name of the disorder in case 8 and as a prefix in the 'wind-induced' disorders of cases 5 (line 3) and 9 (line 3), and, in the light of text structure semantics, probably is an editorial interpolation.[9] Sima Zhen of the eighth century already noted that Pei Yin was mistaken in considering wind to affect the limbs: 'This wind swiftly pierces the five viscera, hence it is called "piercing wind"' (*shi feng ji dong che wu zang, gu yue dong feng* 是風疾洞徹五臟,故曰迵風). While Sima Zhen also takes *dong* as a verb, he speaks of wind affecting the viscera.

Unlike *dong* 迵, *dong* 洞 occurs frequently in medicine. Taki Motohiro quotes *Ling shu* 4, points out that it is called a 'piercing diarrhoea' (*dong xie* 洞泄) in *Zhen jiu jia yi jing* 4,[10] and cites a clause from the *Zheng zhi zhun sheng* 證治凖繩 by Wang Kentang 王肯堂 (1549–1613): 'In the case of an after-dinner diarrhoea, grain and water, without being transformed, come out complete [undigested]' (*can/sun xie zhe, shui gu bu hua er wan*

---

[3] MWD *Huangdi sijing* 'Daoyuan' 道原. See Yu (1993:203).
[4] MWD *Huangdi sijing* 'Daoyuan'. See Yu (1993:203).
[5] *Huainanzi* 21, p. 2126. The above reading is based on Wang Niansun.
[6] *Yu pian* A, p. 99b.
[7] On the 'meronymy' of *mai* 'vessel/pulse' and *jing* 'channel/transition', see case 6, n. 75.
[8] *Shuo wen* 11A (2), p. 8b.
[9] Wind in Yi's case histories is also discussed on pp. 117–18, 211–13, 304–5, 331–2.
[10] *Zhen jiu jia yi jing* 4.2, p. 833.

chu 餐飧泄者 水穀不化而完出).[11] He concludes that *dong feng*, *dong xie* (piercing diarrhoea) and *can/sun xie* (after-dinner diarrhoea) are all comparable disorders.

In order to highlight how wind causes diarrhoea, Taki Motokata cites *Su wen* 17: 'Chronic wind becomes a swill diarrhoea' (*jiu feng wei sun xie* 久風 為飧泄).[12] *Su wen* 42 contains a similar statement: 'If a chronic wind enters and strikes the interior, then it becomes a wind of the intestines and a swill diarrhoea' (*jiu feng ru zhong, ze wei chang feng sun xie* 久風入中 則為腸風飧 泄).[13] Evidently, the commentators interpret *dong feng* as a verb-noun complex, *dong* as 'swift and piercing' and *feng* as wind that can turn into diarrhoea.

In *Ling shu* 4, however, *dong* 洞 can be either, noun or verb: 'In cases of the cavernous, food is not transformed, it [the undigested food] goes down the throat and turns round to get out' (*dong zhe, shi bu hua, xia yi huan chu* 洞者 食不化 下嗌還出).[14] The notion of the 'cavernous' in *Ling shu* 4 comes close to Yi's 'wind of the void' but signs and symptoms differ. Yi spells them out, as though he were introducing a new concept: 'In the case of the wind of the void, drink and food go down the throat,[15] are immediately evacuated, and not retained' (lines 5–6). In the case of *dong* (the cavernous) food and drink 'turn round' (*huan* 還) to get out, but in the case of *dong feng* (wind of the void) food and drink 'instantly' (*zhe* 輒) go out.[16]

Excessive drinking, the cause of the disorder in case 8, gives rise to the 'wind of leakages' in *Su wen* 42, which probably alludes to excessive urination and perhaps also diarrhoea: 'If one drinks wine and wind strikes the centre, then it becomes a wind disorder resulting in leakage' (*yin jiu zhong feng, ze wei lou feng* 飲酒中風 則為漏風). Wang Bing glosses it as 'wind of wine': 'The *Canons* all call it "wind disorder caused by wine consumption"' (*jing ju ming yue jiu feng* 經具名曰酒風).[17]

In summary, the two constituents *dong* and *feng* can be rendered as a verb-noun or a noun-noun compound. The commentators opt for the verb–noun compound, the 'penetrating wind'. By contrast, my translation 'wind of the void' takes account of the cosmological Mawangdui manuscripts, where *dong* 迵 is a noun and means 'the void'; *dong* 洞 in *Ling shu* 4, if translated as 'the cavernous', comes close to it. In all likelihood, *dong* 迵 was the monosyllabic name of the disorder in the assumed medical document of the early second century.

[11] *Zheng zhi sun sheng* 6, p. 12a. The graph *can* 餐, also pronounced as *sun*, is interchangeable with *sun* 飧 and *sun* 殘.
[12] *Su wen* 17, p. 52.   [13] *Su wen* 42, p. 120.   [14] *Ling shu* 4, p. 277.
[15] *yi wei hou xia* 嗌謂喉下 '*yi* is below the throat', according to Pei Yin. Possibly, the gullet.
[16] Biomedically, the former suggests vomiting, for instance, due to a stomach cancer (hence Bridgman's diagnosis), the latter diarrhoea, for whatever reason.
[17] *Su wen* 42, p. 120; HDNJSW 42, p. 86.

han zhong 寒中 – **coldness in the interior (line 3)**   The common doctors speak of 'coldness striking the interior' (line 3), but Yi diagnoses 'wind of the void' (line 4). This suggests the two disorders can easily be confused with one another. The imagery they invoke is a bodily 'interior', likened to 'the void' (*dong* 迵), that *sui generis* is dark and cool like a 'cave' (*dong* 洞). Indeed, in the *Su wen*, the 'piercing diarrhoea' (*dong xie*) occurs twice, once in association with 'wind' and once with 'coldness in the interior'. Thus, *Su wen* 3 gives 'wind' as cause of the 'piercing diarrhoea': 'Therefore, if one is harmed by wind in spring, and if the noxious *qi* remains there and revolves, it eventually becomes a piercing diarrhoea' (*shi yi chun shang yu feng, xie qi liu lian, nai wei dong xie* 是以春傷於風 邪氣留連 乃為洞泄).[18] *Su wen* 4 mentions 'piercing diarrhoea' and 'coldness in the interior' in one and the same sentence: 'In the late summer, one easily gets ill with a piercing diarrhoea and coldness in the interior' (*chang xia shan bing dong xie han zhong* 長夏善病洞泄寒中).[19] In *Su wen* 4, these two disorders may well designate the same condition, but in case 8 Yi draws a clear distinction between the two.

There is a textual anomaly in lines 2–4, hinting at line 3 as a commentatorial interjection: Yi says he was summoned (line 2), then interrupts himself with this comment on *han zhong* (line 3), before he continues with his account on the examination of the patient (line 4). One also wonders why Yi says 'coldness struck the interior' (*han zhong*), which is a technical term in canonical medical texts, and not 'coldness enters and strikes the interior' (*han ru zhong*), as do 'the dull' and the 'wind' in cases 3 (line 2) and 10 (line 2).

Text structure semantics

According to text structure semantics the constituents in the name of the disorder, 'wind of the void' (*dong feng*), should correlate with the pulse qualities. Yi first says the '*mai* came slippery' (*mai lai hua*; line 12), and explains that this is indicative of '*qi* [coming] from a wind of the within' (*nei feng qi*; line 13). In first approximation, one could argue: 'wind *qi*' correlates with the constituent 'wind', *nei* correlates with *dong,* and 'being slippery' is superfluous. If *dong* is a noun meaning 'the void', the term *nei*, which is often used as a verb or adverb meaning 'to enter' or 'internally', may also be a noun. We have already encountered *nei* as a noun in Yi's *Memoir* (e.g. case 1, line 15). Moreover, Zhou dynasty texts like Confucius' *Lun yu* use *nei* as a noun, in the sense of 'the private within'.[20] Perhaps *nei* 'the within' and *dong* 'the void' alluded to a body internal cavity.

---

[18] *Su wen* 3, p. 15.   [19] *Su wen* 4, p. 16.
[20] Graham (1989:26) quotes *Lun yu* 4, p. 2471c; 5, p. 2475b; 12, p. 2503a.

In the canonical medical literature, *nei* 內 and *dong* 迵 are mostly used as verbs and adverbs.[21] When the term *nei* refers to sexual activity, it can be interpreted either as verb or noun, meaning 'inner chambers' or 'private parts', as in *Su wen* 42: 'If after entering into the bedchamber, one sweats and is struck by wind, then this becomes a "wind of the inner [chambers]"' (*ru fang han chu zhong feng, ze wei nei feng* 入房汗出中風 則為內風).[22] Although *nei feng* tends to be translated as 'internal wind', *nei* is here no doubt a verb or noun as indicated in the translation above.

hua 滑 – **slippery (line 12)**   From the viewpoint of text structure semantics, if *nei* as a noun correlates with *dong* (the void) and *feng qi* with *feng* (wind), no further pulse quality is needed to determine the name. But line 12 mentions the 'slippery' (*hua*) pulse and there is canonical medical evidence for it correlating with 'wind'. Thus, Taki Motokata cites *Su wen* 18: 'If the pulse is slippery, you call it wind' (*mai hua yue feng* 脈滑曰風).[23] To this can be added *Ling shu* 74: 'If the skin of the foot area is slippery, slushy and lubricant, it is wind' (*chi fu hua, qi zhuo ze zhe, feng ye* 尺膚滑 其淖澤者 風也),[24] and *Su wen* 64, where 'being slippery', inter alia, is indicative of 'wind amassments' (*feng shan* 風疝).[25]

'Being slippery' and 'rough', which form a pair in the Zhangjiashan 'Mai shu' (see p. 31), belong among the six standard *mai* of *Ling shu* 4 (quoted on pp. 173–4), for which there is a parallel in *Ling shu* 3: 'There are those who know how to regulate the inch and the foot, the small and large, the lax and intense, the slippery and rough, in order to diagnose what is in disorder' (*you zhi tiao chi cun xiao da huan ji hua se, yi yan suo bing ye* 有知 調尺寸小大緩急滑濇 以言所病已).[26] In *Ling shu* 73, the 'smooth and slippery' are associated with wind and warmth, the 'rough' with coldness, constriction and obstructions.[27]

nei qi 內氣 or *feng qi* 風氣 – *qi* **coming from within or from wind? (line 13)**   In line 12, the mentioning of *mai* in place of *qi* may be taken as a hint of an editorial interpolation or commentatorial interjection, as in case 4 (line 30). It probably is not a commentator's interjection, because rhetorically it fits well into Yi's usual schema (manner 1 in table 4): XYZ *ye, shi* AB *ye* (*mai lai hua, shi nei feng qi ye*).[28] Thus, if on the grounds of the above medical, textual and rhetorical considerations, the pulse quality 'slippery' (*hua*) is made to correlate with the constituent 'wind' (*feng*) in the name of the disorder, then *feng qi* cannot correlate with *feng*, and *feng* in *nei feng qi* must be superfluous and probably is a commentator's interjection. It is more likely that *feng* was interjected (than *nei*), because *feng* occurs in the

---

[21] e.g. *Su wen* 2, p. 11; *Ling shu* 63, pp. 426–7.   [22] *Su wen* 42, p. 120.
[23] *Su wen* 18, p. 55.   [24] *Ling shu* 74, p. 454.   [25] *Su wen* 64, p. 178.
[26] *Ling shu* 3, p. 273.   [27] See also *Ling shu* 4, pp. 276–7; 73, p. 451.
[28] Cases 1, 8 and 10 have no *ye* after XYZ, cases 2 and 7 do.

name (but not *nei*) and because *feng qi* correlates with *feng* as constituent in the name in other cases (cases 5 and 9).

So, in conclusion, text structure semantics suggests '*qi* coming from the within' (*nei qi*) correlates with 'the void' (*dong*), 'being slippery' (*hua*) correlates with 'wind' (*feng*) and *feng* in *nei feng qi* is a scribal error. The intuitive images that both correlations evoke are exceptionally strong, but early and canonical medical parallels in support of them, while existent, are fairly sparse.

The prognostication of death (lines 7–8 and 14–16)

Case 8 is to a large extent concerned with the prognostication of death. Twice reference is made to a 'Model' (*fa*) (lines 7 and 15). This 'Model' is then identified as 'Fen jie fa' (line 16). The meanings of *fen* in the context of prognostication have been explored at length in case 1 (lines 33–40). The compound word *fen jie* 分界 is generally understood as 'limits' or 'boundary'. Its *locus classicus* is *Xunzi* 19: 'When desire is not satisfied, then he cannot be without seeking for satisfaction. When this seeking for satisfaction is without measure or boundary, then there cannot but be contention' (*ren sheng er you yu, yu er bu de, ze bu neng bu qiu, qiu er wu du liang fen jie, ze bu neng bu zheng* 人生而有欲 欲而不得 則不能不求 求而無度量分界 則不能不爭).[29] The same word sequence *fen jie* also occurs in a Dunhuang medical manuscript, but its meaning is unclear.[30] Zhang Shoujie comments *fen* should be read in the fourth tone; it then means 'allotment' or 'share'. Accordingly, 'Fen jie fa' is translated as 'Model of Allotments up to the Boundary [indicative of Death]' or 'The Model for [Calculating] the Limits of one's Share'.

The word *qian* 前 causes some discussion among the commentators. It may either be interpreted as the 'front part', i.e. the first volume, of the 'Model', or it may be part of the title, or it may refer to the 'previously mentioned' (*qian*) 'Model', being used in the same sense as in case 7 (line 20), where Oka Hakku glosses *ru qian* 如前 as 'as said above'. This last reading is the most likely, not least because Yi's prognosticatory calculations are pentic in cases 1 and 6.[31] Despite differences in detail, the time span before death is in both calculated by equating a *fen* on the *mai* (or in the body) to a day. However, if case 7 (line 20) was added by a commentator who used *ru qian* in the same sense as *qian* in case 8 (line 16), this line may also be a commentatorial interjection, and 'Fen jie fa' not an early Han but a later term.

---

[29] *Xunzi* 19, p. 203, translation Dubs (1928:213). See also translation by Knoblock (1994:55).
[30] Dunhuang manuscript P3287, text 5, col. 90 (Ma 1998:20), has an irregularity in the text, which mentions: *yi cun jiu fen jie* 一寸九分界.
[31] See also Osobe Yô (1994:86).

The patient died later than predicted; he lived longer because of his diet: he liked to eat gruel (lines 18–22). Yi's explanation is common sense today. Some of the technical terms that Yi uses are unusual, however. Thus, the term *zhong zang* does not occur in the *Inner Canon*. It may refer, as Osobe Yô proposes, to the 'central viscus', which is the spleen in canonical doctrine.[32] However, considering that *zhong fu*, 'central cavity', occurs in the Mawangdui 'He yinyang',[33] *zhong zang* may be a similarly vague term, meaning the 'viscera in the interior'. Yi says they are 'replete' (*shi*), a term used mostly for pulse qualities in canonical texts, as also in case 10 (line 14). Finally, Yi refers to yet another medical authority, the 'Master' (*shi*), and his 'Saying' or 'Word' (*yan*).[34]

Discussion

Case 8 poses problems for text structure semantics because three constituent pulse qualities, *hua* and *nei feng qi*, are meant to interrelate with two constituents in the name, *dong feng*. Setting up correlations has been difficult because of the wide semantic stretch of the terms involved. Finally, considering that in Yi's case histories *nei* 'the within' can be a noun and that in an early cosmological Mawangdui text *dong* as noun means the 'void', the pulse quality '*qi* [coming] from the within' (*nei qi*) has been made to correlate with the 'void' (*dong*). The 'void' may have been the monosyllabic name of the disorder in the assumed early second-century document. The pulse quality 'being slippery' (*hua*), which qualifies *mai* and may be an editorial interpolation, correlates with 'wind' (*feng*). Intuitively, 'slippery' as an attribute of wind and diarrhoea is easily grasped, even across ages and cultures. More importantly, canonical medical texts explicitly state this correlation. So, *feng* in *nei feng qi* must be a scribal error.

In case 8, the narrative contains many repetitions and Yi invokes medical authorities other than himself more frequently than usual: he mentions the same 'Model' three times (lines 7, 15, 16), and refers to a 'word of the Master' (line 23). The stanza that names the 'Model for [Calculating] the Limits of one's Share' contains apart from its name no new information (lines 14–17). The next stanza (lines 18–20) repeats the information given in the Master's word, by reframing it as a problem of the 'repleteness' of the 'viscera of the interior', and the following one (lines 21–2) repeats this, verbatim. Case 8 forms a pair with case 7, insofar as the former concerns constipation and this one diarrhoea.

---

[32] Osobe Yô (1994:86).
[33] Harper (1998:420). MWD 'He yinyang' (1985:156, S128). See also *Su wen* 27, p. 85.
[34] Kaiho Gembi notes *an* 安 means *an dun* 安頓 'to accommodate'. Takigawa identifies the 'Master' as Master Yang Qing, but, strictly speaking, it is not clear who it is.

19

Case 9

Translation (*Shiki kaichû kôshô* **105, pp. 37–8**)

1. The King of Jibei fell ill.
2. They summoned your servant, Yi. I examined his *mai*.

Name:

3. I <u>said</u>: 'A wind-induced numbness/inversion.
4. The chest feels full.'

5. Forthwith, I prepared a drugged wine.
6. After drinking three *shi*,
7. the illness ceased.

Cause:

8. <u>He contracted it from</u> sweating and lying prostrate on the ground.

Quality:

9. <u>The means whereby I recognised</u> the illness of the King of Jibei were that
10. at the time when your servant, Yi, pressed onto his *mai*, it was wind *qi*.
11. The *mai* [coming] from the heart was murky.

12. According to the 'Model of Disorders',
13. if one excessively makes one's *yang* enter,
14. then, while *yang qi* is exhausted, *yin qi* enters.
15. If *yin qi* enters and expands,
16. then, while cold *qi* ascends, hot *qi* descends,
17. <u>hence</u> the chest feels full.

18. As for the sweating and lying prostrate on the ground,
19. when I pressed onto his *mai*, *qi* was *yin*.
20. In cases of *yin qi*,
21. the illness must have entered and struck the interior.
22. When one expels it, it reaches a degree of swishing water.

1. 濟北王病
2. 召臣意診其脈

3. 曰風蹶
4. 胸滿

5. 即為藥酒
6. 盡三石
7. 病已

8. 得之汗出伏地

9. 所以知濟北王病者

10. 臣意切其脈時風氣也
11. 心脈濁

12. 病法
13. 過入其陽
14. 陽氣盡 而陰氣入
15. 陰氣入張
16. 則寒氣上 而熱氣下
17. 故胸滿

18. 汗出伏地者

19. 切其脈 氣陰
20. 陰氣者
21. 病必入中

22. 出及瀺水也

302

Interpretation

Yi first names the disorder (line 3), with its main concomitant symptom
(line 4). He then reports on successful treatment (lines 5–7), and the cause
of the disorder (line 8). The remainder is medical speculation (lines 9–22).
For explaining the name, Yi mentions pulse qualities (lines 9–11). For
explaining the symptom, he refers to a 'Model of Disorders' (lines 12–17).
Finally, for explaining the cause, he reports on yet another pulse quality,
and outlines his treatment rationale (lines 18–22). The case differs from
others in that Yi gives separate explanations for the name, main symptom,
and cause of the disorder.

Critical evaluation of retrospective biomedical diagnoses

Bridgman suggests pulmonary congestion or chronic exudative pleurisy.[1]
Lu and Needham are silent. From a contemporary Chinese medical viewpoint, indulgence in sexual intercourse leads to '*yang* depletion' (*yang xu*
陽虛).[2] Perhaps this is an early recording of a condition precursory to what
later became known as such. Drastic alcohol consumption certainly would
result in a good night's sleep.

Text structure semantics

Text structure semantics has us expect that the qualities of *mai*, which Yi
mentions in his own vocabulary interrelate with the name of the disorder.
In case 9, this raises the question of whether the name of the disorder is
two-syllabic, 'wind-induced inversion' (*feng jue*; line 3), or four-syllabic,
'wind-induced inversion causing fullness of the chest' (*feng jue xiong man*;
lines 3–4). In what follows, I argue that Yi explains the 'fullness of the chest'
with the 'Model of Disorders' (Bing fa), and that therefore the qualities of
mai should explain the name of the disorder – 'wind-induced inversion/
numbness'.

The first pulse quality, '*qi*' [coming] from wind' (*feng qi*; line 10) correlates nicely with the first constituent of the name – 'wind' (*feng*; line 3). The
question remains as to which pulse quality interrelates with *jue* (numbness/
inversion) in the clause 'the *mai* [coming] from the heart was murky' (line
11). A quick answer would be that the 'pulse [coming] from the heart' (*xin
mai*; line 11) correlates with the 'chest', and 'being murky' (*zhuo*) with *jue*
(lines 3–4). A more considered answer, however, takes into account that
'murky' is an attribute of the 'pulse [coming] from the heart' (*xin mai*). Thus,
in case 1, 'being murky, yet still' (*zhuo er jing*) is an attribute of '*qi* [coming]
from the liver' (*gan qi*) and in case 2, 'murky and hurried, yet [the condition]

---

[1] Bridgman (1955:82).   [2] e.g. Shapiro (1998).

is transient' (*zhuo zao er jing*) is an attribute of '*qi* [coming] from the heart' (*xin qi*). In these two cases we searched for a correlation between the 'liver' and the *ju*-abscess (case 1) and between the 'heart' and the 'disorder of *qi* that is blocked' (*qi ge bing*; case 2). Accordingly, in case 9, '*qi* [coming] from the heart' should correlate with *jue* (inversion). This is indeed a correlation for which there already are parallels in the early medical manuscripts (see pp. 312–18).

To complicate the issue, it is not '*qi* [coming] from the heart' (*xin qi*) but '*mai* [coming] from the heart' (*xin mai*) that is said to be murky. In cases 3, 4, 7 and 8, we took this difference between Yi referring to *mai* instead of *qi* seriously and suggested that sentences that reported on qualifications of *mai* were interpolations by the early first-century editor. In full awareness that Yi qualifies a pulse quality in terms of *qi* later, we note here that the correlation between the heart and *jue* probably reflects the early first-century editor's understanding of *jue*.

So, in case 9, 'wind *qi*' correlates with 'wind', and '*mai* coming from the heart' with *jue* (numbness/inversion). So far, so good. However, the correlation between 'wind *qi*' as pulse quality and 'wind' as constituent in the name of the disorder in cases 5 and 9, as postulated by text structure semantics, is facile (as is the 'lung *qi*' and lungs in case 6 and 'conglomeration *qi*' and the 'conglomeration' in case 7). This should alert our attention to 'wind' as a possible editorial interpolation.

feng 風 – the wind-induced disorder (line 3): an editorial interpolation?   In cases 1–10, Yi mentions three names of disorders that have 'wind' (*feng*) as a constituent: *feng dan ke pao* in case 5, *dong feng* in case 8 and *feng jue* in case 9. The problem with these names is, as already noted, that the correlations between *feng qi* as pulse quality and *feng* as constituent in the name are facile, at least in cases 5 and 9, and, second, that there are no parallels for them in the early and canonical medical literature, or if there are, there are problems.

In case 8 (line 4), there are no early and canonical medical parallels for the name 'wind of the void' (*dong feng*). However, comparison with the signs and symptoms of the 'void/cavernous' (*dong*) in *Ling shu* 4 provides a medical reason why physicians may have wished to differentiate between 'the void/the cavernous', which presented with vomiting, and the 'wind of the void', which involved diarrhoea. Furthermore, the constituent 'wind' correlates with '*mai* that is slippery' (rather than 'wind *qi*'), a correlation, which as others of text structure semantics, is not directly evident, but once established, plausible (see case 8, line 12). In other words, even if the constituent 'wind' in the name of the disorder is an editorial interpolation of the early first century, it is medically motivated.

Cases 5 and 9 concern conditions of utter exhaustion due to sexual over-exertion, excessive sweating, implicitly perhaps an opening of the skin pore pattern which allowed wind to enter, and hence a wind-induced disorder. The names of the disorder in cases 5 and 9 thus contain information about their causes, which in Han China became increasingly body ecological. Accordingly, the prefix 'wind' in the name may reflect developments in medical rationale that date from the early first rather than from the early second century. It furthermore has sexual overtones, as does *feng* in *feng ma* (horse in heat) and as is known from the non-medical early and Han literature, where 'wind' is conceived of as a life-engendering principle, among insects as much as here, by implication, among kings and queens (see case 5, line 3). This suggests that the assumed early second-century medical document had the monosyllabic *dan* (utter exhaustion) and *jue* (numbness) as name of the disorder and that the prefix *feng* was interpolated by the early first-century editor, who had another agenda than a merely medical one.

yin 陰 – the pulse quality that correlates with *jue* (line 19)   In case 9 (line 19), as in case 4 (lines 32–3), a pulse quality mentioned towards the end of the case history qualifies *qi* rather than *mai* and therefore may reflect early second-century medical rationale. Yi says as he pressed onto *mai* he felt that '*qi* is *yin*' (*qi yin*). Text structure semantics thus highlights a correlation between *jue* and *yin qi*, reflecting the understanding of the presumed early second-century author, and between *jue* and the heart *mai*, reflecting that of the early first-century editor. For each, there are parallels in the literature on self-cultivation and medicine.

The name of the disorder (line 3)

Introductory remarks   The term *jue* is an enigma to historians of Chinese medicine, because it is difficult to see what the pathological conditions called *jue* have in common.[3] There is little doubt that the term *jue* has a history, and that its meaning and connotations changed over time. In what follows, I will discuss *jue* based on the above correlations postulated by text structure semantics. I will first search for evidence in favour of reading *jue* in case 9 as a monosyllabic name of the disorder and argue that the early second-century physician considered the pulse quality *qi* is *yin* (line 19) to indicate a *jue* disorder.

I will then argue that *feng qi* and *feng* are interpolations by the first-century editor which changed the name of the disorder to *feng jue*. This will be done by comparing *feng jue* in case 9 with *feng jue* conditions recorded in the *Inner Canon*. It will highlight that *jue* in *Shi ji* 105.1 and *Shi ji* 105.2, as well as *feng jue* in *Su wen* 7, typically arise from *yin yang* inversions.

---

[3] The graphs 厥, 蹶, 瘚 are often used interchangeably, as Lo (1999) suggests, but each has a distinctive basic meaning. See also case 3 (line 2).

Third, I will argue that the early first-century editor considered *jue* to correlate with the heart. Evidence for such a correlation is given in the Mawangdui 'Yinyang vessel text' and the Zhangjiashan 'Maishu'.

Since Chinese medical historians usually define *jue* in the sense it has in the *Shi ming* of 200 CE, finally I will explore *jue* in those chapters of the *Inner Canon* which mention the term in their titles and I will highlight further connotations of *jue*. It has to be borne in mind that the term *jue* took on different shades of meaning over the centuries. The meaning of *jue* in 200 CE is the often quoted but least appropriate for understanding the medical rationale four hundred years earlier around 200 BCE.

jue 厥 – a *yin* disorder in the *Lü shi chun qiu* (line 19)   Text structure semantics suggests that the author of the early second-century document correlated *qi* that is *yin* with *jue* 厥, which then probably designated a 'numbness'. There is compelling evidence from the third century BCE that *jue* was considered a *yin* disorder as in *Lü shi chun qiu* 1: 'If the room is large, then it augments *yin*, if the platform is high, then it augments *yang*. If one augments *yin*, then there is numbness, if one augments *yang*, then there is limpness, these are complaints arising from an imbalance between *yin* and *yang*' (*shi da ze duo yin, tai gao ze duo yang, duo yin ze jue, duo yang ze wei, ci yin yang bu shi zhi huan ye* 室大則多陰 臺高則多陽 多陰則厥 多陽則痿 此陰陽不適之患也).[4] The *Lü shi chun qiu* clearly states that *jue* (numbness) is a *yin* disorder and arises from an imbalance of *yin* and *yang*.

Although the correlation between *jue* and *yin* is not made explicit elsewhere, it may be implicitly given if the head is understood as *yang*, the feet as *yin* in *Lü shi chun qiu* 3: 'If the compressed [*qi*] resides in the head, then it turns into swellings or wind ... if it resides in the feet, then it turns into limpness or numbness' (*yu chu tou ze wei zhong wei feng ... chu zu ze wei wei wei jue* 鬱處頭則為腫為風 ... 處足則為痿為厥).[5] Here wind is associated with the head, and numbness and limpness with the feet. The latter easily get numb. Based on this evidence, it seems that *jue* in the early second century was considered a *yin* disorder, associated with the cold and numbness, and the postulate of text structure semantics that the constituent *jue* (line 3) in the name of the disorder correlates with the pulse quality '*qi* is *yin*' (line 19) is corroborated.

feng jue 風厥 – 'wind inversions' in the *Inner Canon* (line 3)   As suggested above, the first-century editor may have added 'wind' to the names of the

---

[4] *Lü shi chun qiu* 1.3, 'Zhong ji' 重己. Compare with Knoblock and Riegel (2000:69). *jue* 厥 means 'to be stiff', hence its rendering as 'numbness'; *wei* 委 means 'to fall' or 'to hang down' (Karlgren 1957:102, 357a), hence its rendering as 'limpness'.
[5] *Lü shi chun qiu* 3.2. Compare with Knoblock and Riegel (2000:100).

disorders in cases 5 and 9, perhaps primarily for non-medical reasons. The question investigated here is whether or not this editor was aware that *feng jue* was an elite medical term. As will become apparent, this entails the question: what is *feng jue*, and for that matter, what is *jue*? Both involve a *yin yang* imbalance.

Feng jue 'wind inversion' occurs only three times in the *Inner Canon*. Of these, *Su wen* 33 and *Ling shu* 46 parallel case 9, says Taki Mototane, who makes no reference to *Su wen* 7.

In *Ling shu* 46 the aspect of sweating is prominent: 'The Yellow Emperor said: if a person prone to suffer from wind inversion is dripping with sweat, what kind of condition is it? Shao Yu answered: if the flesh is not firm and the skin pore pattern is dredged, then one is likely to get ill from wind' (*Huangdi yue: ren zhi shan feng jue lu han zhe, he yi hou zhi. Shao Yu da yue: rou bu jian, zou li shu, ze shan bing feng* 黃帝曰 人之善風厥漉汗者 何以候之 少俞答曰 肉不堅 腠理疎 則善病風).[6]

Su wen 33 mentions both sweating and feeling upset and full: 'The Emperor said: if one is ill and the body is hot, sweat comes out, one feels upset and full, and if feeling upset and full cannot be released by sweating, what kind of illness is this? Qibo answered: if despite sweating, the body is hot, it is [indicative of] wind. If despite sweating, the feeling of being upset and full is not released, it is [indicative of] an inversion, the name of the disorder is a "wind inversion"' (*Di yue: you bing shen re han chu fan man, fan man bu wei han jie, ci wei he bing? Qibo yue: han chu er shen re zhe, feng ye, han chu [er] fan man bu jie zhe, jue ye, bing ming yue feng jue* 帝曰 有病身熱汗出煩滿 煩滿不為汗解 此為何病 歧伯曰 汗出而身熱者 風也 汗出〔而〕煩滿不解者 厥也 病名曰風厥).[7] In *Ling shu* 46, sweating is the one feature which parallels case 9, while in *Su wen* 33 there are two: sweating and feeling upset and full. There clearly are parallels between *feng jue* in case 9 and the canonical medical literature.

Su wen 7, which is not mentioned by the commentators, discusses *feng jue* in a paragraph on symptoms produced by various *yin yang* imbalances: 'If the second [two] *yang* and the first [one] *yin* develop a disorder, it governs fright and back pain, one is prone to sigh and prone to yawn, the name is "wind inversion"' (*er yang yi yin fa bing, zhu jing hai bei tong, shan yi shan qian, ming yue feng jue* 二陽一陰發病 主驚駭背痛 善噫善欠 名曰風厥).[8] In *Su wen* 7, fright and back pain are best taken as a sign of a disorder in the liver,[9] the sighing and yawning of a disorder in the 'heart'.[10] Wind, which correlates with the 'second *yang*', affects the body architectural liver; *jue*,

---

[6] *Ling shu* 46, p. 388.
[7] *Su wen* 33, p. 96. A textual variation is given in parentheses.
[8] *Su wen* 7, p. 26.
[9] This interpretation is based on Nanjing zhongyi xueyuan (1991:65).
[10] Compare with *Su wen* 23, p. 74, where among the five *qi*, sighing (*yi* 噫) correlates with the heart.

which correlates with the 'first *yin*', affects the body architectural heart. *Su wen* 7 describes an inversion, if one considers the liver to be located in the lower *yin*-part in the body architecture and the heart in its upper *yang*-part. If *yin* that affects the upper *yang* region causes sighing, and *yang* that affects the liver in the abdominal *yin* region causes fright and back pain then *Su wen* 7 concerns a *yin yang* inversion, as does case 9. Perhaps the commentators did not note this parallel of the *yin yang* inversion, because *Su wen* 7 mentions externally observable complaints, which can be recognised as referring to heart and liver only for the initiated?

A note on the dating of the quoted texts is warranted here. In awareness that textual contexts cannot provide a conclusive answer, the conceptions of body they refer to may provide hints. Thus, *Su wen* 7 seems to allude to the bipartite body known from the Warring States period. By contrast, *Su wen* 33 and *Ling shu* 46 focus on sweating as integral to the pathology and therapeutics of the condition discussed, reminiscent of the Eastern Han *Shang han lun* (see pp. 319–22). This suggests that *Su wen* 7 pre-dates the other two texts from the *Inner Canon*. Indeed, case 9 alludes to an early medical bipartite body concept and to *feng jue* as an inversion as given in *Su wen* 7, but additionally it emphasises sweating. This aspect of *feng jue*, massive perspiration, is stressed in *Su wen* 33 and *Ling shu* 46. Why? Did case 9 have an impact on medical history by influencing later medical writers?

feng jue 風厥 – a *yin yang* inversion according to the 'Model of Disorders' (lines 12–17)

The 'Model of Disorders', which in name but not in contents parallels the 'Model for Treating Disorders' in the Zhangjiashan 'Maishu',[11] outlines pathological processes in the body and explains the main concomitant symptom of the King of Jibei's 'wind inversion' which is that the 'chest feels full' (*xiong man*). To anyone familiar with canonical doctrine, the explanations instantly make sense, although some of the processes are described in an unfamiliar wording. Thus, it is worth noting that first an imbalance between *yin* and *yang* is described (lines 14–15), and subsequently one between hot and cold *qi* (line 16). *Yin* and *yang* describe one sort of process: 'while *yang qi* is exhausted, *yin qi* enters'; the cold and hot refer to another one: 'while cold *qi* ascends, hot *qi* descends'. In case 9, the two appear closely related but not identical. This is odd; usually *yin* and *yang* stand for coldness and heat. The expression '*yang qi* is exhausted' (*yang qi jin*) occurs also in *Su wen* 49, and there has the effect that '*yin qi* becomes abundant' (*yin qi sheng* 陰氣盛),[12] a process which Yi describes in a verb-verb idiom as '*yin qi* enters and expands' (*yin qi ru zhang*). Yi seems to imply that *yin qi* could invade the body because the king lay prostrate

[11] ZJS 'Mai shu' (2001:245).
[12] *Su wen* 49, p. 137.

on the [cold] ground. Thus, *yang qi jin* in line 14 is canonical, but not the verb-verb construction in line 15, *yin qi ru zhang*, although the *Inner Canon* describes a similar process in a different vocabulary. So, the processes described in lines 14–15 were known to medical authors.

The expansion of *yin qi*, says Yi, has the effect that 'cold *qi* ascends' (*han qi shang*). In a similar vein, the *Inner Canon* mentions twice 'cold *qi* that ascends', notably, in both cases together with *jue qi* 厥氣 (numb *qi*). This parallels case 9. Thereupon, Yi says, hot *qi* descends (*re qi xia*). However, while the *Inner Canon* mentions this idiom three times, it is not in the context of cold *qi* that ascends nor of *jue qi*.[13] For the combination of these two processes there is thus no textual parallel in the *Inner Canon*.

Incidentally, case 16, where the patient 'is numb above' and 'feels numb in the head' (*jue shang* 厥上, *jue tou* 厥頭), also refers to hot *qi* that is descending, when it states that the 'heat [from the head] has reached [downward] to the shoulders' (*re zhi jian* 熱至肩). A reader familiar with canonical medicine confronted with this final sentence in case 16 instantly thinks of the work of a commentator not well-versed in medicine. Perhaps the same one was at work in case 9 (line 16)?

jue 厥 – a *yin yang* inversion in other case histories of *Shi ji* 105 In Yi's case histories, the term *jue* occurs three times as a constituent of the name of the disorder that Yi diagnoses (cases 9, 11, 16) and twice as a name of the disorder given by the common doctors (cases 3, 23). Yi's concept of *jue* is fairly consistent, while it seems to differ in important ways from that of the common doctors. The term *jue* is also mentioned twice in Bian Que's Memoir. There it refers once to a state where someone has fainted and is numb and lifeless, approximating the state of being dead.[14]

To be precise, in Bian Que's Memoir *jue* is mentioned twice, once as a verb in the phrase 'he suddenly got numb' (*bao jue* 暴厥) and once as a constituent in the term *shi jue* 尸厥 (the corpse is numb), where it probably also figures as a verb, as many early medical terms did (see pp. 246–7). In that context the event described as *bao jue* and the disorder called *shi jue* arise, ultimately, from an inversion between *yin* and *yang*.[15] *Bao jue* and *shi jue* describe a process leading to an apparent (or fake) death. It is likely that *jue* in the phrase *bao jue* means 'being numb'; *jue* in the term *shi jue*, which also means 'being numb', may additionally have had overtones of being 'fake' (see discussion of *jue* in *Ling shu* 24 on p. 318).

---

[13] For *han qi shang*, see *Huangdi nei jing*, p. 1367. See *Su wen* 39, p. 112; *Ling shu* 66, p. 438; and computer printout by Hermann Tessenow (2000 p.c.). For *re qi xia*, see *Huangdi nei jing*, p. 1494. See *Su wen* 70, p. 206; *Ling shu* 66, p. 438; 81, p. 481; and computer printout by Hermann Tessenow (2000 p.c.).

[14] *Shiki kaichû kôshô* 105.1, pp. 8, 13, 15.

[15] However, this *yin yang* inversion is not an attribute of *shi jue* in *Su wen* 63, p. 177, nor of *bao jue* in *Su wen* 28, p. 88; 48, p. 135.

In Yi's Memoir, the common doctors and Yi both diagnose *jue*. As demonstrated in case 3 (line 2), the common doctors might quite literally have referred to *jue* as 'the stone', which appears to have been an epitome of the coarse and crude in the late Zhou and Han.[16] Their concept of *jue* comes close to that of a *yin* disorder, as which 'the stone' and any numbness may well have been perceived, such as that of the numb feet, given in the *Lü shi chun qiu*. The *Shi ji* personage Yi, however, whose medical reasoning already shows more traits of the medical rationale that predominates in the medical canons compiled in the Eastern Han, clearly had a different understanding of *jue*.

The three *jue* Yi diagnoses show some semantic consistency, although one notes again a certain unity among cases 1–10, in that case 9 (lines 19–22) relates to *jue* as a *yin* condition, as may do the common doctors' *jue* in case 3 (line 2). By contrast, cases 11 and 16 both involve heat. In case 9, Yi quotes the 'Model of Disorder' (lines 12–17). It says *jue* arises from an imbalance between *yin* and *yang*. In case 11, he explains the patient suffers from heat and fullness in the feet, which implicitly indicates an imbalance between the hot and cold (feet tend to be cold). And in case 16, he reports that the patient has heat in the head which is cured by clasping cold water onto it and thereby restoring the balance between the hot and cold. Since all three cases of *jue* that Yi diagnoses concern an imbalance within a conceptual framework marked by dual oppositions, *jue* in the rendering of the *Shi ji* personage Yi is best approximated as 'inversion'.[17]

In Yi's understanding, *jue* is thus best conceived of as arising from an inversion of *yin* and *yang*, and the cold and hot. Was *jue*, when understood as 'inversion' of *yin* and *yang* or hot and cold, painful or not? Of the three cases of *jue* mentioned in Yi's Memoir, only one, case 16, alludes to pain, namely a headache (*tou tong* 頭痛). Yet even in case 16, which notably does not belong among cases 1–10, the 'headache' mentioned is one among a whole host of concomitant symptoms which include 'sluggishness' (*wei zhong* 為重), a 'body that feels hot' (*shen re* 身熱) and a 'person who feels upset and oppressed' (*ren fan men* 人煩懣).

The symptom of 'fullness' (*man*) or 'oppression' (*men*) is predominant in all three *jue* cases Yi mentions. In other words, all three *jue* conditions are marked by a feeling of fullness, some in combination with heat, one in combination with coldness. In the two cases where this fullness occurs

---

[16] They also diagnose *jue* in case 23, which Yi considers an 'obstruction' (*bi* 痺). He mentions *ni qi* 逆氣 meaning perhaps 'burping', perhaps 'contravective *qi*'; perhaps a commentatorial interjection? See ch. 7, n. 57.

[17] 'Inversion', as in my 1995 draft (published by Raphals 1998b:24–8), is meant to approximate body conceptions of the Warring States and early Han: it emphasises the duality and complementarity of *yin* and *yang* or hot and cold; *jue* as 'reversal' (Harper 1998:204ff.) or 'reversion' (Lo 1999) conveys the idea of flow of 'contravective *qi*' as given in lexicographic works of the second century CE.

together with heat, Yi applies 'needling' (*ci*): in case 11, he needles three places of each 'foot's heart' (*zu xin* 足心) and in case 16, three places of both the left and right foot's *yang* brightness *mai*. It is worth noting that needling in these cases is not intended to treat pain (as whoever uses acupuncture for pain management today might anachronistically impute into ancient writings).[18] Rather, it reduces the feeling of fullness (which is reminiscent of the way one pricks a balloon to deflate it and let air out).[19]

It has been suggested that throughout *Shi ji* 105 'needling' is applied only to *jue* conditions, which is easily said but, again, not entirely correct. It applies to Bian Que's Memoir, where it is explicitly said that in a case of *shi jue* neither 'decoctions' (*tang ye* 湯液) nor 'unrefined alcoholic drinks' (*li sa* 醴灑) can help, and the recommended treatment is the application of 'stone needles' (*zhen shi* 鑱石), 'exercise' (*jiao yin* 撟引), 'massage' (*an kang* 案抏) and/or 'potent poultices' (*du yun* 毒熨).[20] In Yi's Memoir, it is the case that Yi applies needling twice for treating the *jue* conditions, namely in cases 11 and 16, and that in case 3 the common doctors treat what they diagnose as 'the stone' (*jue*) with needling. However, in case 10, the common doctors aim to treat a 'wind that has entered and struck the interior' (*feng ru zhong*) by means of needling, which Yi diagnoses as a '*qi* amassment' (*qi shan*). The statement that 'needling' is applied only to *jue* conditions in *Shi ji* 105 is simply wrong. The question then arises as to what the conditions treated by needling in Yi's Memoir had in common.

The exceptions are telling: in case 9 Yi diagnoses a condition of *jue* but does not treat it with needling, and in case 10 neither Yi nor the common doctors diagnose *jue*, while the latter are said to have mistakenly treated the patient with needling. Case 10 concerns a condition, which according to Yi is called a '*qi* amassment' (*qi shan*); it manifests in a 'replete' (*shi*) pulse and an 'abdomen that becomes swollen' (*fu zhong*). It thus resembles the three cases Yi diagnoses as *jue* conditions, marked by fullness and oppression, in that it presents with a repletion.

How does such fullness, oppression or repletion arise? The name of the disorder in case 10 hints at the answer. In Yi's case histories, *qi* is not the all-pervasive stuff of the later canonical body ecologic that permeates the universe. In case 10, Yi says *qi* is the stuff that is visiting the bladder. We can thus extrapolate that Yi implies that *qi* is the stuff that causes the *qi* amassment. So, is it *qi* that causes the fullness and oppression in the cases Yi diagnoses as *jue*? Indeed. Once *qi* becomes an integral part of the medical reasoning that explains phenomena of *jue*, the centrality of the

---

[18] See Lo (1999), who is right to note that not all *jue* are needled, but wrong to claim only *jue* are needled.

[19] The concept of the balloon was known, e.g. the dog's bladder in MWD 'Recipes' (1985:56), see p. 218.

[20] *Shiki kaichû kôshô* 105.1, p. 9. Translation based on Yamada (1998:109–10, 130–31), with modifications.

concept *jue* for the history of medicine becomes intelligible, all the more so once *qi* becomes the all-pervasive stuff it is in canonical doctrine.

In the *Shi ji*, Yi needles only patients who suffer from feeling full and hot, namely cases 11 and 16, like pricking a balloon filled with *qi*, but not conditions aggravated by the cold such as case 10. In case 10, the common doctors believe 'wind (which is akin to *qi*) has entered and struck the interior' and attempt to treat it by needling the minor *yang mai*. However, Yi cures the condition by cauterising the dull *yin mai* and administering the broth prepared by careful regulation of fire. It appears the common doctors did not differentiate between feelings of fullness marked by heat or coldness or *yin yang*, while Yi did. Yi does not needle case 9, which involves a feeling of fullness in the chest, but also an explicit expansion of *yin qi*, and, accordingly, coldness.

In summary, in cases 1–10 *jue* is mentioned twice, with connotations of numbness and/or coldness and *yin*. In case 3, the common doctors diagnose 'the stone' (*jue*) and needle it, but Yi diagnoses an amassment and dissolves it with a broth. In case 9, where the pulse quality '*qi* is *yin*' (line 19) has been interpreted as indicative of *jue*, Yi's treatment consists of having the patient drink great amounts of liquid.

jue 蹶 – a disorder of the body architectural heart (line 11)

In case 9 (line 11), Yi states '*mai* coming from the heart was murky'. According to text structure semantics, clearly, the heart correlates with *jue*. Parallels for this are ample in the Mawangdui vessel texts and the Zhangjiashan 'Maishu' of the mid-second century.

jue 蹶 in the Mawangdui 'Yinyang vessel text'

In the Mawangdui 'Yinyang vessel text', which corresponds with parts of the Zhangjiashan 'Maishu',[21] the term *jue* 蹶 is a summarising term at the end of lists of disorders which have in common that they are said to arise when the respective vessel is agitated (*shi dong ze bing* 是動則病): thus, the [foot's] major *yang mai* is said to produce 'ankle *jue*' (*huai jue* 踝蹶) (according to the 'Yinyang vessel text') or 'heel *jue*' (*zhong jue* 踵蹶) (according to the 'Maishu') and the [foot's] *yang* brightness *mai* 'shin *jue*' (*gan jue* 骭蹶), while the arm's major *yin mai* and the arm's minor *yin mai* are both said to produce 'arm *jue*' (*bi jue* 臂蹶). In those four cases, *jue* is modified by a body part of the four extremities: the ankle or heel, the shin, and the arm.

In addition, the [foot's] minor *yin mai*, if agitated, is said to produce a 'bone *jue*' (*gu jue* 骨蹶). Furthermore, since in the Zhangjiashan 'Maishu', the [foot's] minor *yang mai*, if agitated, produces a *yang jue* 陽厥, the contemporary editors of the Mawangdui 'Yinyang vessel text' have accordingly emended the text. This discussion of the names of *jue*, that is, the four

---

[21] See MWD YY (1985:7–13), ZJS MSSW (1989), ZJS (2001:238–42), Gao (1992:35–88).

extremities *jue*, the bone *jue* and the *yang jue*, accounts for *jue* in respect of the agitated *mai* that produce them.[22]

From the above grouping of the vessels a certain regularity becomes evident: *jue* is mentioned in respect of the foot's major *yang* and *yang* brightness *mai* and the arm's major and minor *yin mai* (*ju yang, yang ming, bi tai yin, bi shao yin*), and in those cases it is modified by a body part of the four extremities (ankle or heel, the shin, and the arm). It is not mentioned with regard to the arm's *yang mai*, which are called 'shoulder', 'ear' and 'tooth *mai*' (*jian mai* 肩脈, *er mai* 耳脈, *chi mai* 齒脈). These three *mai* have names that differ ostensibly from other *mai*. *Jue* is furthermore mentioned in respect of the foot's minor *yang* and minor *yin mai*, for reasons that are difficult to know, and then modified by either '*yang*' or 'bone', for reasons that are again not transparent. In summary, *jue* is a condition that arises in *yang mai* of the feet or *yin mai* of the arms that are agitated. In addition, it arises if the foot's minor *yin mai* is agitated.

The above-outlined understanding of *jue* in the Mawangdui vessel texts parallels that of the *Shi ji* personage Yi in two ways. First, considering that in a bipartite body the arms were part of the upper *yang* body part and the feet part of the lower *yin* body part, *jue* in the 'Yinyang vessel text' implicitly alludes to a *yin yang* inversion. As seen above, it occurs only in *yang mai* of the feet and *yin mai* of the arms, except for the 'bone' *jue* of the minor *yin mai* (an anomaly which is difficult to explain).[23]

Second, a *jue* condition arises only when the Mawangdui 'Yinyang vessel text' speaks of agitation (*dong*) in a *mai*. In cases 9, 11 and 16, which the *Shi ji* personage Yi diagnoses as *jue*, it typically presents in feelings of fullness (*man*) and oppression (*men*). This is in line with the well-known finding of Chinese medical history that conditions caused by an agitation in a vessel later started to be conceptualised as conditions of repletion (see also case 10, lines 14, 16). Both 'agitated' (*dong* 動) and 'full' (*man*) become subsumed in later medical writings as an aspect of 'repletion' (*shi* 實).[24]

There is a third common trait, which is that all *jue* cases are curable in *Shi ji* 105 and in the Mawangdui 'Yinyang vessel text'. According to the latter, all disorders of agitated *mai* can be cured. The concluding phrase states this after listing the various disorders to which the agitated vessel gives rise, by indicating that the respective *mai* 'governs the treatment' (*zhu zhi* 主治). This clearly implies that disorders classified as *jue* were considered curable (as were those of *jue* pain in *Ling shu* 24, cited on p. 318).

In the Mawangdui 'Yinyang vessel text', the agitated vessels produce long lists of disorders, which in a summarising statement are said to be *jue*.

---

[22] Compare and contrast with Lo (1999). She tries to make sense of *jue* by investigating the list of disorders enumerated in these paragraphs (and by interpreting them in terms of imputed referential meanings) rather than highlighting that there is a connection between the agitation of *mai* and the production of *jue* conditions.

[23] On the foot's minor *yin mai*, see case 6 (line 35). See also p. 259 and quote on p. 257.

[24] Kuriyama (1999:221).

They all produce 'heart pain' or, perhaps rather, 'heart discomfort'.[25] The 'heart' is in those cases best conceived of as the upper sphere within the bipartite architectural body. And 'discomfort', as will be shown in what follows, is described as a feeling of dissipation and dissolution, a surging or welling, a feeling of the heart becoming numb.

Thus, 'chest pain' (*xiong tong* 胸痛) is attributed to the agitated major *yang mai*[26] and a 'heart [that] dissolves' (*xin chang* 心腸) to the agitated *yang* brightness *mai*.[27] 'Heart pain' (*xin tong* 心痛) is attributed to the agitated arm's minor *yin mai*[28] and a 'heart that is heaving as if it were pain' (*xin pang pang ru tong* 心滂滂如痛) to the agitated arm's major *yin mai*.[29] 'Heart and ribs that are in pain' (*xin yu xie tong* 心與脅痛) are attributed to the agitated minor *yang mai*,[30] and a 'heart [that] dissolves' (*xin dang*) to the agitated minor *yin mai*.[31] All these vessels have in common that they,

[25] Rudolf Pfister (2000 p.c.) kindly inspected the graphs on photographs of the manuscripts, but their discussion conveys my own ideas.

[26] *ji tong* 脊痛 'pain in the spine', according to MWD YY (1985:9, S37). However, Ma (1992:222) specifies that there is a lacuna in the manuscript no. 2 (*yi ben* 乙本). Based on the ZJS 'Maishu', he proposes to read 'chest pain' *xiong tong* 胸痛. The above translation is based on Harper (1998:201), who follows Ma Jixing; 'pain in the spine' is equally possible (Pfister in press).

[27] *xin chang* 心腸 is here read as *xin dang* 心惕, based on Emura (1987:106), who proposes to read *chang* 腸 as *dang* 惕. MWD YY (1985:10, S45) gives *xin chang* 心腸 and proposes to read it as *xin ti* 心惕, rendered by Harper (1998:206) as 'panicky heart'. Ma (1992:235) explains that manuscript no. 2 gives *xin chang*, it is not given in manuscript no. 1. The ZJS 'Maishu' (2001:241–2) reads *xin di di* 心狄狄 as *xin ti*, Gao (1992:48) as *xin dang*. The photographs of MWD (1985) and ZJS (2001) cannot give conclusive evidence.

[28] *xin tong* 心痛, according to MWD YY (1985:13, S71–2). However, Ma (1992:272) explains that manuscript no. 2 gives *xin yong* 心甬, which means 'to surge, to well upward' and is generally transcribed as *xin tong* 心痛; manuscript no. 1 (*jia ben* 甲本) has a lacuna at the slot where one expects the graph *xin*.

[29] *xin pang pang ru tong* 心滂滂如痛 'heart that is heaving as if it were in pain', according to MWD YY (1985:12, S68). Text not defective, but the MWD editors suggest reading *ru* 如 as *er* 而; such an emendation of the text would change its meaning in sensitive ways. Harper (1998:211) explains, following the *Guang ya* 6A, pp. 16b–17a, that *pang pang* suggests the 'quality of surging water'; perhaps it alludes to the sound of the waves of the sea as they beat on the shore, perhaps to surging water masses as the tide comes in. See also *Guang ya* 6A, p. 5b. For explication on the variant *peng peng* 彭彭 in the ZJS 'Maishu', see Harper (1998:211).

[30] *xin yu xie tong* 心與脅痛 'pain in the heart and ribs', according to MWD YY (1985:9, S39). However, Ma (1998:227) points out that the entire phrase is missing in manuscript no. 1. Inspection of the photograph of manuscript no. 2 shows that the character which is now transcribed as 'and' (*yu*) is very difficult to decipher. It is possible that the graph represents 'and' (*yu*) in an abbreviated writing form, which would match the later reading of comparable phrases, given in Ma (1998:227). Nevertheless, the possibility cannot be excluded that the graph may be a verb and the phrase reads: the heart is doing X, the ribs are painful.

[31] *dang* 惕 in MWD YY (1985:12, S63), text not defective; it is glossed as 'to be unrestrained' (*haofang* 豪放) and 'to dissolve, to dissipate' (*fangdang* 放蕩) in HYDCD 7.657; *dang* 惕 is often considered synonymous to *dang* 蕩, and *xin dang* 心蕩 as referring to heart palpitations. See case 2 (line 21), p. 158. The graph 惕 can also be read as *shang*, meaning 'rapid'. For the controversy over the interpretation of the character *chang* 腸, see above case 9, n. 27.

when 'agitated', produce 'discomfort'. Their disorders are classified as *jue*, and like all disorders of 'agitated' vessels, these can be cured. In other words, a curable 'heart pain' is classified as *jue*.[32]

The above could be misunderstood to suggest that the Mawangdui 'Yinyang vessel text' conceives of *jue* as a form of acute pain, namely 'heart pain', diametrically opposed to its early meaning of *jue* 'numb'. However, a close reading of the graphs in the manuscripts shows that in three of the above six cases the editors of the twentieth century have emended a partially defective text to 'heart pain'. None of the other three cases speaks of 'heart pain'. Once, a graph is interpreted as referring to a heart that either 'dissolves' or 'is heaving', and in the remaining two non-defective texts, one clearly says 'the heart dissolves' (*xin dang*) and the other that 'the heart is heaving *as if* it were in pain' (*xin pang pang ru tong*).[33] The 'pain' (*tong* 痛) experience appears here to be associated with 'welling' (*yong* 甬) cold *yin*-waters that invade the body architectural *yang*-heart; an experience of the heart becoming numb.

The 'agitated' *mai* that give rise to disorders classified as *jue* produce fewer pain conditions than the ones that do not give rise to *jue*. This is most conspicuous with regard to the foot's three *yang mai*, which, when 'agitated', give rise to disorders classified as *jue*. Thus, the painful disorders attributed to the foot's three *yang mai* include, when agitated, only one form of 'pain', so-called 'heart welling/pain'. By contrast, we find among the disorders that the foot's three *yang* vessels 'produce' (*qi suo chan bing*) five to seven different forms of localised pain, such as pain in the ankle, the shin, the knee.[34] In other words, the foot's three *yang mai* produce most forms of localised 'pain' (*tong*), but precisely those are not classified as *jue*. In conclusion, in the Mawangdui 'Yinyang vessel text' pain conditions are often mentioned but most are not classified as *jue*. Rather, troubles within the architectural space of the heart region and the chest, which are curable, are classified as *jue*.

jue 蹶 in the *Shuo wen*

In an article on *jue*, Vivienne Lo quotes *Mengzi* 2A: 'Now, *jue* stumbling and hurrying, this is *qi*, and it turns against and agitates the heart' (*jin fu jue zhe, cao zhe, shi qi ye, er fan dong qi xin* 今夫 蹶者 趨者 是氣也 而反動其心) and brings 'stumbling' in connection with a movement of *qi* that 'begins in the feet and ends in the heart'.[35] Indeed, such was the understanding of *jue* by the second century CE, and *jue* as either

---

[32] 'Heart pain' is mentioned also at other instances, we therefore cannot say that if there is 'heart pain' it is a *jue* disorder.

[33] For the three defective texts that have '?chest pain', 'heart ?pain', 'heart ?and rib pain', see case 9, n. 26, n. 28, n. 30. For the inconclusive evidence on *xin chang*, see case 9, n. 27. For the two non-defective texts, see case 9, nn. 29 and 31.

[34] See Hsu (2005a: table 1).

[35] Lo (1999:196). Quote from *Mengzi zhu shu* 3A, p. 21c, translation by Legge (1994.2:188–9).

'being stiff' or 'stumbling' co-occur in the *Shuo wen* definition of *jue* 蹶 with the foot radical: *jue jiang ye* 蹶 僵也, which can be interpreted to mean '*jue* means to be stiff' or '*jue* means to stumble'. The former reading corroborates our reading of *jue* as 'numbness' in the *Lü shi chun qiu* of the third century BCE; the latter is reinforced by the sentence that follows: 'Another one says: to run' (*yi yue tiao/tao*[36] *ye* 一曰跳也).[37] The graph 蹶 with the foot radical can furthermore be pronounced as *gui*, and it then means 'to move rapidly, to stir'.[38]

Mengzi 2A is no doubt important for understanding the relevance of *qi* in early medicine, but not for the reasons Lo gives. She relates a stumbling of the foot to 'heart pain' caused by a stumbling of the heartbeat, which she elucidates in terms of the biomedical angina pectoris and cardiovascular disorders.[39] While Lo is correct to point out that *jue* stumbling is in the first and second century CE explicitly associated with a pattern of movement later known by the idiom of 'contravective *qi*', in my reading the passages surrounding the above quote from *Mengzi* 2A are relevant to early medicine because they associate upward movements of *qi* with the stirring of emotions (see pp. 40–1ff.).

As plausible as the 'heart pain' in the Mawangdui 'Yinyang vessel text' caused by a stumbling heart is for someone who thinks biomedically, the question remains whether or not the *Shuo wen* definition of *jue* 蹶 as 'stumbling' actually explains the notion of *jue* 厥 in the ways the second- and third-century BCE authors conceived of it. Thus, the second-century idiom of a 'dissolving heart', mentioned in a non-defective text, barely invokes an imagery of 'stumbling'. Likewise, even if 'palpitations' instantly come to mind for a reader (for whom the heart, as biomedicine has it, 'beats'), when the heart is said to *pang pang*, this onomatopoetic term may in fact have alluded to other processes, as perhaps to the 'quality of surging water' (which it certainly did in the second century CE).[40] In Bian Que's Memoir, the sudden event of becoming numb is explicitly said to arise from a *yin yang* inversion, which evidently does not allude to the imagery of stumbling. Rather, the upper *yang* body architectural space is understood to be suddenly invaded by *yin*, perhaps by the coldness of surging bodily *yin*-waters, thereby rendering the heart numb.

---

[36] 跳 if pronounced as *tiao* and *tao* means 'to run', while *tiao* can also mean 'to jump', 'to limp'.

[37] *Shuo wen* 2B, 28a. For the *Shuo wen* definitions of other *jue* graphs, see case 3 (line 2).

[38] This is the meaning *jue* has in another *Mengzi* passage, which (mis-)quotes the *Shi jing*: 'Heaven is about to stir, do not chatter so' (*tian zhi fang jue, wu ran xie xie* 天之方蹶 無然泄泄). *Mengzi zhu shu* 7A, p. 53b (translation by Lau 1970:118), compare with the *Shi jing* edition called *Mao shi zheng yi*, 'Da ya', 'Min lao' 民勞, 17.4, p. 281b.

[39] An irregular heartbeat may sometimes lead to a temporary coma, sometimes to palpitations, sometimes to feelings of anxiety and oppression. Incidentally, such heart arrhythmia need not be painful, and is only rarely terminal (Dorin Ritzmann, 1999 p.c.).

[40] See discussion in case 9, n. 29.

jue 瘚 – **contravective** *qi* (*ni qi* 逆氣)   Chinese medical historians typically conceive of *jue* as 'contravective *qi*' (*ni qi* 逆氣). This idea comes close to that of stumbling, given in the *Shuo wen*. However, *ni qi* is not mentioned in Yi's cases 1–10. We traced above how *yin* that moves into a *yang* space becomes conceptualised as *jue*, and how *yin yang* inversions define the concept in the second century BCE. The idea of movement, namely that of a 'contravection', becomes important only after *qi* starts to be conceived of as an all-pervasive medium in medical language. Thus, works of the first century CE and later, the *Shuo wen*, *Yu pian* and other, later lexicographic works define *jue* 瘚 with the illness radical as: '*jue* is contravective *qi*' (*jue ni qi ye* 瘚 逆氣也).[41]

Gao You of the late Eastern Han in his comment on the above-quoted passage of the *Lü shi chun qiu* 1, also speaks of the contravective: '*jue* is a disorder of contravective coldness' (*jue ni han ji ye* 瘚逆寒疾也).[42] This concept of *jue* as 'contravective coldness' parallels the processes described in the 'Model of Disorders' in case 9 (lines 12–17). However, as already noted, the notion *ni qi* is not mentioned in case 9.[43]

The frequently cited but, in fact, rather late *Shi ming* definition of 200 CE gives the following gloss: '*jue* means that contravective *qi* from a numbness in the lower parts rises, goes upward, and enters the heart and ribs' (*jue ni qi cong xia jue qi shang xing ru xin xie ye* 厥逆氣從下厥起上行入心脅也).[44] *Jue* is, according to the *Shi ming*, associated with a movement of contravective *qi* rising upward from the lower parts of the body towards the upper parts of the body. Here, the *yin yang* inversion is only implicitly given, and the movement of *qi* from below upward to the heart region is emphasised.

It is worth noting that modern works mistakenly render the graph for 'ribs' (*xie*) in the *Shi ming* quote as 'vessel' (*mai* 脈).[45] This means that modern authors conceive of the 'heart' (*xin mai*) as a part of the canonical body ecologic.[46] The *Shi ming* definition, which collocates the 'heart' with the 'ribs' (*xin xie*), invokes the bodily architectural heart rather than the body ecological one. Notably, the patient in case 9 suffers from complaints in the architectural space of the chest (line 4).

In summary, the Mawangdui 'Yinyang vessel text' and the corresponding Zhangjiashan passages from the 'Maishu' of the mid-second century provide ample evidence, which in later lexicographic works is corroborated, in

---

[41] *Shuo wen* 7B, p. 29b; *Yu pian* B, p. 8a.

[42] *Shuo wen* 7B, p. 29b. Duan Yucai punctuates Gao You's gloss as follows: '*jue ni* is a cold disorder', but this punctuation is not given in the extant version of the original gloss. See *Lü shi chun qiu* 1.3 (Knoblock and Riegel 2000:69).

[43] The ZJS 'Maishu' (2001:244), emphasises that the sages cooled the head, and prevented heat from moving into the head, but here the rising of coldness is considered pathological.

[44] *Shi ming* 8.26, p. 60b. Wang Niansun quotes it in discussion of case 3 (line 2).

[45] e.g. Ma (1992:224).

[46] *xin cang shen* 心藏神 'the heart lodges the mind'. See *Su wen* 23, p. 76; 62, p. 167.

favour of considering the '*mai* [coming] from the heart' indicative of a *jue* disorder, whereby the heart is the body architectural rather than the canonical medical heart.

jue tong 厥痛 – 'fake pain' in the *Inner Canon*   In Bian Que's Memoir 'numbness' is an important feature of *jue*, perhaps in particular the numbness in the heart which makes a person unconscious and, thereby, a lifeless body similar to a corpse. In Yi's Memoir, in cases 9, 11 and 16, it is the feeling of fullness, which is typical for *jue*. In all three cases, *yin yang* inversions are central to the concept, and pain in none. Careful examination of the graphs in the Mawangdui 'Yinyang vessel text' shows that 'heart pain' (*xin tong*) as *jue* disorder arises mainly from modern editorial interventions. Of the six instances investigated, the only two that are non-defective speak of a heart that is 'dissolving' (*dang*) or of a 'surging' (*pang pang*) in the heart 'comparable to pain' (*ru tong*). Intense pain is a distinctive feature of 'amassments' (*shan*) or 'conglomerations' (*jia*) in Yi's Memoir, or of 'protrusions' (*long* 癃) in the Mawangdui 'Recipes', but not always of *jue*.[47]

With regard to canonical medical texts, a cursory glance at *Ling shu* 24, entitled 'Jue Disorders' (Jue bing 厥病), may again, based on a cursory reading, evoke the impression that *jue* centres on pain conditions.[48] The chapter consists, in Ren Yingqiu's reading, of three paragraphs: the first discusses a '*jue* headache' (*jue tou tong* 厥頭痛), the second a '*jue* heart pain' (*jue xin tong* 厥心痛) and the third an 'ear insensitivity resulting in deafness' (*er long wu wen* 耳聾無聞).[49] However, a careful reading reveals that the '*jue* headache' and the '*jue* heart pain' are discussed in opposition to the 'true headache' (*zhen tou tong* 真頭痛) and the 'true heart pain' (*zhen xin tong* 真心痛): the former conditions can be cured by needling; the latter are lethal. Just as the conditions in Bian Que's Memoir of 'suddenly becoming numb' (*bao jue*) or 'the corpse is numb' (*shi jue*) can be successfully treated, a '*jue* headache' and a '*jue* heart pain' in *Ling shu* 24 can be cured. The condition of '*jue* pain' is opposed to that of 'true pain'; the latter is lethal. As an opposite to 'true' (*zhen*), *jue* takes on meanings in this text of either 'dull/numb' or perhaps even 'fake' (a 'dull' heart pain or 'fake' headache). Perhaps *shi jue* in Bian Que's Memoir may have overtones of saying 'the corpse is fake'.

jue 厥: summary (lines 3 and 19)   The meanings of *jue* changed over time. In the *Lü shi chun qiu* of the third century BCE *jue*, 'being numb', arises

---

[47] For 'amassments', see case 3; for 'conglomerations', see case 7; for 'protrusions', see MWD 'Recipes' (1985:46–8).

[48] *Ling shu* 24, pp. 342–3. In *Su wen* 45, pp. 126–7, entitled 'Treatise on Jue' (Jue lun 厥論), pain is not a prominent feature of *jue*.

[49] In *Su wen* 28, p. 88, 'deafness' (*long*) is also mentioned in the vicinity of *jue*, as an aspect of 'sudden numbness' (*bao jue er long* 暴厥而聾).

when 'one augments *yin*' (*duo yin*). If one, inspired by text structure semantics, considers case 9 in lines 19–22 to relate knowledge from the early second century, one can see a correlation between *jue* and the pulse quality '*qi* is *yin*' (line 19). Probably, the common doctors who diagnosed *jue* 'the stone' in case 3 considered such a condition of numbness a *yin* condition, although it is impossible to ascertain this with the material at hand.

The early first-century editor who gave case 9 its present form (apart from few lines and words that may have been later interjected), by contrast, correlated '*mai* [coming] from the heart' with *jue*. Evidence in favour of this postulate of text structure semantics has been found in the Mawangdui 'Yinyang vessel text' and the Zhangjiashan 'Maishu'. They classified long lists of disorders caused by an agitation of the *mai* as *jue*, among them problems affecting the heart.

In *Shi ji* 105, and also in the Mawangdui 'Yinyang vessel text' and the Zhangjiashan 'Maishu', *jue* typically is associated with an inversion of *yin* and *yang*. In the manuscript texts *jue* conditions are attributed only to agitated vessels, and in Yi's Memoir, paralleling this, all *jue* conditions present with feelings of fullness and oppression (cases 9, 11, 16, 23, except perhaps case 3). Moreover, all *jue* conditions described in all these texts are curable.

The idea that seemingly serious disorders are curable gives rise to *jue* meaning 'fake', as in *Ling shu* 24, where 'true pain of AB' is opposed to '*jue* pain of AB', i.e. 'fake pain of AB': the former is lethal; the latter curable. Accordingly, *shi jue* in Bian Que's Memoir may not only mean 'the corpse is numb' but also 'the corpse is fake'.

Eventually, *jue* is associated with contravective *qi*, a notion that emphasises movement caused by a *yin yang* inversion. In case 9 (lines 12–17), the reasoning recorded in the 'Model of Disorders' comes close to it, as it explains 'fullness in the chest'.

Finally, *feng jue* in case 9 resembles *feng jue* in *Su wen* 7, insofar as it conceives of *feng jue* in terms of *yin yang* inversions within a bipartite body. However, the signs and symptoms they present differ. By contrast, the signs and symptoms of *feng jue* in case 9 are attributed also to *feng jue* in *Ling shu* 46 and *Su wen* 33. The most prominent complaint of *feng jue* in case 9, *Ling shu* 46 and *Su wen* 33 is sweating.

Perspiration as a form of therapy? (lines 8 and 22)

In case 9 (line 8), sweating figures as cause of the disorder: the King of Jibei contracted the illness from 'sweating and lying prostrate on the ground'. A modern reader is inclined to view sweating as a sign of an illness, namely a sign of a fever, but in Yi's case histories sweating is mostly given as cause of a disorder. It indicates a state of overexertion, which weakens the person and allows illness to arise.

What kind of activity caused the state of overexertion in the King of Jibei? One guesses that lying prostrate on the ground and sweating profusely is a sign of extensive sexual intercourse. This is supported by ancient textual evidence, for instance, in the Mawangdui 'Tianxia zhi dao tan' 天下之道談, which describes an outbreak of sweating in the moment of sexual climaxing: 'Sweat flows and reaches the back of the knees' (*han liu zhi guo* 汗流至膕).[50]

Along the lines of canonical texts, which allude to the 'skin's pore pattern' (*cou li*), one could argue that sweating makes it open and thereby lets the essential waters leak out of the body and allows wind to enter. Furthermore, if, when sweating, one lies prostrate on the ground, the open pores make it possible for the cold *yin qi* from the ground, with its earthy *yin*-qualities, to enter the body, expand and ascend. However, even if Yi had ideas akin to those just outlined, he nowhere mentions the 'skin's pore pattern' nor such mechanistic an understanding of the processes involved.[51]

Yi pays much attention to sweating as a cause of all ills, as he seems to consider it indicative of overexertion that makes the body vulnerable to disease. However, he does not consider sweating a cause for the *yin yang* inversion outlined in the 'Model of Disorders' (lines 12–17). In case 9, sweating does not appear to occupy the centrality it has in later conceptualisations of pathological processes and their treatment, particularly in Zhang Zhongjing's *Shang han lun* of the second century CE. Nor is the medical wisdom brought into play that 'enormous sweating causes a loss of *yang*' (*da han wang yang* 大汗亡陽).[52] Rather, the loss of *yang* is explicitly attributed to the fact that 'he [the King of Jibei] excessively caused his *yang* to enter' (*guo ru qi yang*; line 13).[53]

The phrase 'to excessively cause one's *yang* to enter' surprises scholars of the Chinese sexual arts, since *yang* 陽 neither as penis nor as ejaculate, i.e. *yang*-fluids, is attested in other Han texts. The term for penis typically is *yin* 陰,[54] apart from single-syllable terms like 埶 read as *shi* 勢 and *jun* 竣 read as *zui* 朘, and idioms like the 'red infant' (*chi zi* 赤子) or the 'jade whip' (*yu jia* 玉筴).[55] To solve the problem, one could suggest that parts of the 'Model of Disorders' (lines 13–14) are a later interjection. Their reasoning

---

[50] MWD 'Tianxia zhi dao tan' (1985:166, S61). According to *Su wen* 42, p. 120, it was unhealthy.

[51] See also p. 118; case 4, p. 200; case 5, pp. 212–13, 221, 228–9.

[52] *Zhongyi dacidian* (1995:79).

[53] Hübotter (1927:14) translates 'excess entered his *yang*'; Bridgman (1955:34) also makes no sense.

[54] e.g. Harper (1998:402, 425).

[55] e.g. Harper (1998:389, 400, 401, 411).

in terms of *yin yang* is in line with canonical medical doctrine and, as noted on p. 308, at odds with reasoning in terms of the hot and cold in line 16.

However one interprets the incongruencies within the 'Model of Disorders', the phrase *guo ru qi yang* is reminiscent of an early text on the sexual arts, where the verb *ru* also refers to the sexual transfer of a fluid, as in the Mawangdui 'Shiwen': *nai ru qi jing* 乃入其精. So, perhaps, *yang* designates *yang*-fluids here? In the light of the above translation of *guo ru qi yang*, the Mawangdui 'Shiwen' phrase *nai ru qi jing* then means: '[When he is able to move her form and bring forth the five tones], then he enters his essences (semen).'[56] This straightforward rendition of *nai ru qi jing* meets with great opposition from scholars of ancient Chinese sexology, however. They are adamant that the term *ru* in the 'Shi wen' does not refer to ejaculation, but to the absorption of the woman's fluids into the man. This very sentence, *nai ru qi jing*, is one of the most important building blocks in their elaborations that the Chinese sexual arts aim at maximising the man's vitality by absorbing the *qi* and fluids of his woman. However, the above translation of *guo ru qi yang* in case 9 suggests a grammatically correct and semantically equally satisfying interpretation of *nai ru qi jing*.

After explaining why there was a feeling of fullness in the chest by quoting the 'Model of Disorders' (lines 12–17), Yi comments on sweating as cause of the disorder (lines 18–22). He does not say that he attempts to explain 'the means whereby he recognised' it, but simply states in a topic-comment sentence that as far as sweating and lying prostrate on the ground are concerned (line 18), when he pressed on *mai*, he felt that *qi* was *yin* (line 19). It is difficult if not impossible to make sense of this sentence, which from a text critical viewpoint may represent a faultline of two mini-texts. In what follows, I will argue that: line 19 hints at medical rationale prevalent during the third and early second century; lines 20–1 reflect an explanatory editorial voice; and line 22 reports on a therapeutic measure that all commentators consider an induction of sweating. This echoes the sweating mentioned as topic of the entire stanza in line 18.

For making sense of line 22 *chu ji chan shui ye* 出及瀺水也 the commentators suggest that sweating brought about the cure. The key word is *chan* 瀺. Zhang Shoujie cites what Gu Yewang 顧野王 (519–81) is supposed to have said: 'The hands and feet moisten the body' (*shou zu ye shen ti* 手足液身體).[57] In fact, however, the gloss on the graph 瀺 in Gu Yewang's *Yu pian*

---

[56] MWD 'Shiwen' (1985:146). Contrast with Harper (1998:389): 'When able to move her form and bring forth the five tones, then absorb her [the woman's] essence'. On this particular aspect of the Chinese sexual arts, see, for instance, Pfister (in press). In support of their viewpoint, one can argue that *ru* is in early texts an intransitive verb, in later ones a transitive one. Accordingly, line 13 may be a commentatorial interjection.

[57] As Zhang Wenhu points out, Zhang Shoujie's comment is incomplete. It also seems to contain a comment on *zhuo* 汋 (to well up, to well forth), a graph not mentioned in the extant text. Taki Mototane laconically notes that the meaning of *chan shui* remains obscure.

reads: '*chan* is the sound of swishing water' (*chan zhuo shui ye* 瀺灂水也).[58] Zhang Shoujie's quote alludes to sweating, yet the *Yu pian* speaks of the sound of swishing water. But sweating does not produce sound.

One could impute into this ancient text 'sympathetic magic': the King of Jibei had contracted his illness from sweating, so sweating was its cure. The induction of sweating, urinating (and defecating) and vomiting (*han xia tu* 汗下吐) was the common treatment method of the Eastern Han, and perhaps known already to physicians of the Western Han. Indeed, some forms of sweating were hailed as therapeutic, already in the Mawangdui 'Recipes', 'Sweat comes out and reaches to the feet' (*han chu dao zu* 汗出到足),[59] and in *Ling shu* 81 (*han chu zhi zu* 汗出至足).[60] They curiously are reminiscent of the kind of sweating caused by sexual climaxing, which in Yi's Memoir has repeatedly been given as a cause of illness, not only in case 9. However, here a medical manuscript text uses the same idiom to say that sweating is therapeutic! In a similar vein, *Su wen* 32 records sweating as a sign of recovery: 'In all cases where one should sweat, when the day comes for overcoming it [the illness], the sweat will come out in large amounts' (*zhu dang han zhe, zhi qi suo sheng ri, han da chu ye* 諸當汗者 至其所勝日 汗大出 也).[61] *Su wen* 32 invokes a maxim of therapeutics reminiscent of that of crisis days in Greek medicine. So does *Ling shu* 23: 'If in the case of a heat disorder while the *mai* are still abundant and hurried, sweating is not possible, this is the extreme of the *yang mai* and death occurs. If the *mai* are abundant and hurried, and if after being able to sweat, they are still, life continues' (*re bing zhe, mai shang sheng zao er bu de han zhe, ci yang mai zhi ji ye, si, mai sheng zao de han jing zhe sheng* 熱病者 脈尚盛躁而不得汗者 此陽 脈之極也 死 脈盛躁 得汗靜者 生).[62] Yet for a form of therapeutic sweating reminiscent of 'swishing water' (*chan shui*) no parallels have been found.

Likewise, the different kinds of sweating used for diagnostic means make no allusion to 'swishing water'. The Mawangdui 'Yinyangmai sihou' states: 'If sweat comes out like silk [threads], and if while turning round, it does not flow, then blood has died first' (*han chu ru si, zhuan er bu liu, ze xue xian si* 汗出如絲 傳而不流 則血先死).[63] The *Inner Canon* notes: 'Sweat pours out without interruption' (*han chu bu xiu* 汗出不休); 'Sweat comes out in a *zhen zhen* fashion' (*han chu zhen zhen* 汗出溱溱); 'Sweat comes out as if one were bathing' (*han chu ru yu* 汗出如浴).[64] In these passages from the *Inner Canon*, each form of sweating is considered indicative of a specific disorder, but none is like 'swishing water'.

---

[58] *Yu pian* B, p. 71a. HYDCD 6.215 glosses *zhuo* as the 'sound of the rain' (*yu sheng* 雨聲).
[59] MWD 'Recipes' (1985:31, 59).
[60] *Ling shu* 81, p. 481.
[61] *Su wen* 32, p. 94. Consider also *ji qi* (intense time span) in case 7 (line 18), see p. 292.
[62] *Ling shu* 23, p. 340. 'Being abundant, yet hurried' (*sheng er zao*) occurs also in *Ling shu* 9, p. 293.
[63] MWD 'Yinyangmai sihou' (1985:21). See also ZJS MSSW (1989).
[64] *Ling shu* 21, p. 334, *Ling shu* 30, p. 357, *Su wen* 46, p. 130.

Poetry provides a hint, as poets consistently use *chan* for invoking the sound of water: swishing rain, gurgling creeks or roaring torrents. *Chan* is often collocated with *zhuo* 潺, which generally refers to the sound of water.[65] In the *Shuo wen* the term *zhuo* is defined as: '*zhuo* is the tinkling sound of water' (*zhuo shui zhi xiao sheng ye* 潺水之小聲也),[66] and in Guo Pu's 郭璞 (276–324) 'Jiang fu' 江賦 it is glossed as the sound of a waterfall when it hits the ground.[67] In the dictionaries the examples cited for elucidating *chan* are often from times later than the Han,[68] but not exclusively. Thus, *chan* occurs in Ma Rong's 馬融 (79–166) 'Chang di fu' 長笛賦 and Li Shan 李善 (d. 689) glosses it there as: '*chan* is the roaring sound of water' (*chan shui zhu sheng ye* 瀺水注聲也).[69] And *chan zhuo* is mentioned in a *fu*-poem of *Shi ji* 117,[70] where it is glossed in much the same way as *zhuo* (tinkling) in the *Shuo wen*, and in Zhang Heng's 張衡 (78–139) 'Nan du fu' 南都賦, where it describes what a waterfall does.[71] This explains the cure. The sound of a waterfall, whether tinkling or roaring, points to urination, not to sweating.[72]

Considering that Yi (lines 5–7) administers three *shi* of drugged wine, and that one *shi* equalled in Han times about twenty litres,[73] one would expect that the 'swishing water' expelled the 'numbness' through large quantities of liquid. Clearly, three times twenty litres is a considerable amount of drugged wine.[74] Bridgman, however, points out an interesting parallel in *Shi ji* 66: 'Oh, how is it possible that you can drink one *shi*' (*wu neng yin yi shi zai* 惡能飲一石哉).[75] No doubt, the drinking of twenty litres of a fermented slightly alcoholic drink posed a challenge, but it could be done. The masculinity of the sexually very active King of Jibei must have been tripled through his medical treatment, for he must have drunk not only large amounts of beer, but also, for expelling the illness, urinated like a waterfall.[76]

It has to be kept in mind that Yi needles *jue* (inversion) conditions in cases 11 and 16, which are marked by a combination of feeling full and hot, but in this case, which involves *qi* that is *yin* in the body's interior, he administers a drugged wine in large quantities. Perhaps, the alcoholic drink was given because alcohol had a warming effect. It is more likely that in the early second century the drugged wine was consumed in large quantities

---

[65] HYDCD 6.215.   [66] *Shuo wen* 11A, p. 5b.   [67] *Wen xuan* 12, pp. 305–17.
[68] HYDCD 6.215 and HYDZD B.1789.   [69] *Wen xuan* 18, p. 439.
[70] *Shi ji* 117, p. 3017.   [71] *Wen xuan* 4, p. 93.
[72] Urination as a cure; the idea I owe to Robert Hinde (2000 p.c.).
[73] One *shi* 石 equals 19.968 litres (Twitchett and Loewe 1986:xxxviii).
[74] *shi* 石 is replaced by *ri* 日 'day' in Mao's 毛 edition, Takigawa comments, in awareness of this.
[75] Bridgman (1955:81, n. 140), *Shi ji* 66, p. 3199.
[76] In Europe, any schoolboy can tell you about the arch of urine as a sign of masculinity. Among the Mru, who live in the Chittagong Hilltracts on the borders of Myanmar (Burma) and Bangladesh, however, women stand when urinating, men squat (Brauns and Löffler 1986).

in order to rid the body of cold *yin*-waters. If the received text mistakenly recorded the word 'must' (*bi*) in the penultimate instead of the final line, it would explicitly state such a therapeutic maxim: 'If a disorder has entered and struck the interior, for expelling it, it must reach the degree of swishing water' (*bing ru zhong, chu bi ji chan shui ye*).[77]

Perhaps the assumed early second-century medical document had the above therapeutic maxim (lines 21–2), as well as the phrase '*qi* is *yin*' (*qi yin* 氣陰; line 19), which parallels *qi ji* 氣急 (*qi* is intense) in case 3 (line 14) and, perhaps, *qi zhi* 氣至 (*qi* is congested) in case 7 (line 13). Perhaps the first-century editor interpolated line 20, *yin qi zhe*, and changed the text in line 21 from *bing ru zhong* to *bing bi ru zhong*.

Despite the above evidence in favour of interpreting 'swishing water' as referring to urination, the problem of whether these large quantities of an alcoholised beverage induced sweating, or not, cannot be put aside yet: Yamada Keiji maintains that drugged wines have the 'remarkable effect of inducing perspiration',[78] and that this allowed physicians in antiquity to overcome the narrow range of applications that water-based broths originally had, which apparently was limited to diuretics for treating urinary tract infections. In other words, if Yi had wished to increase urination, he would have administered a water-based broth.

This raises the question why Yi administered a drugged wine, if not for the medical reason of inducing sweating. Without intending to imply that medical practice has remained unaltered for over two millennia, it is striking to observe that 'drugged wines' are today still used by 'herbalists' (*cao yi* 草醫), who macerate in alcohol 'supplementing drugs' (*bu yao* 補藥), which have always been precious and expensive. Sometimes these drugged wines have enormous value, like tiger-penis-liquor, both as a medicine and as an aphrodisiac. Today they are administered to patients who suffer from 'depletions'.[79] In the light of this, we are reminded that the King of Jibei was suffering from what would currently be considered a '*yang* depletion' and that the 'drugged wine' had the quality of being 'supplementing'.

Most importantly, a 'drugged wine' may have been chosen as treatment because it matched the king's honourable status. It is interesting that in the *Han Feizi* drugged wine is mentioned as the beverage of kings and sages: 'Indeed, drugged wine and useful advice are what wise men and enlightened sovereigns ought to appreciate in particular' (*fu yao jiu yong yan ming jun*

---

[77] This emendation of the text was undertaken in a seminar held at the University of Heidelberg with Rudolf Wagner (February 2001 p.c.) and his research group.

[78] Yamada (1998:104).

[79] A bottle of clear liquor, within which one could see a macerated tiger-penis (illegally purchased, not hunted), was shown to me by Sichuanese road workers in Xishuang banna, Yunnan province, during a roadside lunch on an exploratory botanical field trip (December 1988).

sheng zhu zhi yi du zhi ye 夫藥酒用言明君聖主之以獨知也).[80] Yi treats a patient of status as high as a king only once in cases 1–10, and he administers drugged wine on this one occasion. Perhaps drugged wine was considered a remedy reserved for kings and sages of high standing only. Apart from the currently well-known warming and supplementing qualities of wine, its suitability for persons of high status may explain why Yi treated the King of Jibei with a drugged wine.

Discussion

Text structure semantics points to two possible readings of case 9: first, in its current form, the name of the disorder must be a 'wind inversion' (*feng jue*) and the 'fullness in the chest' (*xiong man*) a concomitant symptom. The pulse qualities mentioned are 'wind *qi*' (*feng qi*) and '*qi* [coming] from the heart' (*xin qi*). The correlation between 'wind *qi*' and 'wind' is obvious. Given the facile text structural correlation between 'wind *qi*' and 'wind' in cases 9 and 5, it appears that the first-century editor interpolated the constituent 'wind', probably for other reasons than purely medical ones.

This leaves us with the correlation between '*qi* [coming] from the heart' and *jue* meaning 'inversion'. We found that the correlation is corroborated by the Mawangdui and Zhangjiashan manuscript literature, which contains evidence in favour of viewing *jue* as a disorder marked by an inversion of *yin yang*, which is located in the region of the heart, presents with fullness and is curable.

The second reading postulates a correlation between the pulse quality '*qi* is *yin*' (line 19) and the monosyllabic *jue* meaning 'numbness' (line 3). Evidence for this reading is given in the *Lü shi chun qiu* of the third century BCE, where *jue* arises from 'augmenting *yin*' (*duo yin* 多陰). In order to make sense of this second correlation I argue that knowledge contained in lines 3, 5, 19 and 21–2 in case 9 testifies to a document written by a physician of the early second century, while case 9, as it stands, is the work of the first-century BCE editor interspersed with commentatorial interjections.

Nothing can be said about Yi's tactile experience of the *mai* he mentions. Rather, research in this case centres on *jue* meaning 'to be numb and dull' (mostly 厥), 'inversion' (often 蹷) and a 'disorder of contravective *qi*' (often 瘚). Since the first-century editor may have had non-medical motives for adding 'wind' as a constituent to the name of the disorder, the question was explored whether the 'wind-induced inversion' (*feng jue*) in case 9 tallies with understandings of 'wind inversions' (*feng jue*) in medicine. We found that the *feng jue* mentioned in *Ling shu* 46 and *Su wen* 33 have one predominant common feature with case 9, namely perspiration, yet the *feng*

---

[80] *Han Feizi* 11, p. 611. Translation by Liao (1959:2.26). Harper (1982:51) reports on a *yao jiu* in *Shi ji* 69, p. 2265, that was poisonous. Notably, it was offered to a ruler.

jue mentioned in *Su wen* 7, which probably is of an earlier date, describes entirely different signs and symptoms of the disorder, although, implicitly, it is grounded in the same conception of *feng jue* as a *yin yang* inversion.

The disorder *feng jue* in case 9 is marked by feeling full or oppressed in the chest. However, unlike other conditions, which simultaneously present with symptoms of feeling hot, and therefore are treated by needling, *jue* in case 9 clearly has features of *yin qi* expanding. The treatment consists of administering a 'drugged wine' (*yao jiu*), which currently is valued for its warming and supplementing qualities, but at the time probably was chosen primarily as the adequate treatment for patients of high social standing. The King of Jibei consumed it in large quantities, which must have led to an effective expulsion of cold *yin*-waters, roaring royally like a waterfall.

20
Case 10

Translation (*Shiji kaichû kôshô* 105, pp. 38–9)

1. The accredited wife Chu Yu of Beigong, the Officer of Works at Qi, fell ill.
2. All the many doctors took it for a wind that had entered and struck the interior.
3. The host of the disorder resided in the lungs [liver].
4. They needled her foot's minor *yang mai*.
5. Your servant, Yi, examined her *mai* and <u>said</u>:

Name:
6. 'She is troubled by *qi* – an amassment is visiting the bladder –
7. and has difficulties with urinating and defecating. The urine is dark.
8. When the disorder is exposed to cold *qi*, then there is remanent urine.
9. It makes the person's abdomen swollen.'

Cause:
10. <u>Chu Yu's illness was contracted</u> from intending to urinate, but without having the chance to do so,
11. indulging in sexual intercourse.

Quality:
12. <u>The means whereby I recognised</u> Chu Yu's illness were that
13. when I pressed onto her *mai*,
14. they were large, yet replete.
15. They came with difficulty.

16. This is an agitation of the dull *yin*.

17. In cases where *mai* come with difficulty,

1. 齊北宮司空命婦出於病
2. 眾醫皆以為風入中
3. 病主在肺
4. 刺其足少陽脈
5. 臣意診其脈曰
6. 病氣-疝客於膀胱-
7. 難於前後溲 而溺赤
8. 病見寒氣 則遺溺
9. 使人腹腫
10. 出於病得之欲溺不得
11. 因以接內
12. 所以知出於病者
13. 切其脈
14. 大而實
15. 其來難
16. 是蹶陰之動也
17. 脈來難者

327

18. the *qi* of an amassment is visiting the bladder [or: went into . . .].

19. As to the abdomen [or: . . . the abdomen], the reason why it became swollen:

20. it is said that a link of the dull *yin* is knotted to the small abdomen.

21. When the dull *yin* had excess, then the node of the *mai* got agitated.

22. When it got agitated, then the abdomen became swollen.

23. Your servant, Yi, then cauterised her foot's dull *yin mai*.

24. The left and the right one, each at one place.

25. Then, as there was no remanent urine anymore, her urine was clear.

26. The pain in the small abdomen stopped.

27. Forthwith, I additionally prepared the broth [prepared by careful] regulation of fire and had her drink it.

28. After three days, the *qi* of the amassment dissipated.

29. She instantly recovered.

18. 疝氣之 客於膀胱也

19. 腹之 所以腫者

20. 言蹶陰之絡結小腹也

21. 蹶陰有過 則脈結動

22. 動則腹腫

23. 臣意即灸其足蹶陰之脈

24. 左右各一所

25. 即不遺溺 而溲清

26. 小腹痛止

27. 即更為火齊湯以飲之

28. 三日 而疝氣散

29. 即愈

Interpretation

Yi first accuses the common doctors of misdiagnosis (lines 2–3) and mistaken treatment (line 4). He then examines *mai* (line 5), names the disorder (line 6), gives concomitant signs and symptoms (lines 7–9) and states the cause of the disorder (lines 10–11). Thereafter, he engages in medical speculation (lines 12–26), before reporting on treatment in two stages (lines 23–6 and 27–9).

Critical evaluation of retrospective biomedical diagnoses

Lu and Needham do not discuss this case. According to Bridgman, nephrolithiasis (urolithiasis) or vesical schistosomiasis led to the formation of bladder stones. The signs and symptoms – difficulties with urinating and defecating, and pain in the abdomen – point to urolithiasis. What Yi considers the cause of the disorder may in fact be one of its symptoms: acute cystitis is often accompanied by strangury and has the effect that one wishes to urinate but cannot do so.[1] If the stones were small, which would be unusual, the ingestion of a broth that would effect increased urination may have flushed them out.

[1] Bridgman (1955:83).

Comparison with other case histories

The pulse quality 'large' (*da*) is given in cases 3, 5 and 10. Since in case 5 (line 20), Yi explicitly says: 'In cases when it is large, it is *qi* coming from the bladder' and assuming relative consistency in medical rationale across cases 1–10, *da* may also in cases 3 and 10 indicate a bladder disorder. Yet the word for bladder differs in each of the three names of the disorder: case 3 has *yong* 湧 'welling', case 5 *pao* 脬, case 10 *pang guang*.

As noted in case 3 (line 4), *yong* invokes 'welling waters', as in the name of the acupuncture locus called *yong quan* 'welling spring'. In the discussion of *jue* in case 9, we suggested that *xin yong* 心甬 in the Mawang-dui 'Yinyang vessel text' no. 2 alluded to cold *yin*-waters that are welling up and invading the upper bodily cavity, and that they overcome the heart and lead to corpse-like numbness. Comparison with cases 5 and 10 suggests that *yong* 'the welling' pre-dates the concept of 'bladder' as a body part. Like *ge* 鬲 'to separate', which is what the diaphragm does, the 'welling' bladder appears to have been known by its characteristic activity rather than by its structure.

All three cases present with difficulties in urinating and defecating (case 3: *bu de qian hou sou*, case 5: *nan yu da xiao sou*, case 10: *nan yu qian hou sou*), but none of these polysyllabic names has parallels in the medical literature: case 3 concerns a 'welling amassment' (*yong shan*), case 5 a 'wind-induced condition of overexertion' (*feng dan*), case 10, a woman ailing from '*qi* – an amassment that is visiting the bladder' (*qi shan ke yu pang guang*). In all three cases, Yi administers *huo ji tang* (broth prepared over [careful] regulation of fire). In cases 3 and 5, Yi spells out what each dosage of *huo ji tang* effects – it enables urination and defecation – and then he gives a second or third dose, which is said to cure the disorder, but in case 10, treatment has two stages (lines 23–6 and 27–9). The first stage concerns cauterisation, and the second *huo ji tang*. The cauterisation follows the rationale of the early medical manuscripts, and the use of *huo ji tang* may reflect treatment rationale in the assumed early second-century medical document. As in case 9 (lines 21–2), it is mentioned in the last stanza.

Finally, all three cases mention the idiom 'the urine is dark' (*ni chi*). In the very end of cases 3 (lines 21–2) and 5 (lines 4, 21), Yi explicitly states that dark urine indicates heat in the interior, but in case 10, immediately after stating that the urine is dark (line 7), Yi maintains that the disorder is aggravated by exposure to the cold (line 8). This is odd from an early and canonical medical viewpoint. As in cases 3 and 5, *ni chi* probably is a late commentator's interjection, also in case 10.

In summary, there are many parallels between cases 3, 5 and 10. They are all heavily edited, quite apart from interjections of later commentators. This applies, in particular, to case 10.

Incongruencies

Case 10 is riddled with problems. First, the patient: the name is probably a pun (as names can be in cases 11–25) rather than a rhyme (as in cases 1–10) and identification in official rank and gender poses problems (line 1).[2] Second, the common doctors' understanding of bodily processes: the common doctors have more sophisticated body terms (lines 3–4) than the usual one, which is 'the interior' (line 2). Third, gender issues: already in the early medical manuscript literature an 'amassment' is typically a male disorder (line 6), a 'swollen abdomen' a female disorder (line 9) – was the patient male or female? Fourth, hot/cold considerations: dark urine is typically a sign of heat (line 7), but the disorder is said to be aggravated by the cold (line 8). Fifth, body parts: is it the 'abdomen' (lines 9, 19, 22) or the 'small abdomen' (lines 20 and 26) that is affected? Sixth, pulse qualities: are they given in terms of a *dong* agitation (line 16) or in terms of *qi* (line 18)? Seventh, the treatment: it has two stages (lines 23–6, and 27–9) as though two mini-texts had been juxtaposed (as in case 4, lines 20–3 and 24–5).

In consideration of medical rationale, text critical studies and consistency in narrative across cases 1–10 versus cases 11–25, one could argue that case 10, as faultline between two textual sources, recounts two case histories in one. Furthermore, several commentators have been at work.

A semantic continuity can be established between the male 'officer of works at Qi' who after being misdiagnosed, was diagnosed by Yi as suffering from '*qi* [that went into the abdomen]' and difficulties in urinating and defecating. A commentator (or the early first-century editor) may have updated the name to a condition that typically affects men, namely an 'amassment', which as stated in a phrase which with great certainty is a commentatorial interjection, 'is visiting the bladder'. Yi then reports on the pulse qualities he felt and his treatment with *huo ji tang* (lines 1, 2, 5–7, 11, 12–15, 17–18, 27–9). As other patients in cases 1–10, the officer of works was from Qi, indulged in sex, was subject to pulse diagnosis, was found to have, probably, a hernia, and was treated with *huo ji tang*.

Second, case material, which has more affinity with cases 11–25, has been added to the above. Perhaps it concerned an accredited wife Chu Yu from the northern palace, who suffered from a swollen abdomen and was treated by cauterising the foot's dull *yin mai* (lines 1, 9, 10, 23–4). Her name, which probably is a pun, the treatment with moxibustion and the brevity of her case history have more affinity with cases 11–25; for her gender, her disorder and its treatment there are parallels in the early medical manuscripts.

Third, commentators were at work, among whom tentatively five can be identified: on line 7, *ni chi* (the urine is dark) probably was interjected by a commentator, presumably the same who was active in cases 3 and 5;

---

[2] See table 1, d, on p. 54.

his interjections are consistently off the mark, and we called him the confused one (see p. 291, n. 107). On line 8, a grammatically and semantically problematic phrase hints at an interjection; in structure it is reminiscent of case 6 (line 33), in vocabulary *yi ni* (remanent urine) is reminiscent of *yi ji* (remanent stools) in case 7 (line 4), and *xian* (to be exposed), arguably, points also to case 7 (line 14); this commentator used *yi* 遺 in the sense it is used elsewhere in the *Shi ji*, and not in its technical medical sense, and thus was not a medical specialist; he is likely also to have interjected line 25, which has *yi ni*. On line 18, a commentator seems to have interjected *ke yu pang guang ye* and he may have updated the name on line 6 to *shan ke yu pang guang*; it is unlikely that this commentator was the editor himself because line 18 is grammatically odd. Furthermore, either the first-century editor or yet another commentator appears to have added lines 21–2. He speaks of the dull *yin* rather than the dull *yin mai* (line 23), and his medical rationale has much affinity with case 1 (lines 41–3). Finally, in lines 20 and 26 a commentator, well-versed in canonical doctrine, creatively adds elucidating comments on the 'small abdomen'.

By insisting on consistency in medical rationale and narrative across cases 1–10, the text has become a multivocalic fabric. In what follows, medical rationale is explored, which provides the evidence for the above rather audacious suggestions.

The diagnosis and treatment of all the many doctors (lines 2–4)

All the many doctors diagnose 'wind has entered and struck the interior' (line 2).[3] They opine the host of the disorder resides in the lungs [liver] and needle the foot's minor *yang* (lines 3–4). We have already noted that in line 2 they use a similar vocabulary and medical rationale as in cases 3 (line 2) and 8 (line 3), but not in lines 3–4. Three further points are worth noting. First, the common doctors refer to 'wind' (*feng*), but Yi to *qi*. Second, they needle the patient, but Yi cauterises her. Third, they treat the foot's minor *yang*, but Yi the foot's dull *yin*. I will comment on each point in what follows.

In cases 1–10, Yi rarely refers to *qi* as a word on its own, but often to *qi* as a semantic categoriser for describing the qualities of tactile perception he has when examining *mai* (*gan qi* in case 1, *xin qi* in case 2, etc.). The word *qi* is mentioned on its own in case 3 (line 14), case 7 (line 13) and case 9 (line 19), where Yi says, he examined *mai*, and felt that *qi* is 'intense', 'congested' and '*yin*', which may reflect medical rationale of the early second century. Likewise, the name of the disorder of case 2 (line 3), *qi ge bing*, invokes early medical rationale. Accordingly, Yi may state in line 6: 'She is ailing from *qi*. An amassment is visiting the bladder' (*bing qi. Shan*

---

[3] *feng ru zhong.* See discussion of *jue ru zhong* in case 3 (line 2), n. 16.

ke yu pang guang). Probably, 'she is ailing from *qi*' (*bing qi*) was the name of the disorder in the edited early first-century version of case 10, and *shan ke yu pang guang* a commentatorial interjection. The common doctors speak of outdoor 'wind' entering the body, and Yi of *qi* in the body.

The common doctors needle this disorder. Their needling is akin to pricking a balloon in order to let wind out, much like the second-century manuscripts recommend needling for letting pus out of boils.[4] They needle the foot's minor *yang mai* after stating that 'wind entered and struck the interior'. This is in line with Yi's rationale insofar as in case 1 (lines 34–5), pulse qualities felt on the 'minor *yang*' indicate heat in the 'interior' (*zhong*) and in case 6 (lines 31, 34) cauterisation of the 'foot's minor *yang*' and ingestion of a *Pinellia* bolus causes a depletion in the 'abdominal part of the interior' (*fu zhong*). Since in cases 1 and 6 the connection between the 'minor *yang*' and the 'interior' may have been given due to either an editorial interpolation or a commentatorial interjection, the same editor or commentator may have been at work here in case 10 (line 4).

The common doctors needled the minor *yang*; Yi cauterises the dull *yin mai*. Yi's treatment is in line with early medical rationale (see p. 339), and that of the common doctors with no known medical rationale. In canonical doctrine, the foot's dull *yin* and minor *yang* are aspects of one visceral system, that of the liver and its outer aspect the gall bladder, and for conditions marked by coldness, cauterisation is indicated. The commentator who interjected line 4 (and line 8) may have done so for rhetorical reasons, to emphasise the contrast between the common doctors and Yi, being familiar with the basics but not with the intricacies of canonical medicine.

Finally, one may wonder why the common doctors attribute the disorder to the lungs (line 3), although the patient tangibly has a swollen abdomen. Xu Guang points to an edition that renders *fei* 肺 (lungs) as *gan* 肝 (liver). This would enhance consistency in medical reasoning across cases 1–10, considering that both the pre-canonical liver/womb (*gan*) and the minor *yang mai* are mentioned in cases 1 and 6. Nevertheless, *Su wen* 17 reports on an amassment in the architectural space of the heart (inclusive of the lungs) that presents with a bulging abdomen: 'If the name of the disorder is "heart amassment", the minor abdomen must have form' (*bing ming xin shan, shao fu dang you xing ye* 病名心疝 少腹當有形也),[5] and *Ling shu* 26 (quoted on p. 338) speaks of fullness in the small abdomen reaching the heart. Having said this, it is odd that the common doctors refer to viscera, like lungs or liver. In canonical doctrine, the lungs are in charge of breathing and *qi*, and in Yi's case histories, a 'host of the disorder' is otherwise mentioned only in Yi's 'Mai fa' quotes. Possibly, line 3 is also a commentatorial interjection.

---

[4] MWD 'Maifa' (1985:16), ZJS 'Maishu' (2001:144).
[5] *Su wen* 17, p. 52.

Text structure semantics

Line 18 shows textual irregularities and suggests the name of the disorder in the early second-century medical document on which this text elaborates probably was *qi zhi fu* 氣之腹 (*qi* went into the abdomen). This comes to the fore if one slightly alters the word order and punctuation in line 19 and thereby also explains the textual anomaly of the topic 'abdomen' (*fu zhi* 腹 之) in the topic-comment sentence it introduces.

If the name of the disorder is '*qi* went into the abdomen', text structure semantics works well for two constituents in the name: *qi* correlates with 'being replete' and the abdomen/bladder correlates with 'large'. The third pulse quality 'coming with difficulty' is best interpreted as indicative of the concomitant signs and symptoms. Only indirect textual evidence was found to correlate it with the amassment in the name of the disorder. This corroborates the suggestion that 'an amassment is visiting the bladder', *shan ke yu pang guang*, is a commentatorial interjection.

da 大 – large (line 14)   In case 10, Yi says 'it is large yet replete' (*da er shi*); this in contrast to the *mai* that is 'large yet frequent' (*mai da er shuo*) in case 3 or the *mai* that is 'large yet hurried' (*mai da er zao*) in case 5, and it is just possible that 'large yet replete' once described the tactile quality of the swollen abdomen itself. Case 5 (line 20) explicitly states that 'being large' indicates that the bladder is affected, and cases 3 (line 16) and 5 (line 21) that 'being frequent' (*shuo*) and 'hurried' (*zao*) indicate heat. The correlation between 'being replete' and *qi* is well documented in the medical literature (see p. 334), but not that between 'being large' and the 'bladder/abdomen'. Before claiming that in case 10 'being large' indicates a bladder/abdominal disorder as in cases 3 and 5, let us investigate whether being 'large', rather than being 'replete', correlates with *qi*.

'Being large' can be mentioned together with 'being replete' as in *Su wen* 28, 'The pulse is replete and large' (*mai shi da ye* 脈實大也)[6] or in *Su wen* 62, 'Its pulses are firm and large, hence one calls them replete' (*qi mai jian da, gu yue shi* 其脈堅大 故曰實),[7] or in *Ling shu* 12, which says of *yang* brightness: 'If its pulse is large, then there is much blood and *qi* is abundant' (*qi mai da, xue duo qi sheng* 其脈大 血多氣盛).[8] In *Ling shu* 4, 'being large' is opposed to 'being small' (*xiao* 小) and 'rough' (*se* 濇): 'In all cases of [pulses] being large, there is much *qi* and little blood, in the case of them being small, there is both little blood and *qi* ... in [all] cases of [their] being rough, there is much blood and little *qi*, and there is a slight bit of coldness' (*zhu ... da zhe, duo qi shao xue; xiao zhe, xue qi jie shao ... se zhe, duo xue shao qi, wei you han* 諸 大者 多氣少血 小者 血氣皆少 ... 濇者 多血少氣 微有 寒).[9] It is the case that the 'large' pulse indicates repleteness.

---

[6] *Su wen* 28, p. 87.   [7] *Su wen* 62, p. 170.
[8] *Ling shu* 12, p. 312.   [9] *Ling shu* 4, p. 277.

However, 'being large' can also point to a depletion, as in *Su wen* 22: 'In the case of a heart disorder ... if there is depletion then the chest and abdomen are enlarged' (*xin bing zhe ... xu ze xiong fu da* 心病者 虛則胸腹大).[10] And according to *Su wen* 19, a pulse can be: 'large yet depleted' (*da er xu* 大而虛).[11] In *Ling shu* 47, the viscera are said to be steady and at peace, if they are small (AB *xiao ze [zang] an* 小則[臟]安),[12] but if they are large, they are prone to be harmed by the noxious [*qi*].

Since 'being large' indicates both repletions and depletions, it is unlikely that it correlates with *qi*, and almost certain that it correlates, as in cases 3 and 5, with the bladder, although no canonical medical evidence was found for this. If the term '*pang guang* bladder' is a commentatorial interjection for 'abdomen' (*fu*), the correlation between 'being large' as an attribute to the 'abdomen' needs to be established. This poses no problems as it is often given in canonical medicine (e.g. *Ling shu* 26, quoted on p. 338).

shi 實 – replete (line 14)   The 'replete' pulse is frequently encountered in medical texts and belongs among the twenty-four pulses in *Mai jing* 1.1.[13] It is indicative of *qi* in *Ling shu* 3: 'If one speaks of repletion, there is *qi*, if one speaks of depletion, there is no *qi*' (*yan shi zhe, you qi, xu zhe, wu qi* 言實者 有氣 虛者 無氣).[14] A repletion is generally treated by effecting a discharge of *qi*, as advocated in *Ling shu* 9: 'In cases where *mai* are replete, needle deeply into them, in order to discharge their *qi*' (*mai shi zhe, shen ci zhi, yi xie qi qi* 脈實者 深刺之 以泄其氣).[15] This provides scholarly medical evidence for suggesting that the 'replete' pulse correlates with *qi*.

In canonical doctrine, both 'being replete' and 'abundant' are contrasted with 'depleted' (*xu* 虛), as in *Su wen* 25: 'If it is depleted, replete it, if it is full, discharge it' (*xu zhe shi zhi, man zhe xie zhi* 虛者實之 滿者泄之),[16] and in *Su wen* 53: 'When the grains are abundant, *qi* is abundant, and when the grains are depleted, *qi* is depleted, this is their usual state' (*gu sheng qi sheng, gu xu qi xu, ci qi chang ye* 穀盛氣盛 穀虛氣虛 此其常也).[17] However, just as Yi often speaks of the hot but not explicitly in opposition to the cold, he does not explicitly contrast repletion/abundance and depletion. In case 10, 'being replete' certainly correlates with *qi* in the name of the disorder.

qi lai nan 其來難 – they came with difficulty (line 15)   The verb 'to be difficult' (*nan*) is both in Yi's Memoir and in the *Inner Canon* typically used for describing 'difficulties with urinating and defecating' (*bian sou nan*).[18]

---

[10] *Su wen* 22, p. 72.   [11] *Su wen* 19, p. 62.
[12] *Ling shu* 47, pp. 391–4. See also case 7 (line 10).
[13] *Mai jing* 1.1, p. 2.   [14] *Ling shu* 3, p. 273.   [15] *Ling shu* 9, p. 295.
[16] *Su wen* 25, p. 80. See also *Ling shu* 1, p. 264; 3, p. 271. For the expression *mai man* 脈滿 (the vessels are full), see *Su wen* 39, p. 112; 47, p. 139.
[17] *Su wen* 53, p. 144.   [18] e.g. *Ling shu* 26, p. 345 and p. 346.

The *Zhu bing yuan hou lun* mentions disorders like 'difficulties in giving birth' (*nan chan* 難產) or 'difficulties in breastfeeding' (*nan ru* 難乳).[19] In case 18, when the menses do not descend, Yi also speaks of '*mai* coming with difficulty'. All these conditions of 'difficulties' (*nan*) appear to have in common that the flow and expulsion of a bodily product (urine, faeces, menses, milk or a child) is hindered in some way.

'Its coming is difficult' (*qi lai nan*) is not given as a pulse quality in the *Inner Canon* and in case 10 it appears to reflect in an iconic way the patient's 'difficulties with urinating and defecating' (*nan yu qian hou sou*). However, as the text is punctuated in Takigawa's edition, Yi states that 'coming with difficulty' is indicative of '*qi* [coming] from an amassment visiting the bladder' (line 18). This sentence, *shan qi zhi ke yu pang guang ye*, is grammatically odd as it has a superfluous word *zhi* 之. Futhermore, it probably contains a commentatorial interjection *ke yu pang guang ye* (see p. 331).

If 'coming with difficulty' is put in correlation with the constituent 'amassment' (*shan*), this is at variance with case 3 (line 14), where 'being intense' (*ji*) correlates with 'amassment' in the disorder called 'welling/painful amassment'. This problem could be solved by their semantic closeness, as a commentator to the *Guanzi* uses the term *nan* (difficult) to paraphrase *ji* (intense, tense, taut). One could argue that Yi used *nan* as correlate to *shan* (amassment). However, no canonical medical parallels have been found for this correlation. This reinforces the idea that the constituent in the name of the disorder *shan ke yu pang guang* in line 6 is a commentatorial interjection, as is *ke yu pang guang ye* in line 18.

In summary, based on the parallel to cases 3 and 5, 'being large' (*da*) correlates with the bladder/abdomen, and 'replete' (*shi*) with *qi*. Although lines 17–18 explicitly state that coming with difficulties indicates an amassment, establishing a correlation between a pulse quality and the constituent *shan* (amassment) causes problems. 'To come with difficulties' is not actually a pulse quality and in case 3 'being intense' correlates with *shan*, and for that correlation there are many parallels in medical texts. It is thus most likely that the concomitant complaint 'difficulties in urinating and defecating' correlates in an iconic way with *mai* that 'come with difficulty'.

***fu* 腹, *shao fu* 少腹 or *xiao fu* 小腹 – abdomen, minor abdomen or small abdomen? (lines 9, 19, 22; lines 20 and 26)** In case 10, the commentators are not disturbed by the fact that a woman has an 'amassment' in the 'small abdomen', while in case 7, they ponder over whether Pan Manru's pain is in the 'small abdomen' (*xiao fu*) or the 'minor abdomen' (*shao fu*) (line 2).

---

[19] *Zhongyi dacidian* (1995:1329). See *Zhu bing yuan hou lun* 43.1, p. 1227 and 47.75, pp. 1334–5. For *ru* 乳 in the sense of 'giving birth', see ch.7, case 14.

The Mawangdui 'Yinyang vessel text' and the corresponding *Ling shu* 10 specifically refer to the 'minor abdomen' in women: 'In men there are ulcers and amassments [hernias?], in women the minor abdomen becomes swollen' (*zhang fu kui shan, fu ren shao fu zhong* 丈夫癀疝 婦人少腹腫).[20] This sentence testifies to the concept of gender-specific disorders in the early Han; ulcers and amassments affect men, while the 'minor abdomen that is swollen' (*shao fu zhong*) is a typical women's disorder.

However, generally the 'minor abdomen' and 'small abdomen' are used in gender-unspecific ways. Thus, the Mawangdui 'Yinyang vessel text' states that the vessel of the foot's dull *yin* 'comes into contact with the minor abdomen' (*chu shao fu* 觸少腹), while the corresponding text in *Ling shu* 10 states that 'it goes into the pubic hair, passes by the genitals and comes into contact with the small abdomen' before saying that 'it passes along both sides of the stomach,[21] and binds up with the liver' (*ru mao zhong, guo yin qi, di xiao fu, xia wei shu gan* 入毛中 過陰器 抵小腹 挾胃屬肝). As hinted at by the above two quotes and as further research shows, the term 'small abdomen' does not occur in the Mawangdui manuscripts, is hardly mentioned in the *Su wen* and occurs mostly in the *Ling shu*.[22] Differences appear to reflect habits of writing within different medical lineages or time periods, rather than gender-specificity.

In case 10 (line 9), Yi speaks of an 'abdomen' (*fu*) that becomes swollen, not a 'minor abdomen'. He later expands on the reason why it became swollen (lines 19–22), in a stanza within which he mentions the 'small abdomen' (line 20). We can be fairly certain that this stanza was added by someone (see p. 333), who took *fu* (abdomen) as a topic marker (line 19) and ended the stanza with reference to *fu* (abdomen; line 22). The term that the 'abdomen swells' (*fu zhong* 腹腫) rather than 'expands' (*fu zhang* 腹張) or 'becomes full' (*fu man* 腹滿) has parallels in the early manuscript texts (see pp. 336, 338), as does the idiom that *mai* 'have excess' (*you guo* 有過) (see p. 27). This hints at an editor or early commentator of the second or first century BCE. By contrast, the mentioning of the link of the dull *yin* that is knotted to the small abdomen (line 20) reflects canonical medical knowledge and a mechanistic understanding of bodily processes of presumably a late commentator.

Moreover, it is interesting to note a minor difference in expression, which is that in the following stanza (lines 23–6), line 23 has a 'dull *yin mai*' rather than the 'dull *yin*' of lines 20 and 21. In case 1 (lines 41–4), there was no

---

[20] MWD YY (1985:11), *Ling shu* 10, p. 305. See also *Ling shu* 49, p. 402.

[21] *jia* or *xie* 挾 'to clasp something underneath one's arm', i.e. to hold on both sides (Karlgren 1957:168, 630a). Compare with Harper (1998:193).

[22] It is mentioned in *Su wen* 22, p. 73, as opposite of 'large abdomen' (*da fu* 大腹). See *Huangdi nei jing*, p. 582. And occurs in Wang Bing's interpolated *Su wen* 72 and 76. See computer printout by Hermann Tessenow (2000 p.c.).

textual anomaly that would allow us to suggest the work of a commentator, although the peculiar medical rationale in terms of tubular structures was noted. There are striking parallels in technical terminology to this stanza in case 10 (lines 19, 21, 22), namely the mentioning of the 'dull *yin*' (not dull *yin mai*) and 'bright *yang*' (not bright *yang mai*), nodes of the *mai* (*mai jie*) and 'agitation' (*dong*).

jue yin zhi dong 蹶陰之動 – the agitation of the dull *yin* (line 16)   After mentioning that the three pulses were 'large' yet 'replete' and 'come with difficulty' (lines 14–15), Yi says: 'This indicates an agitation of the dull *yin*' (*shi jue yin zhi dong ye*; line 16). He does not say it is '*qi* [coming] from one of the viscera', as in cases 1–9 (see table 5), although in the following line he repeats that in the case of *mai* coming with difficulty, it indicates '*qi* [coming] from an amassment that is visiting the bladder' (lines 17–18).

It is possible that line 16 on the agitation of the dull *yin* is an interjection by the same commentator who added the stanza on postulated processes in it (lines 19, 21, 22), which provide the rationale for his exclamation in line 16. Without the interjection, the text would follow the rhetoric of manner 2 (in table 4): XYZ.Z *zhe*. AB *ye* (lines 15, 17–18). However, it is equally possible that line 16 was written by the editor, who added the stanza on treatment (lines 23–4) into case 10, since the text also fits into the standard rhetorical figure of manner 1: XYZ. *shi* AB *ye* (lines 15–16).

Yi speaks of 'being replete' (*shi*) and of an 'agitation' (*dong*). The Mawangdui 'Yinyang vessel text' makes a distinction between *mai* which 'if agitated, then give rise to disorders' (*shi dong ze bing* 是動則病) and those that have 'disorders that they produce' (*qi suo chan bing* 其所產病). This distinction is considered an early precursor of medical rationale which differentiates between 'repletion patterns' (*shi zheng* 實證) and 'depletion patterns' (*xu zheng*) in later medical texts.[23] This shows that even if line 16 is a commentatorial interjection, it is in line with early and canonical medical knowledge. Likewise, line 21, which states the dull *yin* 'has excess' is in line with the above passage from the Mawangdui 'Yinyang vessel text' (quoted on p. 336), which says: 'If this one is agitated' (*shi dong ze bing*), 'in men there is a drooping amassment, in women then the minor abdomen is swollen and painful'.[24]

The interrelation between a swelling of the minor/small abdomen and the dull *yin* is also given in canonical texts,[25] although the 'swelling' is there mostly rendered as an 'expansion' or 'fullness'. *Ling shu* 10,[26] for instance, elaborates on the above-quoted manuscript text: 'If there is a numbness of

---

[23] MWD YY (1985:9–13). See also *Ling shu* 10, pp. 299–306, and *Nan jing* 22 (Unschuld 1986a:278).
[24] MWD YY (1985:11).
[25] Hermann Tessenow, computer printout (2000 p.c.).
[26] *Ling shu* 10, p. 305.

the dull *yin*, then the minor abdomen is swollen and painful' (*jue yin zhi jue, ze shao fu zhong tong* 厥陰之厥 則少腹腫痛),[27] a passage that is also found in *Su wen* 45. *Su wen* 41 speaks of an abdominal fullness that is best treated by needling the dull *yin*: 'If the minor abdomen feels full, needle the dull *yin*' (*shao fu man, ci zu jue yin* 少腹滿 刺足厥陰).[28] So does *Ling shu* 26: 'If the small abdomen feels full and large, and [this condition] rises to the stomach and reaches the heart, if gradually the body feels at times chills and hot flushes, if urinating is not successful: [for treatment] choose the foot's dull *yin*' (*xiao fu man da, shang zou wei, zhi xin, xi xi shen shi han re, xiao bian bu li, qu zu jue yin* 小腹滿大 上走胃 至心 淅淅身時寒熱 小便不利 取足厥陰).[29] These canonical texts all make the dull *yin mai* responsible for an expansion of or fullness in the small abdomen.

The 'link of the dull *yin*' (*jue yin zhi luo*) of line 20 is presumably the same as the canonical 'small link of the dull *yin*' (*jue yin xiao luo*) in *Ling shu* 19: 'If the small abdomen is painful and swollen, and if one cannot urinate, the noxious resides in the binding of the triple burner: [for treatment] take the large link of the major *yang*. If one observes that the linking vessels, after getting knotted up with the small link of the dull *yin*, bleed, and that the swelling rises and reaches the stomach pit: [for treatment] take the *san li* [today an acumoxa *locus*]' (*xiao fu tong zhong, bu de xiao bian, xie zai san jiao yue, qu zhi tai yang da luo, shi qi luo mai yu jue yin xiao luo jie er xue zhe, zhong shang ji wei wan, qu san li* 小腹痛腫 不得小便 邪在三焦 約 取之太陽大絡 視之絡脈與厥陰小絡結而血者 腫上及胃脘 取三里).[30] The commentator who interjected line 20 and probably also line 26 was evidently guided by the rationale in *Ling shu* 19, also when he brings up the issue of 'pain in the small abdomen' in line 26.

While the interrelation between the 'abdomen that is swollen' and the 'agitation in the dull *yin*' is well documented in early and canonical medical texts, it is not given for amassments in the bladder. This is one of the reasons why case 10 reads as though two originally unrelated case histories have been collated into one. As the text reads now, the 'abdomen's swelling' (*fu zhong*) is explicitly said to be caused by exposure to the cold and 'remanent urine' (*yi ni*; line 8), and not by *qi* visiting the abdomen, or, if so, only indirectly. The sentence, which mentions 'remanent urine', is grammatically odd, however. 'While ailing, being exposed to cold *qi*' (*bing er* 病而 ... *xian han qi* 見寒氣) would be more acceptable than *bing xian han qi*.[31] It is also semantically odd because *yi ni* is medically defined as 'enuresis'.[32] This

---

[27] *Su wen* 45, p. 127.   [28] *Su wen* 41, p. 118.

[29] *Ling shu* 26, p. 346.   [30] *Ling shu* 19, p. 331.

[31] Compare with textual anomaly in case 6 (lines 33–4).

[32] Compare with case 7 (line 4), pp. 278–9, where *yi ji* is interpreted as 'remanent stools'. For *yi ni* 'enuresis', see Wiseman (1990:327), *Huangdi nei jing*, p. 1531. See also MWD 'Tai chan shu' (1985:136, S22). For *yi* in the sense of 'to remove', see MWD 'Yangsheng fang' (1985:106, S77), Harper (1998:341).

grammatically and semantically odd sentence makes use of vocabulary reminiscent of what we identified as interjections in case 6 (lines 33–4) and case 7 (lines 4 and 14) by a commentator familiar with canonical medicine but not expert in it. It unambiguously makes case 10 into a condition marked by coldness, which according to canonical medical understanding warrants cauterisation.

There is a connection between the small abdomen and bladder in that both occupy the same body architectural space. Thus, the bladder is situated in the midst of the 'minor abdomen' in *Su wen* 52: 'If one needles the bladder in the midst of the minor abdomen, urine comes out' (*ci shao fu zhong pang guang ni chu* 刺少腹中膀胱 溺出);[33] and also in *Su wen* 43: 'The obstruction of the bladder: the bladder in the minor abdomen, if you press onto it, it is painful inside' (*pao bi zhe, shao fu pang guang, an zhi nei tong* 胞痺者 少腹膀胱 按之內痛).[34] In contrast to the '*pao* bladder' in case 5, located in the innermost 'interior/centre', these two canonical *Su wen* passages locate the '*pang guang* bladder' inside the 'minor abdomen'. Yi is not explicit about the location of the bladder in case 10, but he is explicit about the location of the swelling caused by the waters of the bladder in the 'abdomen' (*fu*) and the 'small abdomen' (*xiao fu*).

In summary, there is ample evidence in the early and canonical medical literature for the interrelation between 'swellings in the abdomen' and the 'agitation/excess of the dull *yin*'; there is none for one between an 'amassment in the bladder' and 'agitation of the dull *yin*'. Meanwhile there is canonical evidence that the '*pang guang* bladder' and 'small abdomen' inhabit the same body architectural space.

More on huo ji tang *(lines 27–9), cauterisation and needling (lines 23–6)*

The first treatment, cauterisation of the foot's dull *yin mai*, is entirely in line with the recommendations in the Mawangdui 'Yinyang vessel text': cauterisation is indicated for treating any condition on any *mai* that is 'agitated' (*dong*). In canonical medicine, cauterisation was used for warming the patient, as in *Su wen* 12: 'If one of the viscera gets cold and gives rise to a disorder of being bloated, for its cure it is appropriate to cauterise and heat it' (*zang han sheng man bing, qi zhi yi jiu ruo* 臟寒生滿病 其治宜灸焫).[35] One wonders, therefore, whether the grammatically and semantically odd sentence in line 8 was interjected by a commentator, who thought along similar lines as the authors of *Su wen* 12. But needling and cauterising need not be framed in hot/cold complementarities; *Su wen* 41 (quoted on p. 338) recommends treating the 'small abdomen' by needling the dull *yin*, regardless of whether the condition is hot or cold.

---

[33] *Su wen* 52, p. 143.   [34] *Su wen* 43, p. 122.   [35] *Su wen* 12, p. 40.

In the final stanza of case 10, Yi says the ingestion of *huo ji tang* effected that after three days the *qi* of the amassment had dissipated (*shan qi san*; lines 27–9). This is interesting to a medically trained reader. How is this dissipation of *qi* effected? If *huo ji tang* was a 'fire-regulatory broth', one would expect it to reduce heat. However, *qi* does not usually dissipate if it is cooled down, at least not according to canonical medical texts. In general, *qi* congeals and accumulates into amassments if it is cold, and dissipates as it is heated. Thus, if Yi's treatment were framed in hot/cold complementarities in case 10, *huo ji tang* should not be administered to reduce the heat in the patient, but rather to warm her up and thereby dissipate the amassed *qi*.

However, amassed *qi* can be dissipated by other means than by warming up a patient.[36] It is unlikely that in the early second century *huo ji tang* treated disorders framed in a rationale of hot/cold complementarities (see case 5, line 7). It probably meant 'broth [prepared by careful] regulation of fire', as it was simmered over a small fire, which is a characteristic feature of decoctions. Case 10 provides verbatim evidence that *huo ji tang* effected a cure through the dissipation of [accumulated] *qi*.

Discussion

The name of the disorder, 'ailing from *qi* – an amassment is visiting the bladder – and difficulties with urinating and defecating' (*bing qi, shan ke pang guang, nan yu qian hou sou*), has four constituents and Yi mentions three pulse qualities. Text structure semantics works well with regard to two. Comparison with cases 3 and 5 suggests 'being large' (*da*) correlates with the constituent 'bladder', or 'abdomen', and comparison with canonical passages, particularly *Ling shu* 3, suggests a correlation between 'being replete' (*shi*) and *qi*. The third quality, 'coming with difficulty' (*qi lai nan*) is not a canonical medical pulse quality and perhaps it correlates in an iconic way with the signs and symptoms mentioned as part of a very long name: difficulties with urinating and defecating. Yi provides no explicit indications of any tactile qualities, but 'large, yet replete' may comment on the tactile perception of the swollen abdomen itself.

There are no textual parallels for the name of the disorder elsewhere, and minor grammatical problems in lines 18 and 19, and in line 6, suggest that *shan ke yu pang guang* is a commentatorial interjection. The assumed second-century document probably had '*qi* went into the abdomen' (*qi zhi fu*).

It was primarily the treatment in two stages which hinted at the possibility that case 10 conflates two case histories into one. Initially, the two treatments appeared incompatible. Cauterisation is in canonical medicine often

---

[36] e.g. Yamada (1998). Needling, for instance, is still today a method for dissolving amassments.

used for conditions marked by coldness but *huo ji tang*, if translated as 'fire-regulatory broth', would presumably be meant to regulate the fire of a heat condition. However, *huo ji tang* is best translated as 'broth [prepared by careful] regulation of fire' and cauterisation is in the Mawangdui 'Yinyang vessel texts' used for treating disorders arising on 'agitated' *mai*, irrespective of whether they are framed in complementarities of the hot and cold. If case 10 is not marked by reasoning in terms of the hot and cold, as is evident from Yi's treatment, *ni chi* (the urine is dark) on line 7, and the entire line 8 which claims the condition is aggravated by the cold, are with great certainty interjections by two different commentators.

Case 10 shows semantic continuities between *qi* that went into the abdomen, difficulties with urinating and defecating, the pulse qualities and *huo ji tang*, on the one hand, and between the swollen abdomen and its treatment by cauterising the dull *yin*, on the other. From a text critical viewpoint, it may represent the faultline between two documents, i.e. the end of the assumed early second-century medical document on cases 1–10 and the beginning of the stories assembled around it in cases 11–25. The text has thus many layers. Parts of it reveal the hand of the early second-century author and the first-century editor of cases 1–10. In addition, various phrases and sentences are best interpreted as interjections of at least four different commentators. On reflection one commentator may have made so many changes to the text that he needs to be regarded as a second editor. Perhaps there was one such editor who put all cases 1–25 together and worked on the texts after Sima Qian's recasting of, perhaps, cases 1–10? Case 10 points to a multitude of writers who have led to the text in its present form – so many that it calls for a reading more sensitive to the multivocalic fabric of the *Shi ji* case histories than initially expected.

21

Discussion of the medical case histories 1–10 in the Memoir of Chunyu Yi

This study explored the first ten medical case histories in Chunyu Yi's Memoir in the second part of the 105th chapter of the *Shi ji* from a comparative vantage point, with themes in mind that are central to medical anthropology and the anthropology of sensory experience. It therefore risks focusing on questions imposed by Western scholarship. Medical anthropology, as variously pointed out, unduly relies on biomedical interpretations of bodily processes and illness events,[1] and the anthropology of the senses tends to mistake modern European ideas about the senses as biological facts.[2]

Admittedly, this text caught my attention precisely because the *Shi ji* personage Chunyu Yi, much like any contemporary biomedical doctor, systematically attended to names, causes and key qualities of illness events. However, I took precautions so as to be sure not to have imputed this into the ancient text. Names, causes and key qualities are introduced by linguistic markers, which give Yi's case histories a formulaic structure (see p. 112). Based on this insight, an interpretive method was developed, 'text structure semantics', that I used together with other considerations, for unpacking early medical rationale in Yi's cases 1–10.

The study has shown that, indeed, the naming of illness and the attribution of blame, discussed above under 'name of the disorder' and 'cause of the disorder', are important to contemporary medicines and early Chinese medicine alike. However, the key qualities investigated differ. Diagnosis in biomedicine systematically investigates signs and symptoms, which in institutionalised hospital settings are more easily identified and, according to some, became decisive elements in the diagnostic process with the emergence of hospitals in modern Europe.[3] Pathogenesis and disease aetiology, indispensable for a complete biomedical diagnosis, are derived from these signs and symptoms. By contrast, Yi's cases 1–10 only concomitantly mention signs and symptoms, but systematically report on 'examining *mai*'

---

[1] Nichter and Lock (2002). See also Hsu (2005c).
[2] Ingold (2000:243–87), Geurts (2003).   [3] e.g. Foucault (1963), Bynum and Porter (1993).

(*zhen mai*), through 'pressing onto *mai*' (*qie mai*), sometimes at the 'opening of the right *mai*' (*you mai kou*). The key qualities of the illness event Yi attended to were their tactile qualities.

Strictly speaking, these tactile qualities of *mai* mattered to Yi perhaps less in a context of 'pulse diagnosis', as the subtitle of this study has it, than in one of 'pulse prognostics'. It needs to be kept in mind that Yi's main concern lay in prognostication, in particular, of death. In cases 1–10, his calculations of the time period before death were grounded in numerologies of five (cases 1, 6, 8) and three (arguably two, in case 7) for predicting the day of death. They show continuity with other prognosticatory arts performed in early and medieval China, have faint parallels in a few select passages of *Su wen* 17 and 19 (see p. 142), and differ from those prognostications grounded in the five agents doctrine found in cases 12, 15 and 21.[4] To be sure, Yi's Memoir is a multivocalic text, and the *Shi ji* personage Yi makes use of various methods of diagnosis and prognostication. The method at the centre of Yi's cases 1–10, *zhen mai*, specified as *qie mai*, differs from those known from other early Han texts that involve, for instance, the visual inspection of *mai* and *se*, or physiognomy,[5] in that it reports primarily on tactile experiences during the clinical encounter.

What can a highly elaborate tactile method of prognostication achieve? Touch expresses and causes closeness.[6] It can have the effect that a patient starts to speak, and by speaking reveals information that is crucial for making a prognosis/diagnosis. However, touch can be valued as a quality in itself in that it causes presence and 'makes real'. What you can touch often appears more 'real' than what is seen from afar (the disciple Thomas had to touch Christ's wound to believe in his resurrection). Tactile experiences of *mai* are difficult to identify, distinctions are subtle and participant experience makes evident that the procedure of palpating *mai* puts the doctor into a position of great uncertainty.[7] Such uncertainty may well be an artificially construed one, as Susan Whyte has emphasised with regard to the uncertainties created in the divination séances she studied in rural Uganda.[8] Perhaps all divinatory, prognosticatory or diagnostic procedures have in common the development of culture-specific, sophisticated techniques of generating uncertainty. Perhaps all these techniques are meant to deconstruct widely held assumptions among the people involved in the procedure and in an unprejudiced way heighten attentiveness to the present (as any contemporary scientific enquiry should do as well). Touch in the medical encounter not only elicits speech but also enhances somatic attentiveness to unspoken cues from the patient and his or her social entourage. It attends to the 'atmospheric', which ranges from latent dispositions

---

[4] Harper (2001) discusses case 21. See also Kalinowski (2003).   [5] e.g. Despeux (2005).
[6] e.g. Merleau-Ponty (1962), Mazis (1979).
[7] Ethnographic fieldwork in Kunming (1988–9).   [8] Whyte (1997).

and interpersonally constituted emotions to weather-specific, seasonal and climatic change, or in terms of Chinese medicine, to *qi*.

The discussion in what follows will focus on findings relating to the three main themes that were outlined in the introductory part and which provided the framework for this study of Yi's cases 1–10: terms of tactile experience; the concept of *qi*, the motivations for integrating it into medical language and the consequences this had for body conceptions; and beliefs about illness causation in medical theory and practice. Before embarking on those, we need to review the dating of Yi's Memoir.

The dating of cases 1–10 in Chunyu Yi's Memoir

Yi's Memoir is of foremost importance to the historian of Chinese medicine, because it recounts the biography of an early physician, records individual medical case histories, contains a fairly extensive account of pulse diagnosis, i.e. the examination of *mai* that detects qualities of *qi*, and provides information both on therapeutics, particularly in cases 10/11–25, and on the transmission of knowledge, particularly in the two opening and the closing sections. There is little doubt that it relates medical learning of eastern China, especially of the kingdom of Qi, at a period which pre-dates the compilation of the extant version of the *Su wen* (which according to Unschuld happened in the first century and according to Keegan before the mid-third century CE).[9]

While Loewe considers the Memoir the composition of a single author who wrote it in the mid-second century, between 167 and 153 BCE,[10] this study emphasises that it is a multivocalic text, a compilation of textual materials from different currents of learning that were then subject to the hand of at least one creative editor. If the text is as multivocalic as this study suggests, the material presented in it cannot be taken as evidence of early Han medical reasoning without circumspection. The text in its present form reflects knowledge from different time periods: certain phrases reflect knowledge of an assumed early scholarly medical document; others may have been composed/interpolated by an eloquent author/editor, who was not a medical specialist; and several were interjected by later commentators. These layers were detected on the assumption that Yi's medical rationale is fairly consistent across cases 1–10 and on the basis of textual and semantic irregularities.

Two dates are mentioned in the Memoir: 180 BCE is given in both introductory sections as the date when Yi started to devote himself full-time to the study of medicine and 176 BCE is the year he was accused by a patient whom he refused to treat, which resulted in his trip to the Imperial capital where he was to be punished by mutilation. Fan Xingzhun

---

[9] Unschuld (2003:5), Keegan (1988:17). See ch. 1, n. 5.   [10] Loewe (1997).

considers Yi, once amnestied, to have written all twenty-five medical case histories then and there.[11] This study suggests that he did not write all, but only wrote terse notes on the first ten.

Some of Yi's body concepts and conceptions of illness in cases 1–10 due to similarities with the medical manuscripts unearthed from tombs closed in Mawangdui and Zhangjiashan in 168 and the mid-second century respectively, can be interpreted as dating from the early second century, e.g. 176 BCE or earlier. Thus, case 1 and particularly case 2 refer to a bipartite body. Case 1 implicitly alludes to a centrally positioned liver as responsible for blood dynamics and case 2 to the heart as an upper bodily cavity in which *qi* can be trapped. The concepts of the 'welling' (*yong*) waters from the bladder in case 3 and of the 'void' (*dong*) in case 8 allude to early cosmological conceptions contained in the Guodian *Laozi* and the Mawangdui *Huangdi sijing*. The *qi* that went to the abdomen (*qi zhi fu*) in case 10 (line 18), if this interpretation of the anomalous text passage is correct, was not the all-pervasive stuff of the universe as known from the canonical medical texts, but stuff inside the body that moved about and could wander, expand or contract. And the notion *jue* of the common doctors in case 3 and of Yi in case 9 (line 19) has much affinity with the idea that *jue* occurs 'if *yin* augments', as recorded in the third-century BCE *Lü shi chun qiu*.

Heat is pathological in all ten cases, but not mentioned in cases 7 and 8, which concern constipation and diarrhoea respectively. However, it is usually mentioned at the end of the case histories and some of these passages refer to strikingly similar tubular structures, which mention either the bright *yang* or dull *yin* (cases 1, 6, 10). This study has shown, however, that with the exception of the 'heat disorder' (*re bing*) mentioned in case 4 and, arguably, the 'lung consumption' (*fei xiao dan*) in case 6, heat became an aspect of the case histories later, in all likelihood, due to either editorial amendments or commentatorial interjections (in cases 1, 2, 3, 5, 9, 10). Early nosological terms such as the 'welling', the 'void', '*jue*-stones' and the '*jue*-numbness' with *yin* characteristics, and also 'accumulations' and 'conglomerations', point to the cold and cool as pathological (cases 3, 7, 8, 9).

In the received text, the medical case histories are formulaic in structure, and they contain many medical terms that reflect the medical rationale of the *Inner Canon*. Although in each of the first ten cases a few phrases were found that this study identified as testimony to the early second century, the text in the main probably dates from the early first century, which is the date of the composition of the entire *Shi ji*. While the possibility is not to be discarded entirely that the text was repeatedly edited throughout the second century, and perhaps also in the first century after Sima Qian's death

---

[11] Fan (unpubl.).

(d. ca 86 BCE), no attempt has been made to identify systematically multiple early stages of editing.

It is possible that Sima Qian himself rewrote the source material freely, personalising it and making it spicier, sometimes in politically telling ways.[12] Due to contradictions in medical rationale within several case histories and minute recurrent textual anomalies (for instance, consistent reference to either *mai* or *qi* when discussing pulse qualities), there is little doubt that he based his writings on textual source material and incorporated certain idioms verbatim. Since he interwove medical reasoning of his own times (presumably from the early first century) with earlier medical thinking, and added perhaps popular medical understandings to it, as any intellectual who is not specialised in medicine would do, the resultant case histories in the received text cannot be read as a compact early medical document but must be viewed as a document that is framed mostly, but not exclusively, in medical rationale.[13]

Finally, certain words, phrases and paragraphs are best interpreted as interjections of commentators who were inspired by Yi's Memoir and creatively added their ideas.[14] Thus, the last one or two lines in some cases often allude to medical ideas quite unrelated to what is said in the previous paragraphs or they contain unnecessary repetitions or outright misinterpretations:[15] testimony to a creative but disconnected commentator? Case 3 (lines 21–2), case 5 (lines 19–21, end of line 4) and case 10 (end of line 7), which turn the respective cases into heat pathologies, are best interpreted as commentatorial interjections. Moreover, the medical rationale in case 4 shows blatant discontinuities to that otherwise present in cases 1–10, while its vocabulary has striking continuities with case 15. Possible implications of this observation, which points in the direction of yet another Han editor after Sima Qian's death, have not been further pursued.[16]

In summary, due to the multivocality of Yi's Memoir, its medical terms do not all date from the second century BCE. Even in a context of medical rationale from the early second century, an interpolation from the early first century or an interjection of a later commentator, a *caveat* is given,

---

[12] See discussion of causes of the disorder on pp. 57, 117–18, wind as an editorial interpolation in cases 5 and 9 on pp. 211–13, 229, 304–5, names as rhymes and puns on pp. 55–6, and problems surrounding status and privileges of the man in charge of the woman in case 10 in table 1 on p. 54.

[13] e.g. *yi ji* (remanent stools) in case 7 (line 4) and *yi ni* (remanent urine) in case 10 (line 8).

[14] Henderson (1991). See also Lloyd (1991) on Galen's creative commentary on the Hippocratic corpus and Hsu (1999:125–6) on a senior doctor's 'creative mode of interpretation'.

[15] See cases 1 (lines 45–6), 2 (line 26), 4 (line 37), 7 (lines 19–20 or just line 20), and accordingly case 8 (line 16), perhaps case 9 (line 13). See also case 7, n. 107.

[16] Note semantic continuities in case 1 (lines 34–5) with case 6 (line 31 and the possibly interjected line 34) and with case 10 (line 2, and interjected lines 3–4), discussed on p. 332. Note parallel grammatical structure in case 6 (line 33) and case 10 (line 8), discussed on pp. 261 and 338–9. Note the *yang* brightness and the dull *yin* mentioned solely in the end of cases 1 (lines 41–4), 6 (lines 39–42) and 10 (lines 23–6).

because sometimes not only sentences and paragraphs, but also single idioms and terms, appear to have been retained, omitted or added by the editor and later commentators.

Terms of tactile experience

What did Yi feel when he examined *mai*? How did he put his tactile experiences into words and communicate them to others? Can the terms he chose be related to other life experiences, and, if so, to which ones? In full awareness that it is impossible to know their exact referential meaning, is it nevertheless possible to establish sense relations between them? Are there recurrent features that certain terms have in common, and, if so, what are they?

The tactile perception of qi

One of this study's most important findings is that Yi describes his tactile experiences in the language of *qi*. He speaks of *qi* [coming] from the liver, heart, lungs, spleen, bladder and kidneys; the 'within' and the five viscera; conglomerations; wind and water. Yi's Memoir alone among all extant sources, reports for the first time in medical history on a doctor who palpates *mai* and speaks of *qi* coming[17] from the viscera (*zang* 藏). This suggests that the *Shi ji* personage Yi conceived of all *mai* as connecting to the viscera, as they do in *Ling shu* 10 and throughout medical history thereafter, while only a few do so in the mid-second-century medical manuscripts (see p. 42). The significance of attributing to *qi* such centrality in medical language will be explored in more depth in the following section. This section discusses *qi* only in respect of its tactile qualities as perceived in the course of examining *mai*.

One of the first questions in this context is whether Yi actually perceives *qi* or whether he comments, after pressing onto *mai*, that what he felt is indicative of a certain quality of *qi*. Strictly speaking, even in those cases where Yi's wording can be translated 'to have perceived *qi*', it is not entirely certain whether he actually speaks of his tactile experience or comments on the meaning of the tactile perception. The text is ambiguous and, generally, both interpretations are possible (see Box 1).

The *Shi ji* personage Yi related to *qi* in different ways. In the light of the possible heterogeneous provenance of single passages in each case, it is worth noting that the static verbs which, according to this study, may testify to the early second-century document, relate to *qi* as a tactually felt process

---

[17] The *mai* in the 'Mai fa' and *Inner Canon* come and go, but Yi mentions only *mai* that come. See case 2 (lines 16–18).

Box 1: Did Chunyu Yi say he perceived qi or speak of the meanings implied by his tactile perception?

Case 1 (line 13) is perhaps the only one in which Yi can be interpreted unambiguously to perceive liver *qi* when he says he '*got qi* [coming] from the liver'. In case 2 (line 13), he says 'it *was qi* [coming] from the heart', which can be interpreted that he tactually felt it, but could also be a phrase that communicates his interpretation of a tactile perception that is not described further.

In the beginning of case 3 (line 14), Yi can be translated to have felt *qi* when he says its quality is 'intense' (*ji*) and this applies also to the end of case 4 (lines 32–3) when he qualifies the '*qi* [coming from the kidneys]' with static verbs, namely 'being murky, yet still'. Yet in case 3, the sentence that states 'the *mai* did not have *qi* [coming] from the five viscera' may report either on a tactile experience or on Yi's interpretation of a tactile experience not further described. The grammar allows for both interpretations. Likewise, in case 4 (lines 33–4), after reporting on the tactile quality 'being thin', when Yi states 'this is a case of water *qi*', the text reads as though Yi considered 'being thin' indicative of water *qi*, not that he tactually perceived water *qi* (but line 35 probably is a commentatorial interjection).

In case 5 (line 13), Yi can be translated to have felt 'wind *qi*', but not when he explains his tactile perception in a topic-comment sentence (line 20), saying that the pulse quality 'large' is indicative of 'bladder *qi*'.

In case 6 (line 16), the text reads as though Yi perceived the tactile quality *qi* [coming] from the lungs, when he qualifies it with a static verb, namely 'being hot'.

In case 7 (line 13), likewise, when Yi speaks of *qi* and qualifies it with static verbs, he can be interpreted as perceiving it. Yet in lines 10–12, he describes his tactile perception with static verbs, which in my reading he considered indicative of spleen *qi*; i.e. he did not sense the spleen *qi* himself.

In case 8 (line 12), Yi describes his perception of *mai*, with a static verb, 'being slippery', and in line 13 says 'this is wind *qi* [coming] from within'. In its given form, the text reads as though Yi considered the tactile quality 'slippery' indicative of the *qi* in question.

In case 9 (line 10), Yi may or may not have felt wind *qi* but in line 19, when he qualifies *qi* as *yin*, there is little doubt that he speaks of a felt perception.

In case 10 (line 18), there is a grammatical anomaly and at one stage the text may have read, 'the *qi* went to the abdomen' (*qi zhi fu*), which probably referred to a comment on a perception rather than the perception itself. In the preceding line 16, which may or may not have been interjected by a later commentator, Yi does not speak of *qi* but of an 'agitation of the dull *yin*' (*jue yin zhi dong*), which appears to be inferred from the tactile perceptions described with verbs of touch in the previous sentence(s).

or entity;[18] this is in contrast to phrases, presumably from a later period, that state 'this indicates a certain kind of *qi*'.[19] It suggests that in the context of examining *mai* the conception of *qi* changed over time. What in the early second century was a directly perceived tangible *qi*, had become a more abstract entity, known only indirectly, among later physicians.

Recent research has highlighted that *qi* in Warring States texts primarily referred to body internal processes, often in the context of discussing feelings and emotions (i.e. in allusion to a sentimental body, see pp. 13–14). In the received text, Yi does mention 'water *qi*' and 'wind *qi*', which give it body ecological dimensions, but in general Yi's use of *qi* in cases 1–10 provides further evidence that in early Western Han medicine *qi* was used primarily in the context of referring to body internal processes (table 5).

Table 5: Qualities of *mai* in terms of *qi* (Yi's vocabulary)

gan qi 肝氣 – *qi* [coming] from the liver	case 1
xin qi 心氣 – *qi* [coming] from the heart	case 2
qi ji 氣急 – *qi* was intense *wu wu zang qi* 無五臟氣 – no *qi* [was coming] from the five viscera	case 3
shen qi [腎]氣 – *qi* [coming] from the kidneys [*shui qi* 水氣 – water *qi*][a]	case 4
feng qi 風氣 – wind *qi* *pang guang qi* 膀胱氣 – *qi* [coming] from the bladder	case 5
fei qi 肺氣 – *qi* [coming] from the lungs	case 6
pi qi 脾氣 – *qi* [coming] from the spleen ?[*jia qi* 瘕氣 – *qi* [coming] from conglomerations]	case 7
nei [*feng*] *qi* 內[風]氣 – *qi* [coming] from [wind of] the inside	case 8
feng qi 風氣 – wind *qi* *qi yin* 氣陰 – *qi yin*	case 9
?[*jue yin zhi dong* 厥陰之動 – the agitation of the dull *yin*][b] [*shan*] *qi zhi . . . fu* [疝]氣之 . . . 服 – *qi* of the amassment went to . . . the abdomen	case 10

[a]In square brackets are what this study identified as commentatorial interjections: *shui qi* in case 4 (line 34) and *feng* in case 8 (line 13); perhaps also cases 7 (line 14) and 10 (lines 16 and 18).
[b]Case 10 (line 16), which may or may not be a commentatorial interjection, mentions 'agitation' (*dong*) instead of *qi*; one expects the two terms to report on the same kind of (tactile) experience. Was *qi* an entity that flows inside *mai*, as it is today, or was it an event like an agitation or resonance?

[18] See case 1 (line 13); case 2 (line 13); case 4 (lines 32–3); case 5 (line 13); case 6 (line 16); case 9 (line 19); case 10, unclear; but in cases 3 (line 14) and 7 (line 13), the *qi* that is felt at the 'right opening', which parallels the canonical *qi kou*, may reflect a canonical understanding.

[19] See case 4 (line 34) and case 7 (line 12). However, in case 7 (line 14), Yi explicitly says he perceived it (*xian qi*).

Verbs of touch

The terms on the tactile qualities of *mai* are heterogeneous. My reading of the case histories started to make sense once I considered Yi an eclectic who juxtaposed knowledge from diverse strands of medicine. As argued earlier, Yi compares knowledge recorded in the 'Mai fa' with his own findings. In general, most 'Mai fa' terms occur in the *Inner Canon* and *Mai jing*. By contrast, Yi's vocabulary is more heterogeneous. Some terms may well testify to traditions of medical learning that have since fallen into oblivion; others, which may have been interpolated by the first-century author-editor, have more affinity with canonical works. They all have one aspect in common, which is that they generally occur in pairs or phrases. In this respect they contrast with the monosyllabic twenty-eight standard pulse images in contemporary Traditional Chinese Medicine, and show continuities with other early classification systems as, for instance, that of plants in Renaissance Europe, which were assessed in long descriptive phrases before Linnaeus created the binomial system that combined 'genus' and 'species' in one name.

Verbs of touch in the 'Mai fa'

The 'Mai fa' pulses have each been discussed in the respective case histories, and most are known to us from canonical medicine.

Table 6: Verbs of touch mentioned in the 'Mai fa'

chang 長 – elongated (standard *Mai jing* pulse) *xian* 弦 – strung (standard *Mai jing* pulse) given as: *[mai] chang er xian*	case 1
lai 來 – to come (canonical pulse quality) *shuo* 數 – frequent (standard *Mai jing* pulse) *ji* 疾 – swift (canonical pulse quality) *qu* 去 – to leave (canonical pulse quality) *nan* 難 – with difficulty (canonical term, not a pulse quality) *bu yi* 不一 – not one (no textual parallels except in *Shi ji*) given as: *[mai] lai shuo ji qu nan er bu yi*	case 2
yin yang jiao 陰陽交 *yin* and *yang* intermingle (canonical term, not a pulse quality)	case 4
chen 沈 – sunken (standard *Mai jing* pulse), but here a body technique: sinking *fu* 浮 – floating (standard *Mai jing* pulse), but here a body technique: floating *jian* 堅 – firm (canonical pulse quality) *jin* 緊 – tight (standard *Mai jing* pulse) given as: *chen zhi er da jian, fu zhi er da jin*	case 5
bu ping 不平 – uneven (*ping*: canonical pulse quality) *bu gu* 不鼓 – not drumming (*gu*: canonical pulse quality)	case 6

In case 1, the 'Mai fa' pulses 'being elongated' (*chang*) and 'strung' (*xian*), which qualify *mai*, reflect canonical medical knowledge that invokes a body ecological understanding not present in the other passages of case 1.

In case 2, the 'coming' and 'going' of *mai* reflect canonical medical knowledge. 'Being frequent' (*shuo*) is a standard pulse in *Mai jing* 1.1; 'swift' (*ji*) frequently occurs in the *Nei jing*; while the other idioms *nan* (difficult) and *bu yi* (not one) are not canonical pulse qualities. All qualify *mai*, and they describe a movement that is hook-like (*gou* 鉤) – the characteristic movement of the canonical heart *mai*.

In case 4, the phrase '*yin yang* intermingle' probably does not describe a tactile quality but a postulated process inside the body, although the phrase appears in a place where text structure semantics would expect the 'Mai fa' to speak of a quality of *mai*. This textual anomaly is best explained by considering lines 26–31, and with them the 'Mai fa' quote, an interjection by a commentator rather than part of the editor's text.

In case 5, 'sinking' and 'floating' probably designate a body technique of palpation at two different pressure levels on the *mai* or, perhaps, on the buttocks; in later medical writings, they describe tactile qualities of *mai*, 'sunken' and 'floating'. 'Being firm' occurs in the *Nei jing* and 'tight' is one of the standard pulses in *Mai jing* 1.1. Commentators emphasise that they express in this context a tactile quality.

'Being even' and 'drumming' designate qualities of *mai* in canonical texts, but in case 6 Yi uses them in a slightly different, not exactly idiomatic sense. This nuance in shades of meaning is worth noting for it appears characteristic of other situations where a technical term is used in colloquial speech in a slightly different sense. It is just possible that the 'Mai fa' quote in case 6, which does not specify whether *mai* or *qi* is qualified, concerns knowledge on the interface of popular and scholarly currents of medicine.

Yi's verbs of touch

The verb Yi uses most frequently is 'murky' (*zhuo*), which in other writings is often opposed to 'being cool' or 'clear' (*qing*).[20] *Qing* and *zhuo*, written with a water radical, probably referred to clear and muddy waters before being used generically in cosmology. However, there is reason to argue that *zhuo* is not the early second-century pulse diagnostic term. Xu Guang notes in all four cases where 'murky' occurs (cases 1, 2, 4, 9) that in another edition the text reads 'to be clogged up' (*meng* 甿).[21] 'Clogged up' can be understood to convey a tactile perception, and in cases 1 and 9 can be taken as an iconic or indexical sign of the 'abscess' (*ju*) and 'numbness' (*jue*) Yi diagnoses. Chances are that 'being murky' is a commentatorial interjection.

One of the most striking findings with regard to Yi's verbs is that most are in some way linked to what they signify. In what follows, I suggest to

---

[20] Graham (1986). [21] *Shiki kaichû kôshô*, pp. 24, 27, 31, 37.

interpret them as signs that relate in an indexical and/or iconic way to body internal processes. Qualities of *mai* are not arbitrarily linked to bodily processes, as are signifier and signified in de Saussure's linguistics.[22] Rather, the aspect of Peirce's theory of signs that differentiates between the iconic, indexical and symbolic seems useful in this context.[23]

Whereas Peirce's 'symbol', just like de Saussure's linguistic sign, relates to what it signifies by virtue of a more or less arbitrary convention,[24] the indexical and iconic signs are linked to what they signify, albeit in different ways. An iconic sign represents its object mainly by virtue of its similarity, regardless of whether it is ontologically related to it. 'A pure icon can convey no positive or factual information; it affords no assurance that there is any such thing in nature. But it is of the utmost value for enabling its interpreter to study what would be the character of such an object should it exist.'[25] An icon exists by virtue of its characteristics on its own, regardless of whether any such object exists or not. It makes no claim to positive knowledge but speaks in a 'potential mood'.[26]

An index, however, is ontologically linked to what it represents: 'It refers to the Object that it denotes by virtue of being really affected by that Object.'[27] To be sure, an index does not make a claim to positive knowledge either. 'Anything which focuses the attention is an index. Anything which startles us is an index, in so far as it marks the junction between two portions of experience. Thus a tremendous thunderbolt indicates that *something* considerable happened, though we may not know precisely what the event was.'[28] Peirce comments elsewhere: 'Were an index so interpreted, the mood must be imperative, or exclamatory.' In contrast to symbols, which are 'declarative', Peirce maintains that 'icons and indices assert nothing'.[29] Icons express potentialities and indices are imperatives. It is important to keep this in mind with regard to Yi's qualities of *mai*. He may be speaking in terms of potentialities and imperatives rather than making statements in the indicative mood.

An indexical relation postulates very clearly that both the sign, which in Peirce's words is called 'representamen', and what it designates, the 'object', are part of a given reality, even if the reality in question is primarily one accepted by general opinion and socially constructed.[30] To be sure, Peirce's realism is not a positive one, as he is acutely aware of how the observer is involved in the meaning-making process. Reality is not out there for the observer to investigate from a bird's-eye view. Rather, Peirce emphasises

---

[22] De Saussure (1916).
[23] See, in particular, his writings of 1885, 1893 and 1902–3 (Short 2004), in his *Collected Papers* 2.274–308 and 2.247–9 (Peirce 1932:156–73 and 143–4).
[24] 'All words, sentences, books, and other conventional signs are symbols' (Peirce 1932; *CP* 2.291).
[25] Peirce (1932.4:359; *CP* 4.447).   [26] Peirce (1932.2:169; *CP* 2.291).
[27] Peirce (1932.2:143; *CP* 2.248).
[28] Peirce (1932.2:161; *CP* 2.285).   [29] Peirce (1932.2:169; *CP* 2.291).
[30] Daniel (1984:16).

that for interpreting any sign one must take account of the basically triadic structure between the 'representamen', the 'object' (which need not be a material thing, but can be an idea, a process or postulated reality) and the sign it creates in the mind of a person, which he calls the 'interpretant'.[31] This triadic structure of the sign was already invoked in Peirce's early writings in 1866–7, when his division was different;[32] it is fundamental to his theory of signs and one of the main reasons for its current attractiveness to anthropologists.

Anthropologists, who advance Peirce's semiotics in an attempt to avoid working with a notion of culture that, like de Saussure's notion of *langue*, is conceived as a closed and idealistic system of interdependent elements, have emphasised the openness of Peirce's theory of signs in the constitution of reality and his awareness of the position whence a person engages in the meaning-making process. They have stressed the importance of the indexical relationship between representamen and object, for interpreting personhood as an aspect of ranked substances in South Asia,[33] for highlighting identity-marking processes in an informal conversation in the United States, in Thai animal classification and in wine tasting notes of a professional connoisseur,[34] and for pointing out identity-building aspects of magic and healing in post-socialist Russia.[35]

One could interpret Yi's verbs of touch as indicative of a tactile perception standing in an indexical relation to internal bodily processes (see tables 7–9). One could provide a rationale for this by pointing out that the tactually perceived *qi* on the body surface was a process or entity that in a 'real' way linked ('physically linked', we would say) to changes inside the body, just as smoke is an indexical sign of fire and is the substance produced by it. Another possibility would be to highlight the iconic relation between the qualities of *mai* Yi senses on the body surface and the internal bodily processes they signify. Thus, in case 3, the verb *ji*, if translated as 'being taut', indicates an indexical relation to the acute pain that constricts and tightens muscle and flesh, while *ji* 'being intense' emphasises an iconic relation between what Yi took as a diagnostic sign and the 'intense' pain inside the body (that was then considered a principal feature of urinary retentions, *shan*).

The translation of *ji* 急 as 'being taut' makes the tactile quality of *mai* more intelligible to a modern reader; it understands the tactile perceptions of the qualities of *mai* to stand in an indexical relation to internal bodily processes. However, although a modern reader may query how an 'intense' touch feels, this should not be taken as reason to dismiss the translation of *ji* as 'intense'. Given the ambiguities of the vocabulary and grammar in literary Chinese, it is impossible to decide whether *ji* is an indexical or iconic

---

[31] See, in particular, Peirce (1932; *CP* 2.274–308; 2.247–9). See also Almeder (1980).
[32] Short (2004:223).   [33] Daniel (1984).   [34] Silverstein (2004).   [35] Lindquist (2005).

Table 7: Verbs of touch that qualify *qi* in Chunyu Yi's vocabulary

zhuo 濁 – murky (cosmological term) *jing* 靜 – still (canonical pulse quality) given as: *[gan qi] zhuo er jing*	case 1
ji 急 – intense (canonical pulse quality) given as: *qi ji*	case 3
zhuo 濁 – murky (cosmological term) *xi* 希 – thin (manuscript term, but not a known pulse quality) given as: *[shen qi] you shi jian zhuo . . . er xi*	case 4
re 熱 – hot (canonical term, not a known pulse quality) given as: *[fei qi] re*	case 6
zhi 至 – congested (not a known pulse quality) or – extremely, or to arrive (common in canonical contexts) *jin* 緊 – tight (standard *Mai jing* pulse) *xiao* 小 – small (canonical pulse quality) given as: *[qi] zhi jin xiao*	case 7
yin 陰 – yin (cosmological term, but not a known pulse quality) given as: *[qi] yin*	case 9

Table 8: Verbs of touch that qualify *mai* in Chunyu Yi's vocabulary

da 大 – large (canonical pulse quality) *shuo* 數 – frequent (standard *Mai jing* pulse) given as: *mai da er shuo*	case 3
shuai 衰 – weak (canonical pulse quality) given as: *mai shao shuai*	case 4
shun 順 – being smooth (canonical term, not only pulse quality) *qing* 清 – clear (canonical term, not only pulse quality) given as: *mai shun qing er yu*	
da 大 – large (canonical pulse quality) *zao* 躁 – hurried (canonical pulse quality) given as: *mai da er zao*	case 5
hua 滑 – slippery (standard *Mai jing* pulse) given as: *mai lai hua*	case 8
zhuo 濁 – murky (cosmological term) given as: *xin mai zhuo*	case 9
nan 難 – difficult (canonical term, not a known pulse quality) given as: *mai lai nan*	case 10

sign of intense pain. We have to acknowledge the indeterminacy of the phenomenon and its description.

The 'coming with difficulty' (*qi lai nan* 其來難) is another idiom with which Yi described a quality of *mai*, which was perhaps tactile, perhaps not, if we acknowledge the indeterminacy of the situation and its description, as recommended above. 'Coming with difficulty' probably related in an iconic way to difficult processes of expulsion, like urinating or birthing, but

Table 9: Verbs that are indefinite and may or may not qualify *mai* or *qi* in Chunyu Yi's vocabulary

huo or *he*和 – blending or being harmonious (*he*: canonical pulse quality) *dai* 代 – alternating (canonical pulse quality)	case 1
zhuo 濁 – murky (probably commentatorial interjection) *zao* 躁 – hurried (canonical pulse quality) given as: *zhuo zao er jing*	case 2
bing yin 并陰 – a paired *yin* (not a known pulse quality)	case 4
shi 溼 – damp (canonical term, not a known pulse quality)	case 5
bu ping 不平 – uneven (*ping*: canonical pulse quality) *dai* 代 – alternating (canonical pulse quality) given as: *bu ping er dai*	case 6

dai described as: *shi san ji bing zhi* 時三擊並至 –
  from time to time three strikes arrive together
  zha zao zha da 乍躁乍大 – at once hurried, at once large	

shen 深 – deep (canonical term) *xiao* 小 – small (canonical pulse quality) *ruo* 弱 – soft (standard *Mai jing* pulse) given as: *shen xiao ruo*	case 7
qia qia 合合 – confused (no textual parallel) given as: *qi zu ran qia qia*	
ju tuan 俱搏 – altogether united (canonical pulse quality) *bu ju tuan* 不俱搏 – not altogether united (no textual parallel) *yi tuan yi dai* 一搏一代 – once united, once alternating (no textual parallel) *san yin bo* 三陰搏 – three strikes (canonical pulse quality)	
da 大 – large (canonical pulse quality) *shi* 實 – replete (standard *Mai jing* pulse) given as: *da er shi*	case 10
nan 難 – difficult (canonical term, not a known pulse quality) given as: *qi lai nan*	

if, for instance, *qi* ('physically', we would say) linked the two events to each other, it may have been an indexical sign. Likewise, 'being still' (*jing* 靜) in case 1 indicates in a similar iconic/indexical manner that the general state of a person's condition is one of stillness, regardless of whether this stillness is equated with lifelessness and death or considered a positive attribute of an emotionally unperturbed person. And in case 9, where Yi states that *qi* was *yin* 陰, *qi*'s quality of *yin* could have been either iconic or indexical of the king's overall condition identified as a 'numbness' (*jue* 蹶) rising from the cool ground.

It is also possible that 'being strung' (*xian* 弦) originally was an iconic/indexical sign for the womb/liver/bladder. It is possible that in an iconic way the quality 'strung' was thought to resemble the string of the navel cord that is indexical of the womb. In canonical medical writings, 'being strung' became the quality par excellence of the liver, which, as seen above, in early medicine probably was thought to be located centrally, in the region of the womb, and in canonical doctrine retained its reproductive functions, particularly in women, as a blood depot. Likewise, the quality 'thin' (*xi* 希) may have referred to water in an iconic/indexical way, which as an aspect of the 'major *yin*' was associated either with the lungs, kidneys or, in Yi's Memoir, the bladder. If the *pao* 脬 'bladder', as argued in case 5, was indeed conceived of as a large and flabby bag, and if its *yong* 勇 'welling' alluded to the great cosmogonic waters, as in case 3, the 'large' (*da* 大) *mai* would stand in an iconic or indexical relation to the bladder.

In case 7, the verbs 'being deep' (*shen* 深) and 'congested' (*zhi* 至) could in a similar iconic/indexical way have related to the 'spleen' (*pi*), located deep inside the body, and to the congestions that 'conglomerations' (*jia*) are, although the possibility that these verbs were used in an adverbial sense is not to be excluded, meaning 'very' and 'extremely' (or 'to arrive'). 'Being soft' (*ruo* 弱) is how flesh feels in its unhealthy state, and thus can be viewed as an indexical and iconic sign for an adversely affected spleen, and the corresponding accumulations, and the onomatopoetic *qia qia* 合合 can be interpreted as directly or iconically relating to stomach rumbling; 'being small' (*xiao* 小) and 'tight' (*jin* 緊) describes characteristics of hardened pellets, perhaps of stools, and thus can be considered an indexical or iconic sign of conglomerations. In summary, many verbs Yi uses can be interpreted to have an indexical/iconic relation to the body internal processes they signify.

Some verbs, like 'being damp' (*shi* 濕) in case 5 and 'hot' (*re* 熱) in case 6 may refer in an indexical fashion to the overall state of the person or, rather, describe a perception of the skin: a 'damp' skin from profuse sweating (case 5) and a 'hot' one from the characteristically only slightly elevated temperature of consumption patients (case 6). In case 10, the tactually felt 'repletion' refers probably to the tactile perception of the swollen abdomen itself or, if it is a pulse quality, to an indexical sign. Wind and *qi* appear to have been perceived to fill the interior of the abdomen like air fills a balloon and makes it replete.

Finally, some verbs seem to invoke a tactile perception, which cannot be directly related to the body internal processes Yi describes. Thus, 'being frequent' (*shuo* 數) hints at frequent pulsations, and 'alternating' (*dai* 代), 'being uneven' (*bu ping* 不平) and 'not drumming' (*bu gu* 不鼓) may have referred to irregular ones (i.e. what biomedicine calls arrhythmic pulses). Other verbs suggest that Yi felt not just one movement at a time, but several, for instance, when he says 'from time to time three beats arrived together' (*shi san ji bing zhi* 時參擊並至) or 'once united, once intermittent' (*yi tuan yi dai* 一搏一代) or speaks of *mai* that are 'mixed' (*huo* 和) or 'not one' (*bu yi* 不一) or 'not altogether united' (*bu ju tuan* 不具搏). Some of the verbs, such as 'being smooth' (*shun* 順) or 'slippery' (*hua* 滑), seem to allude to a flowing motion; others, such as 'being hurried' (*zao* 躁) or 'swift' (*ji* 急), to rapid movement. These verbs, one surmises, allude to the flows and movements of *mai*, as known from canonical texts and medieval medical manuscripts. In Yi's cases 1–10 none of them qualifies *qi*. Those that qualify *qi* relate an indexical/iconic sign of body internal processes.

The language of *qi* in medical reasoning

In cases 1–10, *qi* is mentioned mostly in association with the five viscera, as is evident from table 5. The viscera and *qi* figure prominently in Yi's medical reasoning. In several cases, a viscus is the aspect in the body whence Yi senses *qi* coming. This suggests, I argue, that *qi* was thought to be stored in the viscera, and that it started to flow in the *mai*, once physicians linked the *mai* to the viscera, as systematically recorded in Yi's Memoir for the first time in the extant medical literature.

To my knowledge, no medical historian so far has suggested that the viscera became prominent in medical language as storage places for *qi*. Traditional Chinese Medicine authors, Japanese scholars and also Western researchers usually mention the five viscera when they talk about anatomical knowledge. Without denying the possibility of viewing the viscera as 'proto-anatomical' entities, known perhaps primarily through animal sacrifice, this study highlights the simultaneous increased occurrence of the notions *zang* (viscera) and *qi* in Western Han medicine and therefore proposes that the medical doctors' interest in integrating the 'viscera' into medical language may not have been primarily anatomical.

In order to understand why the viscera were conceived of as storage places for *qi*, one has to combine the observation found in the non-medical literature of pre-dynastic China, where the heart invariably is referred to as the seat of all emotions and storage place for feelings, with the findings in nurturing life texts of the third and second centuries BCE. The latter texts referred to the body as a visible 'form' (*xing*) that was thought to harbour those aspects of personhood that human beings know from experience but which are invisible. In the context of discussing these subjectively felt but outwardly invisible aspects of personhood – feelings and emotions, the will, thinking and spiritual dispositions – they spoke of *qi*. In contrast to the understanding of *qi* as the all-pervasive stuff of the universe, as known from canonical medical texts, this study highlights that in some medical and nurturing life texts of the late Warring States and early Han, *qi* related to body internal aspects of personhood.

This study suggests that the concepts of *qi* and the viscera became prominent in medical language as physicians became interested in systematising how emotional distress caused illness. As the investigation of the more than sixty occurrences of the term *bing* (disorder/illness) in the *Zuo zhuan* revealed, the term did not only allude to ideas of disorder in the body politic, as is widely known in the field of Chinese Studies, but often also referred to distress caused after, say, a dispute which resulted in feelings of being aggrieved. These occurrences of *bing* in the *Zuo zhuan* show that in the Warring States people were well aware of emotion-induced distress and illness. The language of *qi*, together with that of the viscera (*zang*), which probably were conceived of as seats of emotion and, hence, storage places of *qi*, provided physicians with a vocabulary to psychologise medical problems. Considering that music and its modulation of emotion and morality in ritual was widely discussed during the late Warring States, not least with regard to the sentiment joy (*le*), it makes perfect sense that also physicians of the Warring States increasingly attended to feelings and emotions, i.e. the 'sentimental body'.[36]

How can a physician know about sentiment in the person? The contemporary world has institutionalised Cartesian dualism in the medical domain such that physicians send a patient to a psychiatrist or psychologist if emotions are considered the underlying problem of his or her distress. In psychotherapy one aims to get access to the emotions primarily through talking. As in biomedicine, which has been said to build primarily on a visual inspection of the body that distinguishes between soma and psyche, in currents of medicine of the Warring States period a primarily visually known outward form was distinguished from invisible *qi* inside it. Rulers of the Warring States were admonished to govern not so much through oration, but through ritual and music. Their aim was to modulate sentiment in the populace. Physicians, it appears, attended to individuals, their sentiments and *qi* through touch.

In cases 1–10, Yi reports on tactually perceiving *qi* agitations of *mai* coming from internal viscera. In other words, by palpating *mai* on the body surface, Yi identified a wide range of disorders. Before the state widely promulgated Confucian learning, physicians may have palpated not only *mai* but also other body parts. The verbs of touch 'being firm' (*jian*) and 'soft' (*ruo*) were also used to describe qualities of the flesh and viscera as healthy or diseased. This would suggest that physicians in the late Warring States and early Han had experience with palpating the flesh, the buttocks and lower back, and also the flesh above the abdomen, perhaps in order to detect in an indexical manner whether the viscera inhabiting the internal spaces underneath were firm or not;[37] *qi* fixed within, said the *Guanzi*, made the outward form firm and glowing (see p. 30).

Based on a thematic consideration, namely that non-medical texts in the late Warring States were concerned with the modulation, if not manipulation, of the emotions through music, it seems reasonable to suggest that physicians started to attend simultaneously to feelings and emotions of their clientele, i.e. to the sentimental body. As explained in the introduction and in case 2, this sentimental body was bipartite, framed in the *yin yang* cosmology that seems to have dominated much of medical thinking in the third

---

[36] Nylan (2001), Csikszentmihalyi (2004).   [37] Hsu (2005a).

and early second centuries BCE. The heart often designated the entire upper *yang* sphere above the diaphragm, inclusive of the stomach; and the liver, the lower *yin* sphere. The heart was the seat of morality and all emotions, inclusive of anger; from the liver anger erupted invariably.[38] However, by the mid-Western Han, when the early first-century editor of Yi's Memoir was at work, the interest of the physicians, perhaps not unaffected by the changes in government from a more feudal to a more bureaucratic order, seems to have shifted away from predominantly psychological problems among the nobility to diseases that affected society at large. The latter typically occur in tandem with seasonal change. As argued elsewhere,[39] medical concern with the seasonality of illness led to a systematising of medical knowledge according to the five agents doctrine, which probably raised the prestige of medicine (just as statistics in medicine does so today). As a consequence, the meanings of *qi* shifted. While still attending to the atmospheric, *qi* was no longer imbued primarily with meanings of the atmospheric caused by emotions and feelings. Rather climatic, seasonal and weather-dependent change became the focus of physicians' attention. This medicine framed bodily processes as aspects of the 'body ecologic'.

In Yi's Memoir, cases 1 and 2 obviously differ from all others. First, they strictly differentiate between the notions of *qi* and *mai* in the context of pulse diagnosis. Secondly, the terms 'liver' and 'heart' are best read as referring to an aspect of an architectural body rather than the body ecologic. The liver in case 1 (line 13) is associated with blood physiology and probably refers to a central internal and/or abdominal region of the body architecture and it differs from the seasonality sensitive body ecological liver mentioned in the 'Mai fa' quote (lines 17–19). Likewise, the heart in case 2, within which *qi* is trapped, undoubtedly also refers primarily to an architectural space – the upper bodily sphere.

The above is said in awareness that case 2 contains allusions to all three bodies: the architectural body, the sentimental body and the body ecologic. Thus, the heat (case 2, line 19) can be understood to hint at the aspect of 'fire' that the heart explicitly has in the body ecologic, and the 'infantile irritability' alludes to the heart as a seat of emotion, which it is in the sentimental body. That 'heat' is related to 'infantile irritability' in the 'upper body architectural space' highlights the close relatedness of the heart in all three bodies.

Yi speaks of the 'heart' and 'liver' also in the context of calculating the date of death in case 6. Why should he mention the heart rather than the aforementioned 'lungs'? The disorder is a 'lung consumption' in line 3. Why then does he speak of 'heart' and 'liver' in line 44? The puzzle can be solved if one assumes that the name of the disorder alludes to a body ecologic, but Yi's calculations for prognosticating death allude to the older body concept

---

[38] See pp. 34–41, 109–12, 161–5, 240–1.
[39] Hsu (2007b).

of a bipartite body architecture, which differentiates only between the heart (to which belong the lungs) and liver. Incidentally, when Yi says that the illness wandered from the one on high to the distant one (line 19a) and speaks of two links being severed (line 23), he probably refers to a movement from the body architectural heart to the liver, rather than from the canonical lungs to the canonical liver (a movement that is not elsewhere documented in medical texts).

In cases 3–10, Yi speaks, apart from the 'liver' and 'heart', also of the 'kidneys', 'bladder', 'lungs', 'spleen' and 'five viscera'; he uses the idiom 'five viscera' but mentions six. As shown in case 5, the *pao* bladder (line 3) was conceived of as a flabby bag in the centre of the body, much like the womb; in early medical texts, it had *yin*-qualities. The canonical *pang guang* bladder (line 20), by contrast, has *yang*-qualities and is the outer aspect of the canonical kidneys.

Although I argue that the late Warring States and early Han physicians developed an interest in the viscera because they were conceived of as seats of emotion rather than as proto-anatomical entities, the evidence for arguing this is not ample in Yi's Memoir. He blames the emotions only twice, in cases 2 and 6.[40] Even though the viscera initially may have been integrated into medical language in order to talk about emotions, this aspect of the viscera, which has persisted to the present day,[41] has become subordinate to others in the body ecologic. Ohnuki-Tierney, in the context of speaking of physiomorphism, goes so far as to say that contemporary *kanpo*, within which the notion of *ki* (cognate to *qi*) is central, focuses on diet and climate rather than on the emotions.[42] Finally, it is truly ironic that Arthur Kleinman interpreted complaints among modern Taiwanese that made use of this Chinese medical visceral language as a form of 'somatising' psychological problems,[43] when from a historical viewpoint the integration of the viscera into medical language happened precisely because ancient doctors psychologised medical problems. Notably, it is a study on touch and pulse diagnosis that has led to the finding that physicians framed bodily processes in respect of a sentimental body during the late Warring States and early Han, although it is only implicitly given in canonical medical texts and Yi's cases 1–10.

Re-evaluation of Bridgman's correlations between mai and the viscera

Bridgman, who did the first extensive study on Yi's Memoir, highlighted blatant differences between the correlations of the viscera with the six qualifications of *mai* (*yang* brightness, major *yang*, minor *yang*, major *yin*, minor *yin* and dull *yin*) in Yi's Memoir and canonical doctrine.[44] This study

---

[40] The twenty-five case histories have neither spirits (*shen* 神) nor essences (*jing* 精) stored in the canonical heart and kidneys; in section 4.1, Yi once mentions *shen qi* 神氣.
[41] Ots (1990b).   [42] Ohnuki-Tierney (1984:75–88).
[43] Kleinman (1980).   [44] Bridgman (1955:142–5).

proves Bridgman right in pointing out discrepancies, but they are not as arbitrary as he sees them. In particular, there is insufficient evidence to postulate that Yi had a full-fledged system of twelve *mai* that corresponded to the canonical viscera. Furthermore, Bridgman's 'Tableau des méridiens selon Chouen-yu Yi' is not only based on mistaken body conceptions, but also on quick and speculative readings. So, it is not only dated, but also wrong and misleading.

The minor *yang* is mentioned in cases 1 (line 29), 6 (line 31) and 10 (line 4). In case 1 (line 13), liver *qi* indicates an abscess (*ju*) and Yi prognosticates death after examining the minor *yang*, which connects to the interior (*zhong*). In case 6 (lines 31, 34), the Grand Physician cauterises the foot's minor *yang* and thereby depletes the abdominal parts of the interior. In case 10 (lines 2–4), the common doctors opine that wind has entered and struck the interior and that the host of the disorder is in the lungs, or according to another edition, in the liver, and they needle the minor *yang*.

It is important to recognise that the liver in cases 1 and 6 is not the canonical liver but has at least in parts traits of a pre-canonical one. In case 1, the liver/womb has been shown to be in charge of blood dynamics and in case 6 (line 44) it is explicitly contrasted with the heart, which hints at a liver of a bipartite body inhabited by only two viscera, the heart and the liver. As the text reads now, the minor *yang* connects also to a rather undifferentiated 'interior' (*zhong*), but this connection may have arisen due to commentatorial interjections of, arguably, *zhong re* 'the interior is hot' in case 1 (line 35) and *fu zhong xu* 'the abdominal part of the interior was depleted' in case 6 (line 34), and where *feng ru zhong* 'wind has entered and struck the interior' is unproblematic in case 10 (line 2), the following reference to lungs/liver and minor *yang* was presumably interjected (lines 3–4). These text excerpts draw attention to a liver located in the interior/centre of the body. In canonical doctrine, the minor *yang* correlates either with the triple burner, which incidentally is located in the trunk of the body, i.e. its interior, or with the gall bladder, which is the outer aspect of the liver, i.e. it takes on the qualities of the liver/womb in Yi's Memoir. Thus, the minor *yang*'s correlation with the 'liver' and the body's 'interior' in Yi's Memoir does not blatantly contradict its canonical correlations.

Here a note is warranted: Yi's Memoir and canonical doctrine attribute inversed *yin yang*-qualities to the bladder, kidneys and liver. The liver in case 1 correlates with the minor *yang*, which canonical doctrine attributes to its outer aspect, the gall bladder, while correlating the liver itself with the dull *yin*. In Yi's Memoir the dull *yin* is connected to a 'swollen abdomen' and a 'small abdomen' (as it is in *Ling shu* 10, but there discussed within the entry on the liver). The *pao* bladder, which in case 5 correlates with the major *yin*, correlates as *pang guang* bladder in canonical doctrine with the major *yang*, which is the quality of the kidneys in Yi's case 17. Finally, the Mawangdui 'Yinyang vessel text' correlates the stomach with the major *yin*, which in canonical doctrine is an attribute of the spleen, while the spleen's outer aspect stomach becomes associated with *yang* brightness. Evidently, newly introduced outer or inner aspects of the viscera – the gall bladder, *pang guang* bladder and spleen – take on the qualities of the well-established ones. Changes are drastic, but not entirely arbitrary.

The major *yin* is mentioned twice, in case 5 (line 12) in the clause 'when I pressed onto the opening of the major *yin*' (*qie qi tai yin zhi kou*) and in case 4 (line 33) in the phrase 'at the opening of the major *yin*' (*zai tai yin mai kou*), but the latter probably is in a commentatorial interjection. These phrases remind one of the 'opening of the major *yin*' in *Su wen* 15, which has been interpreted to correlate either with the 'canonical major *yin* lungs' or with the 'pre-canonical major *yin* stomach' in the Mawangdui 'Yinyang vessel text' or with the 'early medical innermost interior' before medical doctors differentiated between the five viscera – the '*pao* womb/bladder'. As explained in detail in case 4, Bridgman was quick to see a correlation between the major *yin* and the kidneys, but then Yi would not pursue a coherent line of argumentation. The commentator who interjected the phrase certainly considered the major *yin* to refer to the canonical lungs.

Yang brightness is mentioned in cases 1 (line 41) and 6 (lines 39–42). Bridgman, guided by canonical considerations, correlates it in case 1 with the intestines and stomach (by jumping from a statement in line 41 to line 6) and in case 6 with the lungs (leaping from line 42 to line 3). Bridgman's interpretation makes Yi appear inconsistent in argumentation and arbitrary in comparison to canonical doctrine. On the grounds of the peculiar medical rational in both stanzas, it is likely that they were interjected by a commentator who correlated *yang* brightness with the canonical stomach. In case 6, as in early and canonical medicine, damage to the *yang* brightness leads to madness.

The dull *yin* is mentioned in case 10 (lines 16, 21, 23). Bridgman correlates it with the *pang guang* bladder, and thereby stresses how arbitrary the difference is from canonical doctrine, where the bladder correlates with the major *yang* and the liver with the dull *yin*. His interpretation is not compelling. Line 23 states that the foot's dull *yin* is cauterised to treat the swollen abdomen. The correlation between the dull *yin* and swollen abdomen, on which Yi dwells, is given also in the Mawangdui 'Yinyang vessel text' and the *Nei jing*.

The minor *yin* is mentioned once in case 6 (line 31). Bridgman considers the Grand Physician to have cauterised the hand's minor *yin*, which in canonical doctrine correlates with the heart. However, it may also have been the foot's minor *yin*, since Yi says it harmed the liver, which in a bipartite body is located in the lower sphere. Notably, the minor *yin* connects to the liver also in the Mawangdui 'Zubi vessel text'.

In cases 1–10, it is unlikely that Yi ever refers to *mai* of the forearm. This is said in awareness that he certainly does so in case 13, where he treats a decaying tooth by cauterising what in the Mawangdui 'Yinyang vessel text' is called the 'tooth *mai*' (*chi mai* 齒脈), which passes along the arms. A researcher interested in highlighting the experiential validity of early Chinese medical rationale will guess that this happened at the location today called *he gu* 合谷, and still today is used for such purposes. Since this acupuncture *locus* is recorded in medieval manuscript texts and arguably the Mawangdui 'Recipes',[45] this is an educated guess and not a simple anachronism. Cases 1–10, however, seem to refer only to the foot *mai*.

In summary, Bridgman's interpretation emphasises the arbitrariness of correlations and by implication renders Chinese medical rationale inconsistent and, lastly, experientially unfounded. However, with one exception, the correlations he postulates are not compelling and, as scrutiny of the text shows, they are wrong. Admittedly, in the 1950s the early medical manuscripts had not yet been excavated, but Bridgman's chief mistake was attitudinal and conceptional. He failed to see that Yi's body conceptions differed from canonical medical understandings and that the same technical term – for example, 'liver' or 'heart' – may have different implications, depending on the body conception to which it alludes.

The above comparison with Bridgman's efforts highlights how important it was to develop the 'sentimental body', the 'architectural body' and the 'body ecologic' as a heuristic device in the course of this study. Fairly indisputable correlations in cases 1–10 are those of the 'minor *yang*' with a pre-canonical liver/womb (*gan*), in a not very clearly defined bodily 'interior/centre', and of the 'major *yin*' with the innermost interior, the 'womb/bladder' (*pao*). Since Yi's rationale can be related to other Han currents of medical learning, discrepancies with canonical understandings are not entirely arbitrary. The comparison of Yi's with canonical rationale cannot be used to deny that there are continuities between early and canonical medicine. Nor can it undermine the validity of the experiential realities they describe.

Illness causation

In biomedicine, the signs and symptoms and the cause are crucial for determining the name of a disease. While Yi does, concomitantly, mention the signs and symptoms of his patients, and also informs us on the 'cause of the disorder', he determines the name of the disorder primarily by examining the tactile qualities of *mai*. In what follows, a short summary of the 'causes' Yi mentions is given, followed by a longer discussion of how Yi's qualities of *mai* relate to the naming of the disorders.

[45] Li (1999).

Cases 1–10 blame wine and women, with two exceptions. Beyond doubt, Yi points to debauchery among the nobility of Qi in a coded language. He speaks of indulgence once in 'wine', once in 'women', twice in 'wine and women', twice as inappropriate conduct during sexual congress, and twice as of excessive perspiration (the perspiration is that of royalty and euphemistically refers to their sexual indulgences). Only once, in case 4, is the 'cause of the disorder' framed in hot/cold complementarities and body ecological considerations.

In two cases emotional distress is given as 'cause'. In case 2, it is 'infantile irritability' (*you* 憂), and in case 6, great 'anger' (*nu* 怒) during sexual intercourse. In case 6, the disorder, identified as 'consumption' or 'wasting heat' (*xiao dan* 消癉) is said to arise from an emotional imbalance – anger. By contrast, a related disorder known from canonical doctrine – 'wasting thirst' (*xiao ke* 消渴) – is attributed to an unbalanced food intake. Yi points out a psychological illness cause, anger, while the canonical text on 'wasting thirst' is concerned with food intake, an aspect of the body ecologic. Case 6 highlights that the rubric concerned with the 'cause of the disorder', like the Greek *aitia*, is best interpreted as attributing blame to improper conduct. Over time such improper conduct became increasingly medicalised, but in Yi's Memoir, it is mentioned in a rubric separate from the diagnostic reasoning which focuses on *mai*.[46]

Yi explicitly says that he examined *mai* to distinguish between different disorders in his reply to question one in the Memoir's section four. This raises the question which qualities of *mai* indicated which disorder. This study, in contrast to an earlier one (Hsu 2001a), has demonstrated that text structure semantics can highlight interrelations between specific qualities of *mai* and constituents in the name of the disorder in all cases 1–10. It does so in an additive way. Therefore, text structure semantics cannot claim to provide insights on how Yi himself thought about the process of diagnosis and is best valued as a heuristic device.

A glance at table 10 shows that interrelations between the name of the disorder and the qualities of *mai* are not always straightforward, but text structure semantics has highlighted correlations that otherwise would not have been detected. Irregularities were encountered, particularly in cases 3, 4, 7 and 8, but careful analysis did not prove wrong the principle of text structure semantics. Rather, it alerted us to possible commentatorial interjections.

In case 1, text structure semantics postulated that '*qi* [coming] from the liver' was indicative of a '*ju*-abscess'. This correlation, which to someone familiar with canonical medicine initially seemed unlikely, started to make sense once texts were found in the received and manuscript literature,

---

[46] One could, of course, consider pulse qualities the proximal cause, and habits, emotional imbalances and lifestyle the distal one, but this is not how Yi framed the issue.

Table 10: Interrelations between the name of the disorder and Chunyu Yi's pulse qualities

	Case 1
	4. Then I went outside and solely informed Cheng's brother Chang <u>saying</u>:
Name:	5. 'This one is ailing from a *ju-abscess*.'[a]
Quality:	11. <u>The means whereby I recognised</u> Cheng's illness were that
	12. when your servant, Yi, pressed onto his *mai*,
	13. I got *qi* [coming] from the liver.
	Case 2
Name:	3. I reported by <u>saying</u>: 'It is a **disorder of *qi* that is blocked**.'
Quality:	12. <u>The means whereby I recognised</u> the youngest son's illness were that
	13. when I examined his *mai*, it was *qi* [coming] from the heart.
	Case 3
Name:	4. Your servant, Yi, examined him and <u>said</u>: 'It is a **welling amassment**.'
Quality:	12. <u>The means whereby I recognised</u> Xun's illness were that
	13. at the time when I pressed onto his *mai*,
	14. at the right opening, *qi* was **intense**.
	15. The *mai* did not have *qi* [coming] from the five viscera –
	16. At the right opening the *mai* were **large**, yet **frequent**.
	17. In cases of the frequent, the interior and lower parts are hot – yet there was a **welling**.
	Case 4
	2. I entered [the palace] to examine his *mai* and formally announced <u>saying</u>:
Name:	3. 'It is the *qi* of a **heat disorder**.
	4. So, you **sweat** [as one does] from summer-heat.'
Quality:	26. <u>The means whereby I recognised</u> Xin's illness were that at the time when I pressed onto his *mai*, there was a paired *yin*.
	...
	32. *qi* [coming] from the kidneys [lungs] was sometimes for a moment **murky**,
	33. at the opening of the major *yin mai*, however, it was **thin**.
	34. This is a case of water *qi*.
	35. The kidneys certainly govern water.
	Case 5
Name:	3. I <u>said</u>: '**A wind-induced condition-of-overexertion is visiting the bladder**.'
Quality:	10. <u>The means whereby I recognised</u> the illness of the queen dowager of the King of Qi were that
	11. when your servant, Yi, examined her *mai*, and
	12. when I pressed onto the **opening of the major *yin***,
	13. it was **damp**. In spite of this, there was **wind *qi***.
	Case 6
	2. Your servant, Yi, examined his *mai* and <u>said</u>:
Name:	3. 'It is a **lung consumption**.
Quality:	15. <u>The means whereby I recognised</u> Shanfu's illness were that
	16. when your servant, Yi, pressed onto his vessels, the *qi* [coming] from the lungs was hot.
	Case 7
	3. Your servant, Yi, examined his *mai* and <u>said</u>:
Name:	4. 'It is a **conglomeration of remanent accumulations**.'

Continued

Table 10: *Continued*

Quality:	9. <u>The means whereby I recognised</u> Pan Manru's illness were that 10. when I pressed onto his *mai*, they were deep, small and soft, 11. abruptly they were confused, 12. this is *qi* **[coming] from the spleen.** 13. At the right *mai*'s opening, *qi* arrived tight and small, 14. it manifested as *qi* **[coming] from conglomerations.**
	Case 8
Name:	4. Your servant, Yi, examined his *mai* and <u>said</u>: 'It is the **wind of the void.**'
Quality:	10. <u>The means whereby I recognised</u> Zhao Zhang's illness were that 11. when your servant, Yi, pressed onto his *mai*, 12. the *mai* came **slippery.** 13. This is *qi* **[coming] from [the wind of the] within.**
	Case 9
Name:	3. I <u>said</u>: 'A **wind-induced numbness/inversion.**'
Quality:	9. <u>The means whereby I recognised</u> the illness of the King of Jibei were that 10. at the time when your servant, Yi, pressed onto his *mai*, it was **wind** *qi*. 11. The *mai* **[coming] from the heart** was murky. ... 19. When I pressed onto his *mai*, *qi* was **yin.**
	Case 10
	5. Your servant, Yi, examined her *mai* and <u>said</u>:
Name:	6. 'She is troubled by *qi* – an amassment is visiting the **bladder** – 7. **and has difficulties with urinating and defecating.** The urine is dark.'
Quality:	12. <u>The means whereby I recognised</u> Chu Yu's illness were that 13. when I pressed onto her *mai*, 14. they were **large**, yet **replete.** 15. They came **with difficulty.**

a Bold indicates correspondences between constituents in the name of the disorder and pulse qualities as detected by text structure semantics.

which hinted at the interpretation of a liver/womb, located in the interior/ centre of the bodily architecture, in charge of blood dynamics, and of the *ju*-abscess as a coagulation of blood.

In case 2, text structure semantics suggested that '*qi* [coming] from the heart' indicated a 'disorder of *qi* that is blocked' (*qi ge bing*). It is certainly not the canonical 'heart' of the body ecologic that is meant here, but the sphere above the diaphragm in the architectural body. Cases 1 and 2 form a pair, as is obvious from their common structure, the semantic closeness of their body concepts, and textual evidence from a Dunhuang manuscript (quoted on p. 43, discussed on p. 166).

With regard to the 'welling amassment' (*yong shan*) in case 3, *qi* that is 'intense' is best taken as an iconic/indexical sign of the pain of the 'amassment', which according to *Su wen* 18, 19 and 55 typically is marked by intense pain. According to text structure semantics, the 'welling' should correlate with Yi's finding that '*mai* did not have *qi* [coming] from the five viscera' (line 15). However, no textual parallels have been found for this correlation. If *yong* is understood as 'welling', which is an attribute of the cosmogonic cool waters, 'being large' (line 16) correlates with it, as does 'yet there was a welling' (line 17). If 'being frequent' (line 16) is understood in the sense of 'being intense', it also correlates with the 'amassment'. However, no textual parallels for 'being frequent and amassments' have been found. So, in case 3, text structure semantics highlights correlations but cannot be applied without problems.

In case 4, text structure semantics postulates a correlation between the 'joined *yin*' and '*qi* of a heat disorder', which is odd (and highlights, once again, that case 4 differs from all other nine). The joined *yin* is probably not a tactile quality and the *qi* of a heat disorder not a name. As shown in detail in this study, case 4 presumably contains large chunks of textual interjections by a commentator-editor operating at a slightly later time period than the presumed early first-century author-editor (whom we have identified as perhaps Sima Qian). The 'joined *yin*' may well relate to the harm 'double coldness' (*chong han*) does to the lungs, as recorded in *Ling shu* 66, or to the 'double *yin*' (*chong yin*) of *Su wen* 7, which describes the disorder's movement from the lungs to the kidneys. Based on text structure semantics and the finding that there is the disorder 'hot sweat comes out' (*re han chu*) in the Mawangdui 'Zubi vessel text', the pulse qualities 'murky, yet thin' (lines 32–3) that qualify *qi* have been found to correlate with the constituents in the name. 'Being murky' correlates with 'becoming hot' and 'thin' with 'water'. Cases 3 and 4 form a pair in that they both concern water physiologies, marked by excessive coldness and heat respectively.

In case 5, the name of the disorder is a 'wind-induced condition-of-over-exertion lodged in the bladder' (*feng dan ke pao*). The interrelation between 'wind *qi*' and 'wind' is clear. 'Being damp' (*shi*), as the skin is when one sweats, accordingly interrelates with the 'condition-of-overexertion' (*dan*), since the place at which these qualities are felt, namely the 'opening of the major *yin*' probably correlates with the place where the illness is located inside the body, namely in the 'bladder' (*pao*).

Towards the end of case 5, in his comments on the 'Mai fa', Yi explicitly states that the 'large' *mai* is indicative of pathological changes in the bladder and the 'hurried' *mai* of heat. This results in *dan* being indicated by the 'damp' in line 13 and by the 'hot' in line 21. If the 'damp' quality Yi mentions in line 13 testifies to medical rationale in the second century and his comments on *mai* in lines 19–21 are considered a commentatorial interjection, we can see an evolution in the understanding of *dan* from a sweaty tiredness to a heat condition, marked by what in canonical medical reasoning is thought to arise from a loss of the salubrious waters due to perspiration, resulting in the body interior's gradual overheating.

In case 6, text structure semantics elegantly elucidates the 'lung consumption' (*fei xiao dan*), if one considers *dan* to indicate a 'heat condition due to overexertion' and *xiao dan* a bisyllabic constituent of 'wasting heat', i.e. 'consumption'. The quality 'lung *qi*' interrelates with the 'lungs', and 'being hot', with the 'consumption'. The translation 'lung consumption' is meant to invoke similarities to European understandings, but not to be equated with them. Cases 5 and 6 both concern a condition of overexertion, one marked by the dampness of perspiration, the other by wasting heat.

Text structure semantics, as applied to case 7, highlights a textual irregularity. As the name *yi ji jia* is best explained by correlating 'conglomeration *qi*' with 'conglomerations' (*jia*) and 'spleen *qi*' with 'accumulations' (*ji*), as well known from *Ling shu* 66, the constituent *yi* is left with no correlate, meaning either 'remanent' or, more colloquially, 'stools'. It probably is a later commentator's interjection, since *yi ji* echoes *yi ni* in case 10 (line 8), which independently was found to be a colloquialism contained in a sentence that was later interjected (based on context, *yi ni* had to be interpreted as 'remanent urine' rather than as 'enuresis'; the latter is its technical meaning in canonical medical texts). According to text structure semantics, the name of the disorder in case 7 was in the early first century 'accumulations and conglomerations' (*ji jia*).

With regard to the 'wind of the void' (*dong feng*) and the pulse quality *nei feng qi* in case 8, the interrelation between the constitutents 'wind *qi*' and 'wind' would appear straightforward, but a rigorous application of text structure semantics suggests that the pulse quality 'being slippery' (*hua*) correlates with the constituent 'wind' and that *feng* in *nei feng qi* must be a commentatorial interjection. If, contrary to the commentators' viewpoint, but in line with the Mawangdui *Huangdi sijing*, the term *dong* is translated as 'the void', it correlates with *nei qi* '*qi* [coming] from within', where *nei* is taken as a noun referring to a body architectural internal space. Cases 7 and 8 concern constipation and diarrhoea respectively.

In case 9, the interrelation between 'wind *qi*' and 'wind' is straightforward, which as in case 5 probably represents a non-medically motivated editorial addition. In the Mawangdui 'Yinyang vessel text' and Zhangjiashan 'Mai shu', 'inversions' (*jue*) of *yin yang* occur in the body architectural 'heart' and sometimes explicitly are said to arise from a 'welling', presumably of cool *yin*-waters, normally stored in the abdominal *yin* sphere. This must also have been the understanding of the presumed early first-century editor, who made Yi say that *mai*, rather than *qi*, coming from the heart was murky (line 11). However, in the early second century, *jue* in the sense of 'numbness' may have been indicated in an indexical/iconic fashion by the quality of *qi* that was *yin* (line 19).

Case 10 probably is the result of an editorial conflation of material from two case histories, to which were added numerous commentatorial interjections. If, as argued in this study, the name of the disorder contains *shan ke yu pang guang* (an amassment is visiting the bladder) as commentatorial interjection in lines 6 and 18, the text perhaps originally read: '*qi*' or '*qi* went into the abdomen' (*qi zhi fu*). The pulse qualities 'being replete, yet large' correlate with *qi* and the abdomen/bladder respectively, for which there are many textual parallels in the medical canons. 'Coming with difficulty' (*qi lai nan*) is synonymous with 'being intense' in some contexts and could be understood to indicate the 'amassment' (*shan*), but for this correlation no parallels were found in the canonical medical literature. Therefore, 'coming with difficulty' probably correlates with the complaint 'having difficulties with urinating and defecating'. Case 9 has more affinities with case 5 than with case 10; and case 10 shares more parallels with cases 3 and 5 than with case 9.

Evidently, text structure semantics proves useful as a heuristic device. From a medical historical viewpoint, it highlighted consistency of medical rationale across cases 1–10. In combination with text critical considerations, it has furthermore provided a means to recognise early medical terminology and differentiate it from later editorial interpolations and commentatorial interjections.

With regard to the anthropology of the senses, it has highlighted that Yi adheres to medical learning that in a sophisticated way attends to tactile signs for diagnosing illness. These synchronous processes that are relevant to the diagnosis Yi discusses in the rubric on the 'qualities of the disorder' are separate from that on the 'cause of the disorder', where Yi reports on bad habits and past conduct of his patients. Although the 'cause of the disorder' did show continuities to the bodily processes outlined in the rubric on the 'quality of the disorder' (cases 1, 2, 4, 5, 6, 9), it was not crucial for diagnosing the 'name of the disorder'. This is relevant for the medical anthropologist.

Ultimately, this study can be viewed as a sustained argument against the widely held belief among many anthropologists and medical doctors that all diagnosis, and subsequent choice of treatment, requires knowledge of the cause of a person's disorder. This text highlights that already in antiquity there were medical specialists who dealt with the issue of blaming improper social conduct separately from and almost entirely unrelated to the process of medical diagnosis for which they had developed a technical vocabulary. They developed finely tuned diagnostic techniques that attended to the present and were attuned to the atmospheric.

This study points out that biomedicine's emphasis on the cause of the disease, aetiology and pathogenesis ultimately is a highly culture-specific phenomenon and should not be taken as a universally valid schema for understanding all diagnostic endeavour. Text structure semantics has provided ample evidence that Yi adheres to the contrary. His ideology of medical learning is that one can differentiate in a sophisticated way between different patterns of bodily disorders without searching for the cause of the illness in past events. This ideology of diagnosis advocates heightened somatic attentiveness to the present, through tactile examination of *mai*.

A. Modern works and modern editions (alphabetically ordered by the name of author, editor or editorial team)

Ackerknecht E. 1947. 'The Role of Medical History in Medical Education'. *Bulletin of the History of Medicine* 21 (2): 135–45.

Ågren H. 1986. 'Chinese Traditional Medicine: Temporal Order and Synchronous Events'. In J. T. Fraser *et al.* (eds.), 211–18.

Allan S. and Williams C. (eds.) 2000. *The Guodian Laozi.* The Institute of East Asian Studies, University of California, Berkeley.

Alleton V. and Volkov A. (eds.) 1994. *Notions et perceptions du changement en Chine.* Collège de France, Institut des Hautes Études Chinoises, Paris.

Almeder R. 1980. *The Philosophy of Charles S. Peirce: a Critical Introduction.* Basil Blackwell, Oxford.

Atran S. 1990. *The Cognitive Foundations of Natural History: towards an Anthropology of Science.* Cambridge University Press, Cambridge.

Baker P. A. and Carr G. (eds.) 2002. *Practitioners, Practices and Patients: New Approaches to Medical Archaeology and Anthropology.* Oxbow Books, Oxford.

Bates D. (ed.) 1995. *Knowledge and the Scholarly Medical Traditions.* Cambridge University Press, Cambridge.

Bendix R. and Brenneis D. (eds.) 2005. *The Senses. Special Issue. Etnofoor* 18 (1).

Bielenstein H. 1980. *The Bureaucracy of Han Times.* Cambridge University Press, Cambridge.

Bloom A. H. 1981. *The Linguistic Shaping of Thought: a Study in the Impact of Language on Thinking in China and the West.* Lawrence Erlbaum Associates, Hillsdale, NJ.

Bodde D. [1978] 1981. 'Marches in the *Mencius* and Elsewhere: a Lexicographic Note'. In *Essays on Chinese Civilisation.* Princeton University Press, Princeton, 416–25.

Bodde D. 1982. 'Forensic Medicine in Pre-Imperial China'. *Journal of the American Oriental Society* 102 (1): 1–15.

Boltz W. 1993. '*Chou li*' 周禮. In M. Loewe (ed.), 24–32.

Bourdieu P. [1979] 1984. *Distinction: a Social Critique of the Judgement of Taste.* Routledge, London.

Bourdieu P. 1991. *Language and Symbolic Power.* Polity Press, Cambridge.

Boyer P. 1990. *Tradition as Truth and Communication: a Cognitive Description of Traditional Discourse.* Cambridge University Press, Cambridge.

Boyle M. O'Rourke 1998. *Senses of Touch: Human Dignity and Deformity from Michelangelo to Calvin.* Brill, Leiden.

Brauns C.-D. and Löffler L. G. 1986. *Mru: Bergbewohner im Grenzgebiet von Bangladesh.* Birkhäuser, Basel.

Bray F. 1984. *Agriculture.* In J. Needham (ed.), *Science and Civilisation in China.* Vol. 6: *Biology and Biological Technology*, Part 2. Cambridge University Press, Cambridge.

Bray F. 1997. *Technology and Gender: Fabrics of Power in Late Imperial China.* University of California Press, Berkeley.

Bridgman R. F. 1955. 'La médicine dans la Chine antique'. *Mélanges Chinois et Bouddhiques* 10: 1–213.

Brothwell D. and Sandison A. T. (eds.) 1967. *Disease in Antiquity.* Charles Thomas, Springfield.

Bynum W. F. and Porter R. (eds.) 1993. *Medicine and the Five Senses.* Cambridge University Press, Cambridge.

Bynum W. F. and Bynum H. (eds.) 2007. *Dictionary of Medical Biography.* Greenwood Press, Westport, CT.

Cartier M., Elisseff D. and Métailié G. (eds.) 1993. *Les Animaux dans la Culture Chinoise. Thematic Issue. Anthropozoologica* 18 (2).

Chan Tim Wai-keung 1998. 'The *jing/zhuan* Structure of the *Chuci* Anthology: a New Approach to the Authorship of Some of the Poems'. *T'oung Pao* 86: 293–327.

Chang K. C. (ed.) 1977. *Food in Chinese Cultures: Anthropological and Historical Perspectives.* Yale University Press, New Haven.

Chavannes E. 1895, 1897. *Les mémoires historiques de Se-ma Ts'ien.* Vols. I, II. Leroux, Paris.

Chen Chiufen 2002. 'Medicine, Society, and the Making of Madness in Imperial China'. PhD thesis in History. University of London, London.

Cheng A. 1993. '*Ch'un ch'iu* 春秋, *Kung yang* 公羊, *Ku liang* 穀梁 and *Tso chuan* 左傳'. In M. Loewe (ed.), 67–76.

Classen C. 2005. *The Book of Touch.* Berg, Oxford.

Cong Chunyu 從春雨 (ed.) 1994. *Dunhuang Zhongyiyao Quanshu* 敦煌中醫藥全書 (The Complete Book of Dunhuang Medicine). Zhongyi guji chubanshe, Beijing.

Cook S. 1995. 'Yue Ji 樂記 – Record of Music: Introduction, Translation, Notes, and Commentary'. *Asian Music* 26 (2): 1–96.

Cros M. 1990. *L'Anthropologie du Sang en Afrique.* L'Harmattan, Paris.

Crump J. I. 1970. *Chan-Kuo Ts'e.* Clarendon Press, Oxford.

Cruse D. A. 1986. *Lexical Semantics.* Cambridge University Press, Cambridge.

Csikszentmihalyi M. 2004. *Material Virtue: Ethics and the Body in Early China.* Brill, Leiden.

Csordas T. J. 1993: 'Somatic Modes of Attention'. *Cultural Anthropology* 8: 135–56. Reprinted in T. J. Csordas (ed.) 2002, 241–59.

Csordas T. J. (ed.) 1994. *Embodiment and Experience: The Existential Grounds of Culture and Self.* Cambridge University Press, Cambridge.

Csordas T. J. (ed.) 2002. *Body/Meaning/Healing.* Palgrave Macmillan, New York.

Cullen C. 2000. 'The Threatening Stranger: *kewu* 客忤 in Pre-modern Chinese Paediatrics'. In L. I. Lawrence and D. Wujastyk (eds.), 39–52.

Cullen C. 2001. 'Yi'an 醫案: The Origins of a Genre of Chinese Medical Literature'. In E. Hsu (ed.), 297–323.

Daniel E. V. 1984. *Fluid Signs: Being a Person the Tamil Way.* University of California Press, Berkeley.

Daniel E. V. 1991. 'The Pulse as an Icon in Siddha Medicine'. In D. Howes (ed.), 100–10.

Davis C. O. 2000. *Death in Abeyance.* Edinburgh University Press, Edinburgh.

De Martino E. [1948] 1988. *Primitive Magic: the Psychic Powers of Shamans and Sorcerers.* Prism, Dorset and Unity, Lindfield.

De Saussure F. 1916. *Cours de Linguistique Générale.* Payot, Paris.

Deng Tietao 鄧鐵濤 (main ed.) 1984. *Zhongyi zhenduanxue* 中醫診斷學 (TCM Diagnostics). Shanghai kexue jishu chubanshe, Shanghai.

Despeux C. 1985. *Shanghanlun: le Traité des "Coups de Froid".* Éditions de la Tisserande, Paris.

Despeux C. 1987. *Prescriptions d'acuponcture valant mille onces d'or: traité d'acuponcture de Sun Simiao du VIIe siècle.* Éditions Guy Trédaniel, Paris.

Despeux C. 2001. 'The System of the Five Circulatory Phases and the Six Seasonal Influences (*wuyun liuqi*), a Source of Innovation in Medicine under the Song (960–1279)'. In E. Hsu (ed.), 121–66.

Despeux C. 2005. 'From Prognosis to Diagnosis of Illness in Tang China: Comparison of the Dunhuang Manuscript P. 3390 and Medical Sources'. In V. Lo and C. Cullen (eds.), 176–205.

Despeux C. (ed.). In press. *Médecine, religion et société dans la Chine médiévale: les manuscrits médicaux de Dunhuang.* Collège de France, Institut des Hautes Études Chinoises, Paris.

Despeux C. and Obringer F. (eds.) 1997. *La maladie dans la Chire médiévale: la toux.* L'Harmattan, Paris.

Du Halde J. B. 1735. *Description géographique, historique, chronologique, politique et physique de l'Empire de la Chine et de la Tartarie Chinoise.* 4 Vols. Le Mercier, Paris. Transl. R. Brookes 1941: *A Description of the Empire of China and Chinese-Tartary, Together with the Kingdoms of Korea, and Tibet: Containing the Geography and History (Natural as well as Civil) of those Countries.* 2 Vols. Cave, London.

Dubs H. H. 1928. *The Works of Hsüntze.* Arthur Probsthain, London.

Dubs H. H. 1938. *The History of the Former Han. By Pan Ku.* 3 Vols. Waverly Press, Baltimore.

Duden B. [1987] 1991. *The Woman beneath the Skin: a Doctor's Patients in Eighteenth-century Germany.* Harvard University Press, Cambridge, MA.

Durrant S. W. 1995. *The Cloudy Mirror: Tension and Conflict in the Writings of Sima Qian.* State University of New York Press, Albany.

Eifring H. 2004. *Love and Emotions in Traditional Chinese Literature.* Brill, Leiden.

Emura Harutatsu 江村治樹 1987. *Mawangdui chutu yishu zixing fenlei suoyin* 馬王堆出土醫書字形分類索引 (Concordance to the Medical Books unearthed in Mawangdui, according to Kinds of Script). Kansai University, Fukida.

Engelhardt U. 2001. 'Dietetics in Tang China and the First Extant Works of *materia dietetica*'. In E. Hsu (ed.), 173–91.

Epler D. C. 1980. 'Bloodletting in Early Chinese Medicine and its Relation to the Origin of Acupuncture'. *Bulletin of the History of Medicine* 54 (3): 337–67.

Evans-Pritchard E. E. 1937. *Witchcraft, Oracles and Magic among the Azande.* Clarendon Press, Oxford.

Fan Xingzhun 范行準 1989. *Zhongguo bingshi xinyi* 中國病史新義 (Novel Approaches to the History of Disease in China). Zhongyi guji chubanshe, Beijing.

Fan Xingzhun 范行準 (unpubl.). 'Erqian yibai nian qiande yiyu' 二千一百年前的醫獄 (A Medical Lawsuit, Two Thousand One Hundred Years Ago). Manuscript reproduced by Quanguo zuguo yixue zhongxin tushuguan in 1963. 28 p.

Farmer P. 1993. *Aids and Accusation: Haiti and the Geography of Blame.* University of California Press, Berkeley.

Farmer P. 1999. *Infections and Inequalities: the Modern Plagues.* University of California Press, Berkeley.

Farmer S., Henderson J. B. and Witzel M. 2000. 'Neurobiology, Layered Texts, and Correlative Cosmologies: a Cross-Cultural Framework for Premodern History'. *Bulletin of the Museum of Far Eastern Antiquities* 72: 48–90.

Farquhar J. 1994. *Knowing Practice: the Clinical Encounter of Chinese Medicine.* Westview Press, Boulder.

Farquhar J. 2002. *Appetites: Food and Sex in Postsocialist China.* Duke University Press, Durham, NC, and London.

Farquhar J. and Hanson M. (eds.) 1998. *Empires of Hygiene. Special Issue. Positions* 6 (3).

Feng Congde 封從德 2003. 'Les cinq cycles et les six souffles: la cosmologie de la médecine Chinoise selon les sept grands traités du *Suwen*'. Thèse de doctorat en Sciences Religieuses. École Pratique des Hautes Études, Sorbonne, Paris.

Fèvre F. 1993. 'Drôles bestioles: qu'est-qu'un *chong*?' In M. Cartier *et al.* (eds.), 57–65.

Flohr C. 2000. 'Qian Yi: der Begründer der chinesischen Kinderheilkunde?' MA dissertation in Sinology, Universität Göttingen.

Forke A. 1962. *Lun-hêng.* Part I: *Philosophical Essays of Wang Ch'ung.* Part II: *Miscellaneous Essays of Wang Ch'ung.* 2nd ed. Paragon Book Gallery, New York.

Forrester J. 1996. 'If *p*, Then What? Thinking in Cases'. *History of the Human Sciences* 9 (3): 1–25.

Foucault M. [1963] 1989. *The Birth of the Clinic: an Archaeology of Medical Perception.* Routledge, London.

Foucault M. [1975] 1979. *Discipline and Punish: the Birth of the Prison.* Penguin Books, London.

Foucault M. [1976] 1990. *The History of Sexuality.* Volume 1: *an Introduction.* Penguin Books, London.

Fraser J. T., Lawrence N. and Haber F. C. (eds.) 1986. *Time, Science, and Society in China and the West.* University of Massachusetts Press, Amherst.

Furth C. 1999. *A Flourishing Yin: Gender in China's Medical History, 960–1665.* University of California Press, Berkeley.

Furth C., Zeitlin I. T. and Hsiung P.-C. (eds.) 2007. *Thinking with Cases: Specialist Knowledge in Chinese Cultural History.* University of Hawaii Press, Honolulu.

Fuyang Hanjian zhenglizu 阜陽漢簡整理組 1983. 'Fuyang Hanjian jianjie' 阜陽漢簡簡介 (Brief Introduction to the Han Bamboo Strips from Fuyang). *Wenwu* 2: 21–3.

Fuyang Hanjian zhenglizu 阜陽漢簡整理組 1988. 'Fuyang Hanjian "Wanwu"' 阜陽漢簡萬物 (The Han Bamboo Strips from Fuyang on the 'Ten Thousand Things'). *Wenwu* 4: 36–47, 54.

Gansusheng bowuguan 甘肅省博物館 and Wuweixian wenhuaguan 武威縣文化館 (eds.) 1975. *Wuwei Handai yijian* 武威漢代醫簡 (Bamboo Strips on Han Dynasty Medicine from Wuwei). Wenwu chubanshe, Beijing.

Gansusheng wenwu kaogu yanjiusuo 甘肅省文物考古研究所 (eds.) 1991. *Dunhuang Hanjian* 敦煌漢簡 (Han Bamboo Strips found at Dunhuang). Zhonghua shuju, Beijing.

Gansusheng wenwu kaogu yanjiusuo, Qinjian zhengli xiaozu 甘肅省文物考古研究所秦簡整理小組 (eds.) 1989. *Qin Han jiandu lunwenji* 秦漢簡牘論文集 (Collection of Articles on Qin and Han Bamboo Strips). Gansu renmin chubanshe, Lanzhou.

Gansusheng wenwu kaogu yanjiusuo, Qinjian zhengli xiaozu 甘肅省文物考古研究所秦簡整理小組 1989. 'Tianshui Fangmatan Qinjian jiazhong "Rishu" shiwen' 天水放馬灘秦簡甲種日書釋文 (Explanations of the Qin Bamboo Strips Type A 'Calendar Book' from Fangmatan near Tianshui). In Gansusheng wenwu kaogu yanjiusuo, Qinjian zhengli xiaozu (eds.), 1–6.

Gao Dalun 高大倫 (ed.) 1992. *Zhangjiashan Hanjian 'Maishu' jiaoshi* 張家山漢簡脈書校釋 (Explanation of the 'Document on the Study of Mai' on Han Bamboo Strips from Zhangjiashan). Chengdu chubanshe, Chengdu.

Gao Dalun 高大倫 (ed.) 1995. *Zhangjiashan Hanjian 'Yinshu' jiaoshi* 張家山漢簡引書校釋 (Explanation of the 'Document on the Study of Guiding' on Han Bamboo Strips from Zhangjiashan). Bashu shushe, Chengdu.

Geaney J. 2002. *On the Epistemology of the Senses in Early Chinese Thought.* University of Hawaii Press, Honolulu.

Geissler P. W. 1998a. '"Worms are our Life", Part I: Understandings of Worms and the Body among the Luo of Western Kenya'. *Anthropology & Medicine* 5 (1): 63–79.

Geissler P. W. 1998b. '"Worms are our Life", Part II: Luo Children's Thoughts about Worms and Illness'. *Anthropology & Medicine* 5 (2): 133–44.

Gernet J. and Kalinowski M. (eds.) 1997. *En suivant la voie royale: mélanges en hommage à Léon Vendermeersch.* Études Thématiques 7. École Française d'Extrême-Orient, Paris.

Geurts K. L. 2003. *Culture and the Senses: Bodily Ways of Knowing in an African Community.* University of California Press, Berkeley.

Good B. J. 1994. *Medicine, Rationality, and Experience: an Anthropological Perspective.* Cambridge University Press, Cambridge.

Graham A. C. 1981. *Chuang-tzu: the Inner Chapters.* George Allen & Unwin, London.

Graham A. C. 1986. *Yin-yang and the Nature of Correlative Thinking.* Institute of East Asian Philosophies, Singapore.

Graham A. C. 1989. *Disputers of the Tao: Philosophical Argument in Ancient China.* Open Court, La Salle, Ill.

Granet M. 1934. *La Pensée Chinoise.* La Renaissance du Livre, Paris.

Grmek M. D. 1962. 'Les reflèts de la sphygmologie Chinoise dans la médicine occidentale'. *Biologie médicale* 51 (numéro hors série): 1–121.

Han Jianping 韓健平 1999. *Mawangdui gumaishu yanjiu* 馬王堆古脈書研究 (Researches on the Ancient Vessel Texts from Mawangdui). Zhongguo shehui kexue chubanshe, Beijing.

Hanying yixue dacidian 漢英醫學大辭典 (Chinese English Medical Dictionary) 1987. Yixue dacidian bianji weiyuanhui (eds.). Renmin weisheng chubanshe, Beijing.

Harbsmeier C. 1989. 'Humor in Ancient Chinese Philosophy'. *Philosophy East and West* 39 (3): 289–310.

Harbsmeier C. 2004. 'The Semantics of *Qing* 情 in Pre-Buddhist Chinese'. In H. Eifring (ed.), 69–148.

Harker R., Mahar C. and Wilkes C. (eds.) 1990. *An Introduction to the Work of Pierre Bourdieu: the Practice of Theory.* Macmillan Press, Houndsmill.

Harper D. 1982. 'The "Wushier pingfang": Translation and Prolegomena'. PhD thesis in Oriental Languages, University of Berkeley.

Harper D. 1985. 'A Chinese Demonography of the Third Century B.C.'. *Harvard Journal of Asiatic Studies* 45: 459–541.

Harper D. 1996. 'Spellbinding'. In D. S. Lopez (ed.), 241–50.

Harper D. 1998. *Early Chinese Medical Literature: the Mawangdui Medical Manuscripts.* Routledge, London.

Harper D. 1999. 'Warring States Natural Philosophy and Occult Thought'. In M. Loewe and E. Shaughnessy (eds.), 813–84.

Harper D. 2001. 'Iatromancy, Diagnosis and Prognosis in Early Chinese Medicine'. In E. Hsu (ed.), 99–120.

Harrison's Principles of Internal Medicine 1987. E. Braunwald *et al.* (eds.). 11th edition. 2 Vols. McGraw-Hill, New York.

Harvey E. D. (ed.) 2003. *Sensible Flesh: on Touch in Early Modern Culture.* University of Pennsylvania Press, Philadelphia.

Hawkes D. 1959. *Ch'u Tz'u: The Songs of the South: an Ancient Chinese Anthology.* Clarendon Press, Oxford.

He Aihua 何愛華 1984. 'Chunyu Yi shengzunian de tantao' 淳于意生卒年的探討 (Discussion of Chunyu Yi's Dates of Birth and Death). *Zhongguo yishi zazhi* 14 (2): 80–81.

He Sana 何撒娜 1999. 'Jusan zhijian: Naren de sangzang yishi yu jiawu xiangzheng' 聚散之間 納人的喪葬儀式與家屋象徵 (Inbetween Gatherings and Dispersals: Funerary Rites and Symbols of the House). Guoli Qinghua Daxue, renleixue yanjiusuo shuoshi lunwen (MA dissertation, Anthropology Research Unit, National Tsinghua University), Taipei. 129 p.

He Z. G. and Lo V. 1996. 'The Channels: a Preliminary Examination of a Lacquered Figurine from the Western Han Period'. *Early China* 21: 81–123.

Heelas P. and Lock A. (eds.) 1981. *Indigenous Psychologies: the Anthropology of the Self.* Academic Press, London.

Henderson J. B. 1991. *Scripture, Canon and Commentary: a Comparison of Confucian and Western Exegesis.* Princeton University Press, Princeton.

Ho P. Y. 1991. 'Chinese Science: the Traditional Chinese View'. *Bulletin of the School of Oriental and African Studies* 54 (3): 506–59.

Howes D. (ed.) 1991. *The Varieties of Sensory Experience: a Sourcebook in the Anthropology of the Senses.* University of Toronto Press, Toronto.

Howes D. (ed.) 2004. *Empire of the Senses: the Sensual Culture Reader.* Berg, Oxford.

Hsu E. 1987. 'Lexical Semantics and Chinese Medical Terms'. MPhil dissertation in General Linguistics, University of Cambridge.

Hsu E. 1992. 'Transmission of Knowledge, Texts and Treatment in Chinese Medicine'. PhD thesis in Social Anthropology, University of Cambridge.

Hsu E. 1999. *The Transmission of Chinese Medicine*. Cambridge University Press, Cambridge.

Hsu E. 2000a. 'Towards a Science of Touch, Part I: Chinese Pulse Diagnostics in Early Modern Europe'. *Anthropology & Medicine* 7 (2): 251–68.

Hsu E. 2000b. 'Towards a Science of Touch, Part II: Representations of the Tactile Experience of the Seven Chinese Pulses indicating Danger of Death in Early Modern Europe'. *Anthropology & Medicine* 7 (3): 319–33.

Hsu E. 2001a. 'The Telling Touch: Pulse Diagnostics in Early Chinese Medicine. With Translation and Interpretation of 10 Medical Case Histories of *Shi ji* 105.2 (ca. 90 BC)'. Habilitationsschrift im Fachbereich Sinologie, Fakultät für Orientalistik und Altertumswissenschaft, Universität Heidelberg (Habilitation in Chinese Studies, Faculty of Oriental Studies and of the Study of Classical Antiquity, University of Heidelberg). 419 p.

Hsu E. 2001b. 'Pulse Diagnostics in a Western Han Text: how *mai* and *qi* determine *bing*'. In E. Hsu (ed.), 51–91.

Hsu E. (ed.) 2001c. *Innovation in Chinese Medicine*. Cambridge University Press, Cambridge.

Hsu E. 2001d. 'Figuratively Speaking of "Danger or Death" in Chinese Pulse Diagnostics'. In R. Jütte *et al.* (eds.), 193–210.

Hsu E. 2003. 'Die drei Koerper – oder sind es vier? Medizinethnologische Perspektiven auf den Körper'. In T. Lux (ed.), *Kulturelle Dimensionen der Medizin: Ethnomedizin, Medizinethnologie, Medical Anthropology*. Reimer, Berlin, 177–89.

Hsu E. 2005a. 'Tactility and the Body in Early Chinese Medicine'. *Science in Context* 18 (1): 7–34.

Hsu E. 2005b. 'Time inscribed in Space, and the Process of Diagnosis in African and Chinese Medical Practices'. In W. James and D. Mills (eds.), 155–70.

Hsu E. 2005c. 'Other Medicines – Which Wisdom do they Challenge?'. In E. van Dongen and J. P. Comelles (eds.), vol. 20: 169–84.

Hsu E. 2007a. 'The Biography of Chunyu Yi'. In W. F. Bynum and H. Bynum (eds.), vol. 2, 343–8.

Hsu E. 2007b. 'The Biological in the Cultural: The Five Agents and the Body Ecologic in Chinese Medicine'. In D. Parkin and S. Ulijaszek (eds.), 91–126.

Hsu E. 2007c. 'The Experience of Wind in Early and Medieval Chinese Medicine'. In E. Hsu and C. Low (eds.), S115–S132.

Hsu E. 2008a. 'A Hybrid Body Technique: Does the Pulse Diagnostic *cun guan chi* Method have Chinese–Tibetan Origins?' *Gesnerus* 65: 5–29.

Hsu E. 2008b. 脈, 視覺到聽覺再到觸覺診查: 運用「身體感」對漢代早期醫學手稿的新解讀 (From a Visual to an Auditory to a Tactile Examination of *mai*: A New Reading of Han Medical Manuscript Texts based on the Anthropology of Bodily Experiences). Transl. Zhen Yan 甄艷. In 余舜德 (Yu Shuennder) (ed.) 體物入微: 物與身體感的研究 (Engaging Things: Researches on Things and Experiences of the Body). National Tsing-Hua University Press, Taipei, 135–64.

Hsu E. 2009. 'Diverse Biologies and Experiential Continuities: Did the Ancient Chinese know that *Qinghao* had Antimalarial Properties?' In F. Wallis (ed.), 203–13.

Hsu E. In press a. 'The Sentimental Body: Outward Form (*xing*) and Inward *qi* in Early Chinese Medicine'. *Early China*.

Hsu E. In press b. 'Le diagnostic du pouls dans la Chine medievale', with detailed summaries of all the Dunhuang manuscripts texts pertaining to sphygmology: P2115, P3106, P3287, P3477, P3481, P3655, P4093, S79, S181, S202, S5614, S6245, S8289. In C. Despeux (ed.).

Hse E. In press c. In collaboration with F. Obringer '*Qinghao* (Herba *Artemesiae Annuae*) in Chinese *materia medica*'. In E. Hsu and S. Harris (eds.), *Plants, Health, Healing: on the Interface of Medical Anthropology and Ethnobotany*.

Hsu E. and Low C. (eds.) 2007. *Wind, Life, Health: Anthropological and Historical Approaches. Special Issue. Journal of the Royal Anthropological Institute.*

Hsu E. and Nienhauser W. H. (transl. and annotat.) In press. "The Memoirs of Pien Ch'üeh and Ts'ang Kung". In W. H. Nienhauser (ed.).

Hubeisheng Jingsha tielu kaogudui 湖北省荊沙鐵路考古隊 (eds.) 1991. *Baoshan Chu jian* 包山楚簡 (Chu Bamboo Strips from Baoshan). Wenwu chubanshe, Beijing.

Hubeisheng wenwu kaogu yanjiusuo 湖北省文物考古研究所 (eds.) 1995. *Jiangling Jiudian Dong Zhou mu* 江陵九店東周墓 (Eastern Zhou Tombs at Jiudian, Jiangling). Kexue chubanshe, Beijing.

Hübotter F. 1927. 'Zwei berühmte chinesische Ärzte des Altertums: Chouen Yu-I und Hua T'ouo'. *Mitteilungen der deutschen Gesellschaft für Natur- und Völkerkunde Ostasiens* 21A: 3–48.

Hulsewé A. F. P. 1985. *Remnants of Ch'in Law*. Brill, Leiden.

Hulsewé A. F. P. 1993. 'Shi ji'. In M. Loewe (ed.), 405–14.

Hume D. [1748] 2007. *An Enquiry Concerning Human Understanding*. Edited by P. Millican. Oxford University Press, Oxford.

Immerwahr R. 1978. 'Diderot, Herder, and the Dichotomy of Touch and Sight'. *Seminar* 14: 84–96.

Ingold T. 2000. *The Perception of the Environment: Essays in Livelihood, Dwelling and Skill.* Routledge, London.

James W. and Mills D. (eds.) 2005. *The Qualities of Time: Anthropological Approaches.* Berg, Oxford.

Jenkins R. [1992] 2002. *Pierre Bourdien*. Revised edition. Routledge, London.

Jiang Yuren 江育仁 (ed.) 1985. *Zhongyi erkexue* 中醫兒科學 (TCM Paediatrics). Shanghai guji chubanshe, Shanghai.

Jiangling Zhangjiashan Hanjian zhengli xiaozu 江陵張家山漢簡整理小組 (eds.) 1989. 'Jiangling Zhangjiashan Hanjian "Maishu" shiwen' 江陵張家山漢簡 '脈書' 釋文 (Transcript of the 'Document on the Mai' on Han Bamboo Strips from Jiangling Zhangjiashan). *Wenwu* 7: 72–4.

Jiangling Zhangjiashan Hanmu zhujian zhenglizu 江陵張家山漢墓竹簡整理組 1985. 'Jiangling Zhangjiashan Hanjian gaishu' 江陵張家山漢簡概述 (Survey of the Han Bamboo Strips from Jiangling Zhangjiashan). *Wenwu* 1: 9–15.

Jingmenshi Bowuguan 荊門事博物館 (eds.) 1998. *Guodian Chumu zhujian* 郭店楚墓竹簡 (The Bamboo Strips from the Chu Tomb in Guodian). Wenwu chubanshe, Beijing.

Jütte R., Eklöf M. and Nelson M. C. (eds.) 2001. *Historical Aspects of Unconventional Medicine: Approaches, Concepts, Case Studies.* European Association for the History of Medicine and Health Publications, Sheffield.

Kalinowski M. (ed.) 2003. *Divination et société dans la Chine médiévale: Étude des manuscripts de Dunhuang de la Bibliothèque Nationale de France et de la British Library.* Bibliothèque Nationale de France, Paris.

Karlgren B. 1957. *Grammata Serica Recensa. Thematic Issue. The Museum of Far Eastern Antiquities Bulletin* 29.

Kawakita Y. (ed.) 1987. *History of Diagnostics.* Taniguchi Foundation, Osaka.

Keegan D. J. 1988. 'The "Huang-ti Nei-Ching": the Structure of the Compilation; the Significance of the Structure'. PhD thesis in History, University of California, Berkeley.

Kempson R. M. 1977. *Semantic Theory.* Cambridge University Press, Cambridge.

Kern M. 2002. 'Methodological Reflections on the Analysis of Textual Variants and the Modes of Manuscript Production in Early China'. *Journal of East Asian Archaeology* 4 (1–4): 143–81.

Kiple K. F. (ed.) 1993. *The Cambridge World History of Human Disease.* Cambridge University Press, Cambridge.

Kleinman A. 1980. *Patients and Healers in the Context of Culture: an Exploration of the Borderland between Anthropology, Medicine, and Psychiatry.* University of California Press, Berkeley.

Kleinman A. 1988. *Rethinking Psychiatry: from Cultural Category to Personal Experience.* Free Press, New York.

Knoblock J. 1988, 1990, 1994. *Xunzi: a Translation and Study of the Complete Works.* 3 Vols. Stanford University Press, Stanford.

Knoblock J. and Riegel J. 2000. *The Annals of Lü Buwei* 閭氏春秋 [*Lü shi chun qiu*]: *a Complete Translation and Study.* Stanford University Press, Stanford.

Kohn L. (ed.) 2000. *Daoism Handbook.* Brill, Leiden.

Kovacs J. and Unschuld P. U. 1998. *Essential Subtleties on the Silver Sea: the Yin-hai jing-wei, a Chinese Classic on Ophthalmology.* University of California Press, Berkeley.

Kuriyama S. 1986. 'Varieties of Haptic Experience: a Comparative Study of Greek and Chinese Pulse Diagnostics'. PhD thesis in the History of Science, Harvard University.

Kuriyama S. 1987. 'Pulse Diagnosis in the Greek and Chinese Traditions'. In Y. Kawakita (ed.), 43–67.

Kuriyama S. 1993. 'Concepts of Disease in East Asia'. In K. F. Kiple (ed.), 52–9.

Kuriyama S. 1994. 'The Imagination of Winds and the Development of the Chinese Conception of the Body'. In A. Zito and T. E. Barlow (eds.), 23–41.

Kuriyama S. 1995a. 'Visual Knowledge in Classical Chinese Medicine'. In D. Bates (ed.), 205–34.

Kuriyama S. 1995b. 'Interpreting the History of Bloodletting'. *Journal of the History of Medicine and Allied Sciences* 50: 11–46.

Kuriyama S. 1999. *The Expressiveness of the Body, and the Divergence of Greek and Chinese Medicine.* Zone Books, New York.

Laderman C. 1987. 'Destructive Heat and Healing Prayer: Malay Humoralism in Pregnancy, Childbirth and Postpartum Period'. *Social Science and Medicine* 25 (4): 357–65.

Laderman C. and Roseman M. 1996. *The Performance of Healing.* Routledge, London.

Lambek M. and Antze P. (eds.) 2003. *Illness and Irony.* Berghahn, New York.

Lambek M. and Strathern A. (eds.) 1998. *Bodies and Persons: Comparative Perspectives from Africa and Melanesia.* Cambridge University Press, Cambridge.

Latour B. [1993] 2006. *We Have Never Been Modern.* Harvard University Press, Cambridge, MA.

Lau D. C. and Chen F. C. 1992. *The ICS Ancient Chinese Texts Concordance Series.* Commercial Press, Chinese University of Hong Kong, Institute of Chinese Studies, Hongkong.

Lau D. C. 1963. *Lao tzu: Tao te ching.* Penguin, Harmondsworth.

Lau D. C. 1970. *Mencius.* Penguin, Harmondsworth.

Lawrence L. I. and Wujastyk D. (eds.) 2000. *Contagion: Perspectives from Premodern Societies.* Ashgate, Aldershot.

Legge J. 1994 (reprint). *The Chinese Classics.* Vol. 2: *Mencius,* Vol. 4: *The She King,* Vol. 5: *The Ch'un ts'ew with the Tso chuen.* SMC Publishing, Taipei.

Leslie C. (ed.) 1976. *Asian Medical Systems: a Comparative Study.* University of California Press, Berkeley.

Leslie C. and Young A. (eds.) 1992. *Paths to Asian Medical Knowledge.* University of California Press, Berkeley.

Levi J. 1993. '*Han fei tzu*' 韓非子. In M. Loewe (ed.), 115–24.

Levinson S. C. 1983. *Pragmatics.* Cambridge University Press, Cambridge.

Lewis G. 1974. 'Gnau Anatomy and Vocabulary for Illness'. *Oceania* 45 (1): 50–78.

Lewis G. 1975. *Knowledge and Illness in a Sepik Society: a Study of the Gnau in New Guinea.* Athlone Press, London.

Lewis G. 1995. 'The Articulation of Circumstance and Causal Understandings'. In D. Sperber *et al.* (eds.), 557–74.

Lewis G. 1999. *A Failure of Treatment.* Oxford University Press, Oxford.

Lewis M. E. 1990. *Sanctioned Violence in Early China.* State University of New York Press, Albany.

Lewis M. 2006. *Construction of Space in Early China.* State University of New York Press, Albany.

Li Bo 李波 (main ed.) 1997. *Shisanjing xinsuoyin* 十三經新索引 (New Concordance to the Thirteen Classics). Zhongguo guangbo dianshi chubanshe, Beijing.

Li Bocong 李伯聰 1990. *Bian Que he Bian Que xuepai yanjiu* 扁鵲和扁鵲學派研究 (Researches on Bian Que and the Bian Que Current of Learning). Shaanxi kexue jishu chubanshe, Xi'an.

Li Jianmin 李健民 1999. 明堂與陰陽 以'五十二病方' '灸其泰陰泰陽' 為列 (Mingtang and Yinyang: the Case of 'Cauterise the *taiyin taiyang*' in the 'Wushier bingfang' from Mawangdui). *Zhongyang yanjiuyuan lishi yuyan yanjiusuo jikan* 70 (1): 49–118.

Li Jianmin 李健民 2000. *Si shen zhi yu – Zhou Qin Han maixue zhi yuanliu* 死生之域 周秦漢脈學之源流 (The Rhyming of Life and Death – the Origins of Vessel Theory in the Zhou, Qin and Han Periods). Zhongyang yanjiuyuan lishi yuyan yanjiusuo, Taipei.

Li Jianmin 李健民 2003. 'Chugoku Igaku-shi niokeru Kakushin Mondai' 中國醫學史における 核心問題 (Core Problems in the History of Chinese Medicine). *Kikan*

Naikyo (Inner Sutra Quarterly) 151. Translated into Japanese by Midori Arakawa.

Li Xueqin 李學勤 2001. 'Lost Doctrines of Guanyin as Seen in the Jingmen Guodian Slips". *Contemporary Chinese Thought* 32 (2): 55–60. Translation of 'Jingmen Guodian Chujian suojian Guanyin shuo' 荊門郭店楚簡所見關尹說. *Zhongguo zhexue* 20 (1999): 160–64.

Liao W. K. 1939, 1959. *The Complete Works of Han Fei Tzu.* Vol. I: *A Classic of Chinese Legalism*, Vol. II: *A Classic of Chinese Political Science.* Arthur Probsthain, London.

Liao Yuqun 廖育群 1984. 'Yi Yin tangye kao' 伊尹湯液考 (Examination of Yi Yin's Decoctions). *Zhonghua yishi zazhi* 14 (3): 150–51.

Liao Yuqun 廖育群 1991. *Qi Huang yi dao* 岐黃醫道 (The Medical Currents of Qibo and Huang Lao). Liaoning jiaoyu chubanshe, Shenyang.

Lin Peizhen 林培真 1984. 'Chunyu Yi shengzunian he zhiren kaobian' 淳于意生卒年和職任考辨 (Examination of Chunyu Yi's Dates of Birth and Death and his Status). *Zhongguo yishi zazhi* 14 (2): 78–9.

Lindenbaum S. and Lock M. (eds.) 1993. *Knowledge, Power, and Practice.* University of California Press, Berkeley.

Lindquist G. 2005. *Conjuring Hope: Magic and Healing in Contemporary Russia.* Berghahn, Oxford.

Lloyd G. E. R. [1950] 1983. *Hippocratic Writings.* Penguin, Harmondsworth.

Lloyd G. E. R. [1966] 1992. *Polarity and Analogy: Two Types of Argumentation in Early Greek Thought.* Cambridge University Press, Cambridge.

Lloyd G. E. R. 1979. *Magic, Reason, and Experience: Studies in the Origins and Development of Greek Science.* Cambridge University Press, Cambridge.

Lloyd G. E. R. 1987. *The Revolutions of Wisdom: Studies in the Claims and Practice of Ancient Greek Science.* Cambridge University Press, Cambridge.

Lloyd G. E. R. 1991. 'Galen on Hellenistics and Hippocrateans: Contemporary Battles and Past Authorities'. In *Methods and the Problems in Greek Science: Selected Papers.* Cambridge University Press, Cambridge, 398–417.

Lloyd G. E. R. 1995. 'Ancient Greek Concepts of Causation in Comparativist Perspective'. In D. Sperber *et al.* (eds.), 536–56.

Lloyd G. E. R. 1996. *Adversaries and Authorities: Investigations into Ancient Greek and Chinese Science.* Cambridge University Press, Cambridge.

Lo V. 1999. 'Tracking Pain: *Jue* and the Formation of a Theory of Circulating *Qi* through the Channels'. *Suddhoffs Archiv* 83: 191–211.

Lo V. 2000. 'Crossing the *Neiguan* 內關 "Inner Pass": a *Nei/wai* 內外 "Inner/Outer" Distinction in Early Chinese Medicine'. *East Asian Science, Technology and Medicine* 17: 15–65.

Lo V. 2001. 'The Influence of Nurturing Life Culture on the Development of Western Han Acumoxa Therapy'. In E. Hsu (ed.), 19–50.

Lo V. 2002. 'Lithic Therapy in Early Chinese Body Practices', in P. A. Baker and G. Carr (eds.), 195–220.

Lo V. and Cullen C. (eds.) 2005. *Medieval Chinese Medicine: the Dunhuang Medical Manuscripts.* RoutledgeCurzon, London.

Lock M. M. 1980. *East Asian Medicine in Urban Japan.* University of California Press, Berkeley.

Lock M. M. 1993. *Encounters with Aging: Mythologies of Menopause in Japan and North America*. University of California Press, Berkeley.

Lock M. and Farquhar J. (eds.) 2007. *Beyond the Body Proper: Reading the Anthropology of Material Life (Body, Commodity, Text)*. Duke University Press, Durham.

Lock M. and Kaufert P. A. (eds.) 1998. *Pragmatic Women and Body Politics*. Cambridge University Press, Cambridge.

Loewe M. A. N. 1960. 'Orders of Honour'. *T'oung Pao* 48: 97–174.

Loewe M. A. N. 1967. *Records of Han Administration*. 2 Vols. Cambridge University Press, Cambridge.

Loewe M. (ed.) 1993. *Early Chinese Texts: a Bibliographical Guide*. Society for the Study of Early China and the Institute of East Asian Studies, University of California, Berkeley.

Loewe M. A. N. 1997. 'The Physician Chunyu Yi and his Historical Background'. In J. Gernet and M. Kalinowski (eds.), 297–313.

Loewe M. 2000. *A Biographical Dictionary of the Qin, Former Han and Xin Periods (221 BC–AD 24)*. Brill, Leiden.

Loewe M. 2004. *The Men Who Governed Han China: Companion to a Biographical Dictionary of the Qin, Former Han and Xin Periods*. Brill, Leiden.

Loewe M. and Shaughnessy E. L. 1999. *The Cambridge History of Ancient China: from the Origins of Civilization to 221 BC*. Cambridge University Press, Cambridge.

Lopez D. S. (ed.) 1996. *Religions of China in Practice*. Princeton University Press, Princeton.

Lu G.-D. and Needham J. 1967. 'Records of Disease in Ancient China'. In D. Brothwell and A. T. Sandison (eds.), 222–37.

Lu G. D. and Needham J. 1980. *Celestial Lancets: a History and Rationale of Acupuncture and Moxa*. Cambridge University Press, Cambridge.

Lucas A. 1982. *Chinese Medical Modernization*. Praeger, New York.

Lyons J. 1977. *Semantics*. 2 Vols. Cambridge University Press, Cambridge.

Ma Boying 1994. *Zhongguo yixue wenhuashi* 中國醫學文化史 (A History of Medicine in Chinese Culture). Shanghai renmin chubanshe, Shanghai.

Ma Jixing 馬繼興 1990. *Zhongyi wenxianxue* 中醫文獻學 (Study of Chinese Medical Texts). Shanghai kexue jishu chubanshe, Shanghai.

Ma Jixing 馬繼興 (ed.) 1992. *Mawangdui guyishu kaoshi* 馬王堆古醫書考釋 (Explanation of the Ancient Medical Documents from Mawangdui). Hunan kexue jishu chubanshe, Changsha.

Ma Jixing 馬繼興, Wang Shumin 王淑民, Tao Guangzheng 陶廣正, Fan Feilun 樊飛倫 (eds.) 1998. *Dunhuang yiyao wenxian jijiao* 敦煌醫藥文獻輯校 (Collected Collations of the Medical Texts from Dunhuang). Jiangsu guji chubanshe, Nanjing.

Machle E. J. 1992. 'The Mind and the "*Shen-Ming*" in *Xunzi*'. *Journal of Chinese Philosophy* 19: 361–86.

Majno G. 1975. *The Healing Hand: Man and Wound in the Ancient World*. Harvard University Press, Cambridge, MA.

Major J. S. 1993. *Heaven and Earth in Early Han Thought: Chapters Three, Four and Five of the Huainanzi*. State University of New York Press, Albany.

Mathieu, R. 1983. *Étude sur la mythologie et l'ethnologie de la Chine ancienne. Traduction annotée du Shan hai jing.* 2 Vols. Collège de France, Institut des Hautes Études Chinoises, Paris.

Mawangdui Hanmu boshu zhengli xiaozu 馬王堆漢墓帛書整理小組 (eds.) 1985. *Mawangdui Hanmu boshu* 馬王堆漢墓帛書 (The Silk Documents from a Han Tomb at Mawangdui). Vol 4. Wenwu chubanshe, Beijing.

Mazis G. A. 1979. 'Touch and Vision: Rethinking with Merleau-Ponty Sartre on the Caress'. *Philosophy Today* 23 (4): 321–28.

McLeod K. C. D. and Yates R. 1981. 'Forms of Ch'in Law: an Annotated Translation of *Feng-chen shih.*' *Harvard Journal of Asiatic Studies* 41: 111–63.

Merleau-Ponty M. [1945] 1962. *Phenomenology of Perception.* Routledge, London.

Misak E. (ed.) 2004. *The Cambridge Companion to Peirce.* Cambridge University Press, Cambridge.

Miyasita S. 1979. 'Malaria (*yao*) in Chinese Medicine during the Chin and Yüan Periods'. In Yabuuti K. (ed.), 90–112.

Mol A. 2003. *The Body Multiple: Ontology in Medical Practice.* Duke University Press, Durham.

Montagu A. 1971. *Touching: the Human Significance of the Skin.* Columbia University Press, New York.

MWD, see Mawangdui Hanmu boshu zhengli xiaozu 馬王堆漢墓帛書整理小組.

Myers F. R. 1979. 'Emotions and the Self: a Theory of Personhood and Political Order among the Pintupi Aborigines'. *Ethos* 7 (4): 343–70.

Nanjing zhongyi xueyuan 南京中醫學院 (eds.) 1986. *Huangdi neijing Lingshu yishi* 黃帝內經素問靈樞譯釋 (Explanations to the *Yellow Emperor's Inner Canon: Divine Pivot*). Shanghai kexue jishu chubanshe, Shanghai.

Nanjing zhongyi xueyuan 南京中醫學院 (eds.) [1959] 1991. *Huangdi neijing Suwen yishi* 黃帝內經素問譯釋 (Explanations to the *Yellow Emperor's Inner Canon: Basic Questions*). Shanghai kexue jishu chubanshe, Shanghai.

Needham J. 1956. *Science and Civilisation in China.* Vol. 2: *History of Scientific Thought.* Cambridge University Press, Cambridge.

Needham J. 1959. *Science and Civilisation in China.* Vol. 3: *Mathematics and the Sciences of Heavens and Earth.* Cambridge University Press, Cambridge.

Needham J. and Lu G.-D. 1999. *Medicine.* In J. Needham (ed.), *Science and Civilisation in China.* Vol. 6: *Biology and Biological Technology*, Part 6. Cambridge University Press, Cambridge.

Needham J., Wang Ling, Lu Gwei-Djen and Ho Ping-Yü 1970. *Clerks and Craftsmen in China and the West.* Cambridge University Press, Cambridge.

Nichter M. and Lock M. (eds.) 2002. *New Horizons in Medical Anthropology.* Routledge, London.

Nichter M. and Nichter M. (eds.) 1996. *Anthropology and International Health: Asian Case Studies.* Gordon and Breach, Amsterdam.

Nienhauser W. H. (ed.) In press. *The Grand Scribe's Records*, Vol. 7. *The Han Dynasty Memoirs, Part I* [*Chapters 89–112*]. Indiana University Press, Bloomington.

Nylan M. 2001. 'On the Politics of Pleasure'. *Asia Major* 14 (1): 73–124.

Obringer F. 1997. *L'aconit et l'orpiment: drogues et poisons en Chine ancienne et médiévale.* Fayard, Genève.

Obringer F. 2001. 'A Song Innovation in Pharmacotherapy: Some Remarks on the Use of White Arsenic and Flowers of Arsenic'. In E. Hsu (ed.), 192–214.

O'Hara A. R. [1945] 1971. *The Position of Woman in Early China: According to Lieh Nü Chuan 'The Biographies of Chinese Women'*. Meiya Publ., Taipei.

Ohnuki-Tierney E. 1984. *Illness and Culture in Contemporary Japan: an Anthropological View*. Cambridge University Press, Cambridge.

Osobe Yô 1994. *'Hen Jaku Sôkô den' Gen'un chu no houji to kenkyû* '扁鵲倉公傳' 勾雲注翻字研究 (Translation and Study of the Memoir of Bian Que and Canggong as commented on by Gen'un [style of Geshû Jukei 月丹壽桂 1470-1533]). Report completed at 北里研究所 東洋醫學總合研究所 醫史研究部.

Ots T. [1987] 1990a. *Medizin und Heilung in China. Annäherungen an die Traditionelle Medizin*. 2nd revised edition. Reimer, Berlin.

Ots T. 1990b. 'The Angry Liver, the Anxious Heart and the Melancholy Spleen: the Phenomenology of Perceptions in Chinese Culture'. *Culture, Medicine, and Psychiatry* 14: 21–58.

Otsuka Y. Sakai S. and Kuriyama S. (eds.) 1999. *Medicine and the History of the Body*. Ishiyaku EuroAmerica, Tokyo.

Ou Ming (ed.) 1988. *Yinghan zhongyi cidian* 英漢中醫辭典 (Chinese–English Dictionary of Traditional Chinese Medicine). Sanlian shudian youxian gongsi and Guangdong keji chubanshe, Hongkong.

Padel R. 1992. *In and Out of the Mind: Greek Images of the Tragic Self.* Princeton University Press, Princeton.

Parkin D. and Ulijaszek S. (eds.) 2007. *Holistic Anthropology: Emergences and Divergences*. Berghahn, Oxford.

Peirce C. S. 1932. *Collected Papers*. Vols. 1–6. Edited by C. Hartshorne and P. Weiss. Harvard University Press, Cambridge, MA.

Pfister R. 2002. 'Some Preliminary Remarks on Notational Systems in Two Medical Manuscripts from Mawangdui'. *Asiatische Studien – Études Asiatiques* 56 (3): 609–33.

Pfister R. In press. *Sexuelle Körpertechniken im alten China: seimbedürftige Männer im Umgang mit lebens-spenderinnen: drei Manuskripte aus Mawangdui: eine Lektüre*. 3 vols. Books on Demand, Norderstedt.

Poo M. 1999. 'The Use and Abuse of Wine in Ancient China'. *Journal of the Economic and Social History of the Orient* 42 (2): 1–29.

Pool R. 1994. *Dialogue and the Interpretation of Illness: Conversations in a Cameroon Village*. Berg, Oxford.

Porkert P. 1974. *The Foundations of Chinese Medicine: Systems of Correspondence*. MIT Press, Cambridge, MA.

Pregadio F. 2004. 'The Notion of "Form" and the Ways of Liberation in Daoism'. *Cahiers d'Extrême-Asie* 14: 95–130.

Pregadio F. and Skar L. 2000. 'Inner Alchemy (*neidan*)'. In L. Kohn (ed.), 464–97.

Puett M. J. 2001. *The Ambivalence of Creation: Debates concerning Innovation and Artifice in Early China*. Stanford University Press, Stanford.

Puett M. J. 2004. 'The Ethics of Responding Properly: the Notion of Qing 情 in Early Chinese Thought'. In H. Eifring (ed.), 37–68.

Pulleyblank E. G. 1995. *Outline of Classical Chinese Grammar.* University of British Columbia Press, Vancouver.

Qiu Maoliang 邱茂良 (ed.) 1985. *Zhenjiuxue* 針灸學 (Acumoxa). Shanghai kexue jishu chubanshe, Shanghai.

Queen S. 1996. *From Chronicle to Canon: the Hermeneutics of the Spring and Autumn, according to Tong Chung-shu.* Cambridge University Press, Cambridge.

Raphals L. 1998a. *Sharing the Light: Representations of Women and Virtue in Early China.* State University of New York Press, Albany.

Raphals L. 1998b. 'The Treatment of Women in a Second-Century Medical Casebook'. *Chinese Science* 15: 7–28.

Rawson J. 1990. *Western Zhou Ritual Bronzes from the Arthur M. Sackler Collections.* 2 Vols. Arthur M. Sackler Foundation, Washington, D. C.

Reckwitz A. 2002. 'Toward a Theory of Social Practices: a Development in Culturalist Theorizing'. *European Journal of Social Theory* 5 (2): 245–65.

Ren Yingqiu 任應秋1982. '"Huangdi neijing" yanjiu shijiang' 黃帝內經 研究十講 (Ten Lectures on Research on the *Yellow Emperor's Inner Canon*). In Ren and Liu (eds.), 1–99.

Ren Yingqiu 任應秋 and Liu Zhanglin 劉長林 (eds.) 1982. *'Neijing' yanjiu luncong* 內經研究論叢 (Essays on Researches on the *Inner Canon*). Hubei renmin chubanshe, Wuhan.

Rickett W. A. 1985, 1998. *Guanzi: Political, Economic, and Philosophical Essays from Early China.* 2 Vols. Princeton University Press, Princeton.

Rivers W. H. R. 1924. *Medicine, Magic, and Religion.* Kegan Paul, London.

Rosaldo M. Z. 1980. *Knowledge and Passion: Ilongot Notions of Self and Social Life.* Cambridge University Press, Cambridge.

Roseman M. 1991. *Healing Sounds from the Rainforest: Temiar Music and Medicine.* University of California Press, Berkeley.

Rosner E. 1991. *Die Heilkunst des Pien Lu: Arzt und Krankheit in Bildhaften Ausdrücken der Chinesischen Sprache.* Franz Steiner Verlag, Stuttgart.

Roth H. D. 1991. 'Psychology and Self-Cultivation in Early Taoistic Thought'. *Harvard Journal of Asiatic Studies* 51: 599–650.

Samuelsen L. and Steffen V. 2004. 'The Relevance of Foucault and Bourdieu for Medical Anthropology: Exploring New Sites'. *Anthropology & Medicine* 11 (1): 3–10.

Santangelo P. 1994. 'Emotions in Late Imperial China: Evolution and Continuity in Ming-Qing Perception of Passions'. In V. Alleton and A. Volkov (eds.), 167–86.

Schafer E. H. 1977. 'T'ang'. In K. C. Chang (ed.), 85–140.

Scheid V. 2002. *Chinese Medicine in Contemporary China: Plurality and Synthesis.* Duke University Press, Durham.

Scheper-Hughes N. 1992. *Death Without Weeping: the Violence of Everyday Life in Brazil.* University of California Press, Berkeley.

Scheper-Hughes N. and Lock M. 1987. 'The Mindful Body: a Prolegomenon to Future Work in Medical Anthropology'. *Medical Anthropological Quarterly* 1 (1): 6–41.

Shapiro H. 1998. 'The Puzzle of Spermatorrhea in Republican China'. In J. Farquhar and M. Hanson (eds.), 551–96.

Shilling C. 1993. *The Body and Social Theory.* Polity Press, Cambridge.

Short T. L. 2004. 'The Development of Peirce's Theory of Science'. In C. Misak (ed.), 214–40.

Shuihudi Qinmu zhujian zhengli xiaozu 睡虎地秦墓竹簡整理小組 (ed.) 1990. *Shuihudi Qinmu zhujian* 睡虎地秦墓竹簡 (The Bamboo Strips from a Qin Tomb in Shuihudi). Wenwu chubanshe, Beijing.

Silverstein M. 2004. '"Cultural" Concepts and the Language-Culture Nexus'. *Current Anthropology* 45 (5): 621–52.

Sivin N. 1987. *Traditional Medicine in Contemporary China: a Partial Translation of* Revised Outline of Chinese Medicine (1972) *with an Introductory Study on Change in Present-day and Early Medicine.* Center for Chinese Studies, University of Michigan, Ann Arbor.

Sivin N. 1991. 'Change and Continuity in Early Cosmology'. In *Chûgoku kodai kagaku shiron. Zoku* 中國古代科學史論。續 (On the History of Ancient Chinese Science, 2). Kyoto: Institute for Research in Humanities, 3–43.

Sivin N. 1993. '*Huang ti nei ching*' 黃帝內經. In M. Loewe (ed.), 196–215.

Sivin N. 1995a. 'Text and Experience in Classical Chinese Medicine'. In D. Bates (ed.), 177–204.

Sivin N. 1995b. 'State, Cosmos, and Body in the Last Three Centuries B.C.'. *Harvard Journal of Asiatic Studies* 55 (1): 5–37.

Sivin N. 1995c. *Medicine, Philosophy and Religion in Ancient China: Researches and Reflections.* Variorum, Aldershot.

Sivin N. 1995d. 'The Myth of the Naturalists'. In Sivin 1995c, 33p.

Sivin N. 1995e. 'Emotional Countertherapy'. In N. Sivin 1995c, 19p.

Soymié M. 1990. 'Observations sur les caractères interdits en Chine'. *Journal Asiatique* 278 (3–4): 377–407.

Sperber D., Premack D. and Premack A. J. (eds.) 1995. *Causal Cognition: a Multidisciplinary Approach.* Clarendon Press, Oxford.

Sterckx R. 2002. *The Animal and the Daemon in Early China.* State University of New York Press, Albany.

Sterckx R. (ed.) 2005. *Of Tripod and Palate: Food, Politics, and Religion in Traditional China.* Palgrave Macmillan, New York.

Tan Qixiang 譚其驤 (ed.) 1991. *Zhongguo lishi ditu ji* 中國歷史地圖集 (Collection of Historical Chinese Maps). Vol. 2. Sanlian shudian, Hong Kong.

Taylor K. 2005. *Medicine of Revolution: Chinese Medicine in Early Communist China.* Routledge, London.

Trawick M. 1992. 'Death and Nurturance in Indian Systems of Healing'. In C. Leslie and A. Young (eds.), 129–59.

Twitchett D. and Loewe M. (eds.) 1986. *The Cambridge History of China.* Vol. 1: *The Ch'in and Han Empires, 221 BC – AD 220.* Cambridge University Press, Cambridge.

Ulijaszek S. J. and Strickland S. S. (eds.) 1993. *Seasonality and Human Ecology.* Cambridge University Press, Cambridge.

Umekawa S. 2004. 'Sex and Immortality: a Study of Chinese Sexual Activities for Better-Being'. PhD thesis in History. University of London, London.

Unschuld P. U. [1980] 1985. *Medicine in China: a History of Ideas.* University of California Press, Berkeley.

Unschuld P. U. 1982. 'Der Wind als Ursache des Krankseins'. *T'oung Pao* 68: 92–131.

Unschuld P. U. 1986a. *The Classic of Difficult Issues. With Commentaries by Chinese and Japanese Authors from the Third through to the Twentieth Century.* University of California Press, Berkeley.

Unschuld P. U. 1986b. *Medicine in China: a History of Pharmaceuticals.* University of California Press, Berkeley.

Unschuld P. U. 1992. 'Epistemological Issues and Changing Legitimation: Traditional Chinese Medicine in the Twentieth Century.' In C. Leslie and A. Young (eds.), 44–61.

Unschuld P. U. 2003. *Huang Di Nei Jing Su Wen: Nature, Knowledge, Imagery in an Ancient Chinese Medical Text.* University of California Press, Berkeley.

Unschuld P. U., Zheng J. S. and Tessenow H. 2003. 'The Doctrine of the Five Periods and Six Qi in the *Huang Di nei jing su wen*'. Appendix to P. U. Unschuld, 385–488.

Unschuld P. U. and Zheng J. S. 2005. 'Manuscripts as Sources in the History of Chinese Medicine'. In V. Lo and C. Cullen (eds.), 19–44.

Van der Geest S. and Whyte S. R. (eds.) 1988. *The Context of Medicines in Developing Countries.* Kluwer, Dordrecht.

Van Dongen E. and Comelles J. P. (eds.) 2005. *Medical Anthropology, Welfare State and Political Engagement. Thematic Issue. Antropologia and Medicina: Rivista della Società Italiana di Antropologia Medica*: 19–20.

Wallis F. (ed.) 2009. *Medicine and the Soul of Science: Essays in Memory of Don Bates. Special Issue. Canadian Bulletin of the History of Medicine* 26 (1).

Wang Shaozeng 王紹增 1994. *Yiguwen baipian shiyi* 醫古文百篇釋譯 (Explanations to One Hundred Essays in Classical Chinese for Medics). Heilongjiang kexue jishu chubanshe, Ha'erbin.

Wang Shumin 王叔岷 1983. *Shiji jiaozheng* 史記斠證 (Emendations to the Records of the Historian). Zhongyang yanjiuyuan lishi yuyan yanjiusuo, Taipei.

Wang Zhipu 王致譜 1980. 'Xiaoke (tangniaobing) shi shuyao' 消渴(糖尿病)史述要 (Outline of the History of 'Wasting Thirst' – Diabetes). *Zhonghua yishi zazhi* 10 (2): 73–82.

Ware J. R. 1966. *Alchemy, Medicine and Religion in China of A. D. 320: the Nei P'ien of Ko Hung* (Pao-p'utzu). MIT Press, Cambridge, MA.

Watson B. 1961. *Ssu-ma Ch'ien: Grand Historian of China.* Columbia University Press, New York.

Whyte S. R. 1997. *Questioning Misfortune: the Pragmatics of Uncertainty in Eastern Uganda.* Cambridge University Press, Cambridge.

Wilbur M. 1943. *Slavery in China during the Former Han Dynasty, 206 B.C. – 25 A.D. Anthropological Series* 34. Field Museum of Natural History, Chicago.

Wilms S. 2002. 'The Female Body in Medieval China: a Translation and Interpretation of the "Women's Recipes" in Sun Simiao's *Beiji qianjin yaofang*'. PhD thesis in East Asian Studies, University of Arizona.

Wiseman N. 1990. *Glossary of Chinese Medical Terms and Acupuncture Points.* Paradigm Publications, Brookline.

Woolgar S. 1988. *Science, the Very Idea.* Routledge, London.

Wu H. 1995. *Monumentality in Early Chinese Art and Architecture.* Stanford University Press, Stanford.

Xie Guan 謝觀 [1921] 1954. *Zhongguo yixue dacidian* 中國醫學大辭典 (Comprehensive Dictionary of China's Medicine). 4 vols. Shangye yinshuguan, Shanghai.

Yabuuti K. (ed.) 1979. *Studies in the History of Chinese Science. Special Issue. Acta Asiatica* 36.

Yamada K. 1988. 'Hen Shaku densetsu' 扁鵲傳說 (Discussion of the Memoir of Bian Que). *Toho gakuho* 60: 73–158.

Yamada K. 1998. *The Origins of Acupuncture, Moxibustion, and Decoction.* International Research Center for Japanese Studies, Kyoto.

Yin Huihe 印會河 (ed.) 1984. *Zhongyi jichu lilun* 中醫基礎理論 (TCM Fundamentals). Shanghai keji chubanshe, Shanghai.

Young A. 1995. *The Harmony of Illusions: Inventing Post-Traumatic Stress Disorder.* Princeton University Press, Princeton.

Yu Mingguang 余明光 *et al.* (eds. and transl.) 1993. *Huangdi sijing jinzhu jinyi* 黃帝四經今注今譯 (The Four Canons of the Yellow Emperor, Contemporary Edition and Annotations). Yuelu shushe, Changsha.

Yu Xingwu 于省吾 [1937] 1962. *Shuangjianchi zhuzi xinzheng* 雙劍誃諸子新証 (New Notes to the Shuangjianchi Scholars). 4 Vols. Zhonghua shuju, Beijing.

Yu Yunxiu 余雲岫 1953. *Gudai jibing minghou shuyi* 古代疾病名侯疏義 (Explanation of the Nomenclature of Disease in Ancient Times). Renmin weisheng chubanshe, Beijing.

Zhang Boyu 張伯臾 (ed.) 1985. *Zhongyi neikexue* 中醫內科學 (TCM Internal Medicine). Shanghai guji chubanshe, Shanghai.

Zhang Xiancheng 張顯成 1997. *Jianbo yaoming yanjiu* 簡帛藥名研究 (Study on Terms of Chinese Drugs recorded in Medical Books written on Bamboo Strips and Silk). Xinan Shifan Daxue chubanshe, Sichuan.

Zhang Xiancheng 張顯成 2000. *Xian Qin liang Han yixue yongyu yanjiu* 先秦兩漢醫學用語研究 (Research on the Use of Language in the Medicine of the Pre-Qin and Two Han Periods). Bashu shushe, Chengdu.

Zhangjiashan 247 hao Hanmu zhujian zhengli xiaozu 張家山二四七號漢墓竹簡整理小組 (eds.) 2001. *Zhangjiashan Hanmu zhujian* (247 haomu) 張家山漢墓竹簡 (二四七號墓) (Bamboo Strips from the Han Tomb Zhangjiashan No. 247). Wenwu chubanshe, Beijing.

Zhangjiashan Hanjian Zhenglizu 張家山漢簡整理組 1990. 'Zhangjiashan hanjian "Yinshu" yiwen' 張家山漢簡 '引書' 釋文 (Explanations to the 'Document on the Study of Guiding' on Han Bamboo Strips from Zhangjiashan). *Wenwu* 10: 82–6.

Zhonghua yaohai 中華藥海 (Sea of China's *Materia Medica*) 1993. Ran Xiande 冉先德 (ed.). Ha'erbin chubanshe, Harbin.

Zhongyao dacidian 中藥大辭典 (Dictionary of Chinese *Materia Medica*) [1977, 1986] 1995. Jiangsu xinyi xueyuan 江蘇新醫學院 (eds.). Shanghai kexue jishu chubanshe, Shanghai.

Zhongyi dacidian 中醫大辭典 (Great Dictionary of Chinese Medicine) 1995. Zhongguo Zhongyi Yanjiuyuan中國中醫研究院 and Guangzhou Zhongyiyuan 廣州中醫學院 (eds.). Renmin weisheng chubanshe, Beijing.

Zimmermann F. 1987. *The Jungle and the Aroma of Meats: an Ecological Theme in Hindu Medicine.* University of California Press, Berkeley.

Zito A. and Barlow T. E. (eds.) 1994. *Body, Subject, and Power in China.* University of Chicago Press, Chicago.

ZJS, see Zhangjiashan 247 hao Hanmu zhujian zhengli xiaozu 張家山二四七號漢墓竹簡整理小組.

ZJS MSSW, see Jiangling Zhangjiashan Hanjian zhengli xiaozu 江陵張家山漢簡整理小組.

ZJS YSSW, see Jiangling Zhangjiashan Hanjian zhenglizu 江陵張家山漢簡整理組.

B. Pre-modern works of the received tradition (titles in *pinyin* transcription, alphabetically ordered)

Bao pu zi 抱朴子 (Essays by Master Holding-to-Simplicity). Eastern Jin, 320. Ge Hong 葛洪. References to *Baopuzi neipian jiaoshi* 抱朴子內篇校釋. Annotated by Wang Ming 王明. Zhonghua shuju, Beijing, 1985.

Bei ji qian jin yao fang 備急千金要方 (Essential Prescriptions Worth a Thousand, for Urgent Need). Tang, 650/659. Sun Simiao 孫思邈. Facsimile of the Jianghu Medical School's reprint of a Northern Song edition, which was reprinted in 1307 by the Meixi Shuyuan. Renmin weisheng chubanshe, Beijing, 1955.

Ben cao gang mu 本草綱目 ([Hierarchically] Classified Materia Medica). Ming, 1596. Li Shizhen 李時珍. 4 Vols. Renmin weisheng chubanshe, Beijing, 1977–81.

Cha bing zhi nan 察病指南 (Compass to the Investigation of Disease). Yuan, 13th c. Shi Fa 施發. References to the Japanese edition 中野小左衛門刻 of 1646.

Chu ci 楚辭 (Songs of Chu). References to *Chuci jizhu* 楚辭集注. Annotated by Zhu Xi 朱熹. Facsimile of the Yuan dynasty print from ca 1330. Guoli zhongyang tushuguan, Taipei, 1991.

Cong shu ji cheng 叢書集成 (CSJC, Collected Collectanea). Shangwu yinshuguan, Shanghai, 1935–40.

Dao de jing 道德經 (Canon on the Way and its Power). Warring States–Han, 3rd–1st c. BCE. Attributed to *Laozi* 老子. References to *Laozi zhuyi ji pingjie* 老子注譯及評介. Edited by Chen Guying 陳鼓應. Zhonghua shuju, Beijing, 1984 and to *Laozi Daodejing He Shang gong zhangju* 老子 道德經 河上公 章句 (Mister He Shang's Chapters on Laozi's Daodejing). Edited by Wang Ka 王卡. Zhonghua shuju, Beijing, 1993.

Er ya 爾雅 (Approaching what is Correct). Zhou, 3rd c. BCE. Anon. SBCK.

Gu wei shu 古微書 (Document of Ancient Subtleties). Qing, 17th c. Sun Jue 孫瑴, CSJC.

Guang ya 廣雅 (Broadening what is Correct). Wei, 3rd c. Zhang Yi 張揖. References to *Guang ya shu zheng* 廣雅疏証. Qing, 1788–96. Composed by Wang Niansun 王念孫. Zhonghua shuju, Beijing, 1983.

Guanzi 管子 (Essays by Master Guan). Zhou–Han, 5th c.–1st c. BCE. In ca 26 BCE edited by Liu Xiang 劉向. SBBY.

Han Feizi 韓非子 (Essays by Master Han Fei). Zhou, 3rd c. BCE. References to *Han Feizi jishi*. Edited by Chen Qiyou 陳啟猷. Zhonghua shuju, Beijing, 1958.

Han shu 漢書 (History of the Former Han). Han, 1st c. Ban Gu 班固. Zhonghua shuju, Beijing, 1962.

Han shu bu zhu 漢書補注 (Supplementary Notes to the *History of the Former Han*). Qing, 1900. Wang Xianqian 王先謙. Facsimile of the Xushoutang print. I wen publishers, Taipei, 1955.

HDNJSW, see *Huangdi nei jing Su wen* 黃帝內經 素問.

Hou Han shu 後漢書 (History of the Later Han). Song, 5th c. Fan Ye 范曄. Zhonghua shuju, Beijing, [1965] 1973.

Huainanzi 淮南子 (Essays from the Masters at Huainan). Han, ca 139 BCE. Assembled and edited by Liu An 劉安. References to *Huainanzi jiaoshi*. Annotated by Zhang Shuangdi 張雙棣. 2 Vols. Beijing Daxue chubanshe, Beijing, 1997.

Huangdi nei jing 黃帝內經 (Yellow Emperor's Inner Canon). Zhou to Han, 3rd c. BCE to 3rd c. CE. Anon. References to Ren Yingqiu 任應秋 (ed.) *Huangdi neijing zhangju suoyin* 黃帝內經章句索引. Renmin weisheng chubanshe, Beijing, 1986.

Huangdi nei jing Su wen 黃帝內經素問 (Yellow Emperor's Inner Canon, Basic Questions). Tang, 610. Edited by Wang Bing 王冰. Facsimile reproducing a Ming woodprint by Gu Congde 顧從德 of the Song edition of 1067. Renmin weisheng chubanshe, Beijing, [1956] 1982.

Huangdi nei jing Tai su 黃帝內經太素 (The Yellow Emperor's Inner Canon, the Grand Basis). Sui. Yang Shangshan (fl.666/683). Toyo Igaku Kenkyujo 東洋醫學研究所 (eds.). Facsimile of the 1168 CE edition kept at Ninnaji. Toyo Igaku Zenpon Sosho, Osaka, 1981.

Ji jiu pian 急就篇 (Quick Reference Book in Case of Need). Han, 48–33 BCE. Shi You 史遊. Annotated by Ceng Zhongshan 曾仲冊. Qiulu shushe, Changsha, 1989.

Ji yun 集韻 (Assembled Rhymes). Song, 1039. Ding Du 丁度. Shanghai guji chubanshe, Shanghai, 1983.

Jin gui yao lüe 金匱要略 (Essentials in the Golden Casket). Part of the *Shang han za bing lun* 傷寒雜病論 (Treatise on Cold Damage and Miscellaneous Disorders). Eastern Han, 196–220. Zhang Ji 張機. Divided into three books in the Song, 968–75 and 1064/65. References to *Jingui yaolüe yishi*. Edited by Li Keguang 李克光. Shanghai kexue jishu chubanshe, Shanghai, 1993.

Lei jing 類經 (Canon of Categories). Qing, 1624. Zhang Jiebin 張介賓. Renmin weisheng chubanshe, Beijing, [1965] 1985.

Li ji 禮記 (Records of the Rites). Han, 1st c. CE. Anon. References to *Liji zhengyi* 禮記正義. In *Shi san jing zhu shu* 十三經注疏, vol. 2.

Lie nü zhuan 列女傳 (Biographies of Outstanding Women). Han, 1st, c. CE Anon. Liu Xiang 劉向, attributed compiler. References to *Lie nü zhuan jiao zhu* 列女傳校注. Commentary by Liang Duan 梁端. SBBY.

Ling shu 靈樞, see *Huangdi nei jing* 黃帝內經.

Lü shi chun qiu 呂氏春秋 (The Annals by Mister Lü). Warring States, ca 239 BCE. Lü Buwei 呂不韋. SBBY.

Lun heng 論衡 (Disquisitions Weighed in the Balance). Han, ca 70–80. Wang Chong 王充. References to *Lunheng quanyi*. Guizhou renmin chubanshe, Guiyang, 1993.

Lun yu 論語 (Analects). Zhou, 3rd c. BCE. Anon. References to *Lun yu zheng yi* 論語正義. Qing, 1866. Commentary by Liu Baonan 劉寶楠. Zhonghua shuju, Beijing, 1990.

Mai jing 脈經 (Canon of the Study of the Pulse). Jin, 280 CE. Wang Xi 王熙. References to *Maijing jiaozhu*. Annotated by Shen Yannan 沈炎南. Renmin weisheng chubanshe, Beijing, 1991.

Mawangdui vessel texts, see Mawangdui Hanmu boshu zhengli xiaozu 馬王堆漢墓帛書整理小組 1985 and Ma Jixing 馬繼興 1992 in Bibliography A.

Mengzi 孟子 (Mencius). Zhou. Meng Ke 孟軻, fl. 340 BCE. References to *Mengzi ji zhu* 孟子集注. Song, 1177. Annotated by Zhu Xi 朱喜. Zhonghua shuju, Shanghai, 1936. See also *Mengzi zhu shu* 孟子注疏 in *Shi san jing zhu shu* 十三經注疏, vol. 2.

Nan jing 難經, see Unschuld P. U. 1986a in Bibliography A.

Nei jing 內經, see *Huang di nei jing* 黃帝內經.

Shan hai jing 山海經 (Canon of the Mountains and Lakes). Warring States–Han. Anon. References to *Shanhaijing jiaozhu*. Annotated by Yuan Ke 袁珂. Shanghai guji chubanshe, Shanghai, 1980.

Shang han lun 傷寒論 (Treatise on Cold Damage Disorders). Part of the *Shang han za bing lun* 傷寒雜病論 (Treatise on Cold Damage and Miscellaneous Disorders) of the Eastern Han, 196–220. Zhang Ji 張機. Divided into three books in the Song, 1064–5. Annotated by Cheng Wuyi 成無已. Zhonghua shuju, Beijing, 1991.

Shang shu 尚書 (Book of Documents). Zhou, 11th c. BCE–4th c. CE. Anon. References to *Shang shu zheng yi* 尚書正義, in *Shi san jing zhu shu* 十三經注疏, vol. 1.

Shen jian 申鑒 (Extended Reflections). Eastern Han, 198–200 CE. Xun Yüe 荀悅. *Zhu zi ji cheng* 諸子集成, vol. 8. Zhonghua shuju, Beijing, [1954] 1993.

Sheng ji zong lu 聖濟宗彔 (Sagely Benefaction Medical Encyclopaedia). Song, 1111–17. Zhao Ji 趙佶 2 Vols. Renmin weisheng chubanshe, Beijing, [1962] 1992.

Shennong ben cao jing 神農本草經 (Divine Husbandman's Canon on Materia Medica). Han, 1st c. CE. Anon. References to *Shennong bencaojing jizhu*. Annotated by Ma Jixing 馬繼興. Renmin weisheng chubanshe, Beijing, 1995.

Shi ji 史記 (Records of the Historian). Han, ca 86 BCE. Sima Qian 司馬遷. Zhonghua shuju, Beijing, 1959. See also *Shiki kaichû kôshô* 史記會注考證.

Shi jing 詩經 (Book of Songs). Zhou, 1000–600 BCE. Anon. References to *Mao shi* 毛詩, SBBY; and *Mao shi zheng yi* 毛詩正義, in *Shi san jing zhu shu* 十三經注疏, vol 1.

Shi ming 釋名 (Explicating Names). Han, ca 200 CE. Compiled by Liu Xi 劉熙. SBCK.

Shi san jing zhu shu 十三經注疏 (Commentary to the Thirteen Canons). Qing, 1816. Ruan Yuan 阮元. Reprint in 2 Vols. Zhonghua shuju, Beijing, 1980.

Shiki kaichû kôshô 史記會注考證 (Examination of the Collected Commentaries to the *Records of the Historian*). Edited by Takigawa Kametarô 瀧川龜太郎. Toyo Bunka Gakuin, Tokyo, 1932–34.

Shiki kokujikai 史記國字解 (Explanations of the Characters in the *Records of the Historian*). Edited by Katsura Ison (Koson), Kikuchi Sankurô (Bankô), Matsudaira Yasukuni, Makino Kenjirô (Sôshu). Waseda University Press, Tokyo, 1919–20.

Shuo wen jie zi 說文解字 (Discussing the Patterns and Explicating the Characters). Han, 121. Xu Shen 許慎. References to *Shuo wen jie zi zhu* 說文解字注. Qing, 1776–1807. Commentary by Duan Yucai 段玉裁. Shanghai guji chubanshe, Shanghai, 1981.

Si bu bei yao 四部備要 (SBBY, Essentials of the Four Branches of Literature). Zhonghua shuju, Shanghai, 1936.

Si bu cong kan 四部叢刊 (SKCK, The Four Branches of Literature Collection). Shangwu yinshuguan, Shanghai, 1927.

Si ku quan shu 四庫全書 (SKQS, Collection of the Works from the Four Storehouses). References to *Wen yuan ge Si ku quan shu* 文淵閣 四庫全書. Shangwu yinshuguan, Taipei, 1983.

Su wen 素問, see *Huangdi nei jing* 黃帝內經 or *Huangdi nei jing Su wen* 黃帝內經 素問.

Tai ping yu lan 太平御覽 (Imperial Encyclopaedia of the Taiping Reign Period). Song, 983. Li Fang 李昉. References to Zhonghua shuju, Beijing, [1960] 1985.

Tong ya 通雅 (Understanding what is Correct). Ming, completed in 1636, printed in 1664. Fang Yizhi 方以智. SKQS.

Wen xuan 文選 (Literary Selections). Liang, ?520-?26. Xiao Tong 蕭統. 2 Vols. Wunan tushu chuban youxian gongsi, Taibei, 1991.

Xunzi 荀子. Warring States, 3rd c. BCE. Xun Qing 荀卿. References to *Xunzi jianzhu*. Annotated by Zhang Shitong 章詩同. Shanghai renmin chubanshe, Shanghai, 1974.

Yi shuo 醫說 (Ruminations on Medicine). Song, preface 1189. Zhang Gao 張杲. SKQS.

You ke shi mi 幼科釋謎 (Explaining the Puzzles in Paediatrics). Qing, 1773. Shen Jin'ao 沈金鰲. In *Zhongguo yixue dacheng sanbian* 中國醫學大成三編. Edited by Qiu Peiran 裘沛然. Yuelu shushe, Changsha, 1994.

Yu pian 玉篇 (Jade Tablets). Liang, 543. Gu Yewang 顧野王. References to *Da guang yi hui yu pian* 大廣益會玉篇. Song, 1013. Edited by Chen Pengnian 陳彭年. Facsimile of the 1702 print. Zhonghua shuju, Beijing, 1987.

Zhan guo ce 戰國策 (Plots of Warring States). Warring States – Han, 5th–1st c. BCE. Anon. Compiled by Liu Xiang 劉向. 3 Vols. Shanghai guji chubanshe, Shanghai, 1978.

Zhangjiashan manuscripts, see Zhangjiashan 247 hao Hanmu zhujian zhengli xiaozu 張家山二四七號漢墓竹簡整理小組, Jiangling Zhangjiashan 江陵張家山 and Gao Dalun 高大倫 in Bibliography A.

Zhen jiu jia yi jing 鍼灸甲乙經 (A–B Canon of Acupuncture and Moxibustion). Eastern Jin, 256–82. Huangfu Mi 皇甫謐. References to *Zhenjiu jiayijing jiaozhu*. Annotated by Zhang Canga 張燦玾 and Xu Guoqian 徐國仟. Renmin weisheng chubanshe, Beijing, 1996.

Zheng zhi zhun sheng 證治準繩 (Standards for the Treatment of Distinguishing Patterns). Ming, ca 1603. Wang Kentang 王肯堂. 4 Vols. Xinwenfeng chuban gongsi, Taipei, 1974.

Zhong zang jing 中藏經 (Canon kept at the Palace Repository). Song, 11th c. Attributed to Hua Tuo 華佗 of the 2nd–3rd c. In *Zhongguo yixue dacheng sanbian* 中國醫學大成三編. Edited by Qiu Peiran 裘沛然 *et al.* Yuelu shushe, Changsha, 1994.

Zhou li 周裡 (Rites of Zhou). Late Warning States, 3rd–1st c. BCE. Anon. References to *Zhou li zhu shu* 周裡注疏. In *Shi san jing zhu shu* 十三經注疏, vol. 1.

Zhou yi 周易 (The Changes of the Zhou). Zhou–Han, 9th–2nd c. BCE. Anon. References to *Zhou yi zhengyi*. In *Shi san jing zhu shu* 十三經注疏, vol. 1.

Zhu bing yuan hou lun 諸病源候論 (Treatise on the Origins and Symptoms of Medical Disorders). Sui, 610. Chao Yuanfang 巢元方. References to *Zhubing yuanhoulun jiaozhu*. Annotated by Ding Guangdi 丁光迪. Renmin weisheng chubanshe, Beijing, 1991.

Zhuangzi 莊子 (Essays by Master Zhuang). Zhou–Han, 4th–2nd c. BCE. Ascribed to Zhuang Zhou 莊周. References to *Zhuangzi ji shi* 莊子集釋. Qing, 1894. Commentary by Guo Qingfan 郭慶藩. Annotated by Wang Xiaoyu 王孝魚. Zhonghua shuju, Beijing, [1961] 1985.

Zuo zhuan 左傳 (*Zuo* tradition). Zhou–Han, 3rd–1st c. BCE. Anon. References to *Chunqiu Zuozhuan zhu*. Annotated by Yang Bojun 楊伯峻. 4 Vols. Zhonghua shuju, Beijing, 1981.

INDEX

392

UNIVERSITY OF CAMBRIDGE ORIENTAL PUBLICATIONS PUBLISHED FOR THE FACULTY OF ORIENTAL STUDIES

1. *Averroes' commentary on Plato's Republic*, edited and translated by E. I. J. Rosenthal
2. *FitzGerald's 'Salaman and Absal'*, edited by A. J. Arberry
3. *Ihara Saikaku: the Japanese family storehouse*, translated and edited by G. W. Sargent
4. *The Avestan Hymn to Mithra*, edited and translated by Ilya Gershevitch
5. *The Fuṣūl al-Madanī of al-Fārābī*, edited by D. M. Dunlop (out of print)
6. *Dun Karn, poet of Malta*, texts chosen and translated by A. J, Arberry; introduction, notes and glossary by P. Grech
7. *The political writings of Ogyū Sorai*, by J. R. McEwan
8. *Financial administration under the T'ang dynasty*, D. C. Twitchett
9. *Neolithic cattle-keepers of south India: a study of the Deccan Ashmounds*, by F. R. Allchin
10. *The Japanese enlightenment: a study of the writings of Fukuzawa Yukichi*, by Carmen Blacker
11. *Records of Han administration*. Vol. I, *Historical assessment*, by M. Loewe
12. *Records of Han administration*. Vol. II, *Documents*, by M. Loewe
13. *The language of Indrajit of Orchā: a study of early Braj Bhāṣā prose*, by R. S. McGregor
14. *Japan's first general election, 1890*, by R. H. P. Rosenthal
15. *A collection of Indrajit of Orchā: a study and translation of 'Uji Shūi Monogatari'*, by D. E. Mills
16. *Studia semitica*. Vol. I, *Jewish themes*, by E. I. J. Rosenthal
17. *Studia semitica*. Vol. II, *Jewish themes*, by E. I. J. Rosenthal
18. *A Nestorian collection of Christological texts*. Vol. I, *Syriac text*, by Lusie Abramowski and Alan E. Goodman
19. *A Nestorian collection of Christological texts*. Vol. II, *Introduction, translation, indexes*, by Lusie Abramowski and Alan E. Goodman
20. *The Syraic version of the Pseudo-Nonnos mythological scholia*, by Sebastian Brock
21. *Water rights and irrigation practices in Lajih*, by A. M. A. Maktari
22. *The commentary of Rabbi David Kimhi on Psalms cxx–cl*, edited and translated by Joshua Baker and Ernest W. Nicholson
23. *Jalāl al-dīn al-Suyūtī*. Vol I, *Biography and background*, by E. M. Sartain
24. *Jalāl al-dīn al-Suyūtī*. Vol II, *AI-Tahadduth bini'mat allāh*, Arabic text, by E. M. Sartain

25. *Origen and the Jews: studies in Jewish–Christian relations in third-century Palestine*, by N. R. M. de Lange
26. *The Vīsaladevarāsa: a restoration of the text*, by John D. Smith
27. *Shabbethai Sofer and his prayer-book*, by Stefan C. Reif
28. *Mori Ōgai and the modernization of Japanese culture*, by Richard John Bowring
29. *The rebel lands: an investigation into the origins of early Mesopotamian mythology*, by J. V. Kinnier Wilson
30. *Saladin: the politics of the holy war*, by Malcolm C. Lyons and David Jackson
31. *Khotanese Buddhist texts* (revised edition), edited by H. W. Bailey
32. *Interpreting the Hebrew Bible: essays in honour of E. I. J. Rosenthal*, edited by J. A. Emerton and Stefan C. Reif.
33. *The traditional interpretation of the Apocalypse of St John in the Ethiopian orthodox church*, by Roger W. Cowley
34. *South Asian archaeology 1981: proceedings of the Sixth International Conference of South Asian Archaeologists in Western Europe*, edited by Bridget Allchin (with assistance from Raymond Allchin and Miriam Sidell)
35. *God's conflict with the dragon and the sea. Echoes of a Canaanite myth in the Old Testament*, by John Day
36. *Land and sovereignty in India. Agrarian society and politics under the eighteenth-century Maratha Svarājya*, by André Wink
37. *God's caliph: religious authority in the first centuries of Islam*, by Patricia Crone and Martin Hinds
38. *Ethiopian Biblical interpretation: a study in exegetical tradition and hermeneutics*, by Roger W. Cowley
39. *Monk and mason on the Tigris frontier: the early history of Ṭur 'Abdin*, by Andrew Palmer
40. *Early Japanese books in Cambridge University Library: a catalogue of the Aston, Satow and Von Siebold collections*, by Nozumu Hayashi and Peter Kornicki
41. *Molech: a god of human sacrifice in the Old Testament*, by John Day
42. *Arabian studies*, edited by R. B. Serjeant and R. L. Bidwell
43. *Naukar, Rajput and Sepoy: the ethnohistory of the military labour market in Hindustan, 1450–1850*, by Dirk H. A. Kolff
44. *The epic of Pabūjī: a study, transcription and translation*, by John D. Smith
45. *Anti-Christian polemic in Early Islam: Abū 'Īsā al-Warrāq's 'Against the Trintiy'*, by David Thomas
46. *Devotional literature in South Asia: Current research, 1985–8. Papers of the Fourth Conference on Devotional Literature in New Indo-Aryan Languages*, edited by R. S. McGregor
47. *Genizah research after ninety years: the case of Judaeo-Arabic. Papers read at the Third Congress of the Society of Judaeo-Arabic Studies*, edited by Joshua Blau and Stefan C. Reif
48. *Divination, mythology and monarchy in Han China*, by Michael Loewe
49. *The Arabian epic: Heroic and oral storytelling. Vols. I–III*, by M. C. Lyons
50. *Religion in Japan: arrows to heaven and earth*, edited by P. F. Kornicki and I. J. McMullen
51. *Kingship and political practice in colonial India*, by Pamela G. Price

Printed in the United States
By Bookmasters